District Laboratory Practice in Tropical Countries

Part 1

Second Edition

Monica Cheesbrough

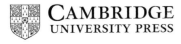

CAMBRIDGE
UNIVERSITY PRESS

CO-PUBLISHED BY THE PRESS SYNDICATE OF THE UNIVERSITY OF CAMBRIDGE
The Edinburgh Building, Cambridge CB2 2RU, UK
AND TROPICAL HEALTH TECHNOLOGY
PO Box 50, Fakenham, Norfolk, NR21 8XB, UK

CAMBRIDGE UNIVERSITY PRESS
Cambridge, New York, Melbourne, Madrid, Cape Town, Singapore, São Paulo

www.cambridge.org

First published by Tropical Health Technology 1998
Reprinted by Cambridge University Press 1999, 2001, 2003, 2004
Second edition first published 2005

Printed in Hong Kong by Sheck Wah Tong Printing Press Ltd.

A catalogue record for this book is available from the British Library

ISBN-13: 978-0-521-67630-4 paperback
ISBN-10: 0-521-67630-4 paperback

Every effort has been made in preparing this book to provide accurate and up-to-date
information which is in accord with accepted standards and practice at the time of
publication. Nevertheless, the authors, editors and publisher can make no warranties
that the information contained herein is totally free from error, not least because clinical
standards are constantly changing through research and regulation. The authors, editors
and publisher therefore disclaim all liability for direct or consequential damages
resulting from the use of material contained in this book. Readers are strongly advised
to pay careful attention to information provided by the manufacturer of any drugs or
equipment that they plan to use.

Part I
Contents

Chapter 6 Clinical chemistry tests

Appendix I

Appendix II

Appendix III

Supplement

Index

Preface

Since the publication of the first edition of Part 1 *District Laboratory Practice in Tropical Countries* the essential role of the laboratory in providing a scientific foundation for district health care and improving the quality of health care to communities, has not changed. The new challenges faced by health authorities however, have led to changes in laboratory practice and a greater emphasis on the need for reliable well managed district laboratories and their rational use in district health care.

In deciding the changes to be incorporated in the new edition of Part 1, the author and those who have helped with the revision have been guided by the views and requests of those using the book in their work and training programmes. The important chapters covering management, quality assurance, health and safety and equipping of district laboratories have been reviewed and updated where needed. For those with internet access and e-mail facilities, the details of equipment manufacturers now include website information and e-mail addresses.

Information on parasitic diseases and their control has been brought up to date. Current knowledge on HIV interaction with parasitic pathogens and new technologies to diagnose parasitic infections have been included. Immunochromatographic tests to diagnose malaria have been described, their limitations discussed, and information on the WHO malaria rapid diagnostic tests website included. Other parasite-related websites and a list of up to date references and recommended reading are given at the end of the parasitology chapter.

Within the clinical chemistry chapter, the text covering diabetes mellitus has been revized to include the current WHO classification of diabetes and guidelines for diabetes diagnosis. Urine strip tests have also been updated. To assist in monitoring HIV/AIDS patients for toxicity to antiretroviral drugs, a colorimetric test kit to measure alanine aminotransferase (ALT) has been included where it is not possible to refer specimens for testing to a regional clinical chemistry laboratory. Information is also given for a colorimetric creatinine test kit.

For many laboratory programmes, the introduction of standard operating procedures for laboratory tests backed by quality assessment schemes has been key to improving the reliability, efficiency and accountability of district laboratory services, motivating laboratory staff and increasing the confidence of laboratory users. Safe laboratory practices now followed in many laboratories have reduced work-related accidents and laboratory-acquired infections. It is hoped that the new edition of Part 1 will continue to help those involved in training and those working in district laboratories, often in difficult situations. It is also hoped that it will encourage health authorities to provide the resources needed to provide a quality laboratory service to the community.

Monica Cheesbrough   May 2005

Acknowledgements

Special thanks are due to all those working in laboratories in tropical and developing countries and those involved in training laboratory personnel who have corresponded and contributed their suggestions for this second edition of Part 1 *District Laboratory Practice in Tropical Countries*.

Gratitude is expressed to all those who have helped to prepare the new edition:

Mr Malcolm Guy, formerly Scientific Administrator MRC Laboratory in the Gambia, for reading through and commenting on chapters covering the organization, management, safe working practices and equipping of district laboratories.

Mr John Williams, Clinical Scientist, Department of Infectious and Tropical Diseases, London School of Hygiene and Tropical Medicine, for helping to update the parasitology chapter.

Mr Anthony Moody, previously Laboratory Manager, Hospital for Tropical Diseases, London, for also assisting in the revision of the parasitology chapter and for contributing text on rapid malaria diagnostic tests.

Professor Claus C Heuck, University Hospital, Duesseldorf, formerly of the World Health Organization Health Laboratory Technology Unit, for reading through and making suggestions for the clinical chemistry chapter.

Mr Robert Simpson, Laboratory Manager, Chemical Pathology, St Thomas Hospital, London, for also assisting in the revision of the clinical chemistry chapter.

Gratitude is also expressed to Dr Geoffrey V Gill, Reader in Tropical Medicine, Liverpool School of Tropical Medicine, for updating the diabetes mellitus text.

Thanks are also due to Dr Peter Hill for commenting on quality assurance in clinical chemistry. The help of Mr Ray J Wood, Laboratory Manager Mengo Hospital, Uganda, is also acknowledged.

The author wishes to thank Fakenham Photosetting for their careful and professional preparation of the new edition.

Acknowledgements for colour artwork: These can be found on page 177 before Chapter 5 Parasitological Tests.

1

Organization and staffing of district laboratory services

1.1 Importance of laboratory practice in district health care

District laboratory services have an essential role in the surveillance, prevention, control, diagnosis and management of diseases of greatest public health importance. In discussing the role of laboratories at district level, the World Health Organization comments that with the scaling up of interventions against HIV/AIDS, tuberculosis and malaria, the need for diagnostic and laboratory services has never been greater.[1]

Meaning of district as used in this manual
The district is designated by the World Health Organization as the key level for the management, growth and consolidation of primary health care (PHC). It is the most peripheral unit of local government and administration that has comprehensive powers and responsibilities.

A typical rural district health system consists of:

- A network of PHC facilities, including village health clinics, maternity centres, health centres and small urban clinics. Mobile health units may also provide some outreach PHC services and support for home-based health care.

- A system for the referral of seriously ill patients needing specialist care.

- The district hospital (first referral hospital).

- Other government health related departments, including social and rehabilitative services, environmental health, nutrition, agriculture, water supply and sanitation.

- Non-government health sector organizations working in the district.

A district health system is usually administered by a district health management team or health council, consisting of representatives from the community, PHC and hospital services, and health related departments such as water and sanitation.

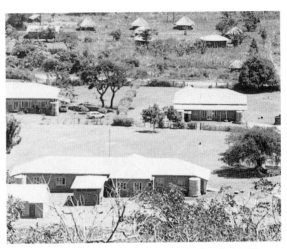

Plate 1.1 Typical community-based district hospital in Kenya.

The growth of district health systems has led to:

- essential health services and health decisions being brought closer to where people live and work.
- communities becoming more aware of health issues and demanding health services that are relevant, accessible, reliable, affordable, and accountable.
- district health councils being formed to identify and assess community health care needs, develop and manage local health services, and ensure district health resources are used effectively, efficiently and equitably.

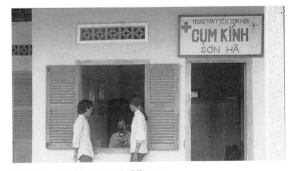

Plate 1.2 Health centre in Vietnam.
Courtesy: RP Marchand, MCNV.

WHY THE LABORATORY IS NEEDED IN DISTRICT HEALTH CARE

The laboratory has an important role in improving the:

- quality,
- efficiency,
- cost-effectiveness,
- planning and management of district health care.

What difference can the laboratory make to the quality of district health care?

■ *Laboratory investigations increase the accuracy of disease diagnosis*

Many infectious diseases and serious illnesses can only be diagnosed reliably by using the laboratory. For example, errors in the diagnosis of malaria have been shown to be particularly high when diagnosis is based on clinical symptoms alone.

Misdiagnosis or late diagnosis can lead to:

- incorrect treatment with misuse and waste of drugs.
- increased morbidity and mortality.
- hospitalization and need for specialist care.
- patient dissatisfaction leading to negative responses to future health interventions.
- underutilization of health facilities.
- lack of confidence and motivation of health personnel.
- increased risk to the community from inappropriate disease management and untreated infectious disease.

■ *The laboratory has an essential role in screening for ill health and assessing response to treatment*

At district level the laboratory is needed to:

- assess a patient's response to drug therapy.
- assist in monitoring the condition of a patient and help to decide when it may be necessary to refer for specialist care.
- screen pregnant women for anaemia, proteinuria, and infections which if not treated may cause disease in the newborn, premature birth, low birth weight, or significant maternal illness.
- screen the contacts of persons with infectious diseases such as tuberculosis and sexually transmitted diseases.
- detect inherited abnormalities such as haemoglobin S as part of district family planning health services.
- screen whole blood and blood products for transfusion transmitted pathogens.

■ *The laboratory is needed to work with others in reducing infection in the community and investigating epidemics rapidly*

The public health functions of a district health laboratory service include:

- detecting the source(s) of infection, identifying carriers, and contact tracing.
- participating in epidemiological surveys.
- assisting in disease surveillance and in the selection, application, and evaluation of control methods.
- helping to control hospital acquired infections.
- participating in health education.
- examining designated community water supplies for indicators of faecal and chemical pollution.
- responding rapidly when an epidemic occurs, including appropriate on-site testing and the collection and despatch of specimens to the Regional or Central Microbiology Laboratory for pathogen identification.

In what ways can the laboratory contribute to achieving efficiency and cost effectiveness in district health care?

■ *The laboratory can help to reduce expenditure on drugs*

When the laboratory is used to improve the accuracy of diagnosis, perform appropriate antimicrobial susceptibility testing, and monitor a patient's response to treatment:

- drugs can be used more selectively and only when needed.
- patterns of emerging drug resistance can be identified more rapidly and monitored.

■ *The laboratory can lower health care costs by identifying disease at an early stage*

Early successful treatment following early correct laboratory diagnosis can help to:

- reduce the number of times a patient may need to seek medical care for the same illness.
- prevent complications arising from advanced untreated disease.
- avoid hospitalization and further costly investigations.

■ *Significant savings can be made when the laboratory participates in local disease surveillance and control*

This is because:

- the spread of infectious disease can be contained more rapidly.
- disease control measures can be selected and targeted more effectively.
- sources of infection and disease carriers can be identified.

What information can the laboratory provide to achieve rational health planning and good health management?

■ *Reliable laboratory test results with relevant patient data, provide information on the health status of a community, health patterns, and disease trends*

This information is needed to establish health care priorities and plan:

- health care programmes and location of health facilities.
- training of district health personnel and delivery of health services.
- treatment schedules and changes in drug usage.
- financing of district health care programmes.

■ *Public health laboratory activities provide accurate epidemiological information for health planning*

This information can help to determine:

- causes of ill health in the community and risk factors contributing to the presence and spread of diseases.
- prevalence and incidence rates of important infectious diseases.
- effectiveness of health care programmes, drug treatments, and immunization programmes.
- which methods have appropriate sensitivity and specificity to be useful.

Further information: Readers are referred to the paper of Mundy *et al*: The operation, quality and costs of a district laboratory service in Malawi.[2]

SUMMARY
Laboratory practice in district health care

● District laboratories form an integral part of good health care planning and delivery.

● Reliable, integrated, and well managed district laboratory services are essential if:
  - an acceptable quality of community health care and district health management are to be achieved and sustained.
  - illness and premature death are to be reduced.
  - the community is to have confidence in its health services.

● Unless the importance of the laboratory in generating valid and objective health data is recognized:
  - district health programmes will be unable to respond adequately to local health care needs and priorities.
  - scarce health resources are likely to be wasted on other less effective interventions.
  - national health planning will lack a scientific foundation on which to develop and evaluate its health strategies.

● For district laboratories to operate effectively, district health authorities must allocate the correct proportion of available resources to:
  - district laboratory practice.
  - training and continuing education of district laboratory personnel.
  - instructing district medical officers and community health workers in the correct and optimum use of laboratory services.

1.2 Structuring of a district laboratory network

A district laboratory service must be integrated in the health system which exists within its district if it is to function as a network, be accessible, and provide a service that is needed by the community and those managing health care in the district.

An example of a laboratory service that has been integrated in a rural district health system is shown in Fig. 1.1. The district laboratory service network consists of:

■ Outreach community-based laboratory facilities located in:
  - comprehensive health centres, staffed by laboratory personnel and able to perform a range of microscopical investigations and other basic tests to assist in the diagnosis, assessment, treatment and prevention of common diseases.
  - maternity health units, with nursing staff

screening for anaemia and proteinuria and collecting blood for appropriate antibody screening in the district hospital laboratory.

■ District hospital laboratory with facilities to service the clinical, epidemiological, and training requirements of a first referral hospital.

■ Specimen collection and transport system to enable:
– patients attending health centres to benefit from the facilities of the district hospital laboratory.
– epidemics to be investigated rapidly.

■ Mobile laboratory work as required by district health needs.

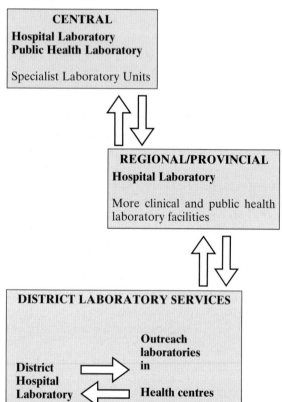

Fig. 1.1 Laboratory service network

COMMUNITY-BASED LABORATORY FACILITIES

A reliable community-based laboratory service is one of the most important ways of improving the quality of PHC and avoiding patients and pregnant women having to travel to the district hospital for essential laboratory tests. To be effective in PHC, community-based laboratory practice must:

– meet the health needs of individuals and the community.
– operate in an acceptable way.
– be accessible to the community and affordable.
– be reliable and sustainable.

Health centres with laboratory facilities are generally better attended and more highly valued by the community because laboratory testing can often be seen to establish the true cause of an illness, enabling correct treatment to be prescribed at a patient's first attendance.

Establishing a health centre laboratory

When deciding whether to site a laboratory in a health centre the following are important considerations:

■ What is likely to be the affect on morbidity and mortality in the area if essential laboratory facilities were to be made available. How will the results of tests be used?

■ Is the health centre sufficiently well attended and what is likely to be the demand for laboratory tests?

■ Is it possible to train local community health workers to use laboratory facilities correctly, particularly in early diagnoses, follow-up, care, and local disease surveillance?

Note: Written *Guidelines on the Use of the Laboratory in PHC* must be provided for community health workers by the district medical officer. Included in the *Guidelines* should be when to order particular tests, type of specimen required, interpretation of test results and appropriate follow-up. Health workers should know the relative costs of tests and average time it takes to perform individual tests.

■ Is there a person trained or can be trained to perform the required tests competently and manage safely and efficiently a health centre laboratory?

■ Can the necessary measures be taken to ensure the safe collection, transport and disposal of specimens?

■ Is it possible for the health centre laboratory to be visited regularly by the district laboratory coordinator or a senior person from the district hospital laboratory?

Important: At no time should a laboratory be established in a health centre unless it can be visited regularly and the work controlled adequately.

■ Is it possible to organize a reliable system for supplying the laboratory with reagents and other essential supplies?

■ Is the cost of running the laboratory affordable, including the cost of supplies, maintaining equipment, and staff salaries? How will laboratory expenditures be met?

■ Can the health centre provide adequate facilities for a laboratory to operate effectively and safely, i.e. can a room be provided that is:

- structurally sound with secure door(s), and burglar proof, insect screened windows that provide adequate light and ventilation.

- sufficiently large to be sub-divided into areas for working, reception of patients and specimens, keeping records, decontamination of infected material and cleaning of laboratory-ware.

- provided with running water.

- provided with separate sinks for cleaning laboratory-ware and hand-washing.

- fitted with facilities for the safe disposal of specimens.

- wired for mains electricity or if unavailable, supplied with an alternative source of power, e.g. battery, rechargeable from a solar panel.

- fitted with appropriate washable working surfaces, seating for patients and staff, secure storage cupboards, and shelving.

Staffing a health centre laboratory

A laboratory in a community health centre will usually be staffed by a laboratory worker or a local community health worker trained to examine specimens microscopically, perform appropriate diagnostic and screening tests, collect and refer specimens for specialist tests, and participate in community health education and disease surveillance. Depending on the workload of the health centre, one or two laboratory aides may also be required.

Activities of a health centre laboratory

■ To investigate by referral or testing on site, important diseases and health problems affecting the local community. Depending on geographical area such investigations will usually include:

Bacterial and viral infections: Tuberculosis, leprosy, meningitis, cholera, gonorrhoea, syphilis, vaginitis, urinary tract infections, respiratory tract infections, bacillary dysentery, and relapsing fever. In the more comprehensive health centres staffed by a laboratory technical officer, it may also be possible to investigate HIV disease and associated infections.

Parasitic diseases: Malaria, schistosomiasis, lymphatic filariasis, loiasis, onchocerciasis, African trypanosomiasis, Chagas' disease, leishmaniasis,

amoebic dysentery, giardiasis, strongyloidiasis, trichuriasis, hookworm disease, and any other locally important parasitic diseases.

Other causes of ill health: Including anaemia, diabetes, renal disease, and skin mycoses.

■ To assist the health worker in deciding the severity of a patient's condition and prognosis.

■ To collect and refer specimens for testing to the district laboratory, including:

- drinking water samples from sources used by the community.

- faecal specimens for the microbiological investigation of major enteric pathogens.

- serum for antibody tests to investigate important communicable diseases.

- specimens for biochemical testing to investigate disorders of the liver and kidney, metabolic and deficiency diseases.

- specimens for culture and antimicrobial sensitivity testing to diagnose important bacterial infections and monitor drug resistance.

■ To notify the district hospital laboratory at an early stage of any result of public health importance and send specimens for confirmatory tests.

■ To screen pregnant women for anaemia, proteinuria and malaria, and refer serum to the district hospital laboratory for antibody screening of sexually transmitted diseases such as syphilis.

■ To promote health care and assist in community health education, e.g. by demonstrating microscopically parasites of public health importance.

■ To keep careful records which can be used by health authorities in health planning.

■ To keep an inventory of stock and order reagents and other supplies in good time..

■ To send an informative monthly report to the district hospital laboratory of the work carried out and results obtained.

Screening for proteinuria and anaemia in maternity health centres

All health units providing antenatal care should be able to test for proteinuria and anaemia. Laboratory staff from the district hospital should train health workers how to collect specimens correctly and how to perform and control the required tests. Maternity centres should be provided with standardized reagents and specimen containers.

A reliable system is also needed for transporting venous blood collected from antenatal women to the district hospital laboratory for appropriate testing.

DISTRICT HOSPITAL LABORATORY

The important functions of a district health system can be found in the 3rd edition, *Principles of Medicine in Africa.*[3]

Depending on the area served by the district hospital, number of hospital beds, and workload of the laboratory, the district hospital laboratory may consist of a number of connecting laboratory units or a subdivided laboratory room.[4,5]

Staff

A district hospital laboratory is usually staffed by at least one experienced laboratory officer and depending on workload, by two to four assistants and several aides. Ideally the district laboratory coordinator and tutor in charge of training should be based at the district hospital.

Note: The training of district laboratory personnel is described in subunit 1.3. The responsibilities of the district laboratory coordinator and involvement of the medical staff in district laboratory services are discussed in subunit 2.1.

Activities of a district hospital laboratory

■ In consultation with the district health management team, public health officers, and clinical staff, to decide which laboratory tests are needed and can be performed at district level (see subunit 2.2).

■ With the district laboratory coordinator, to manage effectively the district laboratory network as explained in subunit 2.1.

■ To prepare and implement standard operating procedures for all district laboratory activities (see subunit 2.4).

■ To support the work of the outreach laboratories by:
  - testing specimens referred from community health centres and maternity health units and returning test results speedily.
  - confirming a test result that indicates serious illness or is of major public health importance.
  - supplying standardized reagents, controls, stains, specimen containers, stationery and other essential laboratory supplies.
  - checking the performance of equipment.
  - implementing and monitoring safe working practices.
  - visiting each outreach laboratory every three months (role of the district laboratory coordi-

nator) to assist staff and monitor work performance and quality of laboratory reports.
  - training health centre laboratory personnel and arranging supervision and continuing training in the work place.
  - organizing a district external quality assessment scheme as described in subunit 2.4.

■ To refer specimens to the regional laboratory that cannot be tested locally or are more economically batch-tested at regional level. Also, to notify the regional Public Health Laboratory of any result of public health importance and to send specimens for confirmatory testing.

■ To participate in external quality assurance programmes organized by the regional or central laboratory.

■ To keep accurate records and send a report every three months to the district management team and director of the regional laboratory, detailing the activities of the district laboratory network, together with suggestions for managing problems and improving the laboratory service to the community.

DISTRICT SPECIMEN COLLECTION AND TRANSPORT SERVICE

An efficient laboratory specimen collection and transport service from the community health centres with a reliable and prompt return of test results, is an important way of extending laboratory facilities throughout the district with the following benefits:

  - improved treatment and follow-up care of patients in the community and better health care of pregnant women.
  - confirmation and further investigation of patients with important abnormal test results.
  - more reliable information on health trends and the causes of disease in the district.
  - more rapid investigation and control of epidemics.
  - opportunities for detecting the emergence of drug resistance and monitoring its spread in the community.

Requirements of a specimen referral system

A specimen referral system will function reliably providing:

■ There is close communication between staff of

the community-based health facilities and the district hospital laboratory.

- Outreach laboratories are supplied with specimen containers and laboratory request forms.
- Community health workers and district laboratory personnel are trained in the correct collection, preservation, and despatch of specimens.
- Correctly completed documentation accompanies all specimens, and careful records are kept of referred specimens and test reports.
- There is a reliable and secure means of transporting specimens throughout the year and returning test results with the minimum of delay.

MOBILE DISTRICT LABORATORY WORK

Basic mobile laboratory services may be required in district health care for the following reasons:

- to support mobile community health programmes usually in areas where communities are nomadic or sparsely distributed.
- to investigate outbreaks of serious disease and identify high risk factors.
- to work with specialist teams to assess the effectiveness of disease control interventions, check the efficacy of immunization programmes, and obtain epidemiological data.
- to assist medical teams in emergencies and disaster situations.
- to provide back-up for health education and the promotion of health activities in the district.
- to monitor community water supplies for pollution.

Mobile laboratory work must be well planned and organized. Most of the difficulties and poor performance associated with mobile laboratory work are due to:

- using inappropriate technologies,
- equipment that is not sufficiently rugged or designed for field use,
- reagents that have deteriorated due to heat, high relative humidity or incorrect storage,
- bypassing quality control procedures because they are too time-consuming or difficult to apply under field situations.

Problems of safety arise when specimens are collected and transported in unsuitable and leaky containers, handled without due care, or disposed of unsafely. Accidents tend to occur more frequently under field conditions due to cramped, unfamiliar or noisy working conditions, unsafe pipetting, limited facilities for handwashing, tiredness, pressure to work rapidly, and lack of supervision.

The cost of mobile laboratory work can be high because in addition to transport costs, heat-sensitive reagents deteriorate more rapidly, equipment needs to be repaired more often, and extra controls are needed in field work. The travelling time of staff needs also to be considered.

Recommendations for mobile district laboratory work

- Establish the reasons and objectives for undertaking mobile laboratory work and the anticipated extent of it. Discuss the data required and how it should be obtained and recorded.
- Assess whether full field-testing is necessary or whether specimens can be collected, stabilized, and brought back to the district hospital laboratory for testing under more controlled conditions.
- Obtain in advance as much information as possible about travelling time and conditions, the community and its customs, location of the work, electricity supplies, water availability and quality.
- Select technologies and instrumentation of proven reliability and acceptability in the field. If this cannot be established, pretest the techniques and equipment under simulated field conditions.
- Decide how to check the performance of instruments and test for reagent deterioration under field conditions.
- Make a detailed check list of every item needed and quantity of each required. Prepare rugged containers for transporting the mobile laboratory, including insulated containers for storing heat sensitive reagents, controls, and specimens.
- Discuss in advance the tasks that each member of the mobile laboratory team will perform and measures to be taken to ensure quality and safety.
- Monitor the cost, information provided, benefits to the community and performance characteristics of any on-going mobile laboratory work.

Note: Further information on mobile laboratory work can be found in the WHO publication *Health laboratory facilities in emergency and disaster situations.*[6]

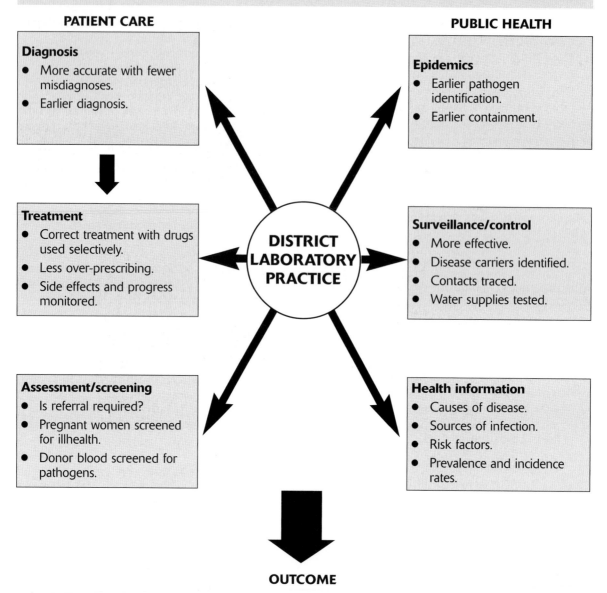

PATIENT CARE

Diagnosis
- More accurate with fewer misdiagnoses.
- Earlier diagnosis.

Treatment
- Correct treatment with drugs used selectively.
- Less over-prescribing.
- Side effects and progress monitored.

Assessment/screening
- Is referral required?
- Pregnant women screened for illhealth.
- Donor blood screened for pathogens.

PUBLIC HEALTH

Epidemics
- Earlier pathogen identification.
- Earlier containment.

Surveillance/control
- More effective.
- Disease carriers identified.
- Contacts traced.
- Water supplies tested.

Health information
- Causes of disease.
- Sources of infection.
- Risk factors.
- Prevalence and incidence rates.

DISTRICT LABORATORY PRACTICE

OUTCOME

- Improvement in the quality of care with:
  - acute illness more rapidly diagnosed,
  - less preventable advanced/chronic illness,
  - reduced mortality.
- Reduced transmission of infectious diseases.
- Lower expenditure on drugs.
- More efficient use of health resources.
- Better health planning and management.
- Greater patient satisfaction.
- Greater motivation of health workers.

Fig. 1.2   **Role of the laboratory in district health care.**

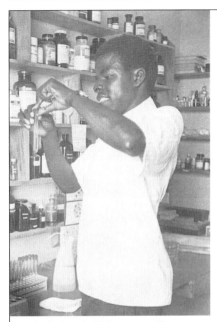

1 District hospital laboratory officer.

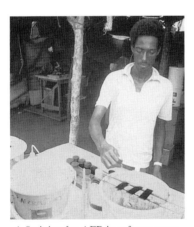

2 Urinary schistosomiasis survey.

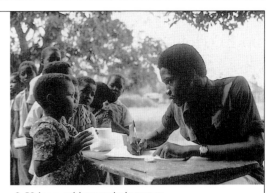

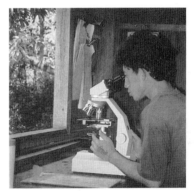

3 Examining malaria smears in a health centre.

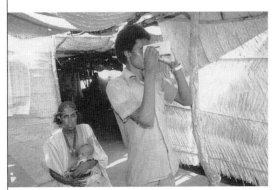

4 Staining for AFB in refugee camp.

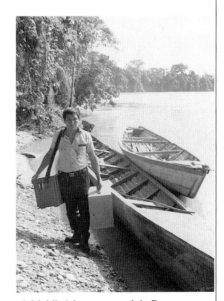

5 Screening for anaemia in refugee camp.

6 Mobile laboratory work in Peru.

Acknowledgements: Plate 2: Courtesy TALC, Plates 4, 5, 6: Courtesy Warren L Johns, Plate 3: Courtesy Graham Mortimer.

1.3 Training and continuing education of district laboratory personnel

In most developing countries the training of medical laboratory personnel is changing in response to:

■ The need for more appropriately trained district laboratory staff to support community-based health care.

■ The need for improved quality, safety, efficiency and management in district laboratory practice to optimize the use of health resources.

■ The need for relevant, better planned, indigenous training programmes with educational objectives that define clearly what trainees need to learn to become competent district laboratory officers.

■ The need for continuing on-site training and education to retain competency and motivation.

A job related approach to the training and continuing education of laboratory personnel is *essential* if district laboratories are to provide a service that is reliable, cost-effective, efficient, and relevant. Inappropriate or inadequate training of laboratory personnel is not only wasteful but also potentially dangerous.

The following are some of the indicators of poor training of laboratory personnel:[8]

– increase in the number of wrong test results.
– delays in issuing reports or loss of reports.
– frequent and serious complaints from those requesting laboratory tests and an increase in requests for repeat tests as confidence decreases.
– increase in the damage to equipment.
– increase in the contamination of reagents and materials and in the amounts of reagents used.
– greater incidence of laboratory-acquired infections and other laboratory-related accidents.
– poorly motivated staff and job dissatisfaction.
– more time needed to supervize new staff.
– increase in laboratory operating costs.

A good learner-centred training programme will help students to learn the right facts, skills, and attitudes in an efficient and integrated way. It will assess whether students have learned the right things and help students to put into practice what they have learned.

The training programme should allow sufficient time both for learning and assessment. Students and tutors need to be assured of progress during training. Becoming aware of learning problems or teaching inadequacies at the end of training is too late.

Teaching students[7]

● The purpose of a training programme is to teach students to do a job.

● Teachers should concentrate on essential facts, skills, and attitudes. It is neither possible nor desirable to teach everything.

● Teachers should base their teaching on the health problems of the community and on the work their students will be expected to do.

● Teachers should plan courses and lessons using situation analysis and task analysis (see Supplement, *Training curriculum for district laboratory personnel*, pages 430–435.

Important: If students can do their job competently at the end of their training, the course has been successful. If students cannot do the work they have been trained for, then the course has failed.

JOB RELATED TRAINING CURRICULUM FOR DISTRICT LABORATORY PERSONNEL

A job related training programme is usually referred to as competency-based or task-orientated and is recommended for the basic training of medical laboratory personnel. It is ideally suited to the training of district laboratory officers in developing countries because it ensures the training is indigenous and relevant to the working situation. It fits a person to do the job that is needed, where it is needed, and to take on the responsibilities that go with the job.

The better a person can do their job the greater will be their effectiveness and satisfaction. Competency and job satisfaction are major factors in achieving and retaining quality of service.

How to design a curriculum for district laboratory personnel

Information on how to design and implement a job-related, i.e. competency-based, training programme can be found in a SUPPLEMENT at the back of this book, see pages 430–435.

CONTINUING EDUCATION OF DISTRICT LABORATORY STAFF

Continuing professional education with support in the workplace are required to retain the competence and motivation of district laboratory staff and prevent a decline in working standards. It is also an effective way of promoting job satisfaction and personal development.

Practising laboratory officers have a professional responsibility to participate in continuing education. Continuing professional education is also necessary for the successful introduction of new technologies and the implementation of changes in standard operating procedures.

Continuing education and updating of district laboratory staff is best provided on-site by the district laboratory coordinator during regular visits (see subunit 2.1). On-going training in the workplace is also one of the most effective ways of upgrading the knowledge, attitudes, technical and management skills of a laboratory worker who may have received only a semi-formal training some years before. Use of continuing education in this situation is often referred to as 'closing the performance gap.'

Value of Newsletters

A further way of promoting continued professional development at district level is to circulate a simple *District Laboratory Newsletter* which has an education section contributed by qualified laboratory personnel and district medical officers. Laboratory workers should be encouraged to stimulate discussion about their work. Such a *Newsletter* could also circulate information about new advances in laboratory practice relevant to community health care and disease control.

For those countries with a Medical Laboratory Association, laboratory personnel will usually be able to continue their professional education through their Association's journal/newsletter and by attending refresher courses, seminars, and professional meetings organized by their Association.

Upgrading and career development

For all laboratory personnel there should be opportunities for upgrading and career development according to an individual's abilities, participation in continuing education, work responsibilities, and the staffing needs and structure of the indigenous laboratory service.

Staffing of a laboratory service must be based on national health needs, organization of national health services, and finance available for operating the service and staff salaries.

The career structure should be flexible to allow for future development. Career prospects should be sufficiently attractive to discourage trained district laboratory personnel leaving the health service and laboratory profession.

Note: The employment of district laboratory staff, contracts of employment, and supervision of newly appointed staff are discusssed in subunit 2.1 *Ensuring a reliable and quality laboratory service.*

1.4 Code of conduct for laboratory personnel and status of medical laboratory practice

A *Code of Professional Conduct for Medical Laboratory Personnel* should include those practices and attitudes which characterize a professional and responsible laboratory officer and are necessary to ensure a person works to recognized standards which patients and those requesting laboratory investigations can expect to receive. It also emphasizes the professional status of medical laboratory practice.

Adopting a *Code of Professional Conduct* helps to remind district laboratory personnel of their responsibilities to patients, duty to uphold professional standards, and need to work with complete integrity.

Note: A suggested *Code of Professional Conduct for medical laboratory personnel* is shown on p. 12.

STATUS OF MEDICAL LABORATORY PRACTICE

Recognition by health authorities of the importance of medical laboratories in health care programmes is key to the development and adequate resourcing of laboratory practice and to laboratory services becoming more accessible to the community.

Such recognition is most successfully achieved when:

■ A Director of Medical Laboratory Services is appointed and is effective in defining clearly laboratory services in the Ministry of Health and collating laboratory data to demonstrate the essential role of laboratory services in epidemiology, diagnosis and treatment of disease, health planning, and management of health resources.

■ District medical officers become more involved in developing laboratory policies and supporting district laboratory personnel.

■ Medical laboratories:
   – are adequately staffed by competent and well motivated personnel.
   – are managed and networked efficiently.
   – follow a professional code of practice which incorporates standard operating procedures (SOPs).
   – provide a service that is reliable, consistent, relevant, and accountable.

■ A national *Association of Medical (Biomedical) Laboratory Sciences* is formed.

NATIONAL ASSOCIATION OF MEDICAL (BIOMEDICAL) LABORATORY SCIENCES

The following are the important functions of an *Association of Medical Laboratory Sciences*:
   – to discuss with health authorities the activities and requirements of laboratories at district, regional, and central level.
   – to promote national legislation regarding the professional registration of laboratory personnel and certification of laboratories to practice.
   – to discuss with health authorities: laboratory training, supervision of trainees, continuing education, staffing needs, employment, working conditions, levels of remuneration, and career development of qualified laboratory officers.
   – to organize laboratory training and qualification, set professional standards, inspect laboratories, assess the appropriateness of new technologies, and provide professional support and continuing education.
   – to establish links with laboratory associations in other countries and with the International Association of Medical Laboratory Technologists (IAMLT).

A professional laboratory association can only function with the active support of its members. An inexpensive, informative news sheet produced quarterly can help to retain the interest of members and increase the status of the medical laboratory profession, particularly if health officials and medical officers are invited to contribute articles.

Code of professional conduct for medical laboratory personnel

● Be dedicated to the use of clinical laboratory science to benefit mankind.*

● Place the well-being and service of patients above your own interests.

● Be accountable for the quality and integrity of clinical laboratory services.*

● Exercise professional judgement, skill, and care while meeting established standards.*

● Do not misuse your professional skills or knowledge for personal gain, and never take anything from your place of work that does not belong to you.

● Be at all times courteous, patient, and considerate to patients and their relatives. Safeguard the dignity and privacy of patients.*

● Do not disclose to a patient or any unauthorized person the results of your investigations and treat with strict confidentiality any personal information that you may learn about a patient.

● Respect and work in harmony with the other members of your hospital staff or health centre team.

● Promote health care and the prevention and control of disease.

● Follow safe working practices and ensure patients and others are not put at risk. Know what to do should an accident or fire occur and how to apply emergency First Aid.

● Do not consume alcohol or take unprescribed drugs that could interfere with your work performance during laboratory working hours or when on emergency stand-by.

● Use equipment and laboratory-ware correctly and do not waste reagents or other laboratory supplies.

● Strive to improve professional skills and knowledge and adopt scientific advances that benefit the patient and improve the delivery of test results.*

● Fulfill reliably and completely the terms and conditions of your employment.

*Taken from the *Code of Ethics* of the International Association of Medical Laboratory Technologists.

REFERENCES

1 *Laboratory services at the district level*. World Health Organization, Department of Essential Health Technologies, 2003, p. 1–4. Website www.who.int/eht (to be found under EHT Advocacy folder)

2 **Mundy CJF et al**. The operation, quality and costs of a district hospital laboratory service in Malawi. *Transactions Royal Society Tropical Medicine and Hygiene*, 2003, 97, pp. 403–408.

3 **Parry E et al**. *Principles of Medicine in Africa*, 3rd edition, 2004. Cambridge University Press. Low price edition is available.

4 *Manual of basic techniques for a health laboratory*. World Health Organization, Geneva, 2nd edition, 2003, pp. 11–12.

5 *Essential medical laboratory services project, Malawi 1998–2002, Final Report*. Malawi Ministry of Health, Liverpool School of Tropical Medicine, DFID. Obtainable from HIV/AIDS Dept, Liverpool School Tropical Medicine, Pembroke Place, Liverpool, L3 5QA, UK.

6 *Health laboratory facilities in emergency and disaster situations*. World Health Organization, 1994 (WHO Regional Publications Eastern Mediterranean Series No. 6). Obtainable from WHO Regional Office, Abdul Razzak, Al Sanbouri Street, Po Box 7608, Nasr City, Cairo, 11371, Egypt.

7 **Abbatt F**, **McMahon R**. *Teaching health care workers – Practical guide*, Macmillan publication, 2nd edition, 1993.

8 **McMinn.** *Design of basic training for laboratory technicians*. Developing Country Proceedings 17th Congress International Association of Medical Laboratory Technologists. Stockholm, 1986, pp. 176–188 (no longer in print).

RECOMMENDED READING

Carter, JY and Kiu OJ. *Clinicians' Guide to Quality Outpatient Diagnosis. A Manual for Tropical Countries*, AMREF, Kenya, 2005.

Manual of basic techniques for a health laboratory. World Health Organization, Geneva, 2nd edition, 2003.

Lewis SM. Laboratory practice at the periphery in developing countries. *International Journal Haematology*, 2002, Aug 76, Supplement 1, pp. 294–298.

Essential medical laboratory services project, Malavi 1998–2002. *Final Report*. Malawi Ministry of Health, Liverpool School of Tropical Medicine, DFID. For availability, see Reference 5.

Carter JY, Lema OE. *Practical laboratory manual for health centres in eastern Africa*, Nairobi, 1994. African Medical and Research Foundation, PO Box 30125, Nairobi, Kenya.

Bedu-Addo G, Bates I. Making the most of the laboratory. In *Principles of Medicine in Africa*, 2004, pp. 1326–1329. Cambridge University Press (available in low price edition).

WEBSITES

www.who.int/eht
This is the WHO website for the Department of Essential Health and Technologies (EHT). It was established in 2002, out of what was formerly the Dept of Blood Safety and Clinical Technology (BCT). Laboratory technology is one of the eight areas that come under the new EHT department. A document entitled *Laboratory services at district level* can be accessed from the website under EHT, Advocacy folder.

This outlines how to provide safe and reliable district laboratory services through a WHO Basic Operational Framework.

www.phclab.com
This website has been established by Gabriele Mallapaty to assist primary health care laboratory workers in developing countries. It carries news features, information on training, total quality management (TQM), equipment resources, and carries links to other relevant websites.

2

Total quality management of district laboratory services

2.1 Ensuring a reliable and quality laboratory service

A reliable and quality laboratory service is achieved and sustained not just by implementing quality control of laboratory tests. This is important but only part of what is needed. Increasingly the term *total quality management* (TQM) is being used to describe a more comprehensive and user-orientated approach to quality. TQM addresses those areas of laboratory practice that most influence how a laboratory service functions and uses its resources to provide a quality and relevant service.

Total quality management in district laboratory practice

TQM includes the following:

● Correct use of the laboratory in district health care.

● Providing a quality service to patients and those requesting tests.

● Management of finances, equipment, and supplies.

● Staffing of district laboratories, training and competence of staff.

● Quality assurance to obtain correct test results.

● Responsibility for TQM.

● Continuing improvement in quality.

TQM incorporates both the technical aspects of quality assurance and those aspects of quality that are important to the users of a laboratory service, such as information provided, its correctness and presentation, time it takes to get a test result, and the professionalism and helpfulness of laboratory staff.

Such a comprehensive commitment to quality is essential to achieve:

– best possible service to patients,
– user confidence,
– effectiveness and efficiency,
– accountability,
– optimal use of resources.

Successful TQM of district laboratory services requires close collaboration between laboratory staff, those who request laboratory tests, district laboratory coordinator, district hospital medical officers, and the district health management team.

CORRECT USE OF THE LABORATORY IN DISTRICT HEALTH CARE

Using the laboratory correctly in district health care involves:

■ Selecting those investigations that are needed in:
    – curative health care to establish or confirm a diagnosis, assess a patient's condition and prognosis, and monitor progress during treatment,
    – disease surveillance and the rapid investigation of epidemics,
    – health protection, health promotion, and health education,
    – health planning.

Note: Guidelines on the selection of laboratory investigations and methods can be found in subunit 2.2.

■ Deciding whether those investigations that are needed can be:
    – afforded,
    – reliably performed in district laboratories (see *Laboratory considerations* in subunit 2.2).

■ Assessing whether those requesting laboratory tests have sufficient training and experience to:
    – order diagnostic tests and epidemiological laboratory investigations appropriately,

- understand the meaning of test results and the limitations of laboratory tests (see sub-unit 2.2).
- use laboratory data appropriately.

■ Reviewing the value of tests performed so that:

- redundant, out-dated tests become replaced by tests that are more cost-effective, rapid, informative, and easier to perform in district laboratories,
- new appropriate technologies are introduced in response to changes in disease patterns, district health priorities, and treatment of diseases.

■ Monitoring the impact and cost-effectiveness of district laboratory practice.

Evaluating district laboratory practice

● Ask the views of those requesting laboratory tests and enquire how the laboratory is understood and rated by the community.

● Find out whether those health centres with laboratories are better attended than those without laboratory facilities.

● Review district morbidity and mortality data and how laboratory tests have been used in patient diagnosis and management.

● Assess whether the causes of illhealth, such as 'fever' are being better diagnosed when the laboratory is used.

● In areas with access to laboratory facilities, determine whether there are fewer patients presenting with complications resulting from incorrect and late diagnoses.

● Assess whether drug prescribing patterns are different in those health centres with laboratory facilities, particularly whether drugs are being used more selectively with fewer antimicrobial and antimalarial drugs being prescribed.

● Evaluate the extent to which district laboratory practice helps to define health priorities, detect disease carriers, identify those at greatest risk, and improve the local management of epidemics.

● Review operating costs and whether opportunities exist for greater efficiency.

● Assess whether laboratory practice is helping to target district health resources more effectively.

PROVIDING A QUALITY SERVICE

Understanding and responding to the needs and expectations of patients and those requesting laboratory tests are key components of TQM.

If users of district laboratories are to receive a quality service, the service provided must be:

- *Reliable and accountable:* with tests performed, using standard operating procedures (SOPs), competently under routine and emergency conditions and reports issued 'on time'.
- *Accessible and available:* through a network of health centre laboratories and an efficient specimen collection and transport system.
- *Professional:* by laboratory staff knowing their job, presenting clear and informative reports, and respecting patient confidentiality.
- *User friendly:* by laboratory staff communicating courteously, informatively, and patiently, particularly when the workload is high and the laboratory is being pressed for test results.
- *Dependable:* by laboratory staff arriving at work on time, not being absent unnecessarily, and not allowing tests to be discontinued because reagents have not been ordered correctly or in good time, or equipment has failed because preventive maintenance has not been carried out or replacement parts ordered.
- *Flexible:* to allow for the introduction of new technologies in response to the needs of users and changing health care strategies.

MANAGEMENT OF FINANCES, EQUIPMENT, AND SUPPLIES

Good management of laboratory finances, equipment and supplies are important functions of TQM.

Managing laboratory finances
The training of district laboratory officers must include accountancy skills and how to keep accurate records of requisitions, expenditures and income.

The financing of district laboratory practice, estimating laboratory operating costs, and ways of controlling laboratory expenditure are discussed in subunit 2.3.

Managing laboratory equipment
Lack of an effective equipment management policy is a major cause of:

■ District laboratories being under-equipped or supplied with inappropriate equipment.

- Equipment being purchased incorrectly, often without a *User Manual* and essential replacement parts.

- Equipment failure due to laboratory staff not being trained to use and care for equipment correctly, and damage to equipment due to unstable electricity supplies.

- Health resources being wasted due to equipment not being repaired.

- Equipment related accidents and risks to staff and others particularly when electrical equipment is not connected or earthed correctly, inspected regularly, and serviced.

- Poor laboratory services to patients and relationships between laboratory and medical staff deteriorating as tests cannot be performed or test results are delayed due to equipment breakdowns.

- Laboratory staff becoming dissatisfied at not being able to do their job.

To avoid such equipment related problems, the management of equipment must include:

- guidelines covering equipment specifications, standards, and purchasing.

- inventory of all the equipment in the laboratory, giving manufacturer, model details, date of purchase and order number, price paid, supplier, power requirements, source of replacement parts with code numbers, checks and maintenance schedules.

- preparation of written standard operating procedures (SOPs) covering the use and maintenance of each item of equipment with safety considerations.

- training of laboratory staff in the use, control, and care of equipment and provision of continuing on-site support.

- procedure for reporting equipment faults and ensuring faulty equipment is not used, and procedure for the rapid repair of equipment.

Note: Guidelines for the selection and purchasing of equipment and how to keep equipment in working order can be found in subunit 4.1. Equipment safety is described in subunit 3.6.

Managing laboratory supplies

Before any district laboratory is established, a reliable system for supplying it must be identified and organized. As mentioned in subunit 2.3, district laboratory costs must be budgeted separately from those of pharmacy with a separate fund allocated and available for the purchase of laboratory items.

A policy covering the regular supply of reagents and other items to district laboratories and a system for monitoring stocks are *essential* if laboratory services are to be available and free from disruption and staff are to remain motivated and not frustrated in their work.

Every district laboratory, with the help of the district laboratory coordinator, should prepare an *Essential Laboratory Reagents and Supplies List* for the items it needs on a regular basis. It is important to purchase chemicals, reagents, test kits, and other supplies from known reliable professional sources to avoid receiving substandard goods, e.g. test kits which have false expiry dates, or manipulated potencies.[1] The quality of supplies must be checked by a trained laboratory worker.

An efficient system is needed to supply outreach laboratories with standardized reliable reagents and other laboratory items. District laboratory staff must keep accurate signed records of all items requisitioned and received. Supplies must be requested correctly. A careful inventory should be kept of all supplies and a workable system for controlling stock levels.

A reliable system must also be established for packing and transporting laboratory supplies, including heat-sensitive reagents, to outreach laboratories. It is often possible to use the same system which exists for the transport of essential drugs to health centres.

STAFFING OF DISTRICT LABORATORIES AND COMPETENCE OF STAFF

The quality of district laboratory practice is directly dependent on the quality of performance of district laboratory personnel. Those in charge of district health care and laboratory services are responsible for:

- Deciding the grades, salary structure, and number of laboratory personnel required to staff the service and the career development of staff.

- Preparing job descriptions for each grade of district laboratory worker and the qualifications each grade requires.

- Ensuring all laboratory personnel are well trained (see subunit 1.3) and supported in their workplace.

- Employing as district laboratory workers only those who are:
  - qualified and competent,
  - interested in district health care,
  - speak the local language and are likely to be accepted by the community.

Before being employed, a laboratory officer must have:
- visited the laboratory in which he or she will work,
- studied the job description and discussed terms of employment,
- produced a valid Certificate of Qualification (to be checked by the employer).

If previously employed, references should be obtained.

Contract of employment
Employers should provide all laboratory personnel with a written contract of employment, detailing grade of worker, responsibilities, salary and method of payment, hours of work, emergency working arrangements, vacation, and any other relevant issues.

Note: For all newly appointed district laboratory staff, there should be a probationary working period of three months.

- Ensuring the working conditions of district laboratory staff are safe and acceptable and staff are paid according to their contract of employment.

- Supervizing adequately the work of newly appointed staff. The district laboratory coordinator has a responsibility to visit all laboratories in the district on a regular basis to discuss the work, motivate staff, address any problems, check the quality of reports and records, and assess working practices and performance standards.

Important: Where trainees perform laboratory tests, their work *must be* supervized. No test result should be issued before it has been verified by a qualified laboratory officer.

- Providing support in the workplace and continuing education for all district laboratory personnel as discussed in subunit 1.3.

QUALITY ASSURANCE TO OBTAIN CORRECT TEST RESULTS

Immediate and long term clinical, public health, and health planning decisions are based on the results of laboratory tests. Incorrect, delayed, or misinterpreted test results can have serious consequences for patients and communities, undermine confidence in the service, and waste scarce district health resources.

Achieving reliability of test results is dependent on:

- Understanding what are the commonest causes of inaccuracy and imprecision in the performance of tests and of delayed or misinterpreted

test results (see subunit 2.4, *Quality assurance and sources of error*).

- Taking the necessary steps to prevent and minimize errors by:
  - implementing *Standard Operating Procedures* (SOPs) with quality control for all district laboratory activities.
  - introducing every month a quality control day and an external quality assessment scheme for outreach laboratories (see later text, *Role of the district medical officer in TQM*).
  - appointing a district laboratory coordinator to monitor the performance of district laboratories (see later text).

- Agreeing with those requesting laboratory tests, policies of work that will enable the laboratory to provide an efficient, safe, cost-effective, and reliable service (see subunit 2.4).

- Maintaining good communications between laboratory staff and those requesting tests.

Note: A definition of quality assurance (QA) and how it is applied in district laboratory practice can be found on pages 31–34. Guidelines on the QA of parasitological tests are described on pages 178–182, clinical chemistry tests on pages 313–333, microbiology on pages 3–6 in Part 2, haematology tests on pages 267–270 in Part 2, and blood transfusion techniques on pages 350–351 in Part 2.

RESPONSIBILITY FOR TQM

In tropical and developing countries few district hospitals have a resident or visiting pathologist or even a medical officer with sufficient knowledge of laboratory practice to assist in the running of district laboratories. In the past this has lead to neglect of district laboratories and poor performance by staff.

With the development of district health care systems, most district laboratory services are now managed locally by a district laboratory coordinator helped by a district hospital medical officer trained in the use of laboratory investigations and basic quality assurance.

Responsibilities of the district laboratory coordinator
The person appointed as a district laboratory coordinator must be a senior well trained medical laboratory officer with management skills and several years experience of district laboratory practice and training

of laboratory personnel. Opportunities must be provided for continued professional development and the learning of management skills.

The most important responsibilities of the district laboratory coordinator are to:

- Assist in the establishment, integration, and management of district laboratories.

- Visit district laboratories at least every three months to help and motivate staff, monitor the quality of laboratory service being provided, discuss problems, and inform staff of important district health activities.

- Help to prepare, apply, and update standard operating procedures (SOPs) for district laboratories.

- Implement and monitor safe working practices and investigate laboratory accidents.

- Promote effective communication between laboratories, and good working relationships between laboratory staff, patients, and those requesting laboratory tests.

- Check whether equipment is functioning well and whether laboratory workers are using, cleaning, controlling/calibrating, and maintaining equipment correctly.

- Make sure essential reagents and other supplies are being ordered correctly and reaching laboratories satisfactorily.

- Examine quality control data, laboratory reports, and records.

- Help laboratory staff to learn new skills and work more efficiently.

- Implement an effective quality assurance scheme to assess the performance of laboratory staff and promote continuous improvement in the quality of district laboratory services.

- Investigate complaints from users of the laboratory and check whether the waiting time for test results is acceptable.

- Review the routine, emergency, and 'on call' workload of district laboratories.

- Evaluate laboratory operating costs and prepare the yearly budget.

- Check whether there is any unauthorized use of district laboratories.

- Make sure specimens are being collected and transported correctly and the system for referring specimens from health centres to the hospital laboratory is working well.

- Ensure district laboratory staff are well trained for their job (see subunit 1.3) and the work of trainees is being adequately supervised.

- Participate in laboratory clinical meetings and district health meetings.

- Every three months prepare a laboratory report for the district health management team, detailing the utilization of district laboratories, tests requested, workload, laboratory expenditures, staff needs and training.

Important: Because of the comprehensive duties of the district laboratory coordinator, it is recommended that the person appointed to do this job is carefully selected and is not already fulltime employed as laboratory officer in charge of the district hospital laboratory. A check list should be prepared of the activities which need to be performed during visits to the district's laboratories and also a list of the tools, spares, reagents, standards, etc, that the coordinator should take.

Role of the district hospital medical officer in TQM of district laboratory services

The medical officer appointed to help in the running of district laboratory services must be a good communicator and 'laboratory-friendly'.[2] The following are practical ways in which a district hospital medical officer with only a limited knowledge of laboratory procedures can help to motivate laboratory staff and contribute to improving the quality of service provided, particularly that of the district hospital laboratory:

- Visiting the laboratory on a regular basis to discuss the workload, any specimen collection problems, and any difficulties which may be affecting the quality of work or well being of the laboratory staff.

- Promoting good communications between the laboratory and the medical and nursing staff and monitoring how the results of tests are being used.

- Monitoring whether test results are being verified and clearly reported on request forms, and whether the target turnaround times for tests are being met and if not how the situation can be improved.

- Checking with the senior laboratory officer whether equipment maintenance schedules are being performed.

- Observing whether essential safety is being practised, e.g. glassware and plasticware are being decontaminated before being washed and reused, specimens are being collected, tested and disposed of safely, laboratory staff are not mouth-pipetting specimens and reagents, the laboratory is being kept clean and tidy, flammable and toxic chemicals are being stored safely, laboratory staff know what to do if there is a fire and are trained in essential First Aid.

- Investigating the reasons for any tests not being performed, particularly if due to supplies not being ordered or delivered.
- Establishing with the help of the district laboratory coordinator, a monthly *quality control day*.

Quality control day: This can best be achieved by the medical officer dividing a few specimens, giving each a different identity and checking whether the results of all the specimens are the same (within acceptable limits). If not, the medi-

cal officer should ask the senior laboratory officer to investigate the likely cause(s), e.g. SOPs not being followed by the staff, an instrument malfunctioning, variable pipetting, deteriorating reagents, staff not having sufficient experience.

To control the reporting of microscopical preparations, the medical officer should obtain stained quality control smears of specimens from the district laboratory coordinator, e.g. smears showing malaria parasites, trypanosomes, AFB, gram negative diplococci, blood cells, etc. The medical officer should ask as many of the staff as possible to examine the preparations.

- Holding monthly clinical meetings with laboratory staff and the district laboratory coordinator to discuss interesting test results and the findings of the *quality control day*.

CORRECT USE OF THE LABORATORY IN DISTRICT HEALTH CARE
see subunits 2.1 and 2.2

PROVIDING A QUALITY SERVICE TO USERS OF THE LABORATORY
see subunit 2.1

TRAINING AND ONGOING SUPPORT OF STAFF IN THE WORK PLACE
see subunits 2.1 and 1.3

TQM

MANAGEMENT OF FINANCES AND BUDGETING
see subunit 2.3

MANAGEMENT OF EQUIPMENT AND SUPPLIES
see subunits 2.1 and 4.1

QUALITY ASSURANCE SOPs, QC, EQA. GOOD COMMUNICATIONS
see subunits 2.1, 2.4, 2.7

Abbreviations: **TQM** Total Quality Management, **QA** Quality Assurance, **SOPs** Standard Operating Procedures, **QC** Quality Control, **EQA** External Quality Assessment.

Continuing improvement in quality

The following are effective ways of monitoring progress and implementing ongoing improvement in the quality of district laboratory services:

- Discussing with the users of district laboratories what changes and improvements are needed and how laboratory tests can be used more cost-effectively and efficiently.

- Regularly reviewing and updating standard operating procedures and laboratory policies.

- Improving the system for supplying district laboratories.

- Monitoring quality control and the effectiveness of the district quality assessment scheme.

- Investigating errors at the time they occur, taking corrective action, and checking whether the action taken has been effective.

- Considering how to improve specimen collection and transport in the district and how to reduce the time patients wait for test results.

- Providing on-site continuing education and support for district laboratory staff.

- Ensuring all laboratories in the district are kept informed of district health programmes.

- Looking ahead, planning, and budgeting realistically for future laboratory needs.

- Promoting the right attitude to quality which has been summarized by Elsenga as 'willing people make failing systems work, unwilling people make working systems fail'.[3]

2.2 Selection of tests and interpretation of test results

The importance of using laboratory investigations correctly in district health care has been outlined in subunit 2.1 (TQM). This subunit covers in more detail the factors that need to be considered when selecting tests and interpreting test reports.

REASONS FOR PERFORMING LABORATORY TESTS

The reasons for performing laboratory tests and follow-up investigations must be clear. The tests performed in district laboratories must reflect the common and emergency health needs of the area and provide information that can be easily interpreted. The tests must also be efficient, i.e. provide sufficient benefit to justify their cost and any risks involved in their performance.

Medical officers should encourage qualified experienced laboratory staff to provide maximum information from laboratory tests and to proceed to further testing when this is obviously indicated and will lead to better and earlier treatment for a patient.

Examples of maximizing information from laboratory tests

- When examining a thick stained blood film for malaria parasites, report also if the neutrophils or eosinophils are significantly increased. If no parasites are found check the preparation for trypanosomes or borreliae if the patient is from an area where these organisms are found.

  Check also for significant background reticulocytosis which may indicate sickle cell disease if the patient (particularly a child) is from a haemoglobin S (Hb S) prevalent area. Perform a sickle cell test and examine a thin stained blood film.

- If many malaria parasites are found in the blood of a young child, measure and monitor the haemoglobin.

- When pus cells are found in the urine from a male patient, Gram stain the urine sediment and look for Gram negative intracellular diplococci, indicative of gonorrhoea.

- When finding glycosuria, measure the fasting blood glucose.

- If red cells and protein are found in urine from a patient living in a schistosomiasis endemic area, examine the urine sediment for S. haematobium eggs.

- If blood and mucus are present in faeces, examine the specimen carefully for the eggs of S. mansoni or motile amoebae with ingested red cells, indicative of amoebic dysentery.

- If faeces appears like rice water, inoculate it in alkaline peptone water and look for vibrio.

- If there is a rapid fall in haemoglobin and a rising ESR in a febrile patient from a trypanosomiasis endemic area, check the blood for trypanosomes.

- When the blood film from an adult shows significant hypochromia and the haemoglobin is low, check the faeces for hookworm eggs.

In deciding which tests and test methods are appropriate it is important to consider:

- the clinical and public health needs of the district,
- wellbeing of patients,
- laboratory technical aspects,
- costs involved.

Relevance of laboratory tests

It is both wasteful and unscientific to perform laboratory tests:

- that provide little useful clinical or public health information,
- that contribute only minimally to patient management and quality of care,
- that are not sufficiently rapid, reliable, sensitive, or specific for the purpose.

Tests should be requested rationally and specifically based on the value of the information they provide and their cost-effectiveness. Ordering several tests that provide similar information cannot be justified. Asking the following questions will help medical officers to request tests appropriately:

- why am I requesting this test?
- is it affordable?
- can the laboratory perform it reliably, and how long will it take to get the result?
- what will I look for in the result?
- how will it affect my diagnosis and my care of the patient?
- ultimately, what will be the benefits to the patient and to the community?

Clinical and public health considerations

Priority diagnostic tests

Priority should be given to selecting those tests that help to diagnose those conditions:

- that are difficult to diagnose accurately from clinical symptoms alone, particularly at an early stage of an illness, when a patient has a secondary infection or has received drugs or herbal medication at home before attending the clinic.
- that require lengthy, high risk, or expensive treatment.
- that can cause epidemics with high mortality or much illhealth and disability.

Tests needed in treatment, disease control and prevention

Other tests will also be required in the treatment, control, and prevention of disease to:

- achieve a more rational and selective use of drugs.
- detect and monitor drug resistance particularly resistance to antimalarials and antibiotics.

- assess the severity of illness and likely outcome of an illness.
- make the treatment and care of a patient safer and help to assess the effectiveness of treatment.
- establish a baseline value for follow-up care.
- assess whether a patient being treated in a health centre needs to be referred to the district hospital for specialist care.
- monitor anaemia or occupational disease.
- monitor the health of pregnant women.
- improve the care of HIV infected persons.
- identify disease carriers and improve case-finding.
- detect carriers of Hb S as part of family planning counselling services.
- monitor microbial pollution of community water supplies.
- prevent blood transmissible infections, particularly those caused by HIV and hepatitis viruses.
- promote community health education.
- increase the validity of disease reporting by providing reliable information on the causes and pattern of illhealth in the community.

Important: Clinicians and public health officers must be kept up to date regarding the availability and relevance of new technologies. Laboratory personnel need to know how tests are used to be able to report tests informatively.

The sensitivity and specificity of tests are explained in subunit 2.2.

Patient considerations

In the selection of tests and test methods the following are important patient considerations:

- Many patients requiring laboratory investigations in tropical and developing countries will be young children, therefore specimen collection techniques must be appropriate.

- Specimen collection techniques for all patients must be safe, respectful of the person, as stress free as possible, and culturally acceptable.

- When several different tests requiring blood are required, the tests should be coordinated to avoid the unnecessary repeated collection of blood from patients.

- A high proportion of patients will be outpatients requiring their test results before receiving treatment, therefore rapid techniques are needed.

- Tests performed must lead to improved quality of patient care and be affordable. Patients should always be advized why a particular test is needed and what is required in providing the specimen(s).

■ Whenever possible patients should not have to travel considerable distances for essential laboratory investigations, e.g. tests required by pregnant women.

Laboratory considerations

The following are important technical considerations in the selection of tests, test methods, and in deciding which tests should be performed in outreach laboratories and in the district hospital laboratory:

■ Competence and experience of local laboratory staff and whether support can be provided on a regular basis.

■ How well a test can be standardized and controlled in the laboratory in which it will be performed.

■ Communication and transport links that exist between outreach laboratories and the hospital laboratory to facilitate the referral of specimens.

■ Reagents, standards, controls, and consummables required to perform tests, including their cost, complexity of preparation or availability as ready-made products, stability and storage and hazards associated with their use particularly in outreach laboratories.

■ Quality and quantity of water required.

■ Equipment needed, including its running cost, power requirements, complexity and safety of use, maintenance, local repair facilities and availability of replacement parts, anticipated reliability and working life.

■ Type of specimen required, including its collection, stability, transport, storage, safe handling and disposal.

■ Performance time of tests and how frequently particular tests are requested.

Cost considerations

The following are important financial considerations when selecting tests and test methods:

■ How expensive is the test, for example:

   – what is the cost of collecting the specimen including the cost of the specimen container, and is there a significant cost in preparing the patient?

   – does the test require the use of inexpensive reagents that can be prepared locally or expensive reagents and controls that have a limited shelf-life and need to be imported?

   – does the test require the use of equipment which is expensive to operate and maintain?

   – is the technique simple and rapid or complex and lengthy, and does it require the skills of a specialist laboratory officer?

Note: Subunit 2.3 describes how to estimate the unit cost of a test based on laboratory operating costs, number of tests performed, and the workload unit value of the test.

■ What are the costs of the different technologies? Can using an expensive technology be justified when there is a reliable cheaper alternative for obtaining the same or similar information? A costly new technology does not necessarily mean that it will have improved performance characteristics and be more appropriate. It may even have important limitations, e.g. a rapid malaria antigen test that is not able to differentiate species.

■ Is it cost effective for district laboratories to use:

   – clinical chemistry kits for frequently performed tests when the reagents and standards can be easily and cheaply made in the laboratory?

   – a diagnostic kit test in district laboratories when the format of the kit is designed for testing large numbers of specimens at one time and the working reagents have poor stability?

   – urine reagent strip tests in areas of high relative humidity when moisture causes the strips to deteriorate rapidly, resulting in significant wastage (and unreliable test results).

■ How will the cost of tests be met? It is essential that tests are ordered only when they are needed and the cost is known of each test when performed in a health centre laboratory and in the district hospital laboratory.

Note: Financing district laboratory services and controlling laboratory costs are discussed in the next subunit (2.3).

How to decide which tests are the most important in community-based health care

Answering the following questions will help medical officers and community health workers to decide which tests are the most important in meeting individual and community health needs:

1 What are the commonest and most life-threatening conditions for which people seek medical care? Make separate lists for infants,

children, men, non-pregnant women, pregnant women.

2   What conditions are the most difficult to diagnose? Which laboratory tests are the most likely to assist in investigating these? Which conditions if misdiagnosed could have serious consequences for an individual and public health?

3   For what symptoms are antibiotics being prescribed and how often? Which laboratory tests could be used to confirm a diagnosis or rule out an infection before prescribing an antibiotic?

4   What is the transmission pattern of malaria? How often are antimalarials being prescribed without confirming the diagnosis microscopically? Is drug resistance a problem?

Misdiagnosis of malaria

An increasing number of surveys show malaria is often misdiagnosed both by experienced and less experienced medical officers and community health workers, leading to costly antimalarial drugs being prescribed unnecessarily, and the true cause of a patients's illness remaining undiagnosed. Misdiagnosis also leads to incorrect reporting of malaria incidence.

5   How many patients are being treated without being diagnosed, e.g. patients with fever of unknown origin, headache, or general body pain? Go back through several months' records to include seasonal influences.

6   How many patients return to see the medical officer or community health worker because the prescribed drugs or other treatment appear not to have worked? Looking back, could any laboratory test if performed at the time of the first visit have helped the patient to receive a more appropriate treatment and prevent their condition worsening.

7   Are there any prevalent infectious diseases in the community which the laboratory could investigate to assist in breaking the cycle of transmission and preventing reinfection?

8   In the last 12 months have there been any serious epidemics which the laboratory could have helped to bring more quickly under control or even helped to prevent?

9   Are there any major health education programmes which the laboratory could make more effective, e.g. demonstrating microscopically the parasites that cause schistosomiasis?

10 How many young children and adults are needing to travel to the district hospital for laboratory investigations? List the tests being requested.

Important: It will not be possible in a community-

based laboratory to perform all the tests that are needed to meet individual and community health needs. Some of the limiting factors are discussed in subunit 1.2.

Further information: Important guidelines on the selection of laboratory tests can be found in a WHO laboratory document: *Laboratory services for primary health care: requirements for essential clinical laboratory tests* (see Recommended Reading).

LABORATORY REQUEST FORM

The format of laboratory request forms should be clear and standardized throughout the district. The layout should be discussed and agreed by laboratory staff and users of the laboratory service.

Whenever possible laboratory request forms, suitable for use in district laboratories should be prepared by a central stationery office. Where forms are not supplied from a central source, simple request forms can be prepared locally. Standardization and clarity in presenting and reporting results can be achieved by the use of rubber stamps (see Fig. 2.1). Adequate ink, however, must be used and the stamp must be positioned carefully.

Information to accompany requests for laboratory tests

The laboratory request form should be dated and provide the following information:

■   Patient's full name, age, and gender.

■   Address or village of patient (valuable epidemiological data).

■   Inpatient or outpatient identification number.

■   Relevant clinical information regarding patient's condition.

■   Details of drugs or local medicines taken by or administered to the patient before visiting the health unit or hospital, and drugs that have been administered by the health unit or hospital prior to collecting the specimen, e.g. antimicrobials, antimalarial drugs.

■   Specific test(s) required.

■   Specimen provided.

■   Origin of request if from an outreach health centre or maternity unit.

■   Name of the medical officer, community health worker, or midwife requesting the test and to whom the report should be sent.

Urgent tests: Only those tests should be requested urgently that are required for the immediate care of a patient or to manage a serious public health situation.

Note: The specimen container must be clearly labelled with the patient's name, identification number, and the date and time of collection.

Patient confidentiality

As soon as request forms and specimens are received by the laboratory the staff have a responsibility to ensure the request forms are not read by unauthorized persons.

Laboratory staff must *never* disclose any information they may learn about a patient or a test result to anyone other than the health personnel caring for the patient. Respecting patient confidentiality must also extend to when laboratory reports are issued. Reports should be delivered in sealed envelopes, labelled CONFIDENTIAL LABORATORY REPORTS, or in labelled sealed folders which can be returned to the laboratory for re-use.

REPORTING AND RECORDING TEST RESULTS

Laboratory staff should provide as much relevant information as possible to assist those requesting tests to interpret the results of tests correctly and use the information in the best possible way to benefit patients and the community. Reports should be clearly and neatly written (particularly figures).

Standardization in reporting test results

Standardization in the presentation of reports and use of units is important because it helps in the interpretation and comparison of results, contributes to the efficiency of a laboratory service, and is of value when patients are referred from one health unit or hospital to another. The use of SI units in the reporting of tests can be found in subunit 2.5.

Laboratory reports in patients' notes

The system sometimes used in district hospitals of 'charting', or transferring, laboratory results from laboratory registers or from laboratory request forms into patients' notes is not recommended. Not only is it time-consuming but it can give rise to serious errors when results are not copied correctly or in their entirety. A patient's notes must contain the signed reports issued by the laboratory.

When resources are limited, an inexpensive reliable way of inserting laboratory reports in patients' notes is to report results on small stamped forms and attach these to a sheet of paper reserved for *Laboratory Reports* in each patient's notes. If the pieces of paper are arranged as shown in Fig. 2.1, several reports can be attached to one sheet.

Keeping laboratory reports in one place in a patient's notes has the added advantage that the latest test result can be quickly compared with a previous result.

Recording results in the laboratory

In district laboratories, records of test results can be kept by retaining carbon copies of reports, using work sheets, or recording test results in registers (exercise books). Whichever system is used it must be reliable and enable patients' results to be found quickly. Test records are also required when preparing work reports and estimating the workload of the laboratory.

If carbon copies or work sheets are used these must be dated and filed systematically each day. If registers are used, backing cards which are headed and ruled can be placed behind pages to avoid having to rule and head each page separately. The cards must be heavily ruled with a marker pen so that the lines can be seen clearly. Separate registers, each with its own cards, can be prepared to record the results of haematological, microbiological, clinical chemistry, urine and faecal tests. Examples of cards which could be used in a Urine Analysis Register are shown in Fig. 2.2.

In smaller district laboratories the registers can also be used to record daily quality control information, e.g. reading of a haemoglobin control. Daily checks on the performance of equipment, e.g. temperature readings should be recorded in a quality control (QC) book or on separate sheets as part of equipment control procedures.

INTERPRETATION OF TEST REPORTS

In the use and interpretation of laboratory test results it is important to understand the limitations of tests, e.g. the ability of tests to indicate when disease is present or absent or whether the value in a report is normal or abnormal for a patient. Reference ranges are required for the interpretation of quantitative test results.

The performance characteristics of tests are also important, e.g. how accurately and precisely (reproducibly) a test can be performed (see subunit 2.4) and for some tests, reader variability can also be important (see later text).

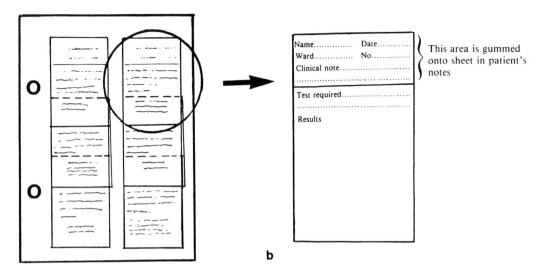

Fig. 2.1   Transfering laboratory results into the hospital notes of a patient.
a) Sheet in patient's notes on to which laboratory report forms are gummed or stapled.
b) Close-up of a simple laboratory form. A rubber stamp can be used to print the upper part of the form.

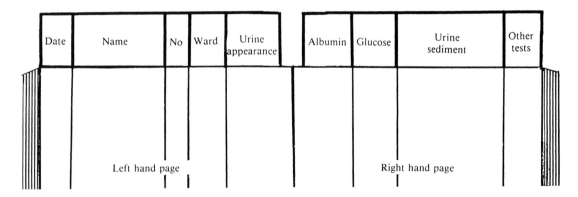

Fig. 2.2   Example of an exercise book with card inserts to record test results. The lines from the ruled cards show through the pages of the book

Ability of diagnostic tests to indicate presence or absence of disease

The ability of a diagnostic test to indicate when a disease is present or absent is dependant on its quality and is described in terms of:

- sensitivity,
- specificity,
- predictive value.

Sensitivity (true positive rate)

This is the frequency of positive test results in patients with a particular disease, e.g. 95% sensitivity implies 5% false negatives. A test which has 100% sensitivity is always abnormal (or positive) in patients with the disease.

Calculating sensitivity

$$\text{Sensitivity} = \frac{\text{total number positive results}}{\text{total number infected patients}}$$

Screening tests should be sensitive to ensure that where possible, a positive test result is obtained in all patients with the disease. The higher the sensitivity of a test, the less likely it is to fail to diagnose a person as having the disease, i.e. the fewer the number of false negative results. For example, it is important to use a high sensitivity HIV serological test when screening blood supplies for HIV antibody.

Analytical sensitivity: this is different to statistical sensitivity as described above. Analytical sensitivity relates to the lowest result which can be reliably differentiated from zero.

Specificity (false positive rate)

This is the frequency of negative test results in patients without that disease. A 95% specificity implies 5% false positives.

Calculating specificity

$$\text{Specificity} = \frac{\text{total number negative results}}{\text{total number uninfected patients}}$$

Definitive tests should be specific to ensure a patient is not incorrectly diagnosed as having the disease, i.e. false positive result. The higher the specificity of a test, the less likely it is to diagnose a person who does not have the disease as having it, i.e. the fewer the number of false positive results.

Examples of tests with high specificity include the Ziehl-Neelsen technique for AFB, and microscopical parasitological diagnostic techniques where parasitic forms can be identified. Sensitivity, however, can vary greatly particularly when pathogens are excreted intermittently or in variable numbers or when only a small amount of specimen is examined.

Neither specificity nor sensitivity is dependent on the prevalence of disease for which the test is being performed.

Analytical specificity: this is different to statistical specificity as described above. Analytical specificity depends on whether only the substance under investigation is measured.

Predictive value of a positive test result

This is the percentage of positive results that are true positives when a test is performed on a defined population containing both healthy and diseased persons. It depends not only on the specificity and sensitivity of the test but particularly on the prevalence of the disease in the population tested as can be shown in the following examples:

$$\text{Predictive \% value of positive test result} = \frac{\text{True positives}}{\text{True positives} + \text{False positives}} \times 100$$

Examples

Low prevalence and predictive value of a positive test.
For example, if a test has 90% sensitivity, 95% specificity (5% false positives), and the condition it detects has a *2% prevalence* in the population it follows that:

- 2% prevalence means, of 1000 persons, 20 have the disease in the population.
- 18 will be detected (true positives), i.e. 90% of 20 based on 90% sensitivity.
- 49 will have false positive tests, i.e. 5% of 980 based on 95% specificity.
- there will be a total 67 positive tests (18 true, 49 false).
- Predictive value of positive test:

$$\frac{18 \text{ (true positives)}}{67 \text{ (all positive tests)}} \times 100 = 27\%$$

The predictive value of a positive test is therefore low when the prevalence is low.

High prevalence and predictive value of a positive test
For example, if the test has 90% sensitivity, 95% specificity and the condition it detects has a *20% prevalence* in the population it follows that:

- 20% prevalence means of 1000 persons, 200 have the disease in the population.
- 180 will be true positives, i.e. 90% of 200.
- 40 will have false positive tests, i.e. 5% of 800.
- there will be a total of 220 positive tests (180 true, 40 false)
- Predictive value of positive test:

$$\frac{180 \text{ (true positives)}}{220 \text{ (all positive tests)}} \times 100 = 82\%.$$

The predictive value of a positive test is therefore high when the prevalence is high.

Predictive values are important diagnostically as they give the probability that an abnormal result comes from someone with disease. The higher the predictive value of a test, the higher the possibility in any population that a positive test means disease.

If a disease has a low prevalence in the population being tested, there will be a higher number of false positive results due to the higher proportion of persons without the disease and therefore a positive result has a lower predictive value.

The positive predictive value of a test for a disease will increase both with the sensitivity of the test and the prevalence of the disease. To be useful, a test's predictive value must be greater than the prevalence of the disease.

Even when a test is highly sensitive and specific there is still a possibility of false positive results when the prevalence of the disease is low. Confirmatory testing becomes important in these situations.

Reader variability

The reader variability percentage gives an indication of how easy it is to report a visually read test. The clearer a test result is to read the lower will be the reader variability. Difficult to read test results will result in greater reader variation.

Reader variability is one of the operational characteristics used by WHO to evaluate HIV test kits when the readings are performed without equipment. The reader variability is expressed by WHO as the percentage of sera for which test results are differently interpreted by different readers. To reduce reader variability, most manufacturers of serological tests include weak positive controls and artwork showing a range of positive test results. Some manufacturers make available instruments to reduce the variability inherent in reading test results visually.

In reporting microscopical preparations, reader variability can be reduced by using reference preparations to assist in the identification of organisms and cells, preparing specimens correctly, and examining preparations for the correct length of time.

Recognizing that some specimens and preparations will always be more difficult to report, reader variability can be minimized by following standardized procedures, using adequate controls and reference materials, and by improving the quality of training and supervision when introducing new tests.

REFERENCE RANGES FOR QUANTITATIVE TESTS

Laboratory staff and those requesting tests should know the accepted reference ranges and clinical significance of the results of the quantitative tests performed in the laboratory. This will ensure that significantly abnormal results are detected, checked, reported, and acted on as soon as possible. Prompt action by laboratory staff may prevent loss of life or lead to an earlier treatment with more rapid recovery for a patient.

Clinical significance of abnormal test results
The clinical significance of abnormal results for the quantitative tests included in this publication can be found at the end of each test method.

Test results are affected both by biological and laboratory analytical factors and these need to be considered when deciding the reference range for each test.

Biological factors

The following are among the biological factors that contribute to differences in test results among healthy people:

- *Age:* e.g. higher plasma urea concentrations are found in the elderly. Alkaline phosphatase activity is higher in growing children compared with adults. Reference values from neonates are very different from those of adults.
- *Gender:* e.g. higher values of haemoglobin, plasma creatinine, urate, and urea are found in men compared with women during the reproductive phase of life.
- *Diet and nutritional state:* e.g. plasma cholesterol and calcium are affected by diet.
- *Time of the day (diurnal variation):* e.g. serum iron levels rise as the day progresses.
- *Posture:* e.g. plasma protein levels are lower in samples collected from patients when they are lying down.
- *Muscular activity:* e.g. the concentration of plasma creatinine rises following exercise.
- *Dehydration:* e.g. haemoglobin, PCV, white blood cells increase due to decrease in plasma volume.

Reference ranges are also affected by weight, phase of menstrual cycle, emotional state, geographical location, rural or city life, climate, genetic factors, cultural habits, smoking, and homeostatic variation.

Some reference values are also altered during pregnancy, e.g. haemoglobin and PCV values decrease and neutrophil numbers increase.

Analytical factors

Among the analytical factors that influence reference ranges the most significant are:

- *Type of sample:* e.g. the concentration of glucose is 12–13% higher in plasma than in whole blood. Small variations also occur between serum and plasma samples for potassium and some other substances.
- *Test method:* e.g. a glucose oxidase enzyme method will give a narrower reference range for blood glucose than a Folin-Wu technique because the enzyme method is specific for glucose.
- *Performance:* Some tests can be performed with less variation than others. The reference ranges for such tests will therefore be narrower.

How reference ranges are established

The reference range for a particular substance is worked out by testing and plotting a graph of frequency of value against concentration. For some assays the graph produced is symmetrical in shape

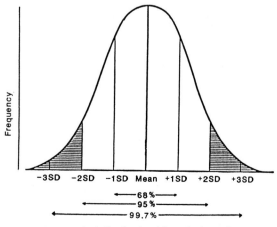

Fig. 2.3 Symmetrical distribution (Gaussian) graph

showing the highest number of people having values around the mean (average) with a gradual decrease in frequency on each side of the mean as shown in Fig. 2.3.

In statistical terms the distribution of values around the mean can be expressed as standard deviation (SD). When the results of a particular test show a symmetrical (Gaussian) type curve, the reference range for the substance being measured is defined by a plus or minus 2 SD from the mean (see Fig. 2.4). This covers 95% of the 'healthy' population (± 1 SD covers 68% of the population, and ± 3 SD covers 99.7% of the population).

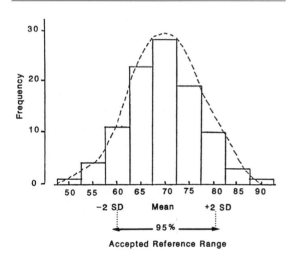

Fig. 2.4 Example of Gaussian distribution of plasma total protein giving a reference range of 60–80 g/l.

Assessing reference (normal) ranges

Because reference ranges are affected by a variety of biological and analytical factors, they should be regarded only as approximate interim reference ranges to be assessed by clinicians and laboratory staff at a later stage when sufficient data becomes available. The central laboratory should assist in confirming reference values for the population.

Note: The reference ranges given in this publication have been compiled from accepted western values and those received by the author from a small number of tropical countries.

Interpretation of results outside the reference range

If a patient's result is outside of the accepted reference range this does not necessarily indicate ill health. The patient may be in the 5% minority healthy group outside the Mean ± 2 SD range.

There can be no clear dividing line between 'normal' and 'abnormal' values. This is one of the reasons why the term reference range is preferred to normal range. To interpret test results adequately, not only should the reference values provided by the laboratory be considered by clinicians, but also the levels of abnormality which are likely to be present in different diseases and in the early and late stages of a disease.

Action to take when results are seriously abnormal

As part of standard operating procedures and QA, laboratories need to decide what procedure should be followed when a result is seriously abnormal or unexpected, e.g. when compared with a previous recent result. For some tests it may be appropriate to define a level of abnormality which leads to immediate action being taken by laboratory staff to check the result and inform the person treating the patient.

Important: Whenever a result is communicated orally, the written report should be issued as soon as possible. Before being issued, *all* reports must be checked (verified) by the most experienced member of the laboratory staff. Verification of reports is particularly important when trainees are performing tests.

2.3 Financing district laboratory services and controlling costs

In most developing countries, district laboratory services are financed centrally by the ministry of health or at district level through district health councils.

In some countries, laboratory and pharmacy services share a common budget. Such a policy, however, is not satisfactory because it frequently leads to under-resourcing of laboratory services as priority is given to purchasing drugs. It is therefore recommended that laboratory services be budgeted and funded separately. To manage laboratory finances efficiently, accurate records must be kept of laboratory expenditures and the workload of the laboratory.

Cost recovery schemes

Increasingly district health expenditures are being met in part by patients contributing towards their health care costs. A partial cost-recovery scheme provides a revolving fund for the purchase of essential supplies.

Local fees for laboratory tests should not be more than can be afforded by patients. Applying an affordable flat standard rate for the laboratory service will help all patients to be tested according to their health need. Most patients recognize that reliable locally accessible laboratory testing improves the quality of their care and often avoids a repeat visit to the health care centre or a longer more expensive journey to the district hospital laboratory.

Resourcing of district laboratory practice
Careful analysis and budgeting of laboratory costs and adequate government resourcing of district laboratory practice are essential to maintain quality of service.

Budgets are more likely to be met when district laboratory services:

● contribute effectively to improving the health status of the community.

● can demonstrate reliability, efficiency, and commitment to continuing improvement in quality.

● provide correct and useful data on infectious diseases.

● respond rapidly and responsibly when epidemics occur.

ESTIMATING LABORATORY OPERATING COSTS

The following need to be included when estimating the yearly variable and fixed costs of operating a district laboratory:

■ Salaries of technical and auxiliary staff.

■ Cost of consummables including:
 – chemicals, control materials, calibrants, stains,
 – culture media and serological reagents,
 – ready-made reagents, diagnostic test kits, reagent strip tests,
 – blood collection sets, collection bags, blood grouping antisera and crossmatching reagents,
 – filter paper and pH indicator papers,
 – coverglasses, microscope slides, pipettor tips,
 – disinfectants, detergents, soap.

■ Cost of services including electricity, gas, kerosene, water supply, water filtration units and communication equipment.

■ Cost of inspecting, maintaining, and repairing equipment and equipment depreciation.

■ Cost of replacing worn or broken items such as:
 – counting chambers
 – pipettes and general glassware and plasticware,
 – cleaning utensils,
 – laboratory linen.

■ Cost of specimen containers, swabs, cotton wool, and dressings.

■ Cost of stationery including:
 – record books,
 – laboratory request forms,
 – labels,
 – pens and markers.

■ Travel and transport costs including the visits of the district laboratory coordinator.

■ Expenditure involved in cleaning and maintaining the laboratory, and keeping it secure.

Variable and fixed costs
The cost of supplies including reagents and consummables are usually referred to as variable costs while salaries, equipment maintenance and depreciation, supervision, and overhead costs are referred to as fixed costs. Careful records of expenditures must be kept.

Financing health centre laboratories
The operating costs of health centre laboratories tend to be low because many of the tests are inexpensive. If, however, the health centre is not well attended the cost of maintaining an underutilized laboratory may be unacceptably high. In an underutilized situation it may be more cost-effective to operate the laboratory on a part-time basis and train a member of the nursing staff to perform the required tests and manage the laboratory. It may also be more cost-effective to send specimens for non-urgent tests to the district hospital laboratory when there are reliable facilities for transporting the specimens and rapid return of test results.

Note: The cost factors that need to be considered when selecting tests and test methods have been discussed in the previous subunit (2.2).

Estimating costs of tests
A method of estimating the cost of tests in district laboratories where the cost of reagents and other supplies tends to be low can be found in the paper of Houang.[4] Individual tests are costed as follows:

1   Estimate the total cost of operating the laboratory over a 1 year period (see previous text).

2   List the tests performed and total the number of each test performed over the year.

3   Estimate the total workload units for each test performed by multiplying the number of each test performed by its laboratory workload unit (LWU). Table 2.2 lists the LWU values frequently assigned to laboratory tests performed in district laboratories and the definition of LWU.

Example: If 523 WBCs are performed in 1 year, the total LWU for WBCs is 523 × 6 = 3138 (where LWU for WBC is 6).

4   Add up the total LWU for each test to give the yearly total workload for all the tests performed.

5   Divide the total laboratory operating cost by the total workload to give the total unit cost.

Example: If the total operating cost is US$ 3131 and the total workload is 20 913, the total unit cost is 3131 ÷ 20 913 = US$ 0.15.

6   To obtain the individual cost of each test, multiply the total unit cost by the unit value for each test.

Examples: If total unit cost is US$ 0.15, a WBC test would cost 0.15 × 6 = US$ 0.90, a differential WBC would cost 0.15 × 11 = US$ 1.65, etc.

Table 2.2   Laboratory workload unit (LWU) values of tests commonly performed in district laboratories

TEST	LWU
Haemoglobin	5
WBC (white cell count)	6
Differential WBC	11
ESR (erythrocyte sedimentation rate)	5
PCV (packed cell volume)	3
Blood grouping: ABO	7
ABO and D	9
Basic urine chemistry (reagent strips tests)	3
Measurement of urine protein	8
Measurement of blood glucose	8
Measurement of blood urea	8
Pregnancy test (rapid test)	2
Rapid plasma reagin (RPR)	2
Ziehl Neelsen	12
Gram	8
Wet faecal preparation	10
Malaria thick film	10
Microscopial examinations for other blood parasites	10

Definition: The laboratory workload unit (LWU) is a standardized unit equal to 1 minute of technical, clerical and aide time. The LWU values in this table may require amending depending on the method used to perform tests in different laboratories. The LWU is not the same as how long it takes to perform a particular test, e.g. ESR is assigned a LWU of 5 not 1 hour.

Note: Further information on how to estimate the cost of running a district laboratory service can be found in the paper of Mundy *et al.*[5]

CONTROLLING LABORATORY COSTS

The following can help to control laboratory costs and minimize waste of laboratory resources:

- If users of the laboratory select tests appropriately as explained in subunit 2.2.

- Advize medical staff and community health workers which tests are more complex to perform and use expensive reagents or equipment that is expensive to operate or maintain. Monitor the use of expensive tests.

- Standardize the technologies and equipment used in district laboratories.

- Purchase new equipment only after considering whether it is appropriate (see subunit 4.1), and whether maintenance costs can be afforded and justified.

- Train laboratory staff to work competently and economically and use equipment correctly (see subunit 1.3). Staff should know the costs of reagents, controls, equipment, and replacement parts.

- Where appropriate, use reusable plasticware instead of glassware. Good laboratory practice can also help to reduce glassware breakages and waste from spillages.

- Before purchasing diagnostic test kits, check the specifications, storage requirements, and shelf-life of the stock and working reagents to make sure the kits can be used cost-effectively.

- Whenever possible use micro-techniques, particularly for clinical chemistry assays, to reduce the volume of reagents, calibrants, and controls needed. Make sure, however, that the total volume of sample is sufficient for reading the absorbance.

- Whenever possible, batch test specimens, particularly clinical chemistry assays, to economize on the use of controls and calibrants and maximize the use of working reagents. This applies more to district hospital laboratory practice.

- Make basic easy-to-prepare reagents in the laboratory instead of buying expensive ready-made products.

- Store chemicals and reagents correctly and take care to avoid contaminating them.

- Collect specimens and perform tests correctly to avoid repeating a test unnecessarily. Supervize adequately the work of trainees and new members of staff.

- Every three months review critically the emergency and routine workload of the laboratory.

- Review whether the layout of the laboratory contributes to an efficient way of working.

- Ensure laboratory buildings, particularly doors, windows, and vents are secure and every measure is taken to discourage break-ins and theft of laboratory equipment and supplies.

- Take precautions to avoid the unauthorized use of laboratory property.

- Keep accurate records of laboratory expenditures.

PRIVATE DISTRICT LABORATORY PRACTICE

In some developing countries, severe government under-resourcing for national laboratory services has led to the growth of private laboratory practice. Private laboratories may be able to perform tests that are either temporarily or permanently unavailable at the district hospital laboratory. For many in the community, however, the fees charged by the privately run laboratories are unaffordable.

Where private laboratory practice is used to compliment community district laboratory services, health authorities have a responsibility to ensure private laboratories:

- are staffed by qualified registered laboratory personnel with a medical officer in attendance,
- do not permit laboratory staff to prescribe drugs,
- have appropriate facilities for the tests being performed,
- operate safely,
- follow standard operating procedures with adequate quality assurance,

- display fees and make these known to patients before performing investigations,
- keep accurate accounts of income and expenditures.

Most private laboratories do not perform essential public health laboratory activities or disease surveillance.

2.4 Quality assurance and sources of error in district laboratory practice

The necessity for total quality management in district laboratory practice has been discussed in subunit 2.1 This subunit covers in detail how to ensure the quality of test results, i.e. quality assurance. The purpose of quality assurance (QA) in laboratory practice is to provide test results that are:

- relevant
- reliable and reproducible
- timely
- interpreted correctly.

QA includes all those activities both in and outside the laboratory, performance standards, good laboratory practice, and management skills that are required to achieve and maintain a quality service and provide for continuing improvement.

Defining quality assurance (QA)
QA has been defined by WHO as the total process whereby the quality of laboratory reports can be guaranteed. It has been summarized as the:

- *right result*, at the
- *right time*, on the
- *right specimen*, from the
- *right patient*, with result interpretation based on
- *correct reference data*, and at the
- *right price*.

Quality control (QC)
The term quality control covers that part of quality assurance which primarily concerns the control of errors in the performance of tests and verification of test results. QC must be *practical*, *achievable*, and *affordable*.

Effective QA detects errors at an early stage before they lead to incorrect test results. Laboratory personnel need to be aware of the errors that can occur when collecting specimens (pre-analytical stage), testing specimens (analytical stage), reporting and interpreting test results (post-analytical stage).

QA is an *essential* requirement of district laboratory practice. Implementing QA requires:

- Preparation and use of *Standard Operating Procedures* (SOPs) with details of QC for all laboratory tests and activities (see later text).

- System for monitoring whether test results are reaching those treating patients at an early enough stage to influence clinical and public health decision making.

- Policies of work, i.e. decisions that are taken in consultation with medical and nursing staff to enable a laboratory to operate reliably, effectively, and in harmony with the other departments of a hospital or units of a health centre. Such policies should cover:
  - laboratory hours and arrangements for emergency testing of specimens outside of normal working hours.
  - range and cost of tests to be performed.
  - tests which can be referred to a specialist laboratory.
  - arrangements for the collection and transport of routine and urgent specimens, and their delivery, to the laboratory.
  - labelling of specimens.
  - laboratory request form and patient information required.
  - time it takes to perform tests, i.e. target turn-around times.
  - reporting of routine and urgent tests and delivery of reports.
  - recording and storing of laboratory data.
  - health and safety regulations.

STANDARD OPERATING PROCEDURES (SOPs)

SOPs, sometimes referred to as the *local laboratory bench manual*, are required for the following reasons:

- To improve and maintain the quality of laboratory service to patients and identify problems associated with poor work performance.

- To provide laboratory staff with written instructions on how to perform tests consistently to an *acceptable standard* in their laboratory.

- To prevent changes in the performance of tests which may occur when new members of staff are appointed. SOPs also help to avoid short-cuts being taken when performing tests.

- To make clinical and epidemiological interpretations of test results easier by standardizing specimen collecting techniques, test methods, and test reporting.

- To provide written standardized techniques for use in the training of laboratory personnel and for potential publication in scientific journals.

- To facilitate the preparation of a list and inventory of essential reagents, chemicals and equipment.

- To promote safe laboratory practice.

Important features of SOPS

SOPs must be:

- Applicable and achievable *in the laboratory in which they will be used.*
- Clearly written and easy to understand and follow.
- Kept up to date using appropriate valid technologies.

Preparing SOPs

SOPs must be written and implemented by a qualified experienced laboratory officer, and followed exactly by all members of staff.

For each SOP it is best to follow a similar format with the information presented under separate headings. Each SOP must be given a title and identification number, and be dated and signed by an authorized person.

A list of staff able to perform the test (unsupervized and supervized) should be identified in the SOP. There should also be an indication of the cost of the test.

The following is a suggested layout for district laboratory SOPs and appendices to be included in the *SOP Manual.*

```
┌─────────────────────────────────────────────┐
│             TITLE OF SOP                      │
│ Authorized signature        Number:          │
│                             Date:             │
├───────────────────────────────────────────────┤
│ Staff able to perform test                    │
│ ●  Unsupervized: List names                   │
│ ●  Under supervision: List names              │
│ Cost of test                                  │
│ Example: Group 1 (high range), Group 2 (medium│
│    range), Group 3 (low range)                │
├───────────────────────────────────────────────┤
│ Suggested headings (see later text for explanation)│
│ VALUE OF TEST                                 │
│ PRINCIPLE OF TEST                             │
│ SPECIMEN                                      │
│ EQUIPMENT                                     │
│ REAGENTS / STAINS                             │
│ CONTROLS                                      │
│ METHOD OF TEST                                │
│ REPORTING RESULTS / INTERPRETATION            │
│ SAFETY MEASURES                               │
│ SOURCES OF ERROR                              │
│ REFERENCES                                    │
└───────────────────────────────────────────────┘
```

```
┌─────────────────────────────────────────────┐
│ Suggested appendices                          │
│ The SOP Manual should include the following   │
│   appendices (see later text):                │
│ APPENDIX A, EQUIPMENT (Items: A/1, A/2, etc)  │
│ APPENDIX B, REAGENTS / STAINS (Items: B/1,    │
│   B/2, etc)                                   │
│ APPENDIX C, SAFETY (Information: C/1, C/2, etc)│
│ ADDITIONAL NOTES                              │
└───────────────────────────────────────────────┘
```

What to write under headings

VALUE OF TEST
State the main reason(s) for performing the test, i.e. clinical and/or public health reasons (consult with medical officer(s).
Example: To detect, identify, and quantify malaria parasites in a person with suspected malaria? (malaria test).
Indicate any relevant limitations of the test.

PRINCIPLE OF TEST
State briefly the technology used.

Examples: 'Microscopical examination of Fields stained thick blood film for malaria parasites (malaria test) ...... or ...... chemical reagent strip test to detect glucose in urine based on glucose oxidase reaction (urine glucose test).

SPECIMEN
State the specimen required and how to collect it, including:
– volume required,
– container and its preparation,
– use of any anticoagulant or stabilizer/ preservative,
– collection procedure (for adult and child) with health and safety notes,
– how container should be labelled,
– stability of specimen and requirements for storage and transport,
– time within which the specimen should reach the laboratory.

Describe the checks to be made when specimen and request form reach the laboratory and criteria which may make it necessary to reject the specimen.

State if the specimen requires priority attention (e.g. c.s.f).

EQUIPMENT
List the items of equipment needed to perform the test. Main items of equipment such as a microscope, centrifuge, colorimeter, incubator, water bath/heat block, etc should be listed in a separate appendix (e.g. Appendix B) at the back of the *SOP Manual* and given a number which can be referenced in each SOP (e.g. B/1, B/2 etc). The information to be included in this appendix is described under *Appendix B* (see later text).

REAGENTS/STAINS
List reagents, stains, reagent strips, etc needed to perform the test. Include the reagents and stains in a separate appendix at the back of the *SOP Manual* e.g. Appendix A and give each a number which can be referenced in the SOP (A/1, A/2, etc). The information which needs to be included in this appendix is described under Appendix A (see later text).

CONTROLS
List controls and source(s) to be used in the test, e.g. positive and negative controls in serological tests, control sera in clinical chemistry assays, positive and negative controls in urine chemical tests, etc.

METHOD OF TEST
Describe in a numbered sequence how to perform the test. For quantitative tests include details of calibration, use of graph or factor, and calculations. Describe how to control the procedure and also the health and safety measures which apply. Full details

of safety procedures should be included in a separate Health and Safety appendix, e.g. Appendix C with each procedure being given a number, (C/1, C/2, etc) which can be referenced in the SOPs.

REPORTING RESULTS/INTERPRETATION
State how the test should be reported, including:

- units to be used and format of reporting (explain any abbreviations).
- accepted reference range for a quantitative test.
- action to take if a result is seriously abnormal or unexpected, e.g. need for verification, additional testing, and, or immediate notification of the result.
- give target turn-around time for issuing the report (routine and urgent).
- interpretation comments that should accompany the test result.

SOURCES OF ERROR
Summarize the important and commonest causes of an incorrect test result.

Examples: Sample not well mixed, smear too thick for staining, inaccurate measurement (pipetting) of a blood or serum sample, clots in anticoagulated blood sample, air bubbles in the solution when using a colorimeter or the sides of the cuvette not being clean and dry, etc.

REFERENCES
List the main source(s) of the information contained in the SOP, e.g. book, journal, published paper, manufacturer's leaflet, WHO guidelines or document, etc.

What should be included in the appendices

APPENDIX A STAINS/REAGENTS
For each stain and reagent, the following information is required:

- method of preparation and performance testing/QC.
- any associated hazard, e.g. chemical that is flammable, toxic, harmful, irritant or corrosive.
- labelling specifications.
- storage requirements and stability ('shelf-life').
- source(s) of chemicals and stains, ordering information (correct name/chemical formula and where possible, catalogue number), and amount of each chemical/stain, etc to be kept in stock.

APPENDIX B EQUIPMENT
For each item of equipment the following information is required:

- name (including model number) and supplier.

- instructions for use, including any safety precautions.
- daily QC, e.g. cleaning, performance checks.
- details of how to replace components such as a lamp, fuse, etc.
- maintenance schedule.
- replacement parts to be kept in stock with part numbers and details of supplier(s).
- trouble-shooting and action to take if the equipment fails.

APPENDIX C HEALTH AND SAFETY
This appendix should include:

- the safe handling and disposal of specimens.
- decontamination procedures, e.g. use of chemical agents (disinfectants), autoclaving, etc.
- safe use of chemicals.
- personal safety measures.
- action to take in the event of a fire.
- First Aid procedures.

Note: Some laboratories may prefer to include the above in a separate Health and Safety Manual.

ADDITIONAL NOTES
Examples of other procedures and information which are commonly included in a district laboratory *SOP Manual* include, laboratory work policies covering laboratory operating times, emergency out-of-hours testing arrangements, specimen collection times, arrangements for the delivery of reports, and also procedures relating to the packing and transport of specimens to the public health laboratory or other specialist laboratory.

Important: SOPs must be kept up to date and reviewed at least annually. Any amendments must be authorized, referenced, dated, signed, and brought to the attention of all members of staff. Users of the laboratory must also receive written amendments to SOPs when these involve changes in the ordering of tests, the collection of specimens and the reporting of tests. No new test should be introduced without an SOP.

SOURCES OF ERRORS IN DISTRICT LABORATORY PRACTICE

As previously explained, the preparation and implementation of SOPs will greatly assist in identifying, monitoring, and minimizing errors that lead to incorrect test results and the waste of resources. Most errors are associated with:

- Misidentifying a patient.

- Collecting or storing a specimen incorrectly.
- Technical imprecision and inaccuracy.
- Reader variability (see subunit 2.2).
- Adverse laboratory working conditions.
- Misinterpreting test reports (see subunit 2.2).

Patient misidentification

In district laboratory practice, the misidentification of a patient is mainly the result of:

- Clerical errors or incomplete identification data, e.g. when names are only used with no check of an outpatient or inpatient identification number at the time a specimen is collected.

- Language difficulties when staff do not speak or understand sufficiently the language or dialect spoken by the patient.

- Specimen containers that are incorrectly labelled or when a specimen is misidentified on a ward because it is first collected in an unlabelled container such as a bedpan or sputum pot. Mistakes can also occur when the writing on a label is illegible or part erased.

- No reliable check-in system when specimens reach the laboratory to ensure that the patient data on the request form is the same as that written on the label of the specimen container.

Faulty specimens

Caused when:

- A specimen is not correct, is inadequate, or collected at an incorrect time.

- The collection technique is not correct, e.g.
  - blood is taken from an arm in which an intravenous (IV) infusion is running.
  - a wet needle and syringe are used to collect a blood specimen, resulting in haemolysis of the red cells.

- A container has not been cleaned properly or dried before being reused, does not contain the correct anticoagulant or preservative, or is not sterile when it should be.

- The container cap is loose resulting in loss, evaporation, or contamination of the specimen.

- A specimen is unsuitable for testing because it has been stored incorrectly, has been left for too long a period in an outpatient clinic, or is too long in transit before it reaches the laboratory.

- Specimens, particularly blood films are not protected from insects, dust, or direct sunlight.

- A specimen contains drugs, herbal medicines, or other substances which can interfere with the performance of a test.

- There is no inspection of specimens when they reach the laboratory.

Imprecision and inaccuracy

Reliable test results depend on laboratory staff keeping errors of imprecision and inaccuracy to a minimum by good laboratory practice and quality control. Consistently reliable results depend on the early detection and correction of errors.

Errors of imprecision

Precision is a measure of reproducibility. Errors of imprecision are often referred to as errors of scatter because they are irregular, or random. Results differ from the correct result by varying amounts as explained in subunit 6.2.

Errors of inaccuracy

Accuracy is defined as the closeness of agreement between a test result and the accepted true value. Errors of inaccuracy are often referred to as errors of bias because they are consistent, or systematic. All the test results differ from their correct result by approximately the same amount as explained in subunit 6.2.

Common causes of imprecision in district laboratory practice

The following are the commonest causes of inconsistent random errors:

- Incorrect and variable pipetting and dispensing caused when:
  - pipetting and dispensing techniques are poor due to inadequate training, no supervision of trainees, or careless working.
  - pipettes with chipped ends or unclear markings are used.
  - pipette fillers are difficult to use.
  - automatic pipettors and dispensers are not used correctly or pipettor tips are not adequately cleaned and dried before reuse (where reuse is possible).

- Inadequate mixing of sample with reagents.

- Samples are not incubated consistently where incubation of tests is required.

- Glassware or plasticware is not clean or dried completely before reuse.

- Equipment malfunction caused when:
  - laboratory staff are not trained in the correct use and maintenance of equipment.
  - instrument readings fluctuate due to unstable power supplies and the equipment is not fitted with a voltage stabilizer.
  - dirty or finger-marked cuvettes are used in

colorimeters or the sample contains air bubbles.

– in hot humid climates, the glass surfaces of lenses and filters become damaged when not protected from fungal growth.

– battery operated equipment performs erratically because the battery is not sufficiently charged.

■ Incomplete removal of interfering substances such as red cells when performing serum assays.

■ Laboratory staff prepare a smear that is too thick for direct microscopical examination or subsequent staining.

■ Incorrect reporting of microscopical preparations and lack of standardization in reporting.

Common causes of inaccuracy in district laboratory practice

The following are the commonest causes of consistent systematic errors:

■ Incorrect or infrequent calibration of a test method or quantitative tests being read at an incorrect wavelength (incorrect filter used).

■ Using an automatic pipettor set at an incorrect volume or one that has been calibrated wrongly.

■ Use of control sera that has been wrongly prepared, incorrectly stored, or used beyond its expiry date.

■ Consistent calculation error.

■ Incubating samples at an incorrect temperature due to the temperature of a waterbath or heat block being wrongly set and not checked.

■ Use of unsatisfactory reagents caused when:

– chemical reagents and stains are not prepared correctly according to SOPs.

– the quality of water used in the preparation of reagents is unsuitable.

– reagents are not prepared from sufficiently pure chemicals.

– new batches of reagents are not tested prior to being used and no controls are used to check the performance of working reagents.

– reagents are used beyond their expiry date without being adequately controlled.

– temperature sensitive reagents deteriorate because they are not stored at the correct temperature, are frequently removed from the refrigerator into a hot environment, or the refrigerator stops working due to a

power failure or running out of gas or kerosene.

– a reagent becomes contaminated when a dirty or wet pipette is used.

– light sensitive reagents become unfit for use because they are not stored in opaque containers and protected from light.

– dry, moisture-sensitive reagents and strip tests deteriorate due to their frequent use in conditions of high relative humidity, or when the container is not tightly closed after use and no desiccant is enclosed.

– stains are used without controls, are not filtered when indicated, or absorb moisture and become unfit for use, e.g. alcoholic Romanowsky stock stains.

■ Staff reporting microscopical preparations incorrectly due to inadequate training with no control preparations being used, particularly to check the ability of staff to report:

– Gram stained smears.
– Ziehl-Neelsen stained smears.
– Thick and thin stained blood films.
– Cerebrospinal fluid, urine and faecal preparations.

Note: Measuring and controlling imprecision and inaccuracy in quantitative serum assays are described in detail in subunit 6.2.

Mistakes made by laboratory staff due to adverse working conditions

Caused when:

■ The workload is too high or too low:

Workload capacity of a laboratory
The workload must be matched to the number of staff and their experience, and to the size of the laboratory and its facilities. Workload is usually measured in terms of time required for a test to be completed. When workload is excessive, the testing of specimens becomes unreliable and safety measures tend to be ignored. Too little work can also lead to unreliable test results due to lack of concentration.

■ The laboratory is small with insufficient or poorly lit working areas and is not sufficiently ventilated or screened from direct sunlight.

■ Laboratory staff become professionally isolated and lack motivation when they receive little support and encouragement.

■ There are too many interruptions or when there is excessive noise from nearby OPD waiting areas or radios.

■ When there are too many urgent test requests.

■ District hospital laboratory staff become fatigued or sick (e.g. with malaria) due to many night emergency calls.

Note: Monitoring the workload and working conditions of district laboratory personnel forms an integral part of health and safety and the total quality management of district laboratory services.

EXTERNAL QUALITY ASSESSMENT (EQA)

Although steps may be taken in a laboratory to ensure test results are reliable, an objective system of assessing a laboratory's ability to do this to a satisfactory standard is recommended, i.e. an external quality assessment (EQA) scheme.

Participation in external quality assessment schemes should always be regarded as additional to internal quality control. EQA must *never* be a substitute for internal QC because it can only assess past performance when test results have already been reported and acted on.

EQA for outreach laboratories

The district laboratory coordinator, with the assistance of the senior district hospital laboratory officer, should implement a basic EQA scheme for outreach laboratories covering the main tests performed, particularly those where errors are more likely to occur such as the reporting of microscopical preparations, measurement of haemoglobin, and testing of urine.

For most outreach laboratories, EQA will be most practically implemented during the regular visit of the district laboratory coordinator. This will give the opportunity for errors to be investigated on-site and corrected rapidly.

EQA for the district hospital laboratory

Comprehensive EQA schemes in which the results from different district hospital laboratories are compared objectively are not yet operating in most tropical and developing countries due to lack of commitment, inadequate resourcing, too few laboratory personnel trained in QA, and difficulties in transporting and mailing pathological specimens.

In recent years, the World Health Organization has issued guidelines on the role of laboratory EQA schemes and how developing countries can participate in WHO International External Quality Assessment Schemes (IEQASs).[6]

In the absence of national EQA schemes, the district laboratory coordinator should prepare control materials for use in district hospital laboratories, particularly control preparations for microscopical

investigations, control serum for clinical chemistry assays, control cultures for microbiology, control blood for checking the measurement of haemoglobin and other haematology tests, and controls for testing the competence of staff in blood typing and compatibility testing.

The district laboratory coordinator should monitor regularly whether SOPs and quality control procedures are being implemented correctly in the district hospital laboratory and also the quality and consistency of reporting and recording test results.

Correcting errors associated with poor work performance

Most of the errors resulting in incorrect test results in district laboratories can be resolved by:

● Using SOPs with adequate QC and reference materials.

● Improving working practices and laboratory management.

● Monitoring laboratory working conditions and workload.

● Supporting district laboratory personnel, i.e. regular visits by the district laboratory coordinator.

● Organizing an effective district quality assessment scheme.

● Changing to competency-based training of laboratory personnel and implementing performance assessment and continuing education of district laboratory staff.

● Improving communication between laboratory staff and those requesting laboratory tests and interpreting test results.

2.5 SI units

Following World Health Organization recommendations, SI units (Système International d'Unités) are used in this publication:

– in test methods,
– preparation of reagents,
– reporting of test results.

The International System of Units has been developed and agreed internationally. It overcomes language barriers, enabling an exchange of health information within a country and between nations to be made without the misunderstandings which arise when each country, or even a separate hospital within a country, uses its own units of measurement for reporting tests. It is therefore important for health authorities and laboratories to adopt SI units.

SI BASE UNITS

The International System of Units is based on the *metre-kilogram-second* system and replaces both the foot-pound-second (Imperial) system and the centimetre-gram-second (cgs) system.

The seven SI base units from which all the other units are derived are as follows:

SI base units	Symbol	Quantity measured
metre	m	length
kilogram	kg	mass
second	s	time
mole	mol	amount of substance
ampere	A	electric current
kelvin	K	temperature
candela	cd	luminous intensity

SI DERIVED UNITS

SI derived units consist of combinations of base units:

SI derived unit	Symbol	Quantity measured
square metre	m^2	area
cubic metre	m^3	volume
metre per second	m/s	speed

Special names have been given to those derived units with complex base combinations:

Name derived unit	Symbol	Quantity measured
Hertz	Hz	frequency
joule	J	energy, quantity of heat
newton	N	force
pascal	Pa	pressure
watt	W	power
volt	V	electric potential difference
degree Celsius	°C	Celsius temperature

SI UNIT PREFIXES

To enable the measurement of quantities larger or smaller than the base units or derived units, the SI Unit System also includes a set of prefixes. The use of a prefix makes a unit larger or smaller.

Example

If the prefix milli (m) is put in front of the metre this would indicate that the unit should be divided by a thousand, i.e. 10^{-3}. The way of expressing this would be 10^{-3} m, or mm.

If however the prefix kilo (k) were used this would indicate that the unit should be multiplied by a thousand, i.e. 10^3. This would be expressed 10^3 m, or km.

The range of SI unit prefixes commonly used in laboratory work are listed as follows:

Prefix	Symbol	Function	
			DIVIDE BY:
deci	d	10^{-1}	10
centi	c	10^{-2}	100
milli	m	10^{-3}	1 000
micro	μ	10^{-6}	1 000 000
nano	n	10^{-9}	1 000 000 000
pico	p	10^{-12}	1 000 000 000 000
femto	f	10^{-15}	1 000 000 000 000 000
			MULTIPLY BY:
kilo	k	10^3	1 000

VOLUME: LITRE (L OR l)

The SI derived unit of volume is the cubic metre (m^3). Because this is such a large unit, the litre (l or L) although not an SI unit, has been recommended for use in the laboratory.

Volume measurements are made in litres or multiples and submultiples of the litre, e.g. dl (10^{-1} l), ml (10^{-3} l), μl (10^{-6} l).

One litre is therefore equivalent to 10 dl, 1 000 ml or 1 000 000 μl. One dl is equivalent to 100 ml, and 1 ml to 1 000 μl.

Old unit	SI unit
100 ml	dl
cc	ml or cm^3
lambda	μl
—	nl
μμl	pl

Useful volume table

1 dl = 10^{-1} l (0.1 l) or 100 cm^3, formerly 100 ml
1 ml = 10^{-3} (0.001 l) or 1 000 μl
1 μl = 10^{-6} (0.000 001 l or 1 mm^3)
1 nl = 10^{-9} l (0.000 000 001 l)
1 pl = 10^{-12} l (0.000 000 000 001 l)
1 fl = 10^{-15}

1 l   = 10 dl
        1 000 ml
        1 000 000 µl
        1 000 000 000 nl

---

1 pint = 0.568 l
1 l   = 1.760 pints or 0.22 gallons

WEIGHT: GRAM (g)

The kilogram (kg) is the SI unit for mass and the gram (g) is the working unit.

Formerly the gram (g) was written gramme, or gm.

Mass measurements are made in grams or in multiples and submultiples of the gram, e.g. mg (10^{-3} g), µg (10^{-6} g), ng (10^{-9}g), pg (10^{-12} g).

One g is therefore equivalent to 1 000 mg, 1 000 000 µg, or 1 000 000 000 ng. One mg is equivalent to 1 000 µg.

Old unit	SI unit
k, kilogramme	kg
gm, gramme	g
mgm	mg
gamma	µg
mug	ng
µµg	pg

Useful weight table

1 kg   = 10^3 g (1 000 g)
1 mg   = 10^{-3} g (0.001 g) or 1 000 µg
1 µg   = 10^{-6} g (0.000 001 g)
1 ng   = 10^{-9} g (0.000 000 001 g)
1 pg   = 10^{-12} g (0.000 000 000 001 g)
1 g   = 1 000 mg
        1 000 000 µg
        1 000 000 000 ng
        1 000 000 000 000 pg

---

1 kg   = 2.205 lb

Tests now reported in g/l include: albumin, total protein, haemoglobin (although dl is still used), mean cell haemoglobin concentration.

LENGTH: METRE (m)

The SI unit for length is the metre (m) and measurements of length are made in metres or in mm (10^{-3} m), µm (10^{-6} m), nm (10^{-9} m).

One m is therefore equivalent to 1 000 mm or 1 000 000 µm and 1 mm is equivalent to 1 000 µm or 1 000 000 nm.

Old unit	SI unit
mµ	nm
µ (micron)	µm

Useful length table

1 dm   = 10^{-1} m (0.1 m)
1 cm   = 10^{-2} m (0.01 m), 10 mm, 10 000 µm
1 mm   = 10^{-3} m (0.001 m), 1 000 µm
1 µm   = 10^{-6} m (0.000 001 m)
1 nm   = 10^{-9} m (0.000 000 001 m)
1 km   =   1 000 m (10^3 m)
1 m   =   10 dm
           100 cm
           1 000 mm
           1 000 000 µm
           1 000 000 000 nm

---

1 m   =   3.281 feet
1 km   =   0.62 137 mile
1 inch   =   2.54 cm

AMOUNT OF SUBSTANCE: MOLE (mol)

The mole (mol) is the SI unit for amount of substance and measurements of the amounts of substances are made in moles, or in mmol (10^{-3} mol), µmol (10^{-6} mol), or nmol (10^{-9} mol).

One mol is therefore equivalent to 1 000 mmol, 1 000 000 µmol, or 1 000 000 000 nmol. One mmol/l is equivalent to 1 000 µmol/l.

Formerly, the results of tests expressed in mmol/l or µmol/l were expressed in mg/100 ml or µg/100 ml. The formula used to convert mg/100 ml to mmol/l is as follows:

$$mmol/l = \frac{mg/100\ ml \times 10}{molecular\ weight\ of\ substance}$$

Where the molecular weight of a substance cannot be accurately determined (e.g. albumin), results are expressed in g/l.

Old unit	SI unit
M	mol
mEq	mmol
µM	µmol
nM	nmol

Useful amount of substance table

1 mmol = 10^{-3} mol (0.001 mol), 1 000 µmol
1 µmol = 10^{-6} mol (0.000 001 mol), 1 000 nmol
1 nmol = 10^{-9} mol (0.000 000 001 mol)
1 mol   = 1 000 mmol
          1 000 000 µmol
          1 000 000 000 nmol

Tests reported in nmol/l, µmol/l, mmol/l include:

nmol/l: thyroxine
µmol/l: bilirubin, creatinine, iron
mmol/l: calcium, glucose, urea, cholesterol, sodium, potassium

Mole per litre solutions (mol/l)

A mole per litre (mol/l) solution contains one mole of solute dissolved in and made up to 1 litre with solvent.

Mole

A mole is defined as the amount of substance of a system which contains as many elementary units (atoms, molecules, or ions) as there are carbon atoms in 0.012 kg of the pure nuclide carbon−12 (^{12}C).

To avoid confusion, mole per litre solutions should not be referred to as molar or M solutions. The internationally agreed meaning of the word molar as used in chemistry is 'divided by amount of substance', i.e. divided by mole. Molar cannot be applied therefore to mole per litre solutions as these refer to mole divided by litre (mol/l). The term molarity should be discontinued.

Conversion of a normal solution into a mol/l solution

To change a normal solution into a mol/l solution, use the formula:

$$\text{mol/l solution} = \frac{\text{Normality of solution}}{\text{Valence of substance}}$$

INTERNATIONAL UNIT (U)

This unit is used to express catalytic enzyme activity corresponding to μmol/minutes. Units for measuring enzyme activity have in the past been given the names of the person who developed the different techniques, e.g. Somogyi, King-Armstrong, Bessey-Lowry, Reitman-Frankel, and Karmen. In an attempt to standardize the reporting of enzyme activity a unit of measurement has been introduced called the International Unit (U)

International Unit

An International Unit of enzyme activity is that amount of enzyme which under defined assay conditions will catalyze the conversion of 1 μmol of substrate per minute. Results are expressed in International Units per litre (U/l).

    In accordance with this definition the assay conditions for enzyme analysis must be specified (see subunit 6.2).

Enzyme activities now expressed in U/l include alkaline phosphatase and aspartate aminotransferase.

PRESSURE AND TEMPERATURE

The SI unit used for measuring pressure is the pascal (Pa).

Approximate conversions

$$\frac{\text{mmHg} \times 2}{15} = \text{kPa}$$

$$\text{lb/sq inch} \times 6.895 = \text{kPa}$$

Temperature

The SI unit for measuring Celsius temperature is degrees Celsius (°C).

Useful conversions

To convert °C to °F:
multiply by 9, divide by 5, and add 32.

To convert °F to °C:
subtract 32, multiply by 5, and divide by 9.

0°C	=	32°F
10°C	=	52°F
20°C	=	68°F
30°C	=	86°F
36.9°C	=	98.4°F
40°C	=	104°F
50°C	=	122°F
100°C	=	212°F

2.6 Guidelines for preparing stains and chemical reagents

As discussed in subunit 2.4, preparing and storing reagents incorrectly are important causes of unreliable test results. This subunit provides guidelines on the correct preparation of stains and chemical reagents to ensure quality of work and prevent waste of resources.

Errors in the preparation of stains and reagents

Most errors that occur in the preparation of stains and reagents are due to:

- Incorrect preparation techniques.
- Calculating incorrectly the weight or volumes of constituents.
- Making dilution errors.

Important: Following the preparation of a stain or chemical reagent, its performance must be checked before it is put into routine use. Standard operating procedures must be implemented for the preparation, control, and safety of reagents used in district laboratories.

Health and safety: Precautions that need to be taken when using *Harmful, Irritant, Toxic, Corrosive,* and *Flammable* chemicals are described in subunit 3.5.

_____

PREPARATION TECHNIQUE

When preparing a solution decide whether the solution requires an accurate volumetric preparation, e.g. a calibrant (standard), or a less accurate method of preparation, e.g. a stain.

Preparing accurate solutions

- Use a balance of sufficient sensitivity (see 4.5). Weigh the chemical as accurately as possible. The chemical should be of an analytical reagent grade. Hygroscopic and deliquescent chemicals need to be weighed rapidly.

Analytical reagents
Errors due to the use of impure chemicals can be avoided by purchasing chemicals that are labelled *Analar, Univar, AR (Analytical Reagent)*, or *GR (Guaranteed Reagent)*. *LG (Laboratory Grade)* reagents are of lower purity but may be suitable for some purposes. *Technical* and *Industrial* grade chemicals, although less expensive, must not be used to prepare calibrants or any reagent which requires a pure chemical.

- Use calibrated, chemically clean glassware.

- Read carefully the graduation marks and other information on flasks and pipettes, for example check whether a pipette is of the containing (rinsing-out) type or of the delivery (non-rinsing-out) type. It is best to use a delivery type. Instructions when using a pipettor can be found in subunit 4.6.

- Use a funnel to transfer the chemical from the weighing container to a volumetric flask. Wash any chemical remaining in the container into the flask with a little of the solvent.

- Make the solution up to its final volume. If warm, make up to volume only when the solution has cooled to the temperature used to graduate the flask (written on the flask).

- To avoid over-shooting the graduation mark, use a Pasteur pipette or wash-bottle to add the final volume of solvent to the flask.

- Make sure the bottom of the meniscus of the fluid is on the graduation mark when viewed at *eye level* (see Fig. 2.5).

- Mix the solution well by inverting the flask at least twenty times.

- Store reagents in completely clean containers that have *leak-proof* airtight screw-caps or stop-pers. Use brown bottles or opaque plastic containers for storing light sensitive reagents. Before transferring a solution to its storage container, first rinse out the container with a little of the solution.

- Label the container clearly with a water-proof marker. Include the full name of the reagent, its concentration, date of preparation and if relevant its expiry date. If it requires refrigeration, state 'Store at 2–8°C'. Protect the label by covering it with clear adhesive tape. If a reagent is *Harmful, Irritant, Toxic, Corrosive*, or *Flammable*, indicate this on the container label (see subunit 3.5).

- Protect all reagents from sunlight and heat. Store light sensitive reagents and stock solutions of stains in the dark.

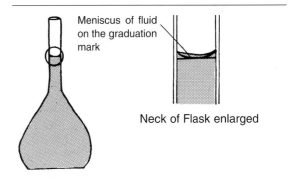

Fig. 2.5 How to read the level of a fluid

Preparation of calibrating solutions (standards)
When preparing calibrants the following are important:

- Always use pure chemicals. The use of impure low grade chemicals can lead to serious errors in test results.

- Avoid weighing a very small quantity of a calibrant substance. Instead prepare a concentrated stock solution which can be diluted to make working solutions.

- Use good quality distilled water. Electrolyte calibrants require deionized water.

- Use calibrated glassware and a volumetric technique as described previously.

- Use a control serum to check the performance of the calibrant solutions.

Whenever possible, calibrants should be prepared and standardized in a regional or control laboratory and distributed with instructions for use to district laboratories.

Preparing stains

There is no need to use expensive volumetric glassware when preparing stains.

- Weigh the dye in a small container and transfer the weighed dye direct to a leak-proof storage container, preferably a brown bottle.

- Add any other ingredients and the volume of solvent as stated in the method of preparation, and mix well. Adding a few glass beads will help the dye to dissolve more quickly. For some stains heat can be used to dissolve the dye (this will be stated in the method of preparation).

  Note: Instead of measuring the volume of solvent each time the stain is prepared, it is more practical to mark the side of the container with the volume which needs to be added.

- Transfer part of the stain to a stain dispensing container, filtering it if required. Always use dispensing containers with tops that can be closed when not in use.

- Label the container in a similar way to that described previously.

- Store as instructed in the method of preparation. Always protect stock containers of stain from direct sunlight.

Water used in preparing solutions and stains

For all the reagents described in Appendix 1, deionized water can be used instead of distilled water.

    For most stains and reagents not used in clinical chemistry tests, boiled filtered rain water or boiled water filtered through a *Sterasyl* candle filter (see subunit 4.4) can be used if distilled or deionized water is not available.

Note: A method of preparing chemically pure water in district laboratories is described in subunit 4.4.

Guidelines for handling chemicals and reagents

- Handle chemicals and reagents with care particularly those that are *Flammable, Toxic, Harmful, Irritant, Corrosive* (see subunit 3.5). Wear appropriate protective clothing.

- Always read the health and safety information on the labels of containers.

- *Do not* mouth-pipette reagents. Instead, use a pipette filler, automatic dispenser or pipettor.

- Always check that an opened bottle of chemical is completely finished before starting a new one.

- Keep containers tightly closed.

- Do not return excess chemical to a stock bottle.

- Make sure all chemicals and reagents are labelled clearly.

- Store chemicals and reagents correctly (see subunit 3.5).

Deliquescent chemicals

Chemicals such as calcium chloride, potassium carbonate, phenol, and sodium hydroxide are very soluble in water and become moist when exposed to damp air. They become dissolved in the moisture and go on taking in moisture until the vapour pressure of the solution equals the pressure of the water in the atmosphere. Such chemicals are said to be deliquescent. They can be used as drying agents (desiccants) in desiccators.

Hygroscopic chemicals

A substance which absorbs water from the air but does not dissolve in the water it absorbs is referred to as hygroscopic, e.g. sodium carbonate.

CALCULATING CORRECTLY

In the preparation of solutions, calculation errors commonly occur due to:

- Simple errors in calculating amounts and volumes, most of which can be prevented by routinely rechecking the calculations.

- Not using the correct formula when preparing a mol/l solution.

- Not using the correct formula when diluting a solution.

Useful table

1 g	= 1 000 mg	1 litre	= 1 000 ml
1 g	= 1 000 000 µg	1 ml	= 1 000 µl
0.1 g	= 100 mg	1 mol	= 1 000 mmol
0.01 g	= 10 mg	1 mol	= 1 000 000 µmol
1 000 µg	= 1 mg	1 mmol	= 1 000 µmol

Preparing mol/l solutions

Based on the fact that chemicals interact in relation to their molecular masses it is recommended that the concentration of solutions be expressed in terms of the number of moles of solute per litre of solution (see subunit 2.5 which describes the use of SI units).

    Only when the relative molecular mass of a substance is not known, should the concentration of such a substance in solution be expressed in terms of mass (weight) concentration, i.e. grams or milligrams per *litre* (per 100 ml should be discontinued).

    To prepare a mol/l solution, use the following formula:

Required mol/l solution × Molecular mass of substance = Number of grams to be dissolved in 1 litre of solution.

When calculating the molecular mass of a chemical it is *important* to check whether it contains water of crystallization. For example, hydrated copper sulphate (blue) has a formula of $CuSO_4 \cdot 5H_2O$, which means it contains 5 molecules of water per molecule. The molecular masses of some hydrated and anhydrous (without water of crystallization) chemicals are listed in Appendix III.

EXAMPLES

■ *To make 1 litre of sodium chloride (NaCl), 1 mol/l:*

Required mol/l concentration = 1
Molecular mass of NaCl = 58.44
Therefore 1 litre NaCl, 1 mol/l contains:
$1 \times 58.44 = 58.44$ g of the chemical dissolved in 1 litre of solvent.

Note: When writing mol/l solutions, the concentration is written after the name of the substance.

■ *To make 1 litre of sodium chloride (NaCl), 0.15 mol/l (physiological saline):*
Required mol/l concentration = 0.15
Molecular mass of NaCl = 58.44
Therefore 1 litre NaCl, 0.15 mol/l contains:
$0.15 \times 58.44 = 8.77$ g of the chemical dissolved in 1 litre of solvent.

■ *To make 50 ml of sodium chloride (NaCl), 0.15 mol/l (physiological saline):*

Required mol/l concentration = 0.15
Molecular mass of NaCl = 58.44
Therefore 50 ml NaCl, 0.15 mol/l contains:
$$\frac{0.15 \times 58.44 \times 50}{1\ 000} = 0.438 \text{ g of NaCl dissolved in 50 ml of solvent.}$$

Note: In some publications the decimal point is written as a comma, e.g. 0.15 would be written as 0,15.

Formula to convert a percentage solution to a mol/l solution

To change a percentage solution into a mol/l solution, use the formula:
$$\text{mol/l solution} = \frac{\textbf{g\% (w/v) solution} \times \textbf{10}}{\textbf{molecular mass of substance}}$$

EXAMPLES

■ *To convert a 4% w/v sodium hydroxide (NaOH) solution into a mol/l solution:*

Gram % solution = 4
Molecular mass of NaOH = 40
Conversion to mol/l: $\dfrac{4 \times 10}{40} = 1$

Therefore 4% w/v NaOH is equivalent to a 1 mol/l NaOH solution.

■ *To convert a 0.9% w/v sodium chloride (NaCl) into a mol/l solution:*

Gram % solution = 0.9
Molecular mass of NaCl = 58.44
Conversion to mol/l: $\dfrac{0.9 \times 10}{58.44} = 0.15$

Therefore 0.9% w/v NaCl is equivalent to a 0.15 mol/l NaCl solution.

Conversion of a normal solution into a mol/l solution

To change a normal solution into a mol/l solution use the formula:
$$\text{mol/l solution} = \frac{\textbf{Normality of solution}}{\textbf{Valence of substance}}$$

EXAMPLES

■ *To convert 0.1 N (N/10) hydrochloric acid (HCl) into a mol/l solution:*

Normality of solution = 0.1
Valence of Cl (in HCl) = 1
Conversion to mol/l: $\dfrac{0.1}{1} = 0.1$

Therefore 0.1 N HCl is equivalent to 0.1 mol/l HCl solution.

■ *To convert 1 N sodium carbonate (Na_2CO_3) into a mol/l solution:*

Normality of solution = 1
Valence of CO_3^{--} (in Na_2CO_3) = 2
Conversion to mol/l: $\dfrac{1}{2} = 0.5$

Therefore 1 N Na_2CO_3 is equivalent to 0.5 mol/l Na_2CO_3 solution.

Note: The relative molecular masses (molecular weights) of some of the more commonly used substances and the atomic masses and valencies of some of the elements, are listed in Appendix III.

DILUTING CORRECTLY

In the laboratory it is frequently necessary to dilute solutions and body fluids. To dilute a solution or body fluid means to reduce its concentration. A weaker solution can be made from a stronger solution by using the following formula:
$$\text{Volume (ml) of stronger solution required} = \frac{\textbf{C} \times \textbf{V}}{\textbf{S}}$$
where:
C = Concentration of solution required
V = Volume of solution required
S = Strength of the stronger solution

EXAMPLES

- *To make 500 ml sodium hydroxide (NaOH), 0.25 mol/l from a 0.4 mol/l solution:*

C = 0.25 mol/l, V = 500 ml, S = 0.4 mol/l
ml of stronger solution required:

$$\frac{0.25 \times 500}{0.4} = 312.5$$

Therefore, measure 312.5 ml NaOH, 0.4 mol/l, and make up to 500 ml with distilled water.

- *To make 1 litre hydrochloric acid (HCl), 0.01 mol/l from a 1 mol/l solution:*

C = 0.01 mol/l, V = 1 litre, S = 1 mol/l
ml of stronger solution required:

$$\frac{0.01 \times 1\,000}{1} = 10$$

Therefore, measure 10 ml HCl, 1 mol/l, and make up to 1 litre with distilled water.

- *To make 100 ml glucose, 3 mmol/l in 1 g/l benzoic acid from glucose 100 mmol/l solution:*

C = 3 mmol/l, V = 100 ml, S = 100 mmol/l
ml of stronger solution required:

$$\frac{3 \times 100}{100} = 3$$

Therefore, measure 3 ml of glucose, 100 mmol/l, and make up to 100 ml with 1 g/l benzoic acid.

- *To make 500 ml sulphuric acid (H_2SO_4), 0.33 mol/l from concentrated sulphuric acid which has an approximate substance concentration of 18 mol/l:*

C = 0.33 mol/l, V = 500 ml, S = 18 mol/l
ml of stronger solution required:

$$\frac{0.33 \times 500}{18} = 9.2$$

Therefore, measure 9.2 ml concentrated H_2SO_4, and slowly *add* it to about 250 ml of distilled water in a volumetric flask. Make up to 500 ml with distilled water.

Diluting body fluids

To prepare a dilution or series of dilutions of a body fluid:

EXAMPLES

- *To make 8 ml of a 1 in 20 dilution of blood:*

Volume of blood required: $\frac{8}{20} = 0.4$ ml

Therefore, to prepare 8 ml of a 1 in 20 dilution, add 0.4 ml of blood to 7.6 ml of diluting fluid.

- *To make 4 ml of a 1 in 2 dilution of serum in physiological saline:*

Volume of serum required: $\frac{4}{2} = 2.0$ ml

Therefore, to prepare 4 ml of a 1 in 2 dilution, add 2 ml of serum to 2 ml of physiological saline.

Calculating the dilution of a body fluid

To calculate the dilution of a body fluid:

EXAMPLES

- *Calculate the dilution of blood when using 50 µl (0.05 ml) of blood and 950 µl (0.95 ml) of diluting fluid:*

Total volume of body fluid and diluting fluid:
50 + 950 = 1 000 µl

Therefore, dilution of blood: $\frac{1\,000}{50} = 20$

i.e. 1 in 20 dilution.

- *Calculate the dilution of urine using 0.5 ml of urine and 8.5 ml of diluting fluid (physiological saline):*

Total volume of urine and diluting fluid:
8.5 + 0.5 = 9.0 ml

Therefore, dilution of urine: $\frac{9.0}{0.5} = 18$

i.e. 1 in 18 dilution.

PROPERTIES OF COMMONLY USED ACIDS AND BASES

An acid is a substance that liberates hydrogen ions in solution and acts as a proton donor (donating H^+).

Acids turn litmus red, and react with carbonates to produce the gas carbon dioxide. When reacted with a base, an acid produces a salt and water. Most acids are corrosive.

Sulphuric acid, nitric acid, and hydrochloric acid are referred to as strong acids because they ionize almost completely in solution with very few intact molecules of the acid remaining. Ionization is the dissociation of a substance in solution into electrically charged atoms known as ions. Lactic acid and glacial acetic acid are referred to as weak acids, because they ionize very little in solution.

The properties of the commonly used acids are as follows:

Sulphuric acid (H_2SO_4): Has a relative density of 1.840, molecular mass 98.08, and concentration 95–97% by weight.

It is very corrosive, viscous, oily, and *reacts violently with water* (hygroscopic). See also subunit 3.5.

Hydrochloric acid (HCl): Has a relative density of 1.190 and molecular mass 36.46. The concentrated acid contains 37% by weight of the gas hydrogen chloride. It is fuming and corrosive. See also subunit 3.5.

Nitric acid (HNO$_3$): Has a relative density of 1.510, molecular mass 63.01, and concentration about 99% by weight. It is fuming, corrosive, stains the skin yellow-brown, and is a powerful oxidizing agent. See also subunit 3.5.

Approximate molarity (mol/l) of some acids

Concentrated acid	Approx. mol/l
Acetic acid, glacial, 99.6% w/w:	17.50
Hydrochloric acid, 1.16, 32% w/w:	10.20
1.18, 36% w/w:	11.65
Nitric acid, 1.42, 70% w/w:	15.80
Sulphuric acid, 1.84, 97% w/w:	18.00

To make approx. 1 mol/l solutions from concentrated acids

Concentrated acid	ml diluted to 1 litre
Acetic acid, (glacial), 99.6% w/w	58 ml
Hydrochloric acid, 32% w/w	98 ml
36% w/w	86 ml
Nitric acid, 70%, w/w	63 ml
Sulphuric acid, 97% w/w	56 ml

BASES

A base is a substance that liberates hydroxide ions in solution and can accept a proton.

Alkaline solutions have a soapy feel, turn litmus blue, and react with an acid to form a salt and water.

The common bases include oxides and hydroxides of metals such as sodium, potassium, calcium, lead, iron, and copper. The oxides of potassium, sodium, and calcium dissolve in water to form alkalis.

Sodium hydroxide and potassium hydroxide are referred to as strong alkalis because they dissociate completely into cations and hydroxide ions in water.

Sodium hydroxide is the most commonly used alkali in district laboratories.

Sodium hydroxide (NaOH)

NaOH (supplied as pellets) is a corrosive deliquescent chemical with a molecular mass of 40.0.

When preparing sodium hydroxide solutions, it is necessary to dissolve small amounts of pellets at a time in water to avoid the production of excessive heat.

Preparation of NaOH solutions of different molarities

NaOH required in 1 litre	Approx. mol/l
4 g	0.1
10 g	0.25
16 g	0.4
40 g	1
200 g	5

Note: The volumes must be made up to 1 litre after the solutions have cooled to room temperature.

ACID BASE REACTIONS

Examples of chemical reactions involving acids and bases include:

Acid		Base		Salt		Water
H^+Cl^-	+	Na^+OH^-	$\rightarrow$	Na^+Cl^-	+	H_2O
Hydrochloric acid		Sodium hydroxide		Sodium chloride		Water
$CH_3COO^-H^+$	+	Na^+OH^-	$\rightarrow$	$CH_3COO^-Na^+$	+	H_2O
Acetic acid		Sodium hydroxide		Sodium acetate		Water

pK OF ACIDS AND BASES

The strength of an acid or base is determined by its pK which is defined as the negative logarithm (to the base 10) of the ionization constant (K):

$$pK = \log_{10}K$$

For example, a strong acid has a low pK value whereas a weak acid has a high pK. The higher the pK value the weaker the acid.

Neutralization reactions

The process of adding an acid to a base, or a base to an acid, to give a neutral solution consisting of a salt and water, is known as neutralization. The neutral solution contains equal numbers of hydroxide and hydrogen ions.

Hydrolysis

Hydrolysis is the chemical decomposition of a substance by water, with the water also being decomposed. Salts of weak acids, weak bases, or both, are partially hydrolyzed to form molecules of weak electrolytes in solution. An ester may be hydrolyzed to form an alcohol and an acid.

pH OF SOLUTIONS

Neutral solutions have equal concentrations of hydrogen ions and hydroxide ions. Pure water is neutral because it ionizes very slightly to give one hydroxide ion and one hydroxide ion for each molecule ionized.

Whether a solution is acidic or alkaline, there are always both H^+ and OH^- ions present. It is the predominance of one type of ion over the other that determines the degree of acidity and alkalinity. When referring to the degree of acidity or alkalinity of solutions it is usual to refer only to the hydrogen ion concentration.

Pure water at 25 °C contains 0.000 000 1 g, or 10^{-7}g, of hydrogen ions per litre.

Because the molecular mass of a hydrogen ion is 1, the hydrogen ion concentration of pure water can be expressed as follows:

$[H^+]$ (Pure water) $= 1 \times 10^{-7}$ mol/l

There is however no SI unit prefix for 10^{-7} and therefore the prefix nano (n) which means 10^{-9} is used. The SI unit formula is written:

$[H^+]$ (Pure water) $= 100 \times 10^{-9}$ mol/l
$= 100$ nmol/l

Normal blood, being slightly alkaline (pH about 7.4), contains fewer hydrogen ions than pure water:

$[H^+]$ (Blood) $\simeq 40$ nmol/l

EXPRESSING HYDROGEN ION CONCENTRATION

As a convenient way of expressing hydrogen ion concentration, the symbol pH was introduced by Sorensen in 1909. pH is defined as the negative value of the logarithm to the base 10 of the hydrogen ion concentration:

$pH = -\log_{10}[H^+]$

The pH of pure water can be expressed as follows:

pH (pure water) $= \log \dfrac{1}{10^{-7}}$
$= 7$ (neutral)

The pH scale is usually expressed from 0 to 14 units, with a pH of less than 7 indicating acidity and a pH above 7 indicating alkalinity:

Acidity	Neutral	Alkalinity
pH 0	pH 7	pH 14

pH can be measured using pH papers which give an approximate pH value, or by using a colorimeter with indicators and a series of coloured standards, or a pH meter which provides the most accurate method of determining pH.

BUFFER SOLUTIONS

Buffer solutions contain a mixture of a weak acid and a salt of a strong base, or a weak base and its salt with a strong acid.

Due to their composition, buffers are able to resist changes in pH. For example, if a small amount of hydrochloric acid is added to a buffer solution the hydrogen ion content does not increase very much because it combines the weak base of the buffer resulting in only a slight decrease in pH.

A buffer has its highest buffering ability when its pH is equal to its pK.

Buffers are used in clinical chemistry when the pH needs to be carefully controlled, e.g. when measuring enzyme activity.

INDICATORS

Indicators are substances that give different colours or shades of colour at different pH values. For example, phenol red changes from yellow at pH 6.8 to a deep red at pH 8.4.

Indicators are used to determine the pH of liquids and the 'end-point' of acid-base titrations. When titrating a strong or a weak acid with a strong base, an indicator is selected which changes colour at an alkaline pH, e.g. phenolphthalein. When titrating a strong or weak base with a strong acid, an indicator is used which changes colour at an acid pH, e.g. methyl orange.

PURCHASING CHEMICALS, REAGENTS, STAINS

Whenever possible, chemicals, reagents and stains for use in district laboratories should be purchased at regional or central level to promote standardization and benefit from bulk-purchasing prices. If this is not possible the following guidelines are recommended when ordering chemicals, reagents and stains.

Ordering chemicals and reagents
- Obtain a catalogue and price list from the manufacturer or local supplier.
- When ordering, use the correct name and whenever possible give the chemical formula. Some chemicals can be obtained in both hydrated and anhydrous form.
- Check that the amount you are ordering is available. Unless a chemical is very expensive, it is unlikely to be available in amounts under 100 g. Many chemicals may only be available in quantities of 250 g or 500 g.
- Check that the shelf-life of the chemical is acceptable and the conditions of storage can be met to ensure stability and safety in transit and in the laboratory.
- If needing to import a chemical, make sure national regulations will permit importation and that the chemical is not listed by the manufacturer as unstable and therefore unsuitable for

export (this information will be in the manufacturer's catalogue).

■ Check the price of the chemical and terms of purchase. Some chemical companies and suppliers have a minimum order value making it unaffordable to buy a single or a few chemicals at a time.

Ordering dyes and ready-made stains
When purchasing dyes and stains it is also important to obtain a supplier's catalogue:

– to ensure the correct name of the dye or stain is used when ordering.

– to know the form available, e.g. powder, liquid concentrate, or liquid ready-made stain, and to know the quantities available.

– to check stability and storage requirements.

Most of the aqueous-based stains used in microbiology and parasitology can be easily prepared locally from powders. The alcohol-based stains used in haematology, however, are less easily made locally when water-free methanol or ethanol are difficult to obtain. In these situations it may be more appropriate and cost-effective to purchase the ready-made stains to ensure quality. Only small volumes of the stains are used in the working solutions.

2.7 Communicating effectively

By definition, communication is the accurate passing on or sharing of information. In district laboratory work there are three main ways of communicating information:

– by writing
– by speaking
– by actions.

WRITTEN COMMUNICATION
To be effective, written communication needs to be:

– presented legibly and neatly,
– expressed clearly and simply.

Writing legibly and neatly
In laboratory work, serious consequences may result when hand-written figures or words are read incorrectly because of poor handwriting or untidy corrections. An illegibly written report may result in

a patient receiving incorrect treatment. The presentation of well-written and neat reports not only avoids errors, misunderstandings, and frustrations, but also inspires confidence in those using the laboratory. Before issue, all reports should be checked by the most senior member of staff. To promote standardization and neatness of reporting, the use of rubber stamps is recommended as described in subunit 2.2. Recording of patient data and the results of tests in laboratory registers must be done with care as also the recording of quality control data.

Importance of communicating effectively
Laboratory staff must be able to communicate well if a laboratory service is to function smoothly and reliably and inspire user confidence.

In communicating it is important to consider:

● nature of the information being communicated.

● person or persons to whom the information is being communicated.

● most effective way of communicating the information.

● whether the communicated information has been understood and responded to appropriately.

Writing clearly and simply
Opportunities for laboratory personnel to develop written skills should be provided during training.

A trained laboratory officer needs to know how to write clear reports and instructions with regard to standard operating procedures, use of equipment, preparation of reagents, safety measures, collection of specimens, laboratory policies, notices (memos), agendas for meetings, work reports, budgets, and requisitioning of laboratory supplies.

Laboratory personnel should be encouraged to contribute to newsletters and journals.

Computer skills: Where facilities exist, laboratory staff should be trained in basic computer skills, including the use of e-mail and how to process data and access information from relevant websites via the internet.

SPOKEN COMMUNICATION
Important aspects of spoken (verbal) communication include:

– clarity of speech and language used.
– tone of voice.
– ability to speak informatively.

Clarity of speech and language used

The main requirement of spoken communication is that the words spoken can be heard distinctly by the person to whom they are addressed in a language and dialect that is clearly understood by the person.

A barrier to effective spoken communication is background noise. Noise should therefore be kept to a minimum when speaking, e.g. reduce the speed of a centrifuge. Radios should not be played in laboratories. Such noise not only interferes with communication but can also be a distraction to persons working in the laboratory leading to errors in work due to loss of concentration.

It is particularly important to speak clearly and politely when addressing patients. Hesitant and mumbled instructions lead to misunderstandings and a lack of confidence by patients.

If the telephone is used to communicate test results, e.g. those needed urgently, it is particularly important to speak clearly to avoid errors. The person receiving the information should be asked to repeat back the name and identification number of the patient, and the test result.

Tone of voice

A kind and understanding tone of voice may greatly help a patient, especially a child, to feel less frightened, whereas a loud and impatient tone of voice may cause fear and add to the suffering of a patient. A laboratory worker should always try to reassure patients by explaining simply the procedure of a test and, without disclosing professional information, seek to answer patients' queries. Try always to have the time to listen.

It is particularly important to communicate well in difficult situations, for example when called to cross-match blood during a night emergency. Under these circumstances it is essential for the laboratory worker not only to function rapidly and reliably but also to reply calmly and patiently to anxious relatives and blood donors.

Spoken communication is influenced by temperament and fatigue, but a greeting and courteous response based on local traditions and a respect for all persons should always be possible.

Ability to speak informatively

The ability to speak competently and informatively is particularly important when giving the results of tests by telephone or directly to a medical officer, community health worker, or nurse. An understanding of the clinical significance of investigations is required.

If a laboratory worker does not have sufficient information to answer a question about a report, the questioner should be referred to a more experienced member of staff. If unable to reply and no other person is available, the laboratory person must advize that he or she is unable to assist. Inaccurate information must *never* be communicated.

The ability to speak informatively is also required when attending hospital interdepartmental meetings to discuss laboratory policies. Always think through what you are going to say before communicating it.

ACTION COMMUNICATION

Communication through a culturally acceptable bodily manner and actions (body language) is particularly important when relating to patients.

A pleasant, friendly, professional manner and a neat clean appearance inspire confidence whereas an impatient, aggressive manner or an untidy appearance can make patients nervous and afraid.

When unable to speak the language of a patient, facial expressions and actions become extremely important in reassuring a patient. In such a situation an interpreter must be used to communicate important information to a patient, obtain confirmation of a patient's identity, and translate what the patient wishes to say. A smile and a caring look and action can inspire trust.

Appropriate action communication is also important among staff members if a pleasant working environment is to be maintained.

REFERENCES
1   **Nwobodo ED**. Medical lab reports: Are we too confident in their results? *Africa Health*, 2002, 3.
2   **Bedu-Addo G, Bates I**. Making the most of the laboratory. *Principles of medicine in Africa*, 2004, p. 1329. Cambridge University Press.
3   **Elsenga WK**. *Introduction of a quality assurance handbook, a guideline for accreditation of medical laboratories.* Paper presented at the 20th World congress of medical technology, Dublin, 1992, July, pp. 26–31.
4   **Houang L**. *Operating costs of the peripheral laboratory and cost of tests. In health laboratories in developing countries. Proceedings of a Workshop*, 1990. Health Cooperation papers No. 10, Associazione Italiana 'Amici di R. Follereau'.
5   **Mundy CJF et al**. The operation, quality and costs of a district hospital laboratory service in Malawi. *Transactions Royal Society Tropical Medicine and Hygiene*, 2003, 97, pp. 403–408.
6   WHO Essential Health Technologies (EHT) Department. *The role of laboratory external quality assessment schemes*, 2004. Accessed from the EHT website www.who.int/eht/main_areas_of_work/DIL/Lab_Tech (listed under Index as External Quality Ass.... 11 Nov 2004).

RECOMMENDED READING

Bates I, Bekoe V, Asamoa-Adu A. Improving the accuracy of malaria-related tests in Ghana. *Malaria Journal*, 2004, 3: 38. Also available online www.malariajournal.com/content/3/1/38

Gadzikwa E. Benchmarking quality in the laboratory. *Mera*, July 2004, pp. vii–viii.

Laboratory services for primary health care: requirements for essential clinical laboratory tests. World Health Organization, WHO/LAB/98.2, 1998. Available from WHO Health Laboratory Unit, WHO, 1211 Geneva, 27-Switzerland.

Basics of quality assurance for intermediate and peripheral laboratories. World Health Organization, Alexandria, 2nd edition, 2002. (WHO Regional Publication, Eastern Mediterranean Series No. 2). Obtainable from WHO Regional Office, Abdul Razzak Al Sanhouri Street, PO Box 7608, Nasr City, Cairo 11371, Egypt.
Website www.emro.who.int

Quality systems for medical laboratories: guidelines for implementation and monitoring. World Health Organization, Alexandria, 1995 (WHO Regional Publication, Eastern Mediterranean Series, No. 14). Obtainable from WHO Regional Office, Abdul Razzak Al Sanhouri Street, PO Box 7608, Nasr City, Cairo 11371, Egypt.
Website www.emro.who.int

Quality assurance of sputum microscopy in DOTs programmes, World Health Organization 2004. Available from WHO, Geneva. Can also be downloaded from www.who.int (use search facility).

3

Health and safety in district laboratories

3.1 Implementing a laboratory health and safety programme

Accidents in the laboratory can result in:

- injury, death, ill health, and disablement of staff, patients, and others.
- work being disrupted with possible discontinuity of laboratory services.
- loss of valuable laboratory equipment, supplies, and records.
- loss of or contamination of specimens with serious consequences for patients.
- damage to the laboratory, adjacent departments and buildings, and to the environment.

If such accidents are to be avoided, a relevant, workable, and affordable laboratory health and safety programme is essential.

Objectives of a laboratory health and safety programme

- To identify hazards in the work place and assess the risk to staff, patients, and others.
- To prepare and implement an effective *Code of Safe Laboratory Practice*.
- To check whether health and safety regulations are being followed.
- To make sure staff know how to work safely, what to do when an accident occurs and how to carry out emergency First Aid.
- To ensure all laboratory accidents are reported informatively and investigated promptly.
- To promote safety awareness.

RISK ASSESSMENT

Before implementing a district laboratory safety programme, it is essential for those in charge of district laboratory services, the district laboratory coordinator, and senior laboratory officers, i.e. district safety committee, to make a careful local risk assessment:

1 Identifying the hazards, i.e. what are the commonest causes of accidents.

2 Deciding what actions can be taken to remove the hazards, e.g. a simple structural repair, changes in the storage of chemicals, or changes to safer working practices.

3 Evaluating for those hazards that cannot be removed what are the associated risks, i.e. what harm can be caused by each hazard.

4 Deciding what safety regulations and safety awareness measures are needed to minimize the risks and prevent accidents occurring.

The district safety committee should:

- prepare a written *Code of Safe Laboratory Practice* based on the findings of the risk assessment.
- circulate the *Safety Code* to all district laboratories and train all laboratory personnel how to apply the *Safety Code* in their workplace.
- appoint a trained safety laboratory officer to manage the laboratory safety programme.

COMMON HAZARDS IN DISTRICT LABORATORIES

The following are important hazards that require assessment and management in district laboratories:

- Unsafe premises
- Naked flames
- Microbial hazards
- Chemical hazards
- Glassware hazards
- Sharps hazards
- Equipment hazards
- Explosions
- Infestation by ants, rodents, cockroaches
- Unreliable water supply

Accidents that can arise from these hazards are summarized in Chart 3.1.

Chart 3.1 Common causes of accidents in district laboratories

HAZARD	ASSOCIATED ACCIDENT
UNSAFE LABORATORY PREMISE	**Burns and inhalation of smoke during a fire:** – when emergency exit routes from the laboratory are blocked by equipment, storage boxes, etc. – when, in a subdivided laboratory, there is only a single exit and staff become trapped in one section. **Staff are injured by falling on a slippery or damaged floor or from broken glass on the floor:** – when the floor is not cleaned properly after spillages or glassware breakages. – when wax or other slippery cleaning substance is applied to the floor. – when damaged areas of the floor are covered with matting. **Risk of infection to staff and others:** – when there is no separate hand basin with a reliable water supply for handwashing. – when no separate rest-room is provided for staff and food and drink are consumed in the laboratory. – when laboratory staff do not leave their protective clothing in the laboratory when leaving the workplace or when the clothing is not laundered frequently enough. – when bench surfaces are not disinfected or cleaned properly each day. – when the working area is not separated from the areas where outpatients are received and blood samples collected. – when the laboratory has no safe systems for decontaminating infective materials, disposing of waste and washing reusable laboratoryware. **Injury from chemicals:** – when chemicals with irritating fumes are used in a laboratory with inadequate ventilation. – when hazardous chemicals are stored on high shelves or on the floor under benches. **Injury from equipment:** – when electrical equipment has faulty earthing or insufficient ventilation. – when unsafe adaptors or extension leads are used because there are insufficient electric wall points. – when the laboratory has no preventive maintenance schedules and equipment is not inspected regularly for defective insulation, corrosion, and loose connections. *Note:* The features of a safe laboratory environment are described in subunit 3.2.
NAKED FLAMES	**Injury from fire caused by lighted bunsen burners, spirit burners, tapers, matches, alcohol swabs, ring burners, stoves:** – when a lighted burner is placed in sunlight, making the flame difficult to see. – when a Bunsen burner, ring burner, match, or taper is lit too close to a flammable chemical. – when sheets of paper or other combustible material are accidentally left over the chimney (burner unit) of a gas or kerosene refrigerator.

– when a lighted taper is carried across the laboratory close to where a flammable stain or reagent is being used or stored.

Note: Fire safety is covered in subunit 3.7.

MICROBIAL HAZARDS

Pathogens are accidentally ingested:
– from contaminated fingers when personal hygiene is neglected.
– when hands are not washed after handling specimens or cultures.
– when specimens or liquid cultures are mouth-pipetted.

Pathogens are accidentally inoculated:
– through needlestick injuries caused by resheathing needles after collecting blood or careless handling of needles and lancets.
– through open uncovered skin wounds.
– through injury from broken contaminated glassware.

Pathogens are accidentally inhaled in airborne droplets (aerosols):
– when snap-closing specimen containers.
– when vigorously dispensing or pouring infectious fluids.
– when sucking up and blowing out fluids from pipettes.
– when specimens are hand-centrifuged in open containers or when a container breaks in an electric centrifuge and the lid is opened before the aerosols have settled.
– when infectious material is spilled following the dropping or knocking over of a specimen container or culture.

Note: Safety measures to prevent accidents associated with microbiological hazards are described in subunits 3.3 and 3.4. Personal hygiene and other personal safety precautions are covered in subunit 3.2.

CHEMICAL HAZARDS

Toxic or harmful chemicals causing serious ill health, injury, or irritation:
– when toxic or harmful chemicals are swallowed by being mouth-pipetted.
– when fumes from irritant chemicals are inhaled in poorly ventilated areas of the laboratory.
– when no protective goggles or gloves are worn and harmful chemicals enter the eye or come in contact with the skin.

Flammable chemicals causing fire:
– when flammable chemicals are used or stored near a naked flame.
– when a lighted 'swab' is used to heat stain in the Ziehl-Neelsen method and ignites nearby flammable chemicals.
– when the neck of a bottle containing a flammable chemical is accidentally flamed.
– when a flammable chemical is spilled near a flame.

Corrosive chemicals causing serious injury and burns:
– when corrosive reagents are ingested by being mouth-pipetted.
– when strong acids are accidentally knocked from shelves or spilled.
– when intense heat is produced during the dilution or dissolving of a strong acid or alkali or when water is added to a concentrated acid.
– when a corrosive chemical comes into contact with the skin, or the eyes are splashed when opening and pouring a corrosive chemical.

Note: Preventing chemical associated accidents is covered in subunit 3.5.

GLASSWARE HAZARDS

Broken glass causing cuts, bleeding, infection:
- when cleaning damaged slides or cover glasses.
- when using pipettes with broken ends that have not been made smooth in a flame.
- when a long pipette is pushed into a pipette filler and 'snaps' because the pipette is gripped near the tip not the top.
- when picking up pieces of glass following a breakage.
- when glass fragments are left on the floor after a breakage.
- when a waste bin containing broken glass is overfilled.
- when glass and other sharp articles are not separated from other refuse or the 'sharps' are discarded in containers that can be easily punctured.

Note: Safety measures to avoid injuries from broken glass are included in subunit 3.6.

EQUIPMENT HAZARDS

Electric shock:
- when equipment is not reliably earthed or electrical circuits are faulty.
- when touching live wires in attempting to repair equipment or replace components, e.g. lamp, without first disconnecting the equipment from the mains.
- when handling electrical equipment with wet hands or standing on a wet floor.

Fire:
- when cables and electrical equipment overheat due to overloading of conductors.
- when there is overheating caused by the overuse of adaptors.
- when insulation is inadequate or becomes damaged.
- when thermostats fail and there is no temperature cut-out device to prevent overheating.
- when electrical sparking or arching causes flammable material to ignite.
- when preventive maintenance is not carried out to check for corrosion, wear, and loose connections.
- when a battery lead becomes accidentally positioned across the opposite battery terminal.

Injury from moving parts:
- when an open hand-centrifuge is used in a part of the laboratory where it can easily injure a person.
- when a person opens a centrifuge lid and tries to stop the motor manually (where the equipment does not have a safety device to prevent this).
- when a centrifuge is not balanced, resulting in the buckets and trunnions spinning off the rotor, particularly when there is corrosion.

Note: The safe use of equipment is covered in subunit 3.6.

EXPLOSION HAZARDS

Injury from explosions:
- when incompatible chemicals explode.
- when leaking gas explodes.
- when bottles of fluid explode inside an autoclave.

Note: The safe use and storage of chemicals and gas cylinders are covered in subunit 3.5 and the correct use of an autoclave in 4.8.

INSECT AND RODENT INFESTATION	**Damaged equipment causing injury:**

Damaged equipment causing injury:
- when insects enter unmeshed ventilation openings, leading to damaged components and electrical faults.
- when rodents damage earthing and insulation around cables causing electric shock and fires.

Damage to structure and furnishings of the laboratory
- when ants and rodents damage wooden window frames, bench supports or shelving.
- when there is no inspection of the laboratory or an infestation is not treated.

UNRELIABLE WATER SUPPLY

Contributing to infection:
- when there is insufficient running water for handwashing and the laboratory has no alternative water supply, e.g. rain water in storage tanks.
- when intermittent water supplies interrupt cleaning of the laboratory, decontamination of infectious material, and washing of laboratoryware.

General factors that contribute to the occurrence of accidents
In addition to identifying the hazards listed in Chart 3.1, the district laboratory safety committee should also address any other environmental or personal factors that can increase the risk of accidents occurring in district laboratories. These include:

- Inexperience and insufficient training and supervision of staff and lack of health and safety awareness by senior laboratory officers.
- Untidy working, allowing the bench to become cluttered and not using racks to avoid spillages.
- Too heavy a workload for the size of laboratory and number of staff.
- Rushing to finish work 'on time'.
- Loss of concentration due to a noisy working environment, constant interruptions, and excessive heat particularly in small poorly ventilated outreach laboratories.
- Fatigue due to frequent emergency work during night hours.

Many of these factors can be remedied by:
- on-going health and safety training in the workplace.
- good laboratory practice and common sense.
- changing the work attitudes of laboratory staff.
- increasing health and safety awareness in the laboratory by frequent discussions on safety issues and displaying appropriate safety symbols and notices.
- monitoring and improving the working con-

ditions of district laboratory personnel as part of total quality management (see Chapter 2).

CODE OF SAFE LABORATORY PRACTICE
After carrying out a careful risk assessment, the district laboratory safety committee should be able to formulate a *Code of Safe Laboratory Practice* that is relevant to the laboratories in its district.

Guidelines for a Code of Safe Laboratory Practice
The following should be included in a *Code of Safe Laboratory Practice* for district laboratories:

SAFE WORKING ENVIRONMENT
- Rules concerning access to the laboratory and displaying of safety signs and notices for staff, patients, and visitors to the laboratory.
- Procedures to follow to maintain local laboratory security.
- How to keep the laboratory clean.
- How to separate and dispose of general waste, broken glass and other 'sharps', contaminated materials, and different specimens.
- Decontamination procedures.
- Washing of reusable specimen containers, needles, syringes, lancets, slides, cover glasses, pipettes.
- Disinfectants and their use in the laboratory.
- Sterilization procedures.
- Ventilation of the laboratory.

- How to check the laboratory for structural damage and wear that may lead to accidents or make the premise less secure.

- Checking for and controlling infestation by ants, cockroaches, rodents.

- Maintenance schedules and routine cleaning of equipment.

- Inspecting electrical equipment for damage to insulation and loose connections in plugs.

- Rules for the storage and labelling of chemicals and reagents and how to keep an inventory of chemicals.

- Regulations covering the safe packing and transport of specimens.

- Procedure for the reporting of faults.

SAFE WORKING PRACTICES
- Personal hygiene measures and wearing of safe footwear.

- Regulations concerning the wearing, storing, decontamination and laundering of protective clothing.

- Preventing laboratory acquired infection including regulations to avoid the accidental:
  - ingestion of pathogens,
  - inhaling of pathogens,
  - inoculation of pathogens.

- What to do when there is a spillage of a specimen or liquid culture.

- Safety rules concerning the handling and storage of chemicals and reagents that are flammable, oxidizing, toxic, harmful, irritant, and corrosive, and how to manage chemical spillages.

- What to do when there is a glass breakage.

- How to pipette and dispense safely.

- Safe operation of manual, electrical, and battery operated laboratory equipment.

- Working tidily, use of racks, and rules to prevent the floor and benches from becoming cluttered and exits obstructed.

- Use of protective gloves, goggles, face shield, dust mask, eyewash bottle.

- How to control noise levels and other causes of loss of concentration.

EMERGENCY FIRST AID
- Contents of a First Aid box.
- First Aid for:
  - cuts, needlestick injuries,
  - poisoning,
  - bleeding,
  - heat burns,
  - chemical burns,
  - fainting,
  - electric shock,
  - resuscitation.

FIRE MANAGEMENT
- Fire prevention.
- What to do if there is a laboratory fire.
- Correct positioning, use, and maintenance of fire fighting equipment and a fire blanket.

REPORTING AN ACCIDENT OR LABORATORY RELATED ILLNESS
- Who should be notified and procedure to be followed.
- Information required for the report and record.

Laboratory accident book
All accidents and laboratory associated illnesses must be reported immediately and recorded in a *Laboratory Accident Book*. The following information is required:
- place, date and time of the accident,
- person or persons involved,
- injuries sustained,
- emergency First Aid given and by whom,
- details of follow-up actions,
- staff comments on the possible reasons for the accident and what should be done to prevent a repetition.

Important: All accidents should be investigated promptly to ensure appropriate treatment is provided and preventive measures are put in place at the earliest opportunity.

PROTECTIVE INOCULATIONS
List those inoculations recommended by the medical officer in charge of district laboratory services (see subunit 3.2).

Note: The following subunits cover laboratory health and safety issues:

3.2 Safe laboratory environment and personal safety measures
3.3 Microbial hazards
3.4 Decontamination of infectious material and disposal of laboratory waste
3.5 Chemical and reagent hazards
3.6 Equipment and glassware hazards
3.7 Fire safety
3.8 Emergency First Aid and contents of a First Aid box

Further information: Detailed information on laboratory biosafety, including a *Safety Checklist* for biomedical laboratories can be found in the WHO, 3rd edition *Laboratory Biosafety Manual* (see Recommended Reading).

Safety equipment for district laboratories

This should include protective clothing for staff, fire blanket, dry chemical type fire extinguisher, eye goggles, face visor, face masks, eyewash bottle, chemical resistant gloves and other types of protective gloves, First Aid box, devices to avoid mouth-pipetting, waste and sharps disposal containers, leakproof specimen containers, and an autoclave (or other sterilizer), and when possible a biological safety cabinet.

DUTIES OF A LABORATORY SAFETY OFFICER

Although it is not possible to achieve absolute safety in the laboratory, a Safety Officer should be appointed and work for the best possible level of health and safety, promote safety awareness, and make provision for continuing education in biosafety.

A system for monitoring safety regulations in the laboratory should be established. A check list should be drawn up and regular (but random) inspections made to:

- Ensure staff are practising their *Safety Code* and know what to do if there is a fire, equipment fault, specimen or chemical spillage, or other accident in the laboratory.

- Make sure test methods are safe, specimens and reagents are being handled and disposed of safely and specimen containers are being decontaminated and cleaned correctly.

- Check that all hazardous chemicals and reagents are marked with the correct hazard label and are being stored and handled safely by staff.

- Make sure that there is no mouth-pipetting and check protective gloves are being worn by staff.

- Observe whether protective clothing is being worn and kept fastened and removed when leaving the laboratory.

- Note whether other safety regulations are being kept such as no smoking, eating, drinking, chewing gum or applying cosmetics in the laboratory. Laboratory fridges should be inspected for food and drink.

- Check whether safety equipment such as the First Aid box, eyewash bottles, eye goggles, sand buckets, fire blanket, and fire extinguishers are in good order and that staff know the locations and how to use the equipment.

- Make sure corridors and exits from the laboratory are not being obstructed and fire doors (where fitted) are being kept closed.

- Check whether the laboratory is being kept clean and that benches are free of books, unnecessary equipment, and personal property.

- Examine equipment for defects and observe whether equipment is being used correctly and maintenance checks are being performed. Check also for cracked or chipped glassware.

- Observe whether safety regulations regarding patients and visitors to the laboratory are being followed and only authorised staff are entering the working area.

- Check for any structural defects in the laboratory or infestation by insects or rodents.

During such inspections, the safety officer should take the opportunity of reviewing and discussing safety regulations with staff and revizing where necessary First Aid and fire regulations. If a laboratory accident has occurred recently, the causes of it should be discussed and if required, new safety measures introduced to help prevent its recurrence. There should follow a written report with recommendations. Laboratory security should also be discussed.

It is the duty of the district safety officer to instruct new members of staff (technical and auxillary) in health and safety regulations. The Safety Officer *must ensure that faults reported by staff concerning safety are investigated promptly*. Careful records must be kept of all laboratory accidents.

3.2 Safe laboratory premise and personal safety measures

Unsafe working premises and staff not following personal health and safety measures are major causes of accidents in district laboratories.

SAFE LABORATORY WORKING ENVIRONMENT

The safety of the working environment must take into consideration:

- Type of work being performed, ie specimens which the laboratory handles and pathogens which may be encountered (mainly Risk Group 2 organisms, see subunit 3.3).

- Working practices including the procedures and equipment used.

- Number of staff and workload.

- Laboratory's location, climatic conditions, and security of premise.

The following are important in making the workplace safe:

- Laboratory premise that is structurally sound and in good repair with a reliable water supply and a safe plumbing and waste disposal system. Drainage from sinks must be closed and connected to a septic tank or to a deep pit.

  Note: If there is a shortage of piped water, provision must be made for the storage of water, e.g. collection of rain water in storage tanks. It is not safe for a laboratory to function without an adequate water supply.

- Adequate floor and bench space and storage areas. The overall size of the laboratory must be appropriate for the workload, staff numbers, storage and equipment requirements.

- Well constructed floor with a surface that is non-slip, impermeable to liquids, and resistant to those chemicals used in the laboratory. It should be bevelled to the wall and the entire floor should be accessible for washing. The floor must not be waxed or covered with matting. Floor drains are recommended.

- Walls that are smooth, free from cracks, impermeable to liquids, and painted with washable light coloured paint.

- When practical, a door at each end of the laboratory so that laboratory staff will not be trapped should a fire break out. Doors should open outwards and exit routes must never be obstructed. Where fitted, internal doors should be self closing and contain upper viewing panes. External doors must be fitted with secure locks.

- Adequate ventilation supplied by wall vents and windows that can be opened. The windows should not face the prevailing winds to avoid excessive dust entering the laboratory in the dry season and the wind interfering with work activities. Windows should be fitted with sun blinds and insect proof screens, and when indicated secure window bars.

- Sectioning of the laboratory into separate rooms or working areas. The area where blood samples are collected from patients must be away from the testing area of the laboratory. Seating should be provided for patients outside the laboratory.

  The specimen reception area must be equipped with a table or hatchway which has a surface that is impervious, washable, and resistant to disinfectants. There should also be a First Aid area in the laboratory containing a First Aid box, eyewash bottle and fire blanket.

Note: A layout of a typical district hospital laboratory and other useful information on how to improve district laboratory biosafety can be found in the *Essential Medical Laboratory Services Project Report: Malawi*, 2002.[1]

- Bench surfaces that are without cracks, impervious, washable, and resistant to the disinfectants and chemicals used in the laboratory.

  Benches, shelving, and cupboards need to be well constructed and kept free of insect and rodent infestation. Benches should be kept as clear as possible to provide maximum working area and facilitate cleaning.

- Suitable storage facilities, including a ventilated locked store for the storage of chemicals and expensive equipment.

- Where required, a gas supply that is piped into the laboratory with the gas cylinder stored in an outside weatherproof, well-ventilated locked store.

- A staff room that is separate from the working area where refreshments can be taken and personal food and other belongings stored safely.

  Wall pegs should be provided *in* the laboratory on which to hang protective clothing.

  Near to the staff room there should be a separate room with toilet and hand-washing facilities. There should be separate toilet facilities for patients.

- A handbasin with running water, preferably sited near the door. Whenever possible, taps should be operated by wrist levers or foot pedals. Bars of soap should be provided, not soap dispensers.

  Ideally paper towels should be used. If this is not possible small cloth hand towels that are laundered daily should be provided.

- Provision of protective safety cabinets and fume cupboards as required and when feasible.

- Safe electricity supply with sufficient wall electric points to avoid the use of adaptors and extension leads (power supplies to district laboratories are covered in subunit 4.2).

- Fire extinguishers sited at accessible points. These need to be of the dry chemical type. Several buckets of sand and a fire blanket are also required.

- As good illumination as possible. Low energy tube lights are recommended. Window screens must be fitted to protect from direct sunlight and glare but these should not make the working areas too dark.

■ Provision of *separate* labelled containers for the decontamination of infected material, discarding of needles, syringes, lancets, glassware for cleaning, broken glass, and general laboratory waste. A warning symbol such as a red triangle can be used to mark containers in which infected material is placed.

Use of safety signs and symbols

Displaying suitable safety signs and symbols is one way of promoting safety awareness. Examples of prohibition (*do not*) signs are shown in Fig. 3.1. They can be easily prepared locally. Prohibition signs are always crossed by a red line. *No smoking* signs should be displayed in the laboratory and adjacent patient waiting areas.

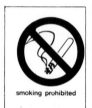 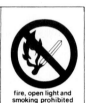 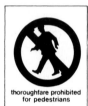

smoking prohibited | fire, open light and smoking prohibited | thoroughfare prohibited for pedestrians

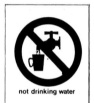 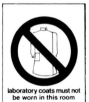 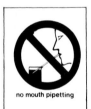

not drinking water | laboratory coats must not be worn in this room | no mouth pipetting

 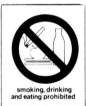 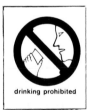

no entry | smoking, drinking and eating prohibited | drinking prohibited

Fig. 3.1　Prohibition signs for wall display

The international biohazard sign as shown in Fig. 3.2 should be displayed on the laboratory door. It indicates that the laboratory handles samples that contain pathogenic microorganisms and therefore access is restricted to authorised persons.

Recommended signs for labelling chemicals and reagents, e.g. *Flammable*, *Toxic*, *Corrosive*, *Harmful*, *Irritant*, *Oxidizing*, and *Explosive* can be found in subunit 3.5.

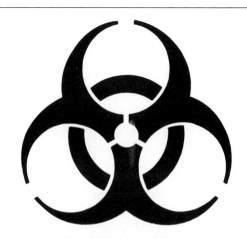

BIOHAZARD

Fig. 3.2　International Biohazard Symbol

PERSONAL HEALTH AND SAFETY MEASURES

Personal health and safety measures include:

– practice of personal hygiene.
– wearing of protective clothing.
– protective inoculations and medical examinations.

Practice of personal hygiene

Laboratory staff *must* practice a high standard of personal hygiene. This includes:

■ Washing hands and arms with soap and water before attending outpatients, visiting wards, after handling specimens and infected material, when leaving the laboratory, and at the end of the day's work. When running water supplies are interrupted, a tip type water container suspended over the sink should be used for handwashing, *not a basin of water. Frequent handwashing is the most effective action a laboratory worker can take to avoid laboratory-acquired infection.*

■ Covering any cuts, insect bites, open sores, or wounds on the hands or other exposed parts of the body with a water-proof adhesive dressing. Irritating insect bites should be treated.

■ Wearing closed shoes and not walking barefoot.

■ Not eating, drinking, chewing gum, smoking, or applying cosmetics in any part of the laboratory and not sitting on laboratory benches.

Note: Food or drink should never be stored in a laboratory refrigerator.

- Not licking gummed labels or placing pens, pencils or other articles near the mouth, eyes, or in hair.
- Avoid wearing jewellery in the working area, particularly pendant necklaces and bracelets.

Important: Staff should know what to do should a laboratory accident occur. An appropriately equipped First Aid box should be accessible (see subunit 3.8).

Protective clothing

Protective overall

An overall (coverall) should be worn over normal clothing or instead of it to protect the major part of the body from splashes, droplets of liquids containing microorganisms, and hazardous chemicals. When indicated a waterproof apron should also be worn.

The protective overall should be made of a fabric such as polycotton that can be bleached and frequently laundered and is suitable for wearing in tropical climates. Ideally the fabric should also be antistatic and flammable-resistant.

The overall *must* be worn with fasteners, buttons, or tape closed. A side closing design with *Velcro* type tape is preferable to a front opening because it gives better protection when working at the bench and enables the overall to be removed quickly should harmful or infectious material be spilt on it.

Soiled clothing should be placed in a special bag and not left in a cupboard or under a bench in the laboratory. Prior to laundering, the clothing and bag should be soaked overnight in 1% v/v domestic bleach. Protective clothing should always be left in the laboratory working area and *never* taken home or worn in a room where refreshments are taken. When attending outpatients or inpatients, a clean overall should be worn.

Gloves

Protective gloves should be worn when taking samples from patients and when handling specimens or cultures which may contain highly infectious pathogens, e.g. Risk Group 3 organisms or specimens from patients who may have hepatitis, HIV infection or haemorrhagic fever. If indicated the work should be undertaken in a biological safety cabinet (see subunit 3.3).

Highly infectious material: This should be handled in a laboratory with adequate containment facilities.

Re-usable gloves must be decontaminated and washed while on the hands and after removal (see subunit 3.4). Heat-resistant gloves should be worn when handling hot objects, e.g. when unloading an autoclave. Chemical resistant gloves should be worn when handling hazardous chemicals. Rubber gloves should be worn when cleaning and washing laboratory-ware.

Safety goggles, face shields, dust masks, respirators

Shatter-proof safety goggles or face shields (visors) should be worn when necessary to protect the eyes and face from splashes, e.g. when handling hazardous chemicals including disinfectants. Safety goggles should fit over spectacles if worn and also have sidepieces. Dust masks can protect against inhaling particles of chemicals that are toxic or irritant. Fabric masks provide only limited protection, particularly against inhaling aerosols or chemical particles. Personal respirators should be considered to protect staff working with *M tuberculosis*.[2]

Protective inoculations and medical examinations

There should be a pre-employment health check for all new members of staff. It is not possible or desirable to vaccinate laboratory workers against all the pathogens with which they may come in contact. The medical officer in charge of the laboratory should decide which vaccinations are required. Protective inoculations are usually given against tuberculosis (when not Mantoux positive), typhoid, diphtheria, tetanus, poliomyelitis, and cholera.

Note: In HIV high prevalence areas, laboratory staff who know that they are HIV positive should be aware of the risk of working with sputum samples that may contain *M. tuberculosis*.

3.3 Microbial hazards

Preventing laboratory associated infections depends on laboratory staff understanding:

- The routes by which infections are acquired in the laboratory. These may be different from 'natural' infections.
- Which organisms are the most hazardous so that time and labour are not wasted on unnecessary precautions.
- Which techniques are the most hazardous so that these may be replaced by those that are safer.

■ How the laboratory worker can reduce direct contact with infectious material and use safe working practices.

LABORATORY ACQUIRED INFECTIONS

Infections may be caused by microorganisms entering the body through the:
- skin,
- eyes,
- mouth,
- respiratory tract.

Infection through the skin and eyes

Organisms can penetrate the skin through cuts and scratches. They can be picked up on the hands from benches and equipment which have been accidentally contaminated by small, usually unnoticed, drops, spills, and splashes. They may be transferred to the face or eyes by the fingers. Eye infections can also occur by sample splashing to the eye.

Infection through the mouth

Microorganisms may be ingested during mouth-pipetting, either by direct aspiration or from the mouth ends of pipettes which have been touched by contaminated fingers. Direct finger to mouth infection is also possible, as is infection by eating food in the laboratory. Food may become contaminated from benches or fingers, or by contact with infected material, for example in a refrigerator.

Organisms may also be transferred to the mouth by cigarettes, cigars, or pipes which are handled or placed on laboratory benches. For some pathogens only a small number of organisms need to be ingested to cause infection, e.g. only a low infective dose is required for *Shigella* infections.

Infection through the respiratory tract

Many common laboratory procedures with microorganisms release aerosols, i.e. infected airborne droplets, into the atmosphere. The larger of these fall rapidly and contaminate hands, benches, and equipment. Small droplets evaporate and leave behind 'droplet nuclei' consisting of bacteria or viruses which are too light to settle. They are moved around a room and even a whole building by small air currents and ventilation systems. If inhaled, particles more than about 10 μm in diameter, will be captured in the nasal passages. Smaller particles, however, particularly those less than 5 μm in size, will not be trapped and may be inhaled right into the lungs where they may start an infection.

Infection of the general public

Microorganisms from laboratories may enter the bodies of members of the general public by the same routes as those affecting laboratory workers, but the sources are different.

The general public may become infected as a result of an 'escape' of microorganisms during the transport of infectious specimens to or between laboratories, for example from health centres to hospitals. Another source of infection can occur if the public comes into contact with infectious waste, discarded or effluent materials from the laboratory, due to a failure of the laboratory to decontaminate such materials.

CLASSIFICATION OF INFECTIVE MICROORGANISMS

Experience has confirmed that some organisms are more hazardous to handle and are more likely to infect laboratory workers than others, e.g. hepatitis viruses. More pathogens are also becoming resistant to available antimicrobials, making the treatment of infections caused by these resistant organisms more difficult.

The World Health Organization classifies infective microorganisms into four Risk Groups 1, 2, 3, and 4.[3]

Agents in each Risk Group

The World Health Organization recommends that the health authorities of each country should make lists of the organisms and viruses in each Risk Group, relevant to their local circumstances so that appropriate precautions may be applied.

No one list will suffice for all countries because circumstances will vary from one region to another. For example, if an organism is widespread in a community, there is no point in taking elaborate laboratory precautions to protect laboratory staff. Again, there will be little need to protect the community if an infection is unlikely to spread because of the absence of vectors or as a result of good sanitation or other public health measures.

Risk Group 1

The organisms in this group present a low risk to the individual laboratory worker and to members of the community. They are unlikely to cause human or animal disease.

Examples include food spoilage bacteria, common moulds, and yeasts.

Risk Group 2

These organisms offer a moderate risk to the laboratory worker and a limited risk to members of the community. They can cause serious human disease but are not a serious hazard. Effective preventive measures and treatment are available and the risk of spread in the community is limited.

Examples include staphylococci, streptococci, enterobacteria (except *Salmonella typhi*), clostridia, vibrios, adenoviruses, polioviruses, coxsackieviruses, hepatitis viruses, *Blastomyces*, *Toxoplasma*, and *Leishmania*.

Risk Group 3

This group contains organisms that present a high risk to the laboratory worker but a low risk to the community should they escape from the laboratory. They do not ordinarily spread rapidly from one individual to another. Again, there are effective vaccines and therapeutic materials for most pathogens in this group.

Examples include *Brucella, Mycobacterium tuberculosis, Salmonella typhi, Francisella, Pasteurella pestis,* many arboviruses, LCM virus, rickettsiae, chlamydia, *Coccidioides, Histoplasma,* human immunodeficiency viruses (HIV).

Risk Group 4

The agents in this group offer a high risk to the laboratory worker and to the community. They can cause serious disease and are readily transmitted from one individual to another. Effective treatment and preventive measures are not usually available.

Examples include viruses of haemorrhagic fevers including Marburg, Lassa and Ebola, equine and other encephalitis viruses, SARS virus, and certain arboviruses.

Classification of laboratories

Work with organisms in different Risk Groups requires different conditions for containment and different equipment and procedures to conduct work safely. Assignment of an agent to a biosafety level for laboratory work must be based on a risk assessment.

There are four Biosafety Levels of laboratory:
- Basic, Biosafety Level 1
- Basic, Biosafety Level 2
- Containment, Biosafety Level 3
- Maximum Containment, Biosafety Level 4

Basic laboratory, Level 1: This is the simplest kind and is adequate for work with organisms in Risk Group 1.

Basic laboratory, Level 2: This is suitable for work with organisms in Risk Group 2. It should be clean and provide enough space for the workload and the staff, have adequate sanitary facilities, especially for handwashing, and be equipped with an autoclave. A biological safety cabinet is desirable.

Containment laboratory, Level 3: This is more sophisticated and is used for work with organisms in Risk Group 3 e.g.

culture work. The principle is to remove from the Basic laboratory those organisms and activities which are particularly hazardous because they are the most likely to infect by the airborne route, ingestion, or injection of very small numbers. The object is to expose as few people as possible to the risk of infection.

The Containment laboratory is therefore a separate room with controlled access by authorized staff only. It should be fitted with an appropriate biological safety cabinet. Its ventilation should be arranged so that air flows into it from other rooms or corridors and out to the atmosphere (e.g. through the filters of the safety cabinet) and never in the reverse direction. This will prevent infectious aerosols which might be released in the Containment laboratory from escaping into other areas.

Maximum Containment laboratory, Level 4: This is intended for work with viruses in Risk Group 4, for which the most strict safety precautions are necessary.

These laboratories are usually separate buildings with strictly controlled access through air locks and exit through decontaminant showers. They have pressure gradients between their various rooms and all air from rooms and safety cabinets is filtered twice before discharge to the atmosphere. All effluents from sinks, lavatories, etc. are decontaminated before discharge into the public sewer. The staff of these laboratories are specifically trained for the work they do.

WORKING SAFELY

Good technique and the practice of personal hygiene as described in subunit 3.2 are the most important ways of reducing contact with infectious material and preventing laboratory related infections.

Special precautions need to be taken when collecting and testing specimens and handling infected material. Careless handling of specimens, cultures and other infected material can result in the:
- contamination of fingers,
- contamination of working surfaces and equipment,
- formation of aerosols (airborne droplets).

Important: Inhaling infected aerosols is a common cause of infection.

How aerosols are formed

The following are the main ways aerosols can be formed in the laboratory:

- Pouring off supernatant fluids, particularly from a considerable height into a discard container.
- Vigorous tapping of a tube to resuspend a sediment.
- Opening cultures and the rapid snap-closing of specimen or culture containers.
- Heating a contaminated wire loop in an open Bunsen burner flame.

- Using a long springy loop which is not properly closed.

- Rapid rinsing of Pasteur pipettes or plastic bulb pipettes, particularly when a discard container is almost full.

- Vigorous shaking of unstoppered tubes in a rack.

- Centrifuging specimens or infected fluids in open buckets, particularly when using a hand operated centrifuge or an angled head centrifuge and the tubes are more than three-quarters full.

- Opening a centrifuge immediately following the breakage of a tube or container of infected fluid before the aerosols have had time to settle.

- Dropping or spilling a specimen or culture.

- Mouth-pipetting and expelling an infected fluid, particularly blowing out the last drop.

Important: It is essential that all laboratory staff know how to work safely to prevent the formation, dispersion, and inhalation of aerosols.

Pouring infectious material safely

When needing to pour infectious fluids, for example in disposing of supernatants that cannot easily be pipetted, the fluids should be poured carefully down the side of a funnel (metal or plastic) with the narrow end of the funnel submerged in disinfectant in a jar or beaker. This prevents splashes and aerosol dispersion. The lip of the tube should then be wiped with absorbent paper soaked in disinfectant.

Opening cultures and ampoules safely

If there is a film of liquid between two surfaces that are parted violently, an aerosol will be produced. Such films containing microorganisms frequently occur between the rims and bottoms of petri dishes, and the stoppers and rims of bottles and tubes. There is no simple solution to this problem apart from care to prevent the films forming, and where possible, opening the containers in a safety cabinet.

Dried material in ampoules (stock cultures) may also be dispersed if an ampoule is opened incorrectly. To open an ampoule safely, etch the glass with a file above a cotton wool wad and then apply a red hot wire to the etching so that the glass cracks gently. After waiting a few minutes to allow air to enter the tube and destroy the vacuum, the ampoule should be held in a wad of cotton wool and gently broken at the crack. Ampoules of Risk

Group 3 organisms should be opened in a safety cabinet.

Inoculating loops and safe looping out

Long, springy, and improperly closed loops all shed their loads easily, releasing aerosols which can be inhaled and droplets which contaminate benches and hands. When a hot loop touches a culture a sizzling noise is heard. This indicates that aerosols are being created.

Care, therefore, is needed in the making and use of wire loops. The length of wire from the loop holder to the loop should be short (6 cm), and the loop itself should be small (2 mm in diameter) and fully closed.

After flaming, loops should be allowed to cool before use. Whenever possible a hooded Bunsen burner should be used (see Plate 3.1). Aerosols can also be dispersed during the inoculation of culture media especially when the surface of an agar plate is rough because it contains air bubbles.

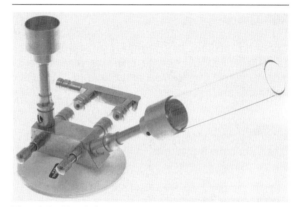

Plate 3.1   Hooded Bunsen burner. Information on suppliers can be found in subunit 4.12

Shaking and homogenizing safely

It is often necessary to shake vigorously cultures and materials containing microorganisms. Unless the caps are very tight, small droplets may escape and contaminate the surroundings. It is therefore good practice to place even tightly capped bottles in plastic bags before shaking.

Less violent mixing is frequently done by sucking a fluid up and down with a pipette (using a rubber teat) but this usually releases aerosols. It is better to use a Vortex mixer (see subunit 4.11). This does a better job more safely.

Avoiding infection from centrifuge accidents

Most centrifuge accidents occur because the contents on each side of a centrifuge are not balanced, the buckets have been neglected and are corroded, have not been placed correctly in the rotor, or the centrifuge tubes are cracked or chipped (see also subunit 4.7).

When tubes break in centrifuges, great clouds of aerosols may be dispersed over wide areas. It is usually obvious from the noise that a tube has broken or a bucket has failed. The motor should be switched off and the staff should leave the room for 30 minutes to allow most of the aerosols to settle or to be removed by natural ventilation. An experienced technician, wearing rubber gloves, should then remove the buckets and debris for autoclaving and swab out the bowl of the centrifuge with a suitable disinfectant.

Even in the absence of accidents or misuse, aerosols can be dispersed from uncapped centrifuge tubes, especially when using a hand operated unprotected centrifuge. All tubes used for centrifuging infectious material should be capped and not filled more than three-quarters full. Sealed centrifuge buckets should be used for Risk Group 3 material.

Avoiding infection from spillages and breakages

Careless handling of pathological material and cultures may result in the contamination of the outside of vessels, the laboratory bench, or floor. Micro-organisms can then be transferred from these surfaces to the fingers and hands, enter the bloodstream through cuts and scratches, or be transferred to the mouth and eyes.

Specimens, culture tubes and bottles should *always* be placed in racks so that they cannot fall over and spill their contents. When culture tubes or bottles are broken, infectious aerosols may be released. The worker should be careful not to breathe the air in close proximity to the breakage (this is difficult, but there is no simple solution).

Spilled material and broken culture vessels should be covered with a cloth soaked in disinfectant, left for 30 minutes, and then cleared up using a metal dust pan and stiff cardboard. These, and the debris should then be autoclaved. Alternatively disinfectant granules can be applied which are able to disinfect the spillage in a shorter time (see subunit 3.4). Rubber gloves should be worn for the clearing up operation.

Safe pipetting and dispensing

Mouth-pipetting has been the cause of many infections, some of which have been fatal. Serious injuries can also occur when mouth-pipetting hazardous chemicals (see subunit 3.5).

Acquiring infection by mouth-pipetting

This can occur when:

– pathogens in fluid specimens and cultures are accidentally sucked up into the mouth,

– aerosols are produced from the fluid as it is being sucked up or expelled,

– a pipette with an end that has been contaminated from fingers or a bench surface, is put in the mouth,

– a pipette with a chipped end causes cuts to the fingers or lips allowing pathogens to enter.

A cotton wool plug in the top of a pipette is not an effective microbial filter. Using a pipette with attached rubber tubing and mouthpiece is also hazardous.

Prohibition of mouth-pipetting
Due to the high risk of infection and injury to laboratory staff, the World Health Organization recommends that mouth-pipetting be banned from all medical laboratories.

There are many inexpensive ways to pipette and dispense safely without mouth-pipetting. These are described in subunit 4.6.

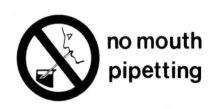

no mouth pipetting

Safe use of syringes and needles

Care in the use of syringes and needles is needed for several reasons. The obvious hazard is pricking oneself or one's colleague with a needle. This may be avoided only by very careful handling. Needle-pricks are a common source of laboratory acquired hepatitis, particularly when the laboratory worker tries to resheath a needle after use or leaves the needle in a collection tray with used cotton wool swabs and other articles instead of placing it in a separate puncture proof container.

The decontamination, cleaning, and sterilization of reusable syringes, and lancets are described in subunit 3.4. Disposable needles and syringes should be incinerated. Prior to incineration they should be discarded into jars or metal cans, not into cardboard boxes because the sharp ends may penetrate the card and prick any person who handles the box. The jars or cans should not be allowed to overfill.

Other hazards arise from aerosols, created if a needle flies off the end of a syringe when pressure is applied to the plunger and the needle is blocked, or when a needle is withdrawn through the rubber cap of a vaccine-type bottle containing micro-organisms. The second situation can be avoided by withdrawing the needle through a swab of cotton wool held over the vaccine bottle cap. This prevents needle vibration and takes care of leakage.

BIOLOGICAL SAFETY CABINETS

Safety cabinets are intended to protect a laboratory worker from aerosols and airborne particles. They will *not* protect the person from spillages and the consequences of mishandling and poor technique. There are three kinds of safety cabinet, Classes I, II, and III.

Class I and Class II cabinets are used in diagnostic and containment laboratories for work with Risk Group 3 organisms. Class III cabinets are used almost exclusively for Risk Group 4 organisms.

Note: In district laboratories the resources for purchasing a safety cabinet and the facilities for installing, using, and maintaining such a cabinet may not be available. It is therefore particularly important for laboratory staff to follow safe working practices.

Class I safety cabinet

A Class I cabinet is shown in Fig. 3.3. It has a front opening. The operator sits at the cabinet, looks through the glass screen, and works with the hands inside. Any aerosols released from cultures or other infectious material are retained because a current of air passes in at the front of the cabinet and sweeps the aerosols up through a HEPA filter which removes all or most of the organisms.

Clean air then passes through the fan, which maintains the air flow, and is exhausted (discharged) to atmosphere where any particles or organisms that have not been retained on the filter are so diluted that they are no longer likely to cause infection if inhaled.

Class II safety cabinet

A Class II cabinet is shown in Fig. 3.4.

In a Class II cabinet about 70% of the air is

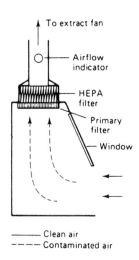

Fig. 3.3   Example of a Class I saftey cabinet
Reproduced from Laboratory Acquired Infections with permission of Butterworth and Co Publishers Ltd.

recirculated through filters so that the working area is bathed in clean (almost sterile) air. The air flow carries along any aerosols produced in the course of the work and these are removed by the filters. Some of the air (about 30%) is exhausted to atmosphere and is replaced by a 'curtain' of room air which

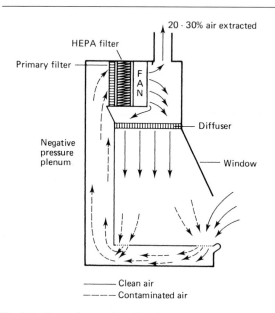

Fig. 3.4   Example of a Class II saftey cabinet
Reproduced from Laboratory Acquired Infections with permission of Butterworth and Co Publishers Ltd.

enters at the working face. This prevents the escape of any particles or aerosols released in the cabinet.

Class III safety cabinet for Risk Group 4 viruses
This type of cabinet is totally enclosed and is tested under pressure to ensure that no particles can leak from it into the room. The operator works with gloves which form part of the cabinet. Air enters through a filter and is exhausted to atmosphere through one or two more filters.

Use of safety cabinets
A safety cabinet should not be loaded with unnecessary equipment or it will not carry out its job properly. Work should be done in the middle to rear of the cabinet, not near the front. The operator should avoid bringing the hands and arms out of the cabinet while working.

After each set of manipulations and before withdrawing the hands, the operator should wait for 2–3 minutes to allow any aerosols to be swept into the filters. After finishing work in a safety cabinet, the hands and arms may be contaminated and should be washed immediately.

Siting and maintenance of a safety cabinet
The efficient working of a safety cabinet depends on its correct siting and proper maintenance. The manufacturer's instruction manual must be studied carefully.

Safety cabinets should be swabbed out with a suitable disinfectant after use and regularly decontaminated with formaldehyde. Decontamination is essential before the filters are changed.

Note: Further information about biological safety cabinets, including specifications, their siting and use can be found in the *WHO Laboratory Biosafety Manual.*[3]

Safety measures are needed to ensure specimens are transported safely and with care:

- from a ward or outpatient (OPD) clinic to the laboratory.
- between laboratories, e.g. from an outreach laboratory to the district hospital laboratory or regional public health laboratory, or from a quality control reference laboratory to laboratories participating in an EQA programme.

Important: All specimens must be collected in leak-proof appropriate containers.

Transporting specimens from wards or OPD clinics
When hand-carrying, place the specimens upright in racks in a closed container. The racks and carrying container should be made of plastic so that they can be easily disinfected and washed between use. The request forms should be placed in a plastic bag that can be sealed (grip type). During the hot season, an insulated container should be used to transport the specimens.

Transporting specimens between laboratories
Make sure the specimen container is tightly closed and the cap is *not leaking*. Wrap each specimen in sufficient absorbent material to absorb it should the container break. Place it individually or with others in a carton or strong plastic bag. Make sure there is sufficient packing material around the specimens to prevent them moving in the container or bag. If sending glass slide preparations, use a plastic reusable slide mailer.

Pack the container or bag of specimens with the sealed plastic bag containing the request forms in a suitable insulated container which will withstand shock and weight pressure. Use sufficient packing material in the insulated container. Insert a freezer pack(s) or ice cubes (in sealed plastic bags) around the container of specimens. Label the outer container 'Biological specimens – Infectious substance', preferably using the biohazard symbol shown in Fig. 3.5. The words KEEP COOL should also be prominently displayed on the container. Fix a clearly written delivery address label to the outer container. A smaller label should show the address of the sending laboratory. Cover the labels with clear adhesive tape.

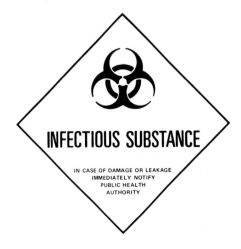

Fig. 3.5 Infections substance label.

Important: Use hospital transport or other reliable carrier to transport specimens.

Postal transport regulations

If using the postal system, laboratories must follow their national postal regulations which apply to the mailing of biological infectious substances. These will be available from the postal service. The postal system is appropriate for sending formol saline preserved biopsies or fixed smears to a histopathological laboratory.

International transport regulations

Strict regulations exist for the transport of infectious materials, including the proper use of packaging materials.[3] Major changes to the transport regulations were introduced in 2003.[4] Guidance can be obtained from WHO[5] and from the International Air Transport Association (IATA).[6]

3.4 Decontamination of infectious material and disposal of laboratory waste

---

It is essential for all district laboratories to operate and sustain safe and effective systems for:

■ Decontamination and disposal of specimens, cultures and other material which may contain infectious pathogens. All specimens should be regarded as potentially infectious.

■ Decontamination of glassware, plasticware, rubber gloves, protective clothing, and equipment used in laboratory testing.

■ Cleaning of reusable items such as specimen containers, other glassware and plasticware, syringes, lancets, rubber gloves, etc.

■ Sterilization of cleaned reusable items where sterility is required before reuse.

Limitations in the use of disposables

Many district laboratory services in developing countries are unable or cannot afford to obtain regular supplies of disposable syringes, lancets, specimen containers, petri dishes, tubes, pipettes, rubber gloves, etc. This subunit provides guidelines on the decontamination, cleaning, and sterilization of reusable items using methods that are feasible in district laboratories.

Responsibility of the laboratory for safe decontamination, recycling, and disposal

Laboratory staff have a responsibility to protect themselves, patients, the community, and environment from injury or damage originating from infectious or toxic laboratory waste and to minimize the hazards involved in decontamination, recycling, and disposal.

Risks can be minimized by laboratory staff:

● practising personal hygiene,
● following safe working practices,
● knowing and following correct methods for:
   – separating infectious materials and laboratory waste,
   – decontaminating and disposing of non-reusable infectious waste,
   – making non-infectious, cleaning, and sterilizing reusable articles.

Important: It is the responsibility of district health authorities to provide the equipment and supplies needed by district laboratories to operate a safe programme of decontamination, disposal, and recycling.

METHODS OF DECONTAMINATION AND DISPOSAL OF LABORATORY WASTE

In microbiological laboratory work, decontamination means the making safe of infectious material or articles that have been in contact with infectious microorganisms prior to their disposal or cleaning and reuse.

Safe processing of infectious laboratory waste and contaminated articles requires the separation of such waste and articles into clearly labelled (preferably colour-coded) discard containers according to method of decontamination, disposal, and associated hazard.

Before being washed and reused, discarded, or leaving the laboratory, all infectious material and contaminated articles should be made non-infectious.

Methods used to decontaminate infectious material in district laboratories include:

■ autoclaving (sterilization)
■ boiling (effective method of disinfection)
■ use of chemical disinfectants

Sterilization

This is the most reliable way of achieving decontamination because it completely destroys microorganisms, including bacterial spores.

Disinfection

This aims to destroy or at least reduce the number of contaminating microorganisms to levels that are no longer regarded as harmful to health. It implies the destruction of vegetative (non-sporing) infectious microorganisms but not necessarily bacterial spores.

Methods used to dispose of laboratory waste in district laboratories include:

- incineration
- burial in a deep covered waste pit or landfill

Note: Chart 3.2 provides guidelines on how to decontaminate and dispose of laboratory waste and make non-infectious those articles that need to be cleaned and reused.

Autoclaving

A district hospital laboratory must have access to a reliable autoclave for decontaminating cultures and other infectious waste. Health centre laboratories should be supplied with a pressure cooker type autoclave and the fuel to run it.

When performed correctly, autoclaving is the most effective method of decontamination because it is capable of *sterilizing* infectious waste, i.e. destroying all bacteria, bacterial spores, viruses, fungi, and protozoa. During autoclaving, pressure is used to produce high temperature steam. A temperature of 121°C and holding time of 15 minutes, timed from when 121°C is achieved *in the load*, is used to sterilize infectious waste.

Agents requiring higher temperatures and holding times

Some transmissible agents, e.g. prions that cause Creutzfeldt Jacob disease (CJD), require autoclaving at 134°C for 18 minutes to be inactivated.

Important: Laboratory staff *must* know how to use an autoclave correctly and be aware of the dangers of its misuse. The operating principle of autoclaves, their correct use and control are described in sub-unit 4.8.

Boiling

Heating in boiling water at 100°C for 20 minutes at altitudes below 600 metres (2 000 feet) is sufficient to kill all non-sporing bacteria, some bacterial spores, fungi, protozoa, and viruses including hepatitis viruses and HIV. Adding 20 g sodium carbonate to every litre of water increases the effectiveness of the disinfection.

Boiling at higher altitudes

Water boils at 100°C at sea level. The temperature of boiling water is reduced by approximately 1°C for every 500 metres above sea level. A boiling time of 30 minutes is therefore recommended when the altitude is greater than 600 metres.

If an electric 'sterilizer' is not available or there is no mains electricity, a large pan or other metal container can be used and the water heated using a charcoal stove, kerosene or gas ring burner (located in a safe place *outside the laboratory working area*). Choose the coolest time of the day to boil and use an autoclave.

When autoclaving is not possible, reusable syringes, lancets, specimen containers and other contaminated glassware and plasticware can be decontaminated by boiling in water for 10–20 minutes before being cleaned for reuse. When boiling, all the items must be completely submerged in the water.

After cleaning and before reuse, syringes and lancets can be disinfected by boiling at 100°C for *20 minutes* if sterilization by autoclaving is not possible. The articles must be allowed to dry before being used to collect blood samples otherwise the water will haemolyze the red cells making the specimen unfit for testing.

Use of disinfectants

Chemical disinfectants are expensive, hazardous to health, and when compared with autoclaving and boiling, chemical disinfection is the least reliable and controllable method for the treatment of laboratory infectious waste. It must also be remembered that no single disinfectant is likely to kill all microorganisms in any sample of infected waste. For example, chlorine releasing disinfectants are highly active against viruses but poorly active against mycobacteria, whereas phenolic agents are effective against mycobacteria but poorly active against viruses.

The laboratory use of chemical disinfectants should be restricted to discard containers on the bench, disinfecting equipment, bench surfaces, and floors, and the treatment of spillages.

Correct dilutions must be used and the dilutions must not be kept beyond their useful life which, according to the disinfectant, will vary from a few hours to a week or more. When used in discard containers, disinfectant solutions must be renewed daily. All disinfectants are to some extent inactivated by protein (particularly hypochlorite solutions), plastics, rubber, hard water, and detergents. Disinfectant solutions must not be overloaded because there is a limit to the amount of material which they can disinfect effectively. The article to be disinfected must be in contact with the disinfectant and not protected by air bubbles, immersion oil, or films of grease.

When emptying discard containers of disposable items, use a plastic strainer to collect the waste. If containing glass, e.g. haematocrit tubes or other sharp items, transfer the waste to puncture-resistant containers for disposal.

Caution: Care must be taken when using disinfectants, particularly when preparing dilutions. Disinfectants are toxic and mostly corrosive and irritant. Safety goggles, plastic apron, and chemical resistant rubber gloves must be worn. When not in use, discard containers should be covered using lids that can be removed easily. The containers should not be placed in direct sunlight.

The following are the most commonly used chemical disinfectants in district laboratories:

- phenolics
- chlorine-releasing products
- peroxygen compounds
- alcohols

Note: None of these substances will kill or even disable microorganisms unless they are properly used and renewed regularly.

Weak disinfectants unsuitable for laboratory use
These include *Dettol*, chlorhexidine products such as *Hibitane*, *Hibisol*, cetrimide compounds such as *Cetevalon*, and hypochlorite solutions sold for treating baby feeding bottles.

Phenolics

Examples of phenolics include *Hycolin*, *Sudol*, *Clearsol*, *Printol*, and *Stericol*. These are active against all non-sporing bacteria including mycobacteria. They do not kill spores and are poorly active against viruses. Phenolics are not markedly inactivated by proteins. At an alkaline pH, their activity is reduced.

Phenolic disinfectants should be used at 2–5% v/v concentration according to the manufacturers' instructions for the 'dirtiest conditions'. Dilutions should not be kept for more than 24 hours. They are useful for decontaminating material which may contain mycobacteria. Phenolics are non-corrosive. They are often used for wiping bench surfaces and floors and when chlorine products cannot be used because of their corrosiveness.

Chlorine-releasing disinfectants

These compounds contain chlorine and work by giving off free chlorine which is highly active against Gram positive and Gram negative bacteria and viruses including HIV and hepatitis B virus. Chlorine-releasing products are used in discard containers and for treating spillages of blood. Against mycobacteria, chlorine products are less effective than phenolics.

In an acid environment, chlorine release is accelerated. Chlorine products are not therefore recommended for use in discard containers into which urine supernatants are poured (phenolics are more appropriate). Chlorine-releasing disinfectants include:

- Sodium hypochlorite solutions sold as bleach solutions for domestic and laundering purposes, e.g. *Chloros, Domestos, Jik, Presept, eau de Javel* and other trade names. These solutions generally contain 5% available chlorine (but always read the label on the container as some 'thin' bleach solutions contain less than 5%).

  Sodium hypochlorite solutions are also sold for commercial use (in dairying and other trades for disinfecting equipment). They usually contain 10% available chlorine and a surfactant.

  Instability of hypochlorite solutions
  Liquid bleach has the disadvantage that in heat and strong light it rapidly deteriorates and looses its chlorine content. This can be a serious problem in tropical countries. To overcome this, the use of a more stable chlorine-releasing compound such as sodium dichloroisocyanurate (NaDCC) is recommended (see following text).

- Calcium hypochlorite granules or tablets which contain about 70% available chlorine.

- Sodium dichloroisocyanurate (NaDCC) available as:
  - a powder containing approximately 60% available chlorine,
  - granules, e.g. *HAZ-TAB* granules containing 57.2–57.8% chlorine (99% by weight NaDCC),
  - tablets containing 1.5 g chlorine per tablet (approx. 2.5 g NaDCC), usually in combination with an effervescent agent,
  - tablets containing 2.5 g chlorine per tablet (approx. 4.6 g NaDCC), e.g. *HAZ-TAB tablets* without an effervescent agent.

Stability and other advantages of using NaDCC
Compared with hypochlorite solutions, NaDCC products are more stable (3–5 y shelf-life) even at high temperatures as along as they are stored in a dry environment. Solutions of NaDCC are less inactivated by protein than hypochlorite solutions and also have greater microbicidal capacity than equivalent bleach solutions.

When treating spillages, the contact time of NaDCC granules with the spillage can be reduced to 2–3 minutes compared to the 30–60 minutes required when using bleach solutions.

NaDCC non-effervescent tablets are easier and safer to use in the laboratory, lighter in weight and therefore easier and cheaper to transport.

Note: Some effervescent NaDCC tablets are expensive. Non-effervescent products such as *HAZ-TAB* tablets and granules made by Guest Medical Trading Ltd (see Appendix II) are recommended. NaDCC is readily soluble in water, no effervescent agent is required.

Use of chlorine-releasing disinfectants in the laboratory: The disinfectant power of all chlorine-releasing compounds is expressed as parts per million (ppm) or percentage of available chlorine (av Cl) according to concentration level as follows:

1 000 ppm = 0.1% (1 g/l)
2 500 ppm = 0.25% (2.5 g/l)
5 000 ppm = 0.5% (5 g/l)
10 000 ppm = 1% (10 g/l)

Note: If expressed in chlorametric degrees (°chloram), 1°chloram is equivalent to approximately 0.3% av Cl.

Chlorine solutions *must* be prepared daily and protected from sunlight and excessive heat. They are strong oxidizing agents, corrosive to metal and may damage rubber. The amount of available chlorine required in solutions depends on the amount of organic matter present. The following solutions are recommended for use in the laboratory:

1 000 ppm (0.1%) av Cl: For routine disinfection of working surfaces and decontamination of soiled hands and gloves.

2 500 ppm (0.25%) av. Cl: For discard containers (use non-metal containers).

5 000 ppm (0.5%) av Cl: For use in emergency situations involving all haemorrhagic fever viruses.

10 000 ppm (1%) av Cl: For treating spillages of infectious material.

Note: Preparation of the commonly used 5% liquid hypochlorites (bleach) and of NaDCC products is given in Table 3.1.

Peroxygen compounds

An example is *Virkon* which when used at 1% w\v concentration has a wide range of bactericidal, virucidal and fungicidal activity. It has variable activity against bacterial spores. A 3% w\v concentration is recommended for *Mycobacterium* species. Neat powder is used for spillages. *Virkon* has a built-in colour indicator and combines cleaning with disinfection. When diluted it is non-irritant and has low dermal toxicity. It can be used to clean centrifuges providing it is washed off. Dilutions are stable for 7 days. It is however expensive when compared to hypochlorite disinfectants. *Virkon* is available in both powder and tablet form from Antec International (see Appendix 11).

Perasafe: Antec International also manufactures *Perasafe* which is a useful disinfectant for sterilizing instruments. It has

Table 3.1 Preparation of chlorine-releasing disinfectants commonly used in district laboratories

PRODUCT	AVAILABLE CHLORINE REQUIRED		
	1 000 ppm	**2 500 ppm**	**10 000 ppm**
Use:	Benches, hands, gloves	Discard jars	Spillages
Sodium hypochlorite *5% solution (bleach)*	20 ml in 1 litre water	50 ml in 1 litre water	200 ml in 1 litre water
10% solution	10 ml in 1 litre water	25 ml in 1 litre water	100 ml in 1 litre water
NaDCC tablets *1.5 g tablet*	1 tablet in 1 litre water	$1\frac{1}{2}$–2 tablets in 1 litre water	2 tablets in 250 ml water
2.5 g tablet (HAZ-TAB)	1 tablet in 2.5 litre water	1 tablet in 1 litre water	1 tablet in 250 ml water

Note: In small laboratories it may be more convenient to dilute a 2 500 ppm solution to obtain a 1 000 ppm solution to disinfect working surfaces: i.e. use 40 ml of 2 500 ppm and 60 ml of water to give 100 ml of a 1 000 ppm solution.

Use of HAZ-TAB NaDCC granules for spillages
While 10 000 ppm NaDCC solution can be obtained from tablets, the use of *HAZ-TAB granules* is recommended because these can be applied direct to the spillage, do not spread the spillage, and have a more rapid action (2–3 minutes).

a rapid action (10 minutes immersion) and does not have the irritant and other health problems associated with the use of glutaraldehyde.

Alcohols

Ethanol and propanol at 70–80% v/v concentration in water are useful for disinfecting skin and surfaces. Penetration of organic matter is poor. Alcohols are highly active against mycobacteria, non-sporing Gram positive and Gram negative bacteria, and fungi. HIV and hepatitis B and C viruses are inactivated. Activity against non-lipid (naked) viruses and bacterial spores is poor. When mixed with hypochlorite their activity is increased.

Aldehydes
These less used disinfectants include:

■ Formaldehyde
■ Glutaraldehyde (glutaral)

Formaldehyde gas is an effective disinfectant against all microorganisms including viruses, except at temperatures below 20°C. A 5% v/v formalin solution (diluted from concentrated formalin solution) is occasionally used as a disinfectant but formalin is too irritant for general use as a laboratory disinfectant. When heated, formaldehyde gas is used to decontaminate safety cabinets. It is non-corrosive. Formalin solution is toxic with an irritating vapour, and may cause sensitivity reactions. It is also a suspected carcinogen. Use only in a well ventilated laboratory.

Glutaraldehyde preparations include *Cidex, Clinicide, Glutarex 3M, Asep, Totacide* and *Triocide*, usually supplied at working concentrations of 2%. It is an expensive disinfectant. An alkaline activator must be added which is usually supplied with the product.

In the laboratory, glutaraldehyde is used mainly to disinfect metal surfaces, e.g. instruments and centrifuge parts where corrosive chlorine products cannot be used and viral contamination is possible. It rapidly inactivates bacteria and viruses including HIV and hepatitis B virus. It is also active against mycobacteria, but its penetration of organic matter is poor. Most glutaraldehyde products remain active for 7–14 days after activation. Cloudy solutions however should be discarded. Glutaraldehyde is toxic, irritant, and mutagenic. Contact with skin, eyes, and respiratory tract should be avoided.

Incineration

In district laboratories, incineration, i.e. destruction by burning, is a practical and effective method of disposing of laboratory waste including contaminated disposables and specimens in non-reusable containers, e.g. faeces. Purpose-built incinerators are rarely available at district level. Open burning is more common. The materials to be incinerated must be carried to the incineration site in closed leakproof puncture resistant containers.

Local construction of a simple incinerator[7]

– Use an empty 300 litre (40 gallon) petrol drum and obtain a metal lid and piece of fine wire

mesh (to replace the lid when burning is in progress).

– Fix a strong metal grating about a third of the way up the drum, inserting steel rods to keep it in place.

– Cut a wide opening below the level of the grating as shown in Fig. 3.6.

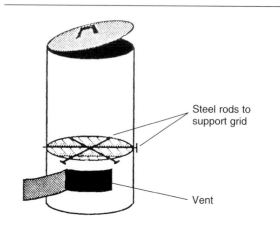

Steel rods to support grid

Vent

Fig. 3.6   Simple field incinerator
Courtesy of the World Health Organization

Use the incinerator as follows:

1 Place the material for incineration on the grating of the incinerator on top of a waste sheet of paper or cardboard (to prevent items falling through the grating). Do *not* overfill. Replace the lid.

2 Fill the bottom of the drum with sticks, wood shavings, and other combustible material.

3 Remove the lid and replace with the fine wire mesh to retain burning fragments and smuts.

4 Light the fire and keep it burning until all the waste has been burnt.

5 When cool, bury the ash in a deep covered pit. Do *not* empty it on open waste ground.

Important: Site the incinerator in a safe place. Surround it with a wire fence to prevent entry of unauthorized persons or animals. Supervize the incineration and bury the ash as soon as it has cooled sufficiently (wear a dust mask and protective gloves).

Brick built incinerator: A simple to construct brick incinerator is described in *Practical Laboratory Manual for health centres in eastern Africa.*[8]

Burial in a deep pit or landfill

Burying laboratory waste prevents it becoming a hazard providing the pit is located in a safe fenced off area, is sufficiently deep (4–5 metres) and wide (1–2 metres), has a strengthened rim, and is *kept* covered. The disposal pit should not be used for items that do not decompose, e.g. plastic laboratoryware. These are best incinerated. Ideally all infectious laboratory waste should be decontaminated or incinerated before it is discarded in a pit or landfill. Once a week the waste should be covered by a layer of quicklime, or if unavailable by soil or leaves.

If a local landfill site is available, local health authority guidelines should be followed regarding its use. (Laboratory waste must never be disposed of with household waste.) Waste must always be transported in *closed*, strong, leakproof containers.

Note: Chart 3.2 summarizes the methods used to decontaminate and dispose of non-reusable infectious material and how to decontaminate and clean reusable articles in district laboratories.

CLEANING AND STERILIZATION OF REUSABLE ITEMS

Decontamination is essential prior to the cleaning and reuse of laboratory-ware. In district laboratories, almost all glassware, many plastic items, and specimen containers will need to be reused. Disposable containers should be used for faecal specimens.

Separate discard containers (preferably plastic), filled with appropriate disinfectant are required for syringes, lancets, slides, cover glasses, pipettes, tubes and specimen containers. Each container should be clearly labelled.

Prior to soaking slides in disinfectant, any oil should be removed using a piece of rag or absorbent paper dampened with disinfectant. Use forceps to wipe the slide and dispose of the rag or tissue.

Most locally available detergents are suitable for cleaning laboratory-ware. After cleaning, each article must be *well rinsed in clean water* to remove all traces of detergent.

Caution: Great care must be taken to avoid injury when handling lancets, scalpel blades, and cover-glasses. When cleaning cover glasses (No 2 thickness are suitable for reuse), lancets, and scalpel blades, use small plastic beakers or jars in which to wash and rinse these items and plastic strainers to collect them after washing and between water rinses to avoid pricks and cuts. Always wear protective gloves when cleaning laboratory-ware.

Sterilization of cleaned laboratory-ware prior to reuse is necessary for microbiology culture work, e.g. specimen containers, petri dishes, tubes, pipettes, etc. Syringes and lancets must also be sterilized before reuse (see subunit 4.8).

Chart 3.2 Processing of infectious and waste material and reuse of non-disposable items in district laboratories

---

SPECIMENS	*Fluid specimens*
In reusable containers:	If the sink has running water and empties into the sewer system or septic tank, pour fluid specimens through a plastic funnel down the sink and rinse the funnel and sink with 2 500 ppm chlorine or 5% v/v phenolic disinfectant. Boil the containers, caps and cap liners for 10 minutes at 100 °C. If this is not possible, immerse the containers, caps, and liners overnight in 5% v/v phenolic disinfectant, 2 500 ppm chlorine disinfectant or 1% w/v *Virkon*.
	Clean each container in detergent, *rinse well in water* and drain dry. If sterile containers are required, autoclave them at 121°C for 15 minutes.
	Urine and other supernatant fluids
	Discard supernatant fluids through a funnel held in the lid of a plastic 1 litre capacity container to which has been added 20 ml of a concentrated phenolic disinfectant. When the fluid level reaches 1 litre, empty the container (do not add supernatant fluids to previously diluted disinfectant solutions). Decontaminate the empty tubes or bottles and clean them as described previously for *fluid specimens*.

Faeces

Use disposable containers for faeces. Dispose of the specimens by incineration.

Sputum

If not liquified, decontaminate sputum by autoclaving at 121°C for 15 minutes or place the container in boiling water and boil at 100°C for 20 minutes. Discard the decontaminated specimen in the latrine or in a deep covered pit and clean the container. If liquified, use the procedure for *fluid specimens.*

In disposable containers: Dispose of the specimens by incineration.

HAEMATOCRIT TUBES   *Immediately after reading,* discard the tubes into a puncture resistant container for incineration or burial in a deep covered pit.

Note: If a capillary tube is found to have broken in the centrifuge, wearing gloves and using forceps, remove the broken glass pieces and clean the centrifuge with a rag soaked in 5% v/v phenolic disinfectant. Place the rag with the pieces of glass in a puncture resistant container for incineration.

SWABS   Immerse swabs in 5% v/v phenolic disinfectant overnight before disposing of them in a deep pit.

CULTURES   Prior to disposal, decontaminate all cultures by autoclaving them at 121°C for 15 minutes.

MICROSCOPE SLIDES   Soak used slides overnight or for at least 1 hour in 2 500 ppm chlorine disinfectant or 1% w/v *Virkon* (detergent as well as disinfectant) in a plastic container. If there is oil on a slide, use forceps and a piece of rag or tissue soaked in disinfectant to wipe off the oil *before* soaking the slide. With care, wash the slides in detergent using a soft brush. Rinse well in water and dry between cotton cloths. When *completely* dry, store the slides in boxes.

COVER GLASSES
Reuse only
when essential

Only No 2 thickness cover glasses should be reused (No 1 cover glasses are too fragile). Using a piece of stick, transfer a cover glass from a slide to a small plastic jar or beaker containing 5% v/v phenolic disinfectant or 1% w/v *Virkon.* Soak overnight or for at least 1 hour.

Use a plastic sieve to collect the contents of the jar or beaker. Transfer a few cover glasses at a time to a container of detergent (not necessary if *Virkon* has been used), and swirl gently. Pour off the detergent and run water on the cover glasses to wash off the detergent. Use a plastic sieve to recover the cover glasses and dry them between two pieces of cotton cloth. Discard any damaged cover glasses into a puncture resistant container.

PIPETTES   *Immediately after use,* soak pipettes for at least 1 hour in 2 500 ppm chlorine disinfectant or 1% w/v *Virkon* in a sufficiently tall container to allow complete immersion of each pipette and the expelling of air bubbles. Do *not* overcrowd the container.

Caution: Use a separate container for glass Pasteur pipettes as the stems of these can be easily broken.

Wash reusable pipettes in detergent (not necessary if Virkon has been used), rinse well in water, and drain dry. Use a rubber bulb to expel the water from each pipette. Bury disposable pipettes in a deep covered pit.

LANCETS
Reuse only
when essential

Immediately after use, immerse the lancets in a small plastic jar or beaker containing 1 000 ppm chlorine or 1% w/v *Virkon*. Soak for 20 minutes. Use a plastic sieve to recover the lancets from the container. Clean as described for cover glasses. Lancets must be sterilized before reuse.

Autoclaving stainless steel lancets

Wrap each lancet in a small piece of non-shiny paper (can be reused). Place the wrapped lancets in a small polypropylene or metal container and with lid removed, sterilize at 121°C for 15 minutes. Replace the lid.

Boiling lancets

If unable to sterilize by autoclaving or because the lancets are part plastic, boil in water at 100°C for 10 minutes together with small glass or polypropylene tubes into which the lancets can be placed after boiling. Use flame sterilized forceps to transfer each lancet to its tube. Plug each tube with non-absorbent cotton wool.

SYRINGES
Reusable glass, nylon, polypropylene syringes
Reuse only
when essential

Immediately after use, rinse through with 1 000 ppm chlorine disinfectant. Remove the plunger from the barrel and immerse plunger and barrel in a container of 1 000 ppm chlorine disinfectant or 1% w/v *Virkon* for 1 hour. Wash and rinse well in several changes of water. The syringes must be sterilized before reuse.

Autoclaving syringes

Wrap each syringe, barrel alongside plunger, in a piece of cotton cloth or non-shiny paper and autoclave at 121°C for 15 minutes.

Boiling syringes

If autoclaving is not possible, boil the syringes in water at 100°C for 10 minutes with a container in which to place the syringes after boiling. Use flame sterilized forceps to remove and assemble the syringes. Use the syringes only when they are *completely* dry.

TUBES

Immerse overnight or for at least 1 hour in a container of 2 500 ppm chlorine disinfectant or 1% w/v *Virkon*. Make sure each tube is fully immersed with air bubbles expelled. Do not overload the container.

Wash in detergent (not necessary if *Virkon* has been used) using a test tube brush, *rinse well in water* and dry tubes facing downwards.

If sterile tubes are required, autoclave at 121 °C for 15 minutes, with caps loosened. Only glass or polypropylene tubes or vials can be autoclaved. If unable to autoclave, boil the tubes with caps and cap liners in water at 100 °C for 10 minutes. Use flame sterilized forceps to remove and cap the tubes when dry.

OTHER GLASSWARE PLASTICWARE

As for tubes.

DISPOSABLE WASTE
Syringes

Incinerate and bury the waste in a deep covered pit.

Contaminated cotton wool, swabs, dressings

Discard into a separate container and cover with a lid. Incinerate and bury the waste in a deep covered pit.

Broken glass, disposable needles, lancets, other 'sharps'
Discard into a puncture resistant container. Incinerate and bury the waste in a deep covered pit.

CLEANING OVERALLS
Prior to laundering, decontaminate laboratory protective clothing and other contaminated clothing by soaking overnight in 1 000 ppm chlorine disinfectant.

REUSING GLOVES
Rinse gloved hands thoroughly in 1 000 ppm chlorine disinfectant followed by several rinses in clean water (do not soak the gloves in disinfectant). Wash gloved hands with soap and water. Remove the gloves and hang them by the cuffs to dry. Wash hands and arms thoroughly.

When dry, examine the gloves for damage. Discard any gloves that are peeling, appear cracked, have punctures or tears, or appear damaged in any other way. Test the gloves for small holes by filling them with water and squeezing. If intact, turn the gloves inside out to dry. When dry sprinkle the inside with talcum powder.

DECONTAMINATING BENCH SURFACES
Use 2 500 ppm chlorine disinfectant to decontaminate work surfaces at the end of each day. Use 5% phenol disinfectant or phenol solution on benches which may be contaminated with mycobacteria.

Spillages
Soak up any spillage of infectious material with *Virkon* powder disinfectant, NaDCC granules or if unavailable use rags soaked in 10 000 ppm chlorine. Always wear protective gloves.

STERILIZING WIRE LOOPS BLADES, ENDS OF FORCEPS
Decontaminate and sterilize by flaming until red hot. Allow to cool before use. Whenever possible, use a hooded Bunsen burner.

Notes
- See Table 3.1 for the preparation of 1 000 ppm, 2 500 ppm and 10 000 ppm chlorine solutions. Wear gloves and a face visor or goggles when preparing all disinfectant solutions.
- When clean running water is not available for rinsing washed laboratoryware, use filtered rain water.
- *Always* wear protective gloves and a plastic apron when decontaminating and disposing of specimens. When disposing of waste from an incinerator, wear a dust mask.

3.5 Chemical and reagent hazards

Hazards associated with the transport, storage, and handling of chemicals include fire, explosion and the effects from toxic (poisonous), harmful, irritating, and corrosive chemicals. In district laboratories the risks associated with the use of chemicals can be minimized by laboratory staff knowing which chemicals are hazardous and how to handle and store them correctly.

In tropical countries it is particularly important to keep chemicals and reagents out of direct sunlight and prevent their overheating in the laboratory or in an outside store. Overheating can decompose many chemicals, causing explosions, fire, or the formation of toxic fumes.

Accurate records *must* be kept of all chemicals in the laboratory. Chemicals and reagents must be labelled clearly. In outreach laboratories those chemicals and reagents that are not required or are not labelled must be sent to the nearest district hospital laboratory for safe storage or disposal. The district laboratory coordinator should supervize the packing and transportation of these chemicals and reagents.

Most manufacturers of chemicals provide comprehensive hazard and safety information with their products. *Before* storing or using a chemical, laboratory staff *must read carefully* the safety (S) and risk (R) phrases written on the label of the container and understand the hazard symbols used by manufacturers to identify chemicals that are:

 Flammable (extremely and highly)

 Irritating

 Oxidizing

 Corrosive

 Toxic

 Explosive

 Harmful

 Dangerous for environment

Hazard identification and classification schemes
The symbols and hazard classification described above are those used by manufacturers and users of chemicals in European Community (EC) countries. Other countries identify and classify chemical hazards differently, e.g. according to type including health, fire, instability, reactivity hazards, and the degree of danger using a scale 0 to 4 where 4 = extreme, 3 = severe, 2 = moderate, 1 = minor and 0 = no unusual hazard.

FLAMMABLE CHEMICALS

A flammable substance is one that readily ignites (catches alight) and burns. Some flammable chemicals are a more serious fire risk than others because they ignite easily. Such chemicals have what is called a low flash point temperature.

Flash point of a chemical: This is the lowest temperature at which the vapour above a liquid can be ignited in air. The lower a chemical's flash point, the higher is the risk of an ignition source igniting it. The most hazardous flammable chemicals are those with flash points below ambient temperature because they evaporate rapidly from open containers. See also Chart 3.3 in subunit 3.7.

Classification of flammable chemicals
The term flammable has the same meaning as inflammable (flammable is preferred).

Extremely flammable: Liquids with a flash point below 0°C and a boiling point of 35°C or below, e.g. acetone, diethyl ether.

Highly flammable: Liquids with a flash point below 21°C, substances which are spontaneously combustible in air at ambient temperature, solids which readily ignite after brief contact with flame or which evolve highly flammable gases in contact with water or moist air. Examples include absolute ethanol and methanol, 70% and above ethanol and methanol, methylated spirit, isopropanol (isopropyl alcohol), toluene, alcoholic Romanowsky stains, acid alcohol, other alcoholic reagents and indicators.

Flammable: Liquids with a flash point of 21°C or more and below or equal to 55°C, e.g. glacial acetic acid, acetic anhydride, xylene.

Safe storage and use of flammable chemicals
Storage

Keep only small quantities of flammable chemicals and reagents on laboratory benches and shelves (not over 500 ml amounts). Store stock supplies of flammable chemicals particularly those that are extremely or highly flammable in a closed steel or thick plywood box at ground level, preferably in an outside locked store that is cool and well ventilated, including ventilation at or near floor level because the vapours of most highly flammable liquids are heavier than air. Label the container *Flammable*. Do not store flammable and oxidizing chemicals together.

Safe use

- Keep the laboratory well ventilated to prevent any build up of flammable gases and vapours.

- Before opening a bottle containing a flammable liquid, always make sure there is no open flame within 2 metres such as that from a Bunsen burner, spirit lamp, kerosene or gas burner. When using ether or acetone allow a distance of 3 metres.

- Ensure stock bottles and dispensing containers of flammable liquids are tightly closed after use.

- Do not light a match or use a lighted taper near to a flammable chemical.

- Do not store ether in a non-spark refrigerator.

- Make sure no one smokes in or adjacent to the laboratory. Display 'no smoking' notices.

- Place dispensing containers of acetone, acid alcohol, methanol, and alcoholic Romanowsky stains well away from the rack used to heat stain on slides in the Ziehl Neelsen technique. Use trays to hold the containers to prevent a flammable liquid spreading should a spillage occur.

- If needing to heat a flammable liquid, use a waterbath. Never heat directly on a hotplate or over an open flame. Do not flame the neck of a bottle or tube containing a flammable substance.

- When transporting Winchester bottles containing flammable chemicals, use strong carriers fitted with handles.

Control of fires involving flammable liquids

Fire caused by a flammable liquid is best controlled by smothering the flames. If the fire is a small one on a bench, cover the container or area with a lid or a fire blanket (see 3.7). If the fire is on the floor, use a dry powder chemical fire extinguisher or smother the flames with a fire blanket, dry sand or earth.

Do not pour water on the flames of a flammable liquid fire because the water will spread the fire, especially if it is caused by a solvent such as xylene which does not mix but floats on the surface of water.

Note: Further information on the fire risks associated with the use of flammable liquids can be found in subunit 3.7 *Fire safety*.

OXIDIZING CHEMICALS

An oxidizing substance is one that produces heat or evolves oxygen in contact with other substances causing them to burn strongly or become explosive or spontaneously combustible. Once a fire is started the oxidizing substance promotes it and impedes fire-fighting.

Oxidizing chemicals include hydrogen peroxide and other strong peroxides, nitric acid, ammonium nitrate, sodium nitrite, perchloric acid, sodium chlorate, chromic acid, potassium dichromate, calcium hypochlorite bleach powder, and potassium permanganate.

Safe storage and use of oxidizing chemicals

Storage

Because oxidizing chemicals can produce much heat when in contact with flammable substances, organic materials and reducing agents, they must be stored well away from such chemicals and other chemicals with which they can react dangerously as indicated in subunit 3.5.

Safe use

Always handle oxidizing chemicals with care. Besides being fire-promoting, most oxidizing substances are dangerous to skin and eyes.

TOXIC, HARMFUL AND IRRITATING CHEMICALS

A *toxic* substance is one that can cause serious acute or chronic effects, even death, when inhaled, swallowed, or absorbed through the skin. The term very, or highly, toxic is used if the substance is capable of causing serious effects.

Toxic chemicals include potassium cyanide, mercury (e.g. from broken thermometers), mercury 11 (mercuric) nitrate, sodium azide, sodium nitroprusside, thiosemicarbazide, formaldehyde solution, chloroform, barium chloride, diphenylamine, and methanol.

A *harmful* substance is one that can cause limited effects on health if inhaled, swallowed, or absorbed through the skin.

Harmful chemicals include barium chloride, benzoic acid, potassium oxalate, saponin, xylene, iodine, and sulphanilic acid.

An *irritating* chemical is one that can cause inflammation and irritation of the skin, mucous membranes, and respiratory tract following immediate, prolonged or frequent contact.

Irritants include ammonia solution, acetic acid, sulphosalicylic acid, potassium dichromate, and formaldehyde vapour.

Safe storage and use of toxic, harmful and irritating chemicals

Storage

Highly toxic chemicals such as potassium cyanide must be kept in a locked cupboard. Stock solutions or solids of harmful and irritating chemicals should be stored safely in a cupboard, not on an open shelf.

Safe use

- Handle toxic, harmful, and irritating chemicals with great care and wash the hands immediately after use. Wear suitable protective gloves, and if indicated a face dust mask, visor or eyeshields, and a plastic protective apron.

- Ensure an eyewash bottle is accessible to rinse the eyes should a toxic, harmful or irritating chemical enter the eye (see Plate 3.2).

- Always lock away highly toxic chemicals immediately after use and never leave such chemicals unattended. Minimize exposure to highly toxic chemicals.

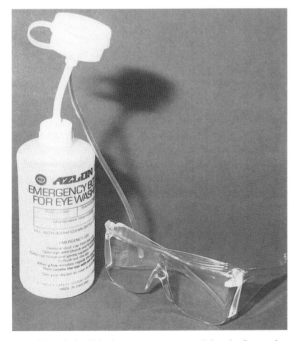

Plate 3.2 *Left:* 500ml emergency eye wash bottle. Squeezing the bottle gently sprays the eye. The waste liquid flows through a tube to the sink or collecting vessel. Instructions for use are printed in green on the bottle. *Right:* Protective eyeshields with closed in sides. The goggles are made from polycarbonate.

- Whenever possible, handle chemicals with an irritating or harmful vapour in a fume cupboard. If this is not possible, ensure the laboratory is well ventilated while the chemical is being used.

- Before opening a chemical with an irritating vapour, place a cloth over the neck of the container and cap.

- Keep containers tightly closed.

- *Never* mouth-pipette any chemical or reagent. Always use a pipette filler, automatic dispenser or pipettor.

Injuries caused by mouth-pipetting chemicals and reagents

The following are the main ways a person can be injured by mouth-pipetting chemicals and reagents.

- accidentally sucking up reagents into the mouth, e.g. when rapidly sucking up in a narrow bore pipette or when a reagent is contained in a brown bottle or opaque plastic container and the level of fluid is low and cannot be seen clearly.

- putting a pipette in the mouth after its end has been in contact with a harmful reagent, disinfectant, or dry chemical picked up from the bench or carried on the fingers.

- inhaling poisonous or irritating fumes, e.g. from acetic acid, concentrated hydrochloric acid, or formalin solution.

Accidents involving toxic, harmful, and irritating chemicals

The First Aid treatment for poisoning and injuries caused by toxic, harmful and irritating chemicals is described in subunit 3.8.

Allergenic, carcinogenic, mutagenic and teratogenic substances

Some toxic chemicals are known to cause or are suspected of causing specific types of disease or of affecting particular organs or functions of the body as follows:

Allergen: Causes in some people allergic or hypersensitivity reactions, e.g. skin contact resulting in dermatitis and inhalation resulting in asthma or related conditions.

Carcinogen: Causes or increases the risk of cancer usually after repeated or long term exposure. Chemicals with proven carcinogenic properties include benzidine, *o*-tolidine, *o*-toluidine, *o*-dianisidine, *alpha*- and *beta*-naphthylamine, nitrosophenols, nitronaphthalenes, and selenite.

Mutagen: Capable of producing mutations of germ cells leading to genetically induced malformations, spontaneous abortion or death of the offspring of an exposed individual. Exposure of a mother to certain mutagenic chemicals during pregnancy may result in cancer developing in her offspring many years later.

Teratogen: Can damage an unborn foetus causing congenital malformations, foetal death, or cancer in the offspring many years later.

Note: Further details regarding the toxicity of chemicals and a list of the reported acute and chronic effects of some chemicals can be found in the *WHO Laboratory Biosafety Manual.*[3] Chemical manufacturers upon request will provide data sheets for the chemicals they produce. Essential safety information can also be found on the labels of containers.

CORROSIVE CHEMICALS

A corrosive chemical is one that when ingested, inhaled, or allowed to come in contact with skin can destroy living tissue and is also capable of damaging inanimate substances.

Examples of corrosive chemicals include phenol, strong acids such as concentrated sulphuric acid, nitric acid, glacial acetic acid, trichloroacetic acid, o-phosphoric acid, caustic alkalis such as sodium hydroxide (caustic soda), and potassium hydroxide (caustic potash), and some concentrated disinfectant solutions.

Safe storage and use

Storage
Corrosive chemicals should be stored at low level to avoid injury which could be caused if such chemicals were accidentally knocked off a shelf. Do not store potassium hydroxide or sodium hydroxide in a bottle having a ground glass stopper because these chemicals absorb carbon dioxide from the air forming carbonates which can cement the stopper in the bottle.

Safe use
- Never mouth-pipette a corrosive chemical (see also previous text). The accidental swallowing of a corrosive chemical can cause severe internal injury.

- Always pour a corrosive chemical at below eye level, slowly and with great care to avoid splashing.

- Wear suitable protective gloves and a face visor or at least eyeshields, when opening a container of a corrosive chemical and when pouring it. Place a cloth over the neck and cap of the container when opening it.

- Dissolve a solid corrosive chemical such as sodium hydroxide in water with great care, mixing in small amounts at a time to dissipate the heat produced.

- When diluting concentrated acids, particularly sulphuric acid, always *add the acid to the water.* NEVER ADD WATER TO ACID. Adding water to sulphuric acid can produce sufficient heat to break a glass container.

- When weighing corrosive chemicals, e.g. phenol, avoid damaging the balance by ensuring the chemical does not spill on the balance pan or other metal parts. Use a suitable weighing container and remove this from the balance pan when adding or removing the chemical.

- Always use a strong carrier to transport bottles of corrosive chemicals.

Accidents involving corrosive chemicals
The treatment of burns caused by corrosive chemicals is described in subunit 3.8. See later text for the management of spillages involving corrosive chemicals.

EXPLOSIVE CHEMICALS

Heat, flame, knocks or friction can cause explosive chemicals to explode. Examples of explosive chemicals include:

- *Sodium azide:* This can form explosive products when in contact with metals such as copper and lead, e.g. in pipes.

- *Perchloric acid:* If allowed to dry on woodwork, brickwork or fabric, this chemical will explode and cause a fire on impact.

- *Picric acid and picrates:* Picric acid must be stored under water. If allowed to dry it can become explosive. This can occur if the chemical is left to dry in pipes without being flushed away with an adequate amount of water.

- *Diethyl-ether and other ethers:* When exposed to air and sunlight, ether can form shock-sensitive explosive peroxides.

Important: Always read carefully the manufacturers' instructions regarding the storage and handling of explosive chemicals. Few techniques in district laboratory work require the use of explosive chemicals.

ENVIRONMENTALLY DANGEROUS CHEMICALS

These are substances that are dangerous for the environment because they can cause immediate or long term harm to aquatic life, fauna and flora, or pollute the atmosphere. Laboratory staff have a duty to avoid chemical pollution of the environment.

Those in charge of district laboratory services must ensure that the drainage and waste disposal systems of district laboratories are safe, adequate and in good repair. Hazardous chemicals and reagents must not be discharged into open drains or disposed of on open ground. Sufficient water must be used when flushing hazardous chemicals and reagents through the plumbing system.

The sewer system should not be used to dispose of highly toxic chemicals, water-immiscible chemicals, or substances that can react with metal drainage pipes to produce dangerously reactive products, e.g. sodium azide or picric acid. Advice should be obtained from a qualified safety officer regarding the disposal of environmentally dangerous laboratory chemicals.

SPILLAGE CONTROL GUIDELINES

In the event of a serious chemical spill, evacuate non-essential personnel from the affected area and proceed as follows:

- If there is personal injury or a hazardous chemical has been spilled on clothing, remove the clothing and immediately wash and immerse the affected part of the body in water. If the injury is serious, apply appropriate First Aid measures and seek medical advice.

- If liquid chemicals (non-flammable) are spilled, place sufficient dry sand or absorbent paper around the spillage to prevent its spread and to soak up the chemical. Wearing chemical resistant gloves and using a plastic dustpan, collect the material, neutralize it if a strong acid or alkali and dispose of it safely.

  ### Neutralization

  Use 50 g/l (5% w/v) sodium bicarbonate or sodium carbonate to neutralize acid spills, and 10 g/l (1% v/v) acetic acid to neutralize strong alkali spills. Clean the spillage area with water and detergent.

- If the spillage is a volatile flammable chemical, immediately extinguish all flames, e.g. from Bunsen and spirit burners. Open the windows and doors to allow the spillage to evaporate. Clean the area with water and detergent.

- If the spillage is a solid chemical, wearing chemical resistant gloves and dust mask if appropriate, collect the chemical in a plastic dustpan and dispose of it safely by dissolving it in an adequate

volume of water and flushing it down the drainage system. If water-immiscible or unsuitable for flushing down the plumbing system, mix the chemical with sand and dispose of it in a deep covered waste disposal pit. Clean the spillage area with water and detergent.

Important: Follow any special spillage control measures recommended by the manufacturer of a chemical and display charts showing how to manage chemical spills.

SAFETY GUIDELINES FOR COMPRESSED AND LIQUEFIED GASES

The use of compressed gases should be avoided whenever possible. Where their use is necessary, the following safety measure should be applied:

- Make sure all cylinders are clearly labelled and correctly colour coded.

- Display warning notices on the doors of rooms where cylinders containing flammable gases are used and stored.

- Do not keep more than one cylinder of a flammable gas in a room at any one time. Store spare cylinders in a locked identified weatherproof store at some distance from the laboratory.

- Fix securely (e.g. chain) a gas cylinder to the wall or a solid bench to avoid it being dislodged.

- Do not locate compressed gas cylinders or liquefied gas containers near to radiators, naked flames or other heat sources, sparking electrical equipment, or in direct sunlight.

- Always turn off the main high-pressure valve when the equipment is not in use and when the room is unoccupied.

- Use a trolley to support compressed gas cylinders when they are being transported (transport with caps in place).

- Do not incinerate single use gas cylinders.

Note: Gases for fixed items of equipment should be connected by a drop level safety cock to permanent pipework using screwed union connectors. Bunsen burners should also be controlled by a safety cock. Installation of piped compressed air, vacuum or gas system must be undertaken by a *qualified* person.

Summary: preventing accidents involving chemicals and reagents

- Identify and list all chemicals kept in the laboratory and stores. Maintain an up to date inventory and information sheets on each chemical including its use, storage requirements, any known risk, and instructions for its safe use. Request safety data sheets from manufacturers.

- Before opening a chemical, always read the safety (S) and risk (R) phrases written on the label. Know the hazard symbols for chemicals.

- Label clearly all reagents with their name, date of preparation, expiry date (if of limited shelf-life), and hazard symbol if indicated. Prepare *written* instructions on how to prepare each reagent safely.

- Store each chemical and reagent correctly, making sure chemicals that can react dangerously together, i.e. incompatible chemicals, are not stored together (see Chart 3.3).

- Store stock containers of liquid acids, alkalis, corrosive and flammable chemicals at floor or low level in drip trays to contain any spillage.

- Keep chemicals and reagents out of direct sunlight and do *not* allow them to overheat.

- Ensure the caps of containers are airtight and tightly closed, particularly of chemicals that are volatile, flammable, hygroscopic, deliquescent or have a toxic or irritating vapour.

- Do not use rubber liners in the caps of bottles containing iodine, ether, xylene or other chemical which attacks rubber. Do not use ground glass stoppers in bottles containing potassium or sodium hydroxide or other chemical that absorbs carbon dioxide from the air.

- When opening a corrosive chemical or one with an irritating vapour, use a cloth over the cap and neck of the container and wear chemical resistant protective gloves.

- Keep the laboratory well ventilated when using hazardous chemicals particularly those that are flammable or have a toxic or irritating vapour. Whenever possible use a fume cupboard.

- When preparing reagents, always mix chemicals with care. Wear appropriate footwear and protective clothing, e.g. laboratory overall, gloves, dust mask, eye goggles or face visor.

- Ensure an eyewash bottle is available and accessible.

- *Never* mouth-pipette, taste, or inhale a chemical or reagent.

- Always wash the hands immediately after handling chemicals.

- Use appropriate hazard symbols on the doors of cupboards storing dangerous chemicals.

- Extinguish all open flames when using flammable and oxidizing chemicals and reagents. Ensure fire fighting equipment is available and accessible.

- Understand how accidents involving chemicals and reagents can occur and know what to do to control and extinguish a chemical fire, treat a chemical spillage (see later text), and apply First Aid.

- Use plenty of water when washing toxic, corrosive, flammable and volatile reagents down the plumbing system, e.g. during staining.
  Mercury from a broken thermometer: Do not discard mercury down the sink. Wearing gloves, carefully collect the mercury using a stiff card and dustpan and discard it in a deep covered waste disposal pit.

- Keep stores and cupboards containing stock and dangerous chemicals securely locked. Do not allow unauthorized persons to enter the laboratory and never leave it unlocked when unoccupied.

Chart 3.3 SAFETY INFORMATION ON SOME CHEMICALS USED IN DISTRICT LABORATORIES

Important: *Not all hazardous chemicals are included in this list. Always read carefully the storage instructions and safety information printed on the container label.* The source of the information in this chart is the BDH/Merck *Laboratory Supplies Catalogue.*

CHEMICAL	MAIN HAZARD	SAFETY PRECAUTIONS
Acetic acid, glacial	Corrosive, causing severe burns. Irritant vapour Flammable, with flash point 40°C.	Protect eyes, skin, clothing, and equipment. Avoid breathing fumes. Use in well ventilated area. Keep away from oxidizers, particularly nitric acid, chromic acid, peroxides and permanganates.
Acetone	*Extremely* flammable and volatile with flash point −18°C.	Keep away from sources of ignition, chloroform, chromic acid, sulphuric acid, nitric acid and other oxidizers. Avoid breathing fumes. Use in well ventilated area. Protect eyes.
Alcohol	See Ethanol	
Ammonia solution	Corrosive Irritant vapour	Protect eyes, skin, clothing, and equipment. Place cloth over cap before removing it or preferably use in a fume cupboard. Keep away from mercury and halogens such as chlorine and iodine.
Barium chloride	Harmful if ingested or inhaled.	Protect against ingestion, inhalation, and skin contact.
Benzoic acid	Harmful if ingested. Irritating to the eyes.	Protect against ingestion, skin and eye contact.
Calcium hypochlorite bleaching powder	Corrosive Contact with acids liberates toxic gas. Oxidizing.	Protect eyes, skin, clothing and equipment. Keep away from acids, flammable chemicals, and combustible materials.
Chlorine solutions	See Sodium hypochlorite solution.	
Chloroform	Harmful if ingested or inhaled. Irritating to the skin. Suspected carcinogen. Volatile with vapour that is anaesthetic. Toxic product formed if heated. Attacks plastics and rubber.	Avoid breathing vapour. Use in a well ventilated area or preferably in a fume cupboard. Protect eyes and skin. Keep away from acetone.

CHEMICAL	MAIN HAZARD	SAFETY PRECAUTIONS
Chromic acid (reagent)	Corrosive	Protect eyes, skin, clothing, and equipment. Keep away from combustible materials, acetone and other flammable chemicals.
	Oxidizing	
Diethylamine	*Extremely* flammable with flash point −39°C.	Protect eyes. Avoid breathing fumes. Use in a well ventilated area or preferably in a fume cupboard.
	Irritant to eyes and respiratory system.	Keep away from sources of ignition and oxidizers. Do not empty into drains.
Diphenylamine	Toxic if ingested, inhaled, or in contact with skin.	Wear appropriate protection. Wash immediately any affected area.
Ethanol, absolute	*Highly* flammable and volatile with flash point 13°C. Harmful if ingested.	Keep away from sources of ignition, silver nitrate, and oxidizers.
Ethanolamine	Harmful if inhaled. Irritant to eyes, respiratory system, and skin. Also corrosive	Protect skin and eyes. Use in a well ventilated area. Keep away from oxidizers.
Ether, diethyl	*Extremely* flammable, with flashpoint −40°C. Volatile with anaesthetic vapour. May form explosive peroxides when exposed to light.	Keep away from sources of ignition, oxidizers, iodine and chlorine. Do not refrigerate. Store in opaque container, not plastic unless polypropylene. Do not use cap with rubber liner. Use in well ventilated area or preferably in a fume cupboard.
Ethylene glycol (Ethanediol)	Harmful if ingested.	Protect against ingestion and skin contact.
Formaldehyde solution	Toxic if ingested, inhaled, or in contact with skin. Causes burns and can cause dermatitis. Probable carcinogen.	Wear appropriate protection. Use in well ventilated area or preferably in a fume cupboard. Wash immediately any affected area. Keep away from hydrochloric acid and oxidizers. Do not store below 21°C. (Keep at 21–25°C).
	Irritating and unpleasant odour.	
Giemsa stock stain (alcoholic stain)	*Highly* flammable with flash point 12°C.	Keep away from sources of ignition. Avoid inhaling fumes and contact with skin.
Glutaraldehyde	Harmful if ingested. Irritating to skin and respiratory system. May cause dermatitis. Can damage eyes.	Wear appropriate protection. Use in well ventilated area. Keep away from oxidizers.

Hydrochloric acid, concentrated		Corrosive, causing severe burns. Irritating to respiratory system. Unpleasant corrosive fumes. Releases toxic fumes in fires.	Protect skin, eyes, clothing, and equipment. Do not breathe fumes. Use in well ventilated area or preferably in a fume cupboard. Keep away from alkalis, chromic acid, potassium permanganate.
Hydrogen peroxide solution		Corrosive	Protect eyes, skin, clothing, and equipment. Store in opaque non-metallic container.
		Irritating to eyes, respiratory system, and skin. Stronger solutions are oxidizing.	Keep out of direct sunlight in a cool dark place away from flammable chemicals and combustible materials.
Iodine		Harmful if ingested, inhaled, or in contact with skin. Irritating to eyes and respiratory system. Evolves toxic fumes in fires.	Avoid skin and eye contact, and breathing in vapour. Store iodine containing reagents in opaque container. Do not use caps with rubber liners. Reacts violently with metals, acetylene, and ammonia.
Iron 111 chloride (Ferric chloride)		Harmful if ingested. Irritating to the skin. Can cause eye damage.	Protect against ingestion, skin and eye contact.
Leishman stock stain		As for Giemsa stain.	
Mercury		Toxic by inhalation. May cause dermatitis. Attacks lead piping and soldered joints. Evolves toxic fumes in fires.	Ventilate area if mercury escapes from broken thermometer (discard in deep covered pit). Avoid skin contact. Keep away from ammonia, bromine, azides, ethylene oxide.
Mercury 11 chloride (Mercuric chloride)		*Very* toxic if ingested. Toxic in contact with skin and can cause burns.	Protect against ingestion and contact with skin. Minimize use. Wash hands immediately after use. Keep in locked cupboard.
Mercury 11 nitrate (Mercuric nitrate)		*Very* toxic if ingested, inhaled, or in contact with skin.	Wear appropriate protection. Minimize use. Wash hands immediately after use. Keep in locked cupboard.
Methanol (Methyl alcohol)	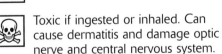	*Highly* flammable with flashpoint 12°C. Volatile and hygroscopic. Toxic if ingested or inhaled. Can cause dermatitis and damage optic nerve and central nervous system.	Keep away from sources of ignition, sodium hypochlorite, nitric acid, chloroform, hydrogen peroxide. Avoid breathing vapour. Protect skin and eyes. Use in a well ventilated area or preferably in a fume cupboard.
Nitric acid, concentrated (fuming)		Corrosive, causing *severe* burns. Has irritating and harmful vapour. Oxidizing	Protect skin, eyes, clothing, and equipment. Avoid breathing fumes. Preferably use in a fume cupboard. Use an eyewash bottle immediately if acid enters eye. Keep away from alkalis, metals, acetic acid, chromic acid, reducing agents, flammable chemicals and combustible materials.

CHEMICAL	MAIN HAZARD	SAFETY PRECAUTIONS
Phenol	Toxic in contact with skin or if ingested or inhaled. Corrosive and hygroscopic. Oxidizes and turns pink on exposure to light.	Protect skin, eyes, clothing, and equipment. Wash immediately any affected area. Keep container tightly closed. Store away from oxidizers.
***o*-Phosphoric acid**	Corrosive Evolves toxic fumes in fires.	Protect skin, eyes, clothing, and equipment.
Picric acid, (solid)	Toxic if ingested, inhaled, or in contact with skin. Evolves toxic fumes in fires.	Wear appropriate protection.
	Explosive when dry. Can form highly explosive salts with many metals and explosive calcium picrate when in contact with concrete.	Ensure chemical is always covered with water. Do not leave chemical to dry in pipes. Keep away from reducing agents. *Note:* If the water on top of the chemical has evaporated, submerge the container in a bucket of water overnight. Loosen cap carefully and fill to the top with water (wear gloves and eyeshields).
Potassium cyanide	*Very* toxic if ingested, inhaled, or in contact with skin. Contact with acid liberates *very* toxic gas.	Wear appropriate protection. Wash immediately any affected area. Keep in a locked cupboard away from acids. Do not empty into drains.
Potassium dichromate	Irritating to the eyes, respiratory system, and skin. May cause dermatitis.	Protect eyes and skin. Avoid breathing dust.
Potassium hydroxide, pellets and solutions	Corrosive Pellets are deliquescent.	Protect skin, eyes, clothing, and equipment. Store away from acids. Do not use reagent bottles with glass stoppers.
Potassium oxalate	Harmful in contact with skin and if ingested.	Avoid contact with skin and eyes.
Potassium permanganate	Oxidizing	Keep away from combustible materials, flammable chemicals, glycerol, ethylene glycol, sulphuric acid.
	Harmful if ingested.	
Salicylic acid	Harmful if ingested. Irritating to skin and respiratory system. Can damage the eyes.	Wear appropriate protection and avoid breathing in chemical.
Saponin powder	Harmful if ingested and in contact with skin.	Wear appropriate protection and avoid inhaling powder.

Silver nitrate		Corrosive and irritating to the eyes and skin. May ignite combustible materials.	Protect skin, eyes, clothing, and equipment. Keep away from ammonia solution, ethanol, charcoal, and combustible materials. Causes brown staining.
Sodium azide		*Very* toxic if ingested, inhaled, or by skin contact. Mutagen. Contact with acids liberates toxic gas. Toxic gas liberated in fires. Violent reaction occurs if water is added to heated solid. Reacts with copper, lead, mercury to form explosive metal azide salts.	Avoid contact by wearing appropriate clothing. Do not inhale dust. Wash immediately any affected area. Keep in a locked cupboard away from acids and metals. Do not flush down copper or lead drainage systems.
Sodium dithionite		Harmful if ingested. Contact with acid liberates toxic gas. May cause fire.	Protect from skin contact. Keep away from acids, flammable chemicals and combustible material.
Sodium fluoride		Toxic if ingested. Irritating to eyes and skin. Liberates toxic gas in contact with acids.	Protect skin and eyes. Keep away from acids.
Sodium hydroxide, pellets and solutions		Corrosive. Causes *severe* internal injury if ingested. Deliquescent (pellets). Heat evolved when mixed with water.	Protect skin and eyes, clothing, and equipment. Store in dry place, away from acids, methanol, and chloroform. Do not use reagent bottles with ground glass stoppers.
Sodium hypochlorite solution		Corrosive and toxic if ingested or inhaled. Irritating vapour. May evolve toxic fumes in fires. Liberates toxic gas in contact with acids.	Protect skin, eyes, clothing, and equipment. Use in well ventilated area. Keep away from acids, methanol and oxidizers.
Sodium nitroprusside*		Toxic if ingested. *sodium nitrosopentacyanoferrate III	Do not breathe dust.
Sodium nitrite		Toxic if ingested.	Protect against skin contact. Keep away from combustible materials and flammable chemicals.
		Oxidizing	
Sulphanilic acid		Harmful if ingested, inhaled, or in contact with skin or eyes.	Avoid contact with eyes and skin. Wear appropriate protection.
Sulphosalicylic acid		Irritating to eyes and skin.	Protect eyes and skin. Use in well ventilated area.
Sulphuric acid		Corrosive, causing *severe* burns. Toxic vapour.	Protect skin, eyes, clothing, and equipment. Avoid inhaling fumes. *Never add water to conc. sulphuric acid.* Keep in dry place away from alkalis, potassium permanganate, perchlorates, chlorates and flammable substances.

CHEMICAL	MAIN HAZARD	SAFETY PRECAUTIONS
o-Tolidine	Toxic and harmful if ingested. Carcinogen.	Minimize exposure. Wear appropriate protection.
Toluene	*Highly* flammable, with flash point 4°C. Volatile. Harmful if ingested, inhaled, or by skin contact. May cause dermatitis. Vapour can be irritating to the eyes.	Keep away from sources of ignition. Wear appropriate protective clothing. Keep away from oxidizers and do not empty into drains.
o-Toluidine solution	Toxic if ingested or inhaled. Carcinogen. Irritating to the eyes. Reacts violently with acids.	Minimize exposure and wear appropriate protection. Keep away from acids.
Trichloroacetic acid	Corrosive and hygroscopic. Unpleasant odour that is irritating to the eyes. May evolve toxic fumes in fires.	Protect skin, eyes, clothing, and equipment.
Wrights stain	As for Giemsa stain.	
Xylene	Harmful if inhaled or in contact with skin. May cause dermatitis. Flammable with flashpoint 25°C.	Protect from skin contact and use in well ventilated area. Do not keep in plastic containers unless polypropylene. Do not use caps with rubber liners.

CHEMICALS AND REAGENTS LISTED BY HAZARD

Extremely flammable
- Acetone
- Diethylamine
- Ether, diethyl

Highly flammable
- Acetone-alcohol
- Acid alcohol
- Alcoholic stains: Giemsa, Leishman, Wrights, May Grunwald
- Ethanol and alcohol reagents
- Methanol
- Methylated spirit
- Toluene

Oxidizing (fire-promoting)
- Calcium hypochlorite
- Chromic acid
- Hydrogen peroxide (strong)
- Nitric acid
- Perchlorates
- Potassium permanganate
- Sodium nitrite

Toxic
- Cadmium sulphate
- Diphenylamine
- Formaldehyde solution
- Lactophenol
- Mercury

Toxic continued
- Mercury 11 chloride (Mercuric chloride)
- Methanol
- Phenol
- Picric acid
- Potassium cyanide
- Sodium azide
- Sodium fluoride
- Sodium nitrite
- Sodium nitrosopenta-cyanoferrate 111 (Sodium nitroprusside)
- Thiomersal
- Thiosemicarbazide
- *o*-Tolidine
- *o*-Toluidine

Harmful
- Aminophenazone
- Ammonium oxalate
- Auramine phenol stain
- Barium chloride
- Benedicts reagent
- Benzoic acid
- Carbol fuchsin stain
- Cetylpyridinium chloride
- Chloroform
- Copper 11 sulphate
- Dobell's iodine

Harmful continued
- Ethylenediaminetetraacetic acid (EDTA)
- Ethylene glycol (Ethanediol)
- Formol saline
- Glycerol jelly
- Glutaraldehyde
- Iodine
- Iron 111 chloride (Ferric chloride)
- Lugol's iodine
- Methylated spirit
- Naphthylamine
- *p*-Nitrophenyl
- Oxalic acid
- Potassium oxalate
- Potassium permanganate
- Salicyclic acid
- Saponin
- Sodium deoxycholate
- Sodium dithionite
- Sodium dodecyl sulphate
- Sodium tetraborate
- Sodium tungstate
- Stains (powder form):
  - acridine orange
  - auramine O
  - brilliant cresyl blue
  - crystal violet

Harmful continued

- Giemsa
- Harris's haematoxylin
- malachite green
- May Grunwald
- methylene blue
- neutral red
- toluidine blue
- Sulphanilic acid
- Thiourea
- Toluene
- Xylene

Irritant

- Acetic acid, glacial
- Ammonia solution
- Calcium chloride

Irritant continued

- Formaldehyde solution
- Hydrogen peroxide
- Lactic acid
- Naphthylethylenediamine dihydrochloride
- Potassium dichromate
- Sodium carbonate
- Sulphosalicylic acid
- Zinc sulphate

Corrosive

- Acetic acid, glacial
- Ammonia solution
- Calcium hypochlorite
- Chromic acid
- Fouchet's reagent

Corrosive continued

- Hydrochloric acid
- Nitric acid
- Phenol
- o-Phosphoric acid
- Potassium hydroxide
- Silver nitrate
- Sodium hydroxide
- Sodium hypochlorite
- Sulphuric acid
- Thymol
- Trichloroacetic acid

Explosive

- Picric acid (when dry)
- Sodium azide

3.6 Equipment and glassware hazards

Fire, electric shock, and injury from moving components are hazards associated with the use of equipment. Most glassware hazards are associated with breakages and the use of damaged glassware.

Equipment related accidents in district laboratories

The safe use of equipment is dependent on:

- equipment being installed and positioned correctly.
- equipment being used as instructed by the manufacturer.
- equipment being cleaned, inspected, serviced and repaired correctly.
- staff being well instructed in the correct use, cleaning and maintenance of equipment.
- the district laboratory coordinator ensuring standard operating procedures (SOPs) and maintenance schedules for equipment exist and are implemented.

PREVENTING EQUIPMENT RELATED ACCIDENTS

Safe positioning and installation of equipment

- When installing and positioning equipment consider both safety and convenience:
  - do not place electrical equipment near to water, in direct sunlight or close to where chemicals and reagents are used or stored.
  - do not position equipment where movement of its components could cause injury.
  - do not locate equipment in a place where access to it or cleaning will be difficult.
  - make sure the equipment is level.
  - do not overcrowd a bench with equipment because this will reduce the working area, and increase the risk of the equipment being damaged from chemical spills and splashes or items being placed on the equipment.

- Make sure ventilation is adequate:
  - follow the manufacturer's instructions.
  - do not cover or obstruct ventilation openings.
  - place wire mesh over ventilation grills to prevent insects and rodents entering.
  - make sure the chimney apertures of gas or kerosene operated refrigerators and the burner aperture of a flame photometer are not obstructed or located under a shelf.
  - provide good ventilation when charging acid rechargeable batteries.

- Use a qualified electrician and follow the manufacturer's instructions when installing electrical equipment. Ensure:
  - the voltage of the new equipment is the same as that of the electricity supply in the laboratory and the voltage selector switch is set correctly.
  - the power required by the instrument does not exceed the power supply circuit of the laboratory.
  - the equipment is wired correctly using a fuse of the correct rating, and the system has a grounded conductor. The laboratory should

have sufficient earthed outlets. Circuit-breakers and earth-fault interrupters should be fitted to all laboratory circuits.*

*Circuit-breakers protect wiring from being over-loaded with electric current. Earth-fault interrupters protect people from electric shock.

- the cable used is not longer than is necessary, has no joins, is well insulated and not positioned near water or hot surfaces.

- the use of multiple adaptors, temporary connections, and extension leads is avoided because these can lead to overheating and bad connections.

Safe use of electrical equipment

■ Do not purchase or accept donated equipment unless accompanied by a manufacturer's instruction manual written in a language that can be understood or accurately translated.

■ Use the equipment correctly:
- whenever possible have new equipment demonstrated by the supplier.
- prepare and display easy to understand instructions and safety precautions near to the equipment.

■ Make sure staff are well instructed and trainees adequately supervised:
- to use and clean correctly the equipment in their care.
- to dry their hands and floor underfoot before using electrical equipment.
- to switch off and disconnect the electricity supply to an instrument by removing the plug at the end of a day's work and during an electric storm (excluding refrigerators and incubators).
- to stop using and report immediately any malfunction of equipment.
- to obtain the help of an electrician to check the electricity circuit should a fuse 'blow'.
- to apply First Aid following an equipment related injury (see subunit 3.8).
- to keep careful records of equipment maintenance, servicing and repair.

Important: District laboratories should be supplied with a dry chemical fire extinguisher to control an electric fire (see also subunit 3.7).

Cleaning, maintenance, inspection and servicing of equipment

■ Perform cleaning, maintenance and servicing as recommended by the manufacturer:
- prepare SOPs and a written maintenance schedule for each piece of equipment with a checklist of the tasks to be performed at specified times.
- always turn off and disconnect equipment before carrying out cleaning, maintenance, and inspections.
- inspect equipment regularly for corrosion, worn components, damaged insulation, frayed cable, loose connections, fungal growth, insect and rodent infestation.

■ Hold stocks of essential components with their part numbers and sources of supply. If unable to obtain spares from the manufacturer make sure the specifications of alternatives are correct, e.g. dimensions, fuse ratings, voltage and wattage of lamps etc. When purchasing spares, always state the model number of the equipment and date it was purchased, and the supplier's part number.

Note: The use and maintenance of different items of equipment can be found in Chapter 4. Publications covering the safety and maintenance of laboratory equipment include *WHO Maintenance and repair of laboratory, diagnostic, imaging and hospital equipment*[9] and the *WHO Laboratory Biosafety Manual,*[3]

PREVENTING GLASSWARE RELATED ACCIDENTS

Although plasticware is increasingly being used in district laboratories, glass pipettes, capillaries, test tubes, specimen containers, flasks, beakers, slides and coverglasses continue to be used because they are easier and cheaper to obtain, clean, and reuse. For some items there are no appropriate plastic alternatives. It is therefore essential for district laboratories to include in their code of safe working practices, effective measures to prevent injury and infection from broken and damaged glassware.

Correct purchasing of glassware

■ Avoid purchasing glassware classified as 'disposable'. Such glassware is usually thin walled and not intended for cleaning and reuse. If needing to reuse cover glasses, purchase thicker No. 2 glasses.

■ Ensure glassware that is to be used at high temperature, or heat sterilized is made from *Pyrex* or other heat resistant glass.

Safe handling of glassware

- Use appropriate plastic containers for soaking and decontaminating used glassware. Minimize damage, breakage, and risk of injury by:
  - not overfilling containers,
  - using separate containers for fragile cover glasses, slides, and sharp ended Pasteur pipettes.

- Before reuse, inspect glassware, particularly tubes, pipettes and specimen containers for cracks, broken and chipped ends.

- Never centrifuge cracked tubes or bottles.

- Flame until smooth the sharp ends of pipettes, and the damaged rims of test tubes.

- Wear protective gloves when cleaning glassware and avoid overcrowding drainage racks.

- Store glassware safely. Do not leave it in open trays or other places where it can be damaged.

- To avoid spillages and breakages, use racks or trays to hold specimen containers and other bottles.

Safe management of breakages

- Wear heavy duty gloves and use forceps to collect broken glass. A piece of plasticine is useful for collecting glass fragments.

- Discard broken glass in a separate puncture resistant waste bin marked 'Sharps' and dispose of the contents safely. Do not allow the bin to overflow.

- Never leave used haematocrit (capillary) tubes on a bench from where they can roll to the floor.

- When a breakage on the bench or floor occurs, immediately collect the broken glass and make sure the area is brushed and cleaned well.

- Wear suitable closed toe footwear. Wear protective gloves when unpacking new glassware. Unpack the glassware in a safe place where any broken glass from packing cases can be safely contained.

- Inspect regularly places where glassware is stored for glass fragments, particularly drawers or containers where glass pipettes, cover glasses, and slides are kept.

- Treat immediately any glass injury and cover cuts with an appropriate dressing (see subunit 3.8).

3.7 Fire safety

A significant fire risk exists in small district laboratories due to the frequent use of matches and open flames in close proximity to highly flammable chemicals and reagents such as acetone, diethyl ether, methanol, methylated spirit, acid alcohol, and stains that are alcohol-based.

Fire may also be caused by overheating in faulty poorly maintained electrical equipment, overloading of electrical circuits, use of adaptors, or overheating of electrical motors due to inadequate ventilation. Gas tubing or electric cables that are worn or too long are also fire risks.

It is *essential* for district laboratory technical and auxiliary staff to receive adequate instruction and training in fire safety and appropriate fire fighting. A local fire fighting service is unlikely to be available in rural district areas.

Injury, damage and loss caused by fire can be minimized when laboratory staff:

- understand how fires are caused and spread.

- reduce the risk of fire by following fire safety regulations at all times.

- know what to do if there is a fire in their laboratory.

- know how to use fire fighting equipment.

- know how to apply emergency First Aid for burns.

Important: Those in charge of district laboratory services must provide adequate training of laboratory staff in fire safety and equip district laboratories with essential fire fighting equipment.

FIRE FIGHTING EQUIPMENT

Fire fighting equipment for district laboratories should include:

- Buckets of water to extinguish paper, fabric and wood fires. Water, however, must *never* be used to extinguish an electrical fire or one caused by a flammable chemical.

- Buckets of sand or dry soil (kept free of refuse) to smother flames and contain and extinguish a free flowing liquid fire.

- Fire blanket(s) made from heavy cotton twill treated with a fire retardant chemical or preferably a manufactured fire blanket made from woven fibre glass sandwiched between a fire retardant material, to extinguish fire on personal clothing or a small fire on the floor or bench.

■ Dry powder chemical fire extinguisher to extinguish electrical fires and fires caused by flammable liquids.

Whenever possible the laboratory should be fitted with a battery operated smoke detector alarm. It should be tested at regular intervals as recommended by the manufacturer.

To alert those in and adjacent to the laboratory of a fire danger, a fire alarm such as a loud handbell or gong should be kept in a prominent place. When facilities allow, a fire alarm system should be installed.

Summary: Guidelines to reduce the risk of fire in district laboratories

- Do not allow smoking in the laboratory or in adjacent outpatient waiting areas or corridors. Display large *No smoking* signs.

- Keep only small amounts of highly flammable chemicals and reagents (classified in subunit 3.5) on laboratory benches and shelves. Whenever possible use plastic dispensing containers that can be closed when not in use. Keep them in a tray to retain the flammable liquid should a spillage occur.

- Store stock flammable chemicals and reagents preferably in an outside cool store, in trays, well away from oxidizing and other incompatible chemicals (see subunit 3.5). If this is not possible store the stock containers at ground level in trays in a metal or thick plywood box with a tight fitting lid.

- When lighting and using a spirit burner, Bunsen burner, or ring burner, always check that there is no flammable chemical or reagent nearby.

- Be particularly careful when heating carbol fuchsin stain on slides in the Ziehl-Neelsen technique. Use only a *small* lighted swab and extinguish it immediately after use. Keep the flame well away from acid alcohol, acetone, methanol, methylated spirits, ether, stains such as Leishman and Giemsa, and other flammable reagents.

- Promote safety awareness by displaying clearly written fire instruction notices in the laboratory, review regularly fire safety rules

and practise every 6 months what to do in the event of a fire.

- Install electrical equipment safely (see subunit 3.6). Inspect and maintain it. Do not allow untrained personnel to repair equipment.

- Keep the laboratory well ventilated, when using flammable chemicals and reagents to prevent any build-up of flammable vapours and gases.

- Keep containers of flammable chemicals and reagents tightly closed to prevent the escape of flammable vapours.

- If the laboratory is fitted with fire doors, keep these closed. Make sure there is a safe unobstructed marked exit route(s) from the laboratory.

- Whenever possible, ask advice from a professional Fire Safety Officer on how to implement and improve fire safety.

Fire hazard of some commonly used chemicals

CHEMICAL	FLASH POINT[8]	CLASSIFICATION
Diethyl ether	−40°C	Extremely flammable Class 1A
Acetone	−18°C	Extremely flammable Class 1B
Toluene	4°C	Highly flammable Class 1B
Methanol	12°C	Highly flammable Class 1B
Ethanol, absolute	13°C	Highly flammable Class 1B
Isopropanol	12°C	Highly flammable Class 1B
Ethanol, 70%	21°C	Highly flammable Class 1B
Xylene	25°C	Flammable Class 1C
Acetic acid, glacial	40°C	Flammable Class 11

Classification terminology: Flash points with boiling points are used to classify liquids by European terminology as *extremely flammable*, *highly flammable* or *flammable* or by United States terminology as flammable *Class 1A*, *Class 1B*, *Class 1C*, or combustible liquids *Class 11* or *Class 111*.

Important fire risk reagents: Acid alcohol, alcohol/acetone decolorizers, and stock alcoholic Romanowsky stains, e.g. Leishman and Giemsa are classified as Highly flammable, Class 1B.

Note: The control of fires involving flammable chemicals is described in subunit 3.5. The emergency treatment of burns in subunit 3.8. Further information can be found in the WHO *Laboratory Biosafety Manual* [3]

3.8 Emergency First Aid

Knowing what to do immediately an accident occurs can help to reduce suffering and the consequences of serious accidents. In some situations, First Aid can be life saving, e.g. by resuscitation or the control of bleeding. It can also prevent an injured person's condition from worsening, e.g. by protecting and treating wounds, placing a person in the best possible position, offering reassurance, and seeking immediate assistance.

TRAINING IN FIRST AID

All laboratory workers should receive a *practical* training in First Aid, with particular attention being paid to the types of accidents that may occur in the laboratory. They should also know what emergency action to take if an outpatient or blood donor collapses in the laboratory.

Training must be given by a person qualified to teach First Aid. A certificate of competence should be issued to those who complete the course successfully. Refresher courses should be held every 3–4 years.

First Aid equipment

An adequately equipped First Aid box and eyewash bottle should be kept in the laboratory in a place that is known and accessible to all members of staff. The First Aid box should be clearly identified by a white cross on a green background. It should be made of metal or plastic to prevent it being damaged by pests and to protect the contents from dust and damp. The contents should be inspected regularly.

Recommended contents of a laboratory First Aid box
- Clear instructions on how to apply emergency treatment of cuts, bleeding, heat burns, chemical burns, chemical injury to the eye, swallowing of acids, alkalis, and other poisonous chemicals, treatment of fainting, electric shock, and how to perform emergency resuscitation (illustrated).
- Sterile unmedicated dressings to cover wounds.
- Absorbent cotton wool.
- Triangular and roll bandages and safety pins.
- Sterile adhesive waterproof dressings in a variety of sizes.
- Sterile eyepads with attachment bandages.
- Roll of adhesive tape.
- Scissors.
- Sodium bicarbonate powder and boric acid powder.
- Equipment for person giving First Aid (mouthpiece, gloves).

Eyewash bottle
An eyewash bottle of the type shown in plate 3.2 (subunit 3.5) is suitable for district laboratories. Clean tap water can be used to wash the eye. If no clean tap water is available, sterile water or isotonic saline should be used (kept next to the eyewash bottle).

EMERGENCY FIRST AID PROCEDURES

First Aid applied to the laboratory should include emergency management of the following:

- Cuts, needlestick injuries
- Bleeding
- Resuscitation
- Fainting
- Electric shock
- Heat burns
- Chemical burns
- Poisoning

A First Aid chart giving the immediate treatment of cuts, bleeding, burns, poisoning, shock and resuscitation should be prepared and displayed in the laboratory.

Emergency treatment of cuts and bleeding

If the cut is small:
- wash with soap and water.
- apply pressure with a piece of cotton wool.
- disinfect the area with a skin antiseptic.
- cover with a water-proof dressing.

Note: If the cut has been caused by contaminated glassware or is a needlestick injury, encourage bleeding before washing well with soap and water. Apply a skin antiseptic and cover the area with a water-proof dressing. Seek medical advice.

If there is serious bleeding from a limb:
- raise the injured limb to reduce the bleeding.
- apply pressure with a clean dressing backed with cotton wool.
- bandage the dressing in position.
- immediately seek medical assistance.

Bleeding from the nose
- seat the person upright with the head slightly forward.
- tell the person to pinch firmly the soft part of

their nose for about 10 minutes and breathe through their mouth.

– if the bleeding does not stop, seek medical advice.

Emergency resuscitation when a person stops breathing

If a person stops breathing following an electric shock or for any other reason, artificial respiration (ventilation) must be applied *as soon as possible* (if the brain is deprived of oxygen for more than about 4 minutes, permanent brain damage will occur). The person may also require heart compression if there is circulatory arrest, i.e. heart is not beating.

Mouth-to-mouth respiration (ventilation)

There are several ways to perform artificial respiration. The most effective is mouth-to-mouth:

1 Lie the unconscious person on the floor. Supporting the neck, tilt the head backwards with the chin pushed upwards as shown in Fig. 3.9(1).

   Important: This position is essential to keep the person's airway open.

2 If the person does not start to breathe, begin immediately mouth-to-mouth respiration:

   – open your mouth wide and take a deep breath.
   – pinch the person's nostrils together with your fingers.
   – press your lips around the person's mouth.
   – blow into the person's mouth (air will pass to the lungs) until the chest is seen to rise.
   – remove your mouth and watch the chest fall as the air escapes from the lungs.
   – repeat the inflation at the normal rate of breathing, i.e. 10–15 breaths per minute.

   Note: Give the first few breaths *rapidly* to saturate the person's blood with oxygen.

If you cannot get air into the person's chest, check that the head is tilted sufficiently far back, you have a firm seal around the mouth, you have closed the nostrils sufficiently, and the airway is not obstructed by vomit, blood, or a foreign body.

Heart not beating

3 If after the first two inflations, natural breathing is not restored, check whether the heart has stopped beating.

Indications that the heart has stopped beating are:

■ person remaining or becoming grey-blue.
■ no carotid pulse being felt (see Fig. 3.10).
■ pupils of the eye appearing widely dilated.

Take immediate action to restart the heart while *at the same time* continuing mouth-to-mouth respiration:

– Begin external heart compression by placing the heel of your hand on the lower half of the person's breastbone and cover this hand with the heel of your other hand as shown in Fig. 3.11 (the palms and fingers of your hand should be raised away from the person's chest so that pressure is not applied over the ribs).

– With your arms straight, press down rapidly on the breastbone (once every second), depressing it about 4 cm ($1\frac{1}{2}$ in) then release the pressure without removing your hands.

– Look to see whether there is an improvement in the person's colour indicating a return of circulation. If there is no improvement, continue compression and mouth-to-mouth respiration.

   If resuscitating by yourself, apply 15 heart compressions followed by 2 quick lung inflations and then repeat.

   If there is someone else to help, apply 5 heart compressions, followed by 1 deep inflation. The person carrying out the mouth-to-mouth respiration should feel for a carotid pulse.

4 Once natural breathing has been restored and the heart is beating, place the person in the recovery position (see Fig. 3.8). This is important because the person may vomit and in this position there will be no danger of choking.

5 Obtain further medical assistance at the earliest opportunity.

Note: Other forms of resuscitation will be required if it is not possible to apply mouth-to-mouth respiration. Alternative methods should therefore be learnt.

Emergency treatment when someone faints

Emergency treatment of a faint is as follows:

– lay the person down and raise the legs above the level of the head (see Fig. 3.7).
– loosen clothing at the neck, chest, and waist.

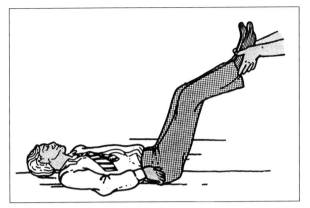

Fig. 3.7   Position in which to place a person who has fainted.

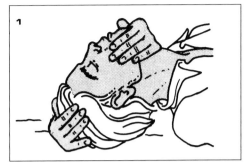

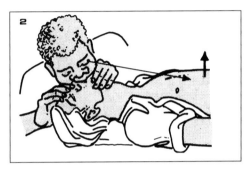

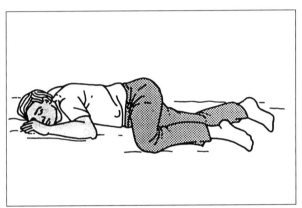

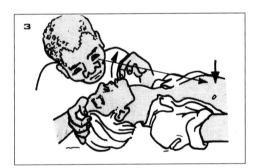

Fig. 3.8   The recovery position.

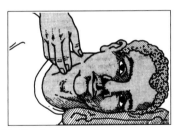

Fig. 3.10   Feeling for the carotid pulse

Fig. 3.9   Mouth to mouth ventilation during emergency resuscitation. If the heart has stopped beating, perform external heart compression (see text for details)

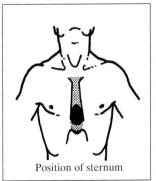

Position of sternum

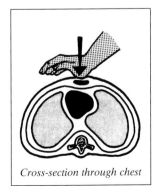

Cross-section through chest

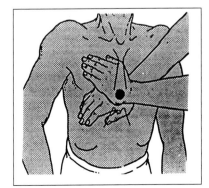

Fig. 3.11   Position of hands over lower breast bone when performing external heart compression.
Acknowledgement: Illustrations are reproduced by permission of St John Ambulance Association

– make sure the room is well-ventilated.

– reassure the person as consciousness is regained.

– gradually raise the person to the sitting position. Sips of drinking water may be given.

Note: If breathing becomes difficult, place the person in the recovery position shown in Fig. 3.8.

Emergency treatment when someone is electrocuted

Carry out the following:

– immediately turn off the electricity from the *mains* if it can be reached easily, otherwise remove the plug or wrench the cable free. DO NOT TOUCH THE PERSON'S FLESH WITH YOUR HANDS until the contact has been broken.

Important: On no account try to free an electrocuted person from the electrical contact without using some form of insulation material, such as a dry *thick* cloth, folded laboratory coat, folded newspapers, wooden or plastic stool or chair. If insulation is not used, the person rescuing will also be electrocuted.

– if the person has collapsed, send immediately for medical help and if the person is not breathing, give artificial respiration until assistance arrives.

– Cool any burns with water.

Emergency treatment of heat and chemical burns

Heat burns

– if clothing is alight, smother the flames using a fire blanket.

– remove the person from the danger area.

– immediately plunge the burnt area into cold water or apply a pad soaked in cold water (or any other non-flammable liquid) to the affected part for 10 minutes.

– cover with a dry dressing.

– remove any constricting articles such as rings or bracelets before the affected area starts to swell and becomes blistered.

– provide frequent small cold drinks.

Note: If more than a minor burn, seek medical treatment immediately. Reassurance of the casualty is important.

Chemical burns of the skin

– wash immediately in running water for several minutes, remove any contaminated clothing.

– neutralize with a suitable chemical as follows:
   If an *acid* burn, neutralize with sodium bicarbonate powder.
   If an *alkali* burn, neutralize with boric acid powder.

– seek medical attention.

Note: Respiratory symptoms may develop if fumes from strong acids and alkalis have been inhaled. Transfer the patient urgently for medical care.

Chemical injury to the eye

– wash the affected eye as quickly as possible under running tap water or with water from an eye wash-bottle.

– neutralize with a suitable chemical as follows:
   If an *acid* injury, neutralize with 5% sodium bicarbonate solution.
   If an *alkali* injury, neutralize with 5% acetic acid or vinegar diluted 1 in 5.

– immediately seek medical attention.

Emergency treatment for poisoning

Swallowing of an acid or alkali

– immediately rinse the mouth well with water.

– neutralize with a suitable chemical as follows:
   If *acid* has been swallowed, neutralize by drinking 8% w/v magnesium hydroxide suspension (milk of magnesia) or milk.
   If an *alkali* has been swallowed, neutralize by drinking lemon juice or 1% acetic acid.

– drink three or four cups of water.

– seek medical attention.

Note: When an acid or alkali has been swallowed, do not encourage vomiting.

Swallowing of other poisonous chemicals

– rinse out the mouth well with water.

– depending on the chemical swallowed, take a suitable chemical antidote under medical supervision.

Note: Always seek medical advice and treatment after swallowing toxic or harmful chemicals.

Swallowing of infected material

– immediately seek medical treatment.

– if required provide follow-up tests.

Mouth-pipetting: This is the main cause of the accidental swallowing of chemicals or infected material in laboratories.

Further information: Full details of emergency First Aid measures can be found in the colour publication: *First Aid Manual* of St John Ambulance, St Andrew's Ambulance Association and Red Cross (see last entry under Recommended Reading).

REFERENCES

1 *Essential medical laboratory services project: Malawi, Final Report*, 2002. Malawi Ministry of Health, Liverpool School Tropical Medicine, DFID. Obtainable from HIV/AIDS Dept, Liverpool School Tropical Medicine, Pembroke Place, Liverpool, L3 5QA, UK.

2 **McNerney R**. Workplace protection from tuberculosis. *Africa Health*, 2002, September, pp. 15–16.

3 *Laboratory Biosafety Manual*, 3rd edition, 2004. World Health Organization, Geneva, NHO/CDS/CSR/LYO/2004.11. Can also be downloaded from the WHO website www.who.int/csr/resources/publications/biosafety

4 *Recommendations on the transport of dangerous goods*, 13th revised edition, 2003. New York and Geneva, United Nations.

5 *Transport of infectious substances*, 2004. World Health Organization, Geneva, WHO/CDS/CSR/LYO, 2004. Can also be downloaded from WHO website www.who.int/csr/resources/publications

6 *Infectious substances shipping guidelines*, 2003. Montreal International Air Transport Association. Can be downloaded from website www.iata.org/ads/issg

7 *Health Laboratory facilities in emergency and disaster situations.* World Health Organization, 1994 (WHO Regional Publications Eastern Mediterranean Series, No. 6). Obtainable from WHO Regional Office, Abdal Razzak, AC Sanhouri Street, PO Box 7608, Nasr City, Cairo 11371, Egypt.

8 **Carter J and Lema O**. *Practical Laboratory Manual for Health Centres in Eastern Africa*, 1994, AMREF, Kenya.

9 *Maintenance and repair of laboratory, diagnostic imaging, and hospital equipment.* Geneva, World Health Organization, 1994.

RECOMMENDED READING

Laboratory Biosafety Manual. Geneva, World Health Organization, 2004, 3rd edition. Can be downloaded from website www.who.int/csr/resources/publications/biosafety

Collins CH. *Laboratory acquired infections: history, incidence, causes and prevention*, 4th edition, 1999. Arnold-Hodder Headline.

Furr AK. *CRC Handbook of laboratory safety*, 5th edition, 2000. Boca Raton FL. CRC Press.

Guidelines for the collection of clinical specimens during field investigations of outbreaks, World Health Organization, WHO/CDS/CSR/EDC/2000.4, 2000.

Transport of infectious substances, World Health Organization, Geneva, 2004. Can be downloaded from the website www.who.int/csr/resources/publications

Guidelines for the prevention of tuberculosis in health care facilities in resource limited settings. World Health Organization, WHO/CDS/TB/99.269, 1999.

Website of the *International Union against Tuberculosis and Lung Diseases*, www.iuatld.org

WHO health-care waste management website: www.healthcarewaste.org

Halbwachs H. Solid waste disposal in district health facilities. *World Health Forum*, 1994, Volume 15, pp. 363–367.

First Aid Manual of St John Ambulance, St Andrew's Ambulance Association and *British Red Cross.* Dorling Kindersley, revised 6th edition, 2004. Supplied with free booklet covering emergency procedures, suitable for First Aid kits. Obtainable from Pearson Educational, Edinburgh Gate, Harlow CM20 2JE, UK, priced £11.99 (2005).

4

Equipping district laboratories

4.1 Selection, procurement and care of equipment

The importance of having an effective equipment management policy has been discussed in subunit 2.1 and equipment safety in subunit 3.6. This subunit covers the selection and purchase of equipment and how to keep it in working order in district laboratories.

SELECTING AND PROCURING LABORATORY EQUIPMENT

The majority of district hospital laboratories will require the basic equipment listed in Table 4.1. The equipment needed by health centre laboratories will depend on the range of tests performed.

Table 4.1 Basic equipment for district hospital laboratories

- Microscope
- Equipment for purifying water
- Balance
- Equipment for pipetting and dispensing
- Centrifuge(s)
- Autoclave
- Incubator (for culturing micro-organisms)
- Water bath and, or, heat block
- Colorimeter
- Mixers and rotator
- General laboratory-ware
- Safety equipment

Note: The specifications, use and care of the above listed equipment are covered in this chapter except safety equipment which is included in Chapter 3. Haemoglobin meters and electrophoresis equipment are described in Chapter 8 in Part 2. Glucose meters are described in subunit 6.5 and flame photometers in subunit 6.10.

Microprocessor controlled equipment

Many items of laboratory equipment are now microprocessor controlled with the user being able to programme different functions (operating modes), e.g. balances, autoclaves, colorimeters, centrifuges, water baths, incubators, heat blocks and mixers. Such microprocessor-based digital display equipment is usually more accurate, versatile, efficient, and has more built-in safety features than traditional analogue electronic equipment. Some microprocessor controlled equipment, however, can be expensive and complex to use, necessitating a longer training to use it correctly. It can also be more difficult to repair in the field.

In this chapter, analogue electronic equipment is included when this is considerably cheaper than microprocessor equipment, meets the required specifications for district laboratory work, and is easily obtainable. Microprocessor controlled equipment is included when this is easy to use, affordable, meets the specifications required, is safer to use, has a proven track record, and is more available.

Standardization of district laboratory equipment

Whenever feasible, equipment for use in district laboratories should be standardized. This can facilitate installation, training of laboratory staff, local maintenance and repair. Also, lower prices are usually available when purchasing equipment and replacement parts in quantity. Ideally the equipment should be available from more than one source for price comparison and ease of availability.

Clearly there are significant benefits in standardizing basic equipment and having a national standard laboratory equipment list but there can also be problems when equipment is not sufficiently tested in the laboratories in which it will be used before the decision to purchase is made. Standardization may also make it more difficult to change technological methods.

Aggressive marketing by suppliers can also be a problem when it becomes known that a bulk purchase is being considered. Attractive discounts and incentives may be offered for a 'quick sale' without the purchaser being given the opportunity to study sufficiently the specifications of the equipment, read the manufacturer's *User Service Manual*, and be assured that spare parts are available and will remain so for an appropriate period of time.

Relevant standardization may be difficult to achieve when equipment is donated, particularly when an overseas donor wishes to supply equipment manufactured in their own country which may not be appropriate for use in the recipient's laboratory. If, however, the equipment is on the national standard equipment list, the donor should respect this and supply the equipment that is specified. This aspect of equipment procurement is covered later in the text (see *Equipment donation guidelines*).

Procurement of laboratory equipment

In developing countries, laboratory equipment is usually procured in one of three ways:

- purchased nationally through a local supplier (agent).
- purchased from an overseas manufacturer or their distributor, often by tender.
- procured through a donor body.

Procurement through a local supplier

Purchasing nationally has the advantage that local currency can be used to buy the equipment and its consumables. The supplier is responsible for importing the equipment and checking it on arrival. Usually it is also possible for the purchaser before buying the equipment to have it demonstrated and ask the supplier about specifications, power requirements, and maintenance. The *User Service Manual* can also be studied. An authorized supplier will usually stock essential replacement parts and local repair facilities will often be available.

The main disadvantages of using a local supplier are that the choice of equipment and range available are usually limited, the cost of the equipment can be high particularly if there is no other local supplier, and the manufacturer's warranty conditions may not be accepted by the supplier.

Note: Whenever possible, before purchasing expensive equipment through a local supplier, the purchaser should check with the manufacturer that the supplier is one that is authorized and recommended.

Procurement from an overseas manufacturer or distributor

This method of equipment procurement is often the only one available to developing countries because there is no local supplier for the equipment that is needed. Advantages in purchasing from overseas include greater choice of equipment and availability of up to date information on new equipment, lower costs (but check also transport, insurance and import charges), and greater opportunity for modifying equipment to meet user requirements, e.g. need for voltage stabilizer, or to use the equipment from a 12 V DC lead-acid battery.

The main disadvantages are the need for foreign currency, no 'hands on' experience before purchasing, no after sales assistance such as help with installation and training of staff in use and maintenance of the equipment, and consumables, spares, and repair facilities may not be available locally. The purchaser also has the responsibility for importing the equipment. If at a later stage a fault develops and the equipment cannot be repaired locally, it can be troublesome and expensive to return the equipment to an overseas distributor.

Procurement through a donor body

While much laboratory equipment is successfully donated and proves to be exactly what is needed, inappropriate equipment may be donated when there is little or no communication between the donor and recipient (see later text).

It is particularly important that equipment is not donated or accepted when its running and maintenance costs are unaffordable, the information it provides is of limited use or difficult to interpret, the equipment is obsolete, no spares are available, or it is unsafe.

Preventing errors when selecting and procuring equipment

The following guidelines can help to avoid resources being wasted due to the incorrect selection and procurement of laboratory equipment:

Before placing an order

- *Discuss and decide what is required* based on:
    - why the equipment is needed, how it will be used, and who will be responsible for its use and maintenance.
    - present and anticipated workload.
    - local power supplies, and climate.
    - available space and ventilation.
    - health and safety considerations.
    - whether the equipment will require any special facilities or additional supplies, e.g. voltage stabilizer, greater purity of water, air conditioning, etc.

■ *Provide the supplier* (manufacturer, distributor, donor) with sufficient information including:

- what functions the equipment needs to perform, and extent of its use, e.g. workload.
- level of skill of the persons who will be using and maintaining it.
- as much detail as possible about local facilities.
- information on the climate and environment, e.g. temperature range, whether problems of corrosion and fungal growth exist due to high relative humidity, or dry dusty conditions prevail.

■ *Ask the supplier* for information and illustrations of the equipment that meets or comes closest to fitting the specifications, including:

- cost of the equipment, replacement parts (spares) and if required, consumables.
- cost of transporting the equipment and insuring it in transit.
- what is the expected working life of replacement parts.
- source(s) of spares, consumables, and details of the nearest authorized repairer.
- what are the power requirements and performance specifications of the equipment.
- how is the equipment used (*detailed instructions* are required).
- installation information.
- what control checks are required.
- what is the maintenance schedule (request a copy of the *Service Manual*).
- are any evaluation reports available.
- has the equipment been field-tested in any tropical country.
- what are the safety features.
- how long has the equipment been in production and how long will the spares remain available.
- what warranty is supplied.

■ *Evaluate and discuss* the information received from the supplier, studying particularly:

- whether the equipment has the features that are needed and any other useful specifications.
- whether the purchase price and anticipated operating and maintenance costs, and reagent costs, can be afforded,
- whether the equipment will be cost-effective to use, compared with existing or alternative technologies.
- whether the equipment appears easy to use

and maintain by laboratory staff and how much training will be needed.
- whether the equipment is of safe design.

Note: Equipment designs are changing rapidly. A purchaser should not hesitate to ask a supplier to explain any unfamiliar terminology or the purpose of any optional feature or accessory.

■ *Select the most appropriate equipment* for the job, i.e. what is relevant and affordable, simplest, and easiest to use and maintain. The simplest design of equipment will often be the most reliable and remain working the longest.

If the supplier is a local supplier:

- request a demonstration of how to use the equipment (including the fitting of replacement parts).
- study carefully the *User Service Manual*.
- ask about any after sales service, particularly staff training, assistance with installation, maintenance and servicing facilities.
- confirm that the equipment is in current production.
- check the conditions of the warranty.
- obtain a written quotation and discuss terms of payment and delivery.

If the supplier is an overseas distributor:

- request a quotation for the equipment.
- indicate how you would like the equipment to be transported e.g. airfreighted, or sent by air parcel post and request a quotation for the transport and in-transit insurance.
- ask how soon after receiving an order and agreeing payment terms, the equipment will be despatched.
- request a copy of the *User Service Manual* to be sent with the quotation for careful study *before* placing an order.

User Service Manual
The *User Service Manual* is important because this will detail (usually with illustrations) the operation of the equipment, its power requirements, temperature range over which the equipment will perform reliably, how the equipment should be controlled, cleaned, and maintained, the recommended replacement parts and their expected working life, and how to identify and correct problems (trouble-shooting). Users, however, should be aware that the *Manual* supplied may describe the use of several different models of similar equipment, not just the model being considered.

- Ask for confirmation that the equipment is a current model and ask for how long the spares will be available.
- Check from the nearest Customs and Excise

Office whether there are any import regulations covering the equipment, whether any import duty and taxes will be charged and whether any documentation is required other than the international Customs declaration and signed commercial invoice which the distributor will send with the goods.

If the goods are airfreighted, a clearing agent will be required to clear the goods through Customs and a fee will be charged by the agent.

Important: Whenever possible, obtain quotations from several different suppliers of the equipment. If prices between suppliers vary greatly, recheck the specifications of the equipment with each supplier. Always question the reason for any unusual discount (possible discontinuity of model).

Placing an order

■ *Never* be rushed into placing an order by a sales person. Take adequate time to evaluate whether the equipment is a *priority* and can be afforded. Always consider and consult adequately.

■ Order correctly in writing, using an order number:
– use the supplier's code numbers as well as descriptions.
– make sure all the items that are needed are clearly specified and ordered, e.g. the rotor and tube holders for a centrifuge or all the optics for a microscope.
– order essential replacement parts (the quantity to order will depend on the anticipated working life of each part and expected use of the equipment in the laboratory).
– for electrical equipment, state the voltage, frequency and phase required (see subunit 4.2).
– state the price you have been quoted for the equipment, its transport and insurance costs, and any other agreed conditions, e.g. terms of payment, despatch/delivery date, training of staff, etc.
– make sure the delivery address is clear.

■ If ordering from an overseas distributor, confirm how you would like the equipment to be transported. Request careful packing to avoid damage in transit. Ask the distributor to airmail in *advance of delivery*, copies of the documentation (signed commercial invoice(s) and packing notes). If an import licence and, or, a *Gift*

Certificate is required, send copies of these to the supplier for sending *with* the equipment.

If the order is being airfreighted, provide a fax number and, or, email address which the distributor can use to fax or email the flight details (airline and flight number, airway bill number, expected date and time of arrival) and an advance copy of the commercial invoice.

Common causes of incorrect equipment selection and procurement in developing countries

● Purchaser having to compromise because the equipment that is needed is not available or will only become available after a long delay.

● Supplier receiving inadequate, non-specific, or confusing information from a purchaser (major cause of error in purchasing).

● Ordering equipment from a brief description in a catalogue or from a promotional leaflet without first obtaining further information, particularly regarding power requirements, availability of spares, use and maintenance of the equipment.

● Discontinued equipment or second-hand equipment being purchased for which replacement parts are not available or are difficult to obtain.

● A procurement officer disregarding the request of the laboratory to buy equipment from a specific manufacturer in favour of a lower price tender without rechecking quality and specifications with laboratory staff.

● Donated funds being used to buy the latest and most complex instrument without due consideration as to exactly what is required and the conditions in which the equipment will be used.

● Microprocessor controlled equipment being selected without knowing the conditions for its use and extent of user training required.

● Analytical equipment being purchased or donated that can only be used with the manufacturer's reagents for which there is no local supplier, and no possibility of importing the reagents on a regular basis due to their high cost and lack of foreign currency.

● Order being placed without consulting laboratory staff, e.g. before staff are appointed to a newly built laboratory.

Page

Considerations when selecting major equipment for district laboratories

NEED

Is the equipment a priority and will it:
- meet district health needs?
- be correct for the workload?
- improve efficiency?

RELIABILITY AND SAFETY

- are any evaluations or field-testing reports available?
- what are the safety features?
- is the equipment in current production?
- is it possible to contact other users?

FACILITIES REQUIRED

Does the laboratory have:
- a suitable power supply?
- sufficient space and ventilation for the equipment?
- adequate quality and quantity of water?

SUPPORT

Who will help to:
- install the equipment?
- train users?
- perform maintenance schedules?

COST OF EQUIPMENT

Can the following be afforded?
- capital cost?
- transport and insurance?
- operating costs?
- cost of training users?

CLIMATIC CONSIDERATIONS

How will performance and durability of the equipment be affected by:
- high temperatures?
- high relative humidity?
- dusty environment?

USE AND MAINTENANCE

How easy is the equipment to:
- use?
- control?
- clean?
- maintain in the workplace?

USER MANUAL AND WARRANTY

Is a *User Service Manual*:
- available to study before purchase?
- adequate and easy to follow?
- what warranty is supplied?

SPARES AND CONSUMABLES

- what are needed and how often?
- who is the supplier?
- what are the current prices?
- can any of the reagents, calibrants or controls be made in the laboratory?

IMPORTED EQUIPMENT

Can regulations and charges be met covering:
- documentation?
- customs duty, import taxes?
- transport and insurance?

Important

A manufacturer, distributor, or donor will not be able to supply equipment of the correct specifications unless the user provides the supplier with sufficient information. To evaluate and order equipment correctly, the user must obtain sufficient and relevant information from the supplier(s).

- Keep a copy of the order and use this when the order arrives to check whether the correct items have been sent. If there are any errors or damage, notify the distributor in writing *as soon as possible*.

Equipment donation guidelines

Donors and recipients need to communicate to establish exactly what is required and to ensure that the equipment supplied is medically, technically, economically and environmentally appropriate and can be operated safely.

Recipient responsibilities

- Have clear policies and specifications of the equipment that is required. Advize a donor if the equipment is on the national standard equipment list.

- Ask the advice of qualified equipment technicians regarding installation of the equipment, its operation and maintenance, training requirements for users, essential parts, and appropriateness of equipment based on running costs and technical design.

- Specify clearly which items should accompany the equipment, e.g. technical documents (*User Service Manual*), reasonable quantity of spares and consumables, and a warranty covering the replacement and, or, repair of new equipment. If only the manufacturer's reagents can be used with the equipment, ask the donor for the prices of each reagent that will need to be imported.

- Make a checklist to ensure a donor is fully informed regarding: specifications of the equipment, functions it needs to perform, staff that will install, use, and maintain the equipment, where the equipment will be located, laboratory conditions e.g. heat, humidity, dust, ventilation, etc., and details of the facilities available including power supply, need for voltage protection, and if applicable details of the water supply and its quality.

- Communicate to the donor alternative preferences, e.g. if a financial contribution would be more appropriate to enable the equipment to be bought in the country in which it will be used (so as to obtain after sales support).

Donor responsibilities

- Communicate with the recipient to obtain a comprehensive description of the required equipment and its expected use. Advize the recipient whether the equipment that can be supplied will be new or reconditioned. Provide details of the model, year of manufacture, and estimated lifespan of the equipment.

- Supply equipment that is in full working order. *Before* sending the equipment, test its performance and safety. Do not supply worn-out, non-functioning, redundant, or unsafe equipment.

- Supply sufficient consumables and spare parts to last at least two years (with the equipment or in stages appropriate to their shelf-life). Include a complete list of spare parts and provide the name and address of the authorized dealer. Do not send equipment for which replacement parts are unavailable or difficult to obtain.

- Ensure the equipment is well packaged in a manageable load(s). Include a full packing list.

- Use the correct procedure and documentation for transporting the equipment. Airmail full copies of the documentation to the donor at the earliest opportunity (fax or email copies in advance).

- Find out about import regulations in the recipient's country and make sure that the recipient will be able to pay the custom duties and any other import charges.

- Offer as much technical assistance as possible, e.g. on-site training for users of the equipment and maintenance personnel.

Note: Above guidelines are based on those published in the newsletter *Contact*[1].

KEEPING EQUIPMENT IN WORKING ORDER

While equipment design faults and the inappropriate purchasing of equipment can lead to premature equipment failure, the commonest causes for equipment not working in district laboratories are:

- incorrect use of equipment.

- no one trained to take responsibility for the care of the equipment and the implementation of equipment standard operating procedures.

- lack of the correct replacement parts.

- no regular cleaning, inspection, and maintenance of the equipment.

- untrained personnel attempting unsuccessfully to correct a fault or replace a component.

- damage to electrical equipment caused by unstable power supplies, e.g. surge of current when power is restored after a power failure, or damage caused by lightning during storms (explained further in subunit 4.2).

Up to 70–90% of all equipment breakdowns are caused by the users of equipment. Non-functioning equipment represents not just a loss of important laboratory services to patients and the community, but also a waste of scarce health resources. As funds to purchase equipment become more difficult to obtain, the need to keep equipment operational and increase its working life has never been greater.

Ways of keeping district laboratory equipment operational

The following are effective ways of preventing damage to equipment and keeping it operational:

- Prepare written standard operating procedures (SOPs) and other relevant information for each item of equipment used in the laboratory, to include:

  - date equipment purchased, name and address of supplier, its cost, and details of the model. e.g. serial number (usually written on a plate on the back of the equipment).

- how to operate the equipment including how to check its performance and calibrate it before use.

- how to clean the equipment and inspect it regularly, e.g. for corrosion, mechanical damage, worn insulation, loose connections in wall plug, etc.

- relevant safety instructions.

- list of essential replacement parts, name of supplier(s), how many of each should be kept in stock, and code number to be quoted when ordering.

- how to maintain the equipment (as recommended by the manufacturer) with a checklist of what needs to be done and when, and a maintenance-job sheet on which to record the date of the maintenance, activities performed, and person who carried out the maintenance.

- name and address of authorized repairer and dated records of repairs to the equipment.

■ Ensure the person in charge of the laboratory:

- is sufficiently well trained to apply equipment SOPs.

- monitors whether equipment is being used, cleaned, and looked after correctly.

- reminds staff of the price and clinical value of equipment (a label attached to the equipment showing its price in local currency can help to remind users of its cost).

■ Locate the equipment in a safe and secure place where it cannot be easily damaged or stolen. Always follow the manufacturer's guidelines regarding installation and ventilation requirements. Use a qualified electrician to assist in the installation of electrical equipment.

■ If a fault develops or a component fails, immediately stop using the equipment. Investigate the fault or replace the component only if qualified to do so. Make sure the replacement part is correct.

■ Report as soon as possible any damage to equipment or fault that cannot be easily put right. The district laboratory coordinator should investigate

Importance of a laboratory equipment preventive maintenance programme
A well organized preventive maintenance programme for laboratory equipment is essential. The important benefits of having effective maintenance are summarized by WHO as:[2]

● Greater safety by preventing hazards resulting from breakdowns.

● Less unexpected shut-down time.

● Improved performance with regard to standard requirements.

● Less need for major repairs and lower repair costs with the elimination of premature replacement.

● Improved effectiveness of laboratory equipment with diminishing cost of tests.

● Identification of equipment with high maintenance costs (and performance problems).

● Improved equipment selection and purchase policy.

Other important benefits include:

● Less waste of reagents and control materials and less time spent repeating tests.

● Improved relationships between the laboratory and those requesting tests as services are maintained and fewer test results are delayed.

● The ability to communicate more informatively with manufacturers regarding what equipment is needed and its specifications.

promptly any report of equipment breakdown or damage, and arrange for the repair as soon as possible.

Important: When damaged equipment is repaired it should *not be put back into operation until measures are taken to prevent it becoming damaged again.*

■ Keep equipment clean and protect it:
- from corrosion and fungal growth, e.g. by sealing a microscope when not in use for several days in a plastic bag containing self-indicating anhydrous silica gel (reusable after drying).

- from insect damage e.g. by covering, but *not blocking*, ventilation grills with appropriate wire mesh.

- from dust and dirt by covering the equipment when not in use with a clean thick cotton cloth (avoid plastic if in high humidity areas).

- from rodent damage by inspecting the laboratory regularly and taking immediate action if there is evidence of infestation.

National equipment workshops and training centres

In recent years an increasing number of developing countries have formulated health care equipment policies and established centres or departments in polytechnical colleges for repairing equipment and training biomedical equipment engineers. Such national centres and workshops can usually provide equipment users with information on how to select appropriate equipment and how to set up equipment preventive maintenance programmes. To find out more about the existence of such centres, readers should contact their Ministry of Health.

Further information on the selection of equipment for district laboratories: Readers are referred to the publication *Selection of basic laboratory equipment for laboratories with limited resources* (see Recommended Reading).

4.2 Power Supplies in district laboratories

In developing countries, district laboratories are often without a mains electricity supply or receive electricity for only a few hours each evening from an on-site generator. The use of a generator enables rechargeable batteries to be used to power essential laboratory equipment.

Even when a laboratory is served by AC mains electricity, the supply may be intermittent and subject to voltage fluctuations. Significant and sudden increases in voltage (spikes and surges), e.g. when mains supplies are restored following a power failure, can damage equipment that is not voltage protected. Significant reductions in voltage (sags or brown-outs) e.g. when the electrical system becomes overloaded, can affect the performance of equipment such as centrifuges, colorimeters, spectrophotometers, electrophoresis equipment, and pH

meters. Some microprocessor-controlled equipment are programmed to cut out when voltage fluctuations become greater than the built in voltage tolerance, e.g. $\pm 10\%$.

Damage to equipment by lightning

Lightning may damage electrical equipment and also injure the operator. Whenever there is an electrical storm, electrical equipment should not be used and electrical plugs should be disconnected from wall sockets (and kept 30 cm from the sockets).

Terminology: Electrical terms used in this subunit are defined at the end of the subunit.

Voltage protection devices

When mains AC electrical supplies are unreliable, unprotected electrical equipment can be used with a voltage protection device such as:

- A voltage protection unit which cuts off the power supply to the equipment when the voltage is significantly increased (usually over 260 V) or decreased (usually below 190 V). Power is restored to the equipment when the voltage returns to acceptable levels. The equipment plugs into the voltage protection unit which is inserted in the wall socket. Such a device is the least expensive way of protecting equipment from damage due to major voltage fluctuations.

- A voltage stabilizer (surge suppressor plus filter) which regulates the voltage supply so that equipment is not damaged particularly by voltage spikes and surges. Although more expensive than a voltage protection unit, a voltage stabilizer is recommended when mains electricity supplies are subject to frequent major changes in voltage. The cost of a stabilizer will depend on its output power, i.e. volt ampere (VA) rating.

- An uninterruptible power supply (UPS) on line unit which in addition to regulating the voltage output in a similar way to a voltage stabilizer, also provides power for a limited period (from a battery) when a mains power failure occurs. This may be sufficient time to complete tests, e.g. - microscopy, colorimetric tests, or centrifuging samples. Like a voltage stabilizer, a UPS is costed by its VA rating.

Note: Further information on how to protect equipment against power surges and power cuts can be found in the publication *Selection of basic equipment for laboratories with limited resources* (see Recommended Reading).

Important: Always consult a qualified electrician or biomedical equipment engineer regarding power supply problems. Before purchasing electrical equipment, ask what is its nominal voltage and level of input voltage variation that the equipment can tolerate.

Handy Mains inverter

The *200 Watt Handy Mains* inverter unit SM 2716, manufactured by Switched Mode Ltd converts DC battery voltage to European mains level voltage and can be used to power some *low power* consumption 240 V mains electrical laboratory equipment from a 12 V DC lead-acid battery e.g. microscope fitted with a 6 V 10 W or 6 V 20 W lamp (see subunit 4.3) or small bench brushed motor variable speed centrifuge having a consumption power of 100 Watt (see subunit 4.7). It is not suitable for high power consumption equipment such as water baths, heat blocks, etc. Always seek the advice of a qualified electrician before using any equipment with the *Handy Mains* inverter. The unit is shown in Plate 4.1.

Important: When used to power equipment in the laboratory the *200 Watt Handy Mains* inverter *must* be used with a residual current device (RCD) safety adaptor (power breaking trip) of the type No. 184-3842.

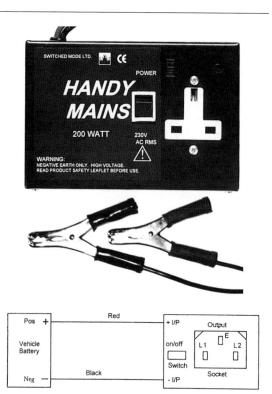

Plate 4.1 SM 2716 Switched Mode *200 Watt Handy Mains Inverter* showing cable and clips for attachment to a 12 V lead-acid battery.

The SM 2716 unit has a 12 V input voltage and is supplied with red and black leads for attachment to a 12 V lead-acid battery. It has an output voltage of 240 V AC via a standard 13 A socket. When used in the laboratory the RCD safety adaptor plugs into the 13 A socket of the inverter and the three pin plug of the equipment plugs into the socket of the RCD adaptor. There is a switch on the unit to enable the output to be turned on and off without disconnecting the unit from the battery. At the end of the day's work the unit must be disconnected from the battery and the equipment unplugged.

The *Handy Mains* 2716 inverter is fitted with an audible warning that sounds when the battery is becoming excessively discharged. The tone begins to sound at around 10.5 V DC and it becomes louder until the unit turns off at around 9.5 V DC to protect the battery (removing the battery connection to the adaptor resets the inverter).

Caution: High voltages exist inside the SM 2716 inverter. It should be treated in the same way as a mains electricity supply. The inverter must not be opened by the user, only by a qualified electrician, e.g. should a fuse need to be replaced. No one should open the unit until it has been disconnected from the battery for at least 2 hours. Lethal voltages may persist inside the inverter for up to 2 hours after disconnection. Before using the SM 2716 read carefully the information that accompanies the unit. Consult a qualified electrician if any part of the manufacturer's literature is not understood, particularly the safety aspects.

Availability of SM 2716 and RCD 184-3842
The *200 W Handy Mains* SM 2716 inverter and RCD safety adaptor No 184-3842 (must be used with the inverter in the laboratory) are available from Durbin plc (see Appendix 11). The SM 2716 inverter has a Durbin catalogue number ER 092 01L and the RCD safety adaptor, catalogue number ER 092 02L.

Further technical information relating to the SM 2716 inverter
Input voltage: 11–15 V DC continuous, 10–18 V DC for 10 seconds. No load current, 0.4 A typical.

Output voltage: 240 V AC rms nominal, 216–255 V AC overload range up to 1.1 A. The output voltage in stepped square waveform, quasi sine wave. Output is by a BS 1363 13 A UK socket.

Output power: The SM 2716 unit has an output power of 250 W short term with a surge capability of up to 500 W and continuous power availability of 200 W.

USE OF BATTERIES

Laboratory equipment that can operate from a DC supply using rechargeable batteries is particularly useful in areas where mains AC electricity supplies are restricted but sufficient for a mains charger to be used to recharge a 12 volt lead-acid battery or rechargeable nickel-cadmium batteries. In developing countries lead-acid batteries are more available and affordable.

In areas where there is no mains AC electricity supply, it may be appropriate to use solar (photovoltaic) energy to recharge 12 V batteries.

Efficient, cost effective, and safe use of equipment from a battery

Achieved by:

- Using low energy consumption equipment and a battery system of adequate capacity.
- Selecting a battery that can withstand deep discharging.
- Controlling the discharge and charge cycle of the battery.
- Maintaining the battery correctly.
- Being aware of the hazards involved, particularly when using 12 V lead-acid batteries.

Calculating energy requirement of equipment and capacity of battery needed

The electrical requirement of equipment (power rating) in watt-hours (Wh) per day is calculated as follows:

Power of equipment (W) $\times$ Expected daily use (h) = Wh/day

The power rating in watts of equipment will usually be written on a plate or label on the back of the equipment or given in the *User Manual*. If only the volts (V) and amps (A) are given, multiply V $\times$ A to obtain wattage (W).

Examples from a district laboratory

- To calculate the Wh/day for two microscopes each with a rating of 10 W and being used for a total of 8 hours each day:
  $2 \times 10 \times 8 = 160$ Wh

- To calculate the Wh/day for a centrifuge with a rating of 96 W and being used for a total of 0.5 hours each day (i.e. ten times for 3 minutes):
  $96 \times 0.5 = 48$ Wh

- To calculate the Wh/day for a colorimeter with a rating of 2 W and being used for a total of 2 hours each day:
  $2 \times 2 = 4$ Wh

Using the above examples the total Wh for the load i.e. all the equipment, is $160 + 48 + 4 = 212$ Wh

To power this equipment, using a 12 V lead-acid battery from which no more than 20% of its energy

is removed and replaced daily, the capacity of battery required can be calculated as follows:

$$\frac{212 \times 100}{12 \times 20} = 88 \text{ Ah}$$

i.e. a battery of capacity 100 Ah would be suitable.

Note: If able to use a deep cycle 12 V lead-acid battery that can be discharged to 50% of its capacity (see later text), the size of battery required would be

$$\frac{212 \times 100}{12 \times 50} = 35 \text{ Ah}$$

In practice the available capacity of a battery depends on the type of battery, its age and condition, and particularly the discharge current i.e. how quickly the battery is used. Both battery efficiency and available capacity are reduced as the discharge current is increased. At lower rates of discharge (C/10 to C/100), efficiency is around 90% whereas at higher rates of discharge (C/1 to C/5), efficiency falls to around 60%.

The capacity of a lead-acid battery is also affected by temperature. At higher temperatures a battery holds more charge. Over about 40 °C, however, battery life is reduced.

Note: Full performance specifications of lead-acid batteries are provided by manufacturers.

Using and maintaining 12 V lead-acid batteries

Understanding how a lead-acid battery works, selecting the most suitable type, and using it correctly are important for the reliable performance of 12 V DC equipment, and for maximizing the life of the battery, and preventing battery related accidents.

How a 12 V lead-acid battery works

Most 12 V lead-acid storage batteries consist of six lead acid-cells joined in series to produce direct current. Each cell contains negative lead (Pb) electrode plates and positive lead dioxide (PbO_2) plates immersed in an electrolyte solution of sulphuric acid (H_2SO_4) having a relative specific gravity of 1.240 (tropical specification).

During discharge, i.e. when the battery is being used, electricity is generated by the electrochemical reactions that take place between the lead plates and the sulphuric acid. Part of the material of both plates is converted to lead sulphate ($PbSO_4$) and the concentration of the electrolyte is reduced as the sulphuric acid is used and water is produced.

During recharge, a battery charger forces electrons through the battery in a direction opposite to that of the discharge process. This reverses the chemical reactions, restoring the electrolyte concentration and electrode materials to their original form.

Battery cycle and depth of discharge

One discharge and charge period is referred to as a battery cycle. A major factor affecting battery life is depth of discharge, i.e. how much the battery is discharged and how often. The depth of discharge of a battery is a measure in percentage of the amount of energy which can be removed from a battery during a cycle. Limiting the depth of discharge will make the battery last longer. If discharged beyond its recommended depth of discharge, the life of a battery will be considerably reduced. The state of discharge of a battery can be measured using a voltmeter or reading the specific gravity of the electrolyte in the cells.

To power 12 V electrical laboratory equipment, a battery that can be deeply discharged is recommended, i.e. *deep cycle battery*. This type of battery is designed to have 40–80% of its charge removed and repeatedly replaced 1 000–2 000 times.

In developing countries, true deep cycling 12 V lead-acid batteries are usually available only from the suppliers of photovoltaic equipment. Other 12 V lead-acid batteries with some of the features of deep cycle batteries may be obtainable locally as portable 'solar' (improved vehicle) batteries, monobloc traction or semi-traction motive batteries (e.g. for powering wheelchairs), and batteries used for leisure activities.

Note: Whenever possible avoid using shallow discharge 12 V lead-acid vehicle (automotive) batteries that have thin plates. They are not designed for stationary use but for supplying a heavy current for a short period followed by immediate recharge from a running vehicle. If such a battery has to be used, no more than 20% of its charge should be removed. It should be charged as soon as possible after discharge, and not overcharged.

Sealed and low maintenance 12 V lead-acid batteries
Sealed batteries are commonly available for use in vehicles but deep cycle sealed gel (captive electrolyte) and absorptive electrolyte type batteries are also obtainable but expensive. Sealed batteries do not leak or spill and require no topping up of electrolyte. They are therefore easily transported and suitable for powering portable equipment.

Compared with vented 12 V lead-acid batteries, sealed 12 V batteries have a shorter life and their discharge and charge cycle require more careful control. A special regulated charger matched to the battery must be used to avoid damage from overcharging. A sealed battery cannot be supplied dry-charged and therefore there is risk of the battery being damaged should it have to be stored or is held in customs for several weeks before it can be charged. Self-discharge will be rapid in temperatures over 40 °C.

What are referred to as low maintenance 12 V lead-acid batteries are also available which require little or no maintenance if discharged and charged correctly. Unlike a sealed battery, the vent caps can be removed to check the level and density of the electrolyte.

Correct and safe use of vented 12 V lead-acid batteries
■ Read the manufacturer's information and in-

structions supplied with the battery. If the battery is supplied dry-charged, i.e. without the electrolyte added, follow carefully the instructions for filling it with electrolyte.

Caution: The electrolyte in lead-acid batteries is a sulphuric acid solution. It is highly corrosive and dangerous. When making a solution of the acid, add the acid to the water, NEVER ADD WATER TO CONCENTRATED SULPHURIC ACID. Wear chemical resistant gloves and protect the eyes, face, and clothing from acid burns (see First Aid, subunit 3.8).

Where to locate a 12 V lead-acid battery
■ Store the battery upright in a secure and dry place, protected from direct sunlight, rain, dew, and excessive dust. Place the battery in a special wooden ventilated battery box or on a block of wood, not directly on the floor, particularly a cement floor.

Make sure the area is well ventilated and kept free from naked flames e.g. from Bunsen burners, matches, lighted tapers. Display 'No Smoking' notices.

Caution: During charging, hydrogen is evolved which can be explosive if allowed to build-up in a non-ventilated place.

Connecting and disconnecting the battery
■ Connect the leads to a battery correctly, i.e. positive (+) lead to the positive terminal (often coloured red), and the negative (−) lead to the negative terminal (often coloured black or blue). Do not allow the lead from one terminal to touch the opposite terminal.

■ Whenever possible use secure clamped battery connections and special DC wall power sockets.

■ Before disconnecting a battery, turn off the equipment the battery is powering.

■ When disconnecting, always remove one lead at a time and DO NOT ALLOW the positive and negative leads or connections to touch. *Touching will cause a dangerous shorting between the terminals.*

■ When in use, make sure the lead from one battery terminal does not lie across the opposite terminal as this will cause the lead to burn.

Shorting between battery terminals.
When an accidental connection is made between the positive and negative terminals of a battery, a path of low resistance is created through which a dangerously high current of electricity can flow which can cause burning, fire, and even explosion of the battery. *Users of batteries must be aware of this serious hazard.*

Caution: As a safety precaution, before touching a battery, always remove any metal objects from the hands, wrists, and neck such as watch straps or jewellery. Also remove metal spatulas and scissors etc, that may fall out of pockets. If using a tool, make sure it has an insulated handle. Never leave metal objects on top of a battery.

Maintenance

- To prevent tracking of electricity on the surface of a battery between terminals, keep the top of the battery dry and dirt-free. Tracking can be dangerous and will increase the self-discharge of a battery.

- To prevent corrosion of the battery terminals and connections, lightly coat the metal surfaces with petroleum grease, e.g. vaseline (do not use oil). If corrosion forms, clean it off using a weak solution of sodium bicarbonate, i.e. about 5 g dissolved in 50 ml of water. Wear rubber gloves and eye protection. Wash off the neutralized acid with water, dry, and apply vaseline to the metal surfaces.

- Inspect regularly (at least once a week) the level of electrolyte in each cell of the battery. The correct level is the top of the level indicator (normally marked). For most 12 V DC vented batteries the electrolyte level should be 9–12 mm above the plates but read the manufacturer's instructions.

- If the level of the electrolyte is below that recommended, top it up using deionized or distilled water (from a non-metallic container) or special 'battery water' available from most garages. Do not overfill as this will cause the electrolyte to overflow during charging. Topping up should be carried out when the battery is fully charged.

  Important: Never use tap water to top up a battery as this will contain impurities that will alter the electrolyte and seriously reduce the efficiency and life of the battery. If the level of electrolyte is consistently low, as shown by excessive gassing (bubbling), this indicates that the battery is being overcharged.

Charging and discharging

- Do not take more energy out of a battery than is recommended. As previously explained, permissible depth of discharge will depend on the type of battery (up to 50% can be removed from deep cycle batteries but only up to 20% from vehicle batteries). The state of charge of a battery should be checked weekly and its depth of discharge controlled to maximize the life of the battery.

- To check the depth of discharge, measure the density (specific gravity) of the electrolyte using a battery hydrometer or the voltage of the battery using a voltmeter.

  Note: The more a battery is discharged, the more dilute the sulphuric acid becomes and the lower will be the specific gravity reading. Voltage also decreases as a battery is being discharged. Measuring the specific gravity is more accurate than measuring the voltage when determining the state of charge of a vented lead-acid battery and its individual cells.

  Interpretation of specific gravity (SG) results for tropical countries

SG	1.230 = 100% charge	SG	1.161 = 50% charge
	1.216 = 90%		1.147 = 40%
	1.203 = 80%		1.134 = 30%
	1.189 = 70%		1.120 = 20%
	1.175 = 60%		

- Recharge a battery as soon as possible after discharge. NEVER leave a battery for a long period in a discharged state because the plates will become permanently damaged. Make sure the area is well ventilated as hydrogen gas is evolved during charging.

- Avoid using a rapid charge at high current as this can damage the battery. Do not charge at a current that is more than one tenth of the rated capacity of the battery. Ideally, charge batteries up to 90 Ah at 3–4 A and higher rated batteries at 5–7 A.

- Use a regulated taper charger. This will ensure the current decreases (tapers down) as the charge progresses. It will prevent the temperature of the electrolyte rising as the battery becomes charged. If the temperature rises to above 38°C, stop charging and wait until the electrolyte cools.

  Charging is complete when the cells are bubbling (gassing) freely.

Important: Repeated overcharging of a battery causes evaporation of the electrolyte and corrosion of the plates which will result in rapid failure of the battery. The charging, particularly of sealed batteries, must be carefully controlled and the correct type of charger used. A battery should not be discharged and charged more than once in 24 hours.

Self-discharge: A 12 V lead-acid battery in good condition will not self-discharge more than about 5% per month. An old battery in poor condition can lose up to 40% of its capacity per month if not charged regularly and kept clean and its surface dry.

Charging from solar panels: When charging a 12 V lead-acid battery from a solar panel, a voltage regulator must be used. Advice on the use of photovoltaic (PV) energy can be obtained from the organization FAKT and Healthlink Worldwide (see Appendix 11).

Nickel-cadmium rechargeable batteries

Nickel-cadmium (NiCd or nicads) are available as:

- Small-capacity sealed batteries (similar in sizes to non-rechargeable dry batteries), e.g. AA size of 300–700 mAh, up to D size of 4 000 mAh (4 Ah) and 5 Ah.
- High capacity NiCd batteries suitable for use in photovoltaic systems.

While sealed NiCd batteries are commonly available, higher capacity NiCd batteries are difficult to obtain particularly in developing countries. They are considerably more expensive than lead-acid batteries but last much longer (up to 20 years).

Important characteristics of vented NiCd batteries

Compared with lead-acid batteries, vented NiCd batteries have several important advantages:

- they can be fully discharged (100% depth of discharge) and left discharged without becoming damaged.
- can withstand overcharging.
- loss of electrolyte is low and therefore topping up is required only occasionally.
- for a given load, the capacity of a NiCd battery can be lower than that needed when using a lead-acid battery (because of its 100% depth of discharge).
- when used in a PV system, a voltage regulator is not required.

Correct use of sealed NiCd batteries

NiCd batteries do not always function reliably in tropical climates. To maximize the cell life and capacity of *sealed* NiCd batteries:

- Allow the batteries to discharge completely before recharging them (do not 'top up' the charge between use).
- Recharge close to the time of use in a *cool dry* place because sealed NiCd batteries rapidly lose their charge during storage particularly in hot humid tropical conditions.
- Use a NiCd charger of the correct capacity and voltage for the batteries being charged. Charge slowly and fully.

- Store recharged batteries (few days only) in a cool dry place, preferably in a refrigerator in a sealed box containing a desiccant.

Note: Further information on the use of batteries and solar energy can be found in the publication *Selection of basic laboratory equipment for laboratories with limited resources* (see Recommended Reading).

Meaning of electrical terms used in this subunit

Voltage: The electrical potential across any two points in a circuit, measured in volts (V). It is the 'push' that makes the electric current flow around a circuit. In Europe and many countries AC supplies are at 220–240 V, whereas in USA and a few other countries, consumer supplies are at 110 V.

Spike: Instantaneous dramatic increase in voltage.

Surge: Short-term increase in voltage

Sag: (brownout): Short-term decrease in voltage levels.

Current: The amount of electricity flowing through any wire or other conductor measured in amperes, or amps (A). There are 1 000 milliamps (mA) in 1 amp. The current may be alternating current (AC) or direct current (DC). If watts (W) and volts (V) are known, amps (A) can be calculated: $A = \dfrac{W}{V}$.

Alternating current (AC or a.c.): Electric current in which the direction of flow changes rapidly all the time.

Frequency: The number of complete cycles per second of an AC supply measured in hertz (Hz), e.g. 50 Hz or 60 Hz.

Phase: The 'live' connections in an AC supply. Three phase supplies are used by large industrial and commercial consumers. Single phase supplies are used for smaller domestic consumers. A single phase will be found in most laboratories fitted with wall sockets.

Direct current (DC or d.c.): Electric current in which the direction of the current does not reverse but remains the same, from the positive to the negative as in a battery system.

Transformer: An AC device which converts power at one voltage to another e.g. 240 V to 110 V or *vice versa*.

Inverter: Device that can convert the DC stored in batteries to mains voltage AC current, enabling mains electrical equipment to be used with a 12 V battery.

Electrical power: Refers to how much work the electricity can do, i.e. the rate of delivery or use of electrical energy. It is measured in watts (W) and is calculated as follows:

Power (W) = Voltage (V) × Current (A), i.e. W = V × A. There are 1 000 W in 1 kilowatt (kW).

Electrical energy: Refers to the total amount of electricity produced or used in a given period. It is measured in watt-hours (Wh) and is calculated as follows:

Energy (Wh) = Power (W) × Time (hours).

There are 1 000 Wh in 1 kilowatt hour (kWh).

Battery capacity in Ah: The total number of amp-hours (Ah) that can be removed from a fully charged battery at a specified discharge rate.

4.3 Microscope

A microscope is the most expensive and important piece of equipment used in district laboratories. Microscopy forms 70–90% of the work.

Microscopy in district laboratories

- malaria
- trypanosomiasis
- leishmaniasis
- onchocerciasis
- lymphatic filariasis
- loiasis
- schistosomiasis
- amoebiasis
- giardiasis
- cryptosporidiosis
- intestinal worm infections
- paragonimiasis
- tuberculosis
- leprosy
- meningitis
- gonorrhoea (male)
- cholera
- urinary tract infections
- trichomoniasis
- vaginal candidiasis
- red cells in anaemia
- white cell changes
- skin mycoses

WORKING PRINCIPLE OF A MICROSCOPE

A microscope is a magnifying instrument. The magnified image of the object (specimen) is first produced by a lens close to the object called the objective. This collects light from the specimen and forms the primary image. A second lens near the eye called the eyepiece enlarges the primary image, converting it into one that can enter the pupil of the eye.

The magnification of the objective multiplied by that of the eyepiece, gives the total magnification of the image seen in microscopes having a mechanical tube length (MTL) of 160 mm. The MTL is the distance between the shoulder of an objective and the rim of the eyepiece.

Examples

Objective magnification	Eyepiece magnification	Total magnification
10×	10×	100 diameters
40×	10×	400 diameters
100×	10×	1 000 diameters

Useful magnification

The objective provides all the detail available in the image. The eyepiece makes the detail large enough to be seen but provides no information not already present in the primary image formed by the objective. The magnification of eyepiece used should therefore be adequate to enable the relevant detail in the primary image to be seen clearly. Increasing

further the magnification will reveal no more detail but only an image that is more highly magnified and increasingly blurred.

Note: The range of total magnifications within which details in the object are seen clearly in the image (useful magnification) is usually taken as between 500 and 1 000 times the numerical aperture of the objective (see following text).

Resolving and defining power of an objective

An objective accepts light leaving the specimen over a wide angle and recombines the diverging rays to form a point-for-point image of the specimen. Objectives of varying magnifications allow a specimen to be examined in broad detail over a wide area, and in increasing detail over a smaller area.

This increase in magnifying power is always linked to an increase in resolving power. The higher the resolving power of an objective, the closer can be the fine lines or small dots in the specimen which the objective can separate in the image.

The resolving power of an objective is therefore of great importance. It is dependent on what is known as the numerical aperture (NA) of the objective. The NA of an objective is an exact figure that has been worked out mathematically from its equivalent focal length and lens diameter. It is not necessary to know the details of this calculation. Both the NA and magnification of an objective are usually engraved on it. The following are the usual NAs of commonly used objectives:

10× objective	NA 0.25
20× objective	0.45
40× objective	0.65
100× (oil) objective	1.25

Working of an oil immersion objective

When a beam of light passes from air into glass it is bent and when it passes back from glass to air it is bent back again to its original direction. This has little effect on low power objectives but with high power lenses this bending limits not only the amount of light which can enter the lens but also affects the NA of the objective and consequently its resolving power.

The bending effect and its limitations on the objective can be avoided by replacing the air between the specimen and the lens with an oil which has the same optical properties as glass, i.e. immersion oil. When the correct oil is used, the light passes in a straight line from glass through the oil and back to glass as though it were passing through glass all the way (see Fig. 4.1). By collecting extra oblique light, the oil provides better resolution and a brighter image. Some 50× objectives and all 100× objectives are used immersed in oil.

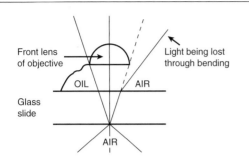

Fig. 4.1 Working principle of an oil immersion objective.

In tropical climates the use of synthetic non-drying immersion oil is recommended.

Chromatic and spherical aberrations

How well an objective is able to define outlines clearly and distinctly depends on how perfectly it has been corrected for chromatic and spherical aberrations. Chromatic aberration is when a biconvex lens splits white light into its component colours and blue light is magnified slightly more than red light so that it comes to a focus nearer to the lens. Spherical aberration is caused by the edge of a lens giving a slightly higher magnification than its centre.

Manufacturers of objectives are able to correct for chromatic and spherical aberrations by combining lenses of different dispersive powers. In recent years a new concept of correction has been developed which includes the entire imaging system as a unit and is referred to as the chromatic-free, or CF system.

Achromats

Achromatic objectives, or achromats, are the most widely used of objectives. In most achromats, chromatic aberrations are corrected for two wavelengths and spherical aberrations are corrected for one wavelength.

Semi-apochromats (fluorite objectives) and apochromats

These objectives are corrected for three wavelengths chromatically and two spherically. They are considerably more expensive than achromats and only required for specialized work. Apochromats have high NAs and therefore the image they produce is sharper but only in focus in the central part of the field due to field curvature. The correct thickness of coverglass must be used. Compensating eyepieces need to be used with apochromats.

Illumination system of the microscope

An adequate, well-aligned, and controllable illumination system is required for good microscopy. This can be achieved by using a microscope with built-in illumination. Whenever possible daylight illumi-nation should be avoided because it is variable, difficult to use, and rarely adequate for oil immersion work.

A substage condenser is used to collect, control, and focus light on the object. It projects a cone of light matching the NA of the objective, controlled by the iris diaphragm. It also projects an image of the light source onto the specimen. The light should just fill the field of view of the eyepiece and back lens of the objective uniformly or the image will not be good.

It is particularly important to avoid glare and reflections in the microscope and to adjust the condenser aperture correctly for each objective and when examining different specimens. To check for glare, the eyepiece can be removed and the inside of the microscope tube inspected. Glare is present if the inside of the tube is illuminated.

How to minimize glare

Glare in the microscope is caused by any light reaching the eye which does not go to make up the perfect image but interferes with it and the ability of the objective to distinguish detail in a specimen.

The following are the most practical ways of reducing glare in routine work:

– Position a microscope with built-in illumination in subdued light, not in front of a window. When this cannot be done, an eyeshade can help to exclude external glare.

– Avoid using a larger source of illumination than is necessary. If using an adjustable light source, adjust the light to illuminate no more than the field of view.

– Reduce condenser glare by reducing the condenser aperture, i.e. adjusting the iris diaphragm, when using low power objectives. This will increase contrast but with some loss of resolving power which is unavoidable.

Some kinds of specimen give more glare than others. A stained blood film or bacterial smear with no cover glass and examined with the oil immersion objective gives little glare and should therefore be examined always with the condenser iris wide open.

Unstained particles suspended in water or physiological saline under a cover glass and examined with the 10× objective, give considerable glare. Preparations such as cerebrospinal fluid, urine, or wet unstained faecal preparations require examination with the condenser iris considerably reduced.

Tungsten and halogen illumination

A quartz halogen illumination is preferred to a tungsten illumination because it gives a consistent bright white illumination. Most modern microscopes with built-in illumination systems use low wattage halogen lamps for transmitted light microscopy e.g. 6 V 20 W or 6 V 10 W.

A tungsten illumination gives a yellow light and its intensity becomes less as the bulb blackens with age. If a tungsten illumination only is available, a *pale* blue filter should be inserted in the filter holder (see following text).

Filters

The following are the main uses of filters in microscopy:

- To reduce the intensity of light when this is required. A ground glass light diffusing filter is used to decrease the brilliance of a light source.

- To increase contrast and resolution. As previously mentioned, a blue daylight filter is commonly used with an electric 'yellow' tungsten lamp. This increases resolution. Green filters also increase resolution.

- To transmit light of a selected wavelength, e.g. an excitation filter used in fluorescence microscopy.

- To protect the eye from injury caused by ultra-violet light e.g. a barrier filter as used in fluores-cence microscopy.

SELECTING A MICROSCOPE FOR USE IN DISTRICT LABORATORIES

The stained smears and wet preparations examined in district laboratories require the use of a standard medical microscope.

Binocular model

Whenever possible a binocular microscope should be available for use in district hospital laboratories and busy health centres. A binocular head enables the user to see the image with both eyes at once. This is more restful particularly when examining specimens for prolonged periods. Using a binocular microscope tends to improve the quality of micro-scopical work.

Increase in magnification when using a binocular head
In some models of binocular microscope the design of the binocular head lengthens the tube length, resulting in an increase in the magnification of the microscope, usually by a factor of ×1.5.

A monocular microscope is suitable for health centres with a low workload or when daylight is the only available source of illumination. When using a binocular microscope the prism system in the

binocular head halves the light, making daylight insufficient when using the 100× oil immersion objective. Whenever possible a monocular micro-scope should be fitted with a viewing aid to prevent the eye not in use from being distracted by light and surrounding objects (see Fig. 4.2). Such a viewing aid can be made locally.

Trinocular head
What is called a trinocular head attachment consists of an inclined binocular with a protruding tube and sliding prism. The additional tube is used for attaching a camera for photo-micrography work.

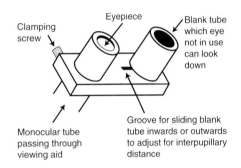

Fig. 4.2 Viewing aid for fitting to a monocular microscope (Elcomatic design).

Eyepieces

The microscope should be supplied with 10× wide-field eyepieces.

7× eyepieces for use with the 100× oil immersion objective: These lower magnification eyepieces produce a brighter and sharper image. For malaria microscopy, the World Health Organization recommends the use of 7× eyepieces.[3, 4]

Compensating eyepieces: These eyepieces are re-quired for use with fluorite and apochromatic objec-tives. Although they can be used with achromatic objectives they are more expensive than other standard eyepieces and not required.

High-eyepoint eyepieces: Some manufacturers equip their microscopes with high-eyepoint eyepieces which help spectacle wearers to use a microscope without removing their spectacles e.g. a person wearing spectacles to correct for astigmatism. High-eyepoint eyepieces also avoid sweating onto the eye lenses and are therefore useful in tropical climates.

Built-in illumination

Whenever possible select a microscope that has:

- A built-in illumination system that uses a 6 V 10 W or 6 V 20 W halogen lamp that can be operated from an AC mains electricity supply and preferably also from a DC battery supply (see later text).

■ A rotary brightness control.

■ A base illuminator that can be easily replaced with a mirror unit (to be supplied with the microscope) should the built-in illumination fail.

Caution: Low cost binocular microscopes with built-in illumination systems are widely available but not all have the same safety standards and use approved reliable electrical components.

It is therefore important to enquire before purchasing a microscope with built-in illumination whether it has any safety certification. If in doubt, have the electrical system checked by a qualified electrician before purchasing and using the microscope. Examine particularly the wiring of the circuitry and whether any live terminals are easily accessible. Check whether the transformer is properly insulated and provides short-circuit protection to avoid it becoming a fire hazard. Also check that the earth connections are adequate and that fuses of the correct rating have been used.

Long life halogen lamps
Several microscope manufacturers use small capsule type halogen lamps as their source of illumination. Halogen illumination provides excellent white light for microscopy. The capsule halogen lamps commonly used for routine transmitted light microscopy are 6 V 10 W and 6 V 20 W. It is best to buy those halogen lamps that give the longest life, i.e. 2 000 average life hours:

– For 6 V 10 W halogen lamps, obtain those coded M42.
– For 6 V 20 W halogen lamps, obtain those coded M34.

Manufacturers include GE (General Electric), Phillips, and Osram.

Operating a mains microscope from a 12 V DC battery
In areas where mains electricity supplies are restricted or intermittent, it is useful to be able to operate a microscope with built-in illumination from both AC mains electricity and a DC 12 V lead-acid battery.

A microscope with built-in illumination using a 6 V 10 W or 6 V 20 W lamp that is normally operated from a mains AC supply can be operated from a 12 V lead-acid battery by using an inverter such as the *200 Watt Handy Mains* inverter unit SM 2716 with a residual current device (RCD) as explained in subunit 4.2. Alternatively the microscope can be rewired by an electrician to operate directly from a 6 V battery.

Note: As explained in subunit 4.2, a 12 V lead-acid battery will require regular charging.

Battery and mains power microscope
The *Tropical Medicine Microscope* manufactured by Gillet and Sibert Elcomatic is one of the few microscopes that has been designed for use with both AC mains electricity and a 12 V lead-acid battery. It has a 6 V 10 W halogen built-in illumination system, and is fitted with battery terminals. Battery leads are supplied.

A 12 V sealed lead-acid battery with charger and regulator, and a solar panel to charge the battery are available as accessories.

Availability of the Tropical Medicine Microscope
The mains and battery powered binocular *Tropical Medicine Microscope* model GS-10B is available from Elcomatic Ltd (see Appendix 11). It is equipped with 10× widefield eyepieces and 10× 40× and 100× achromatic objectives.

Objectives
The following objectives are required for district laboratory work:

■ 10× achromatic objective
■ 40× achromatic objective
■ 100× oil immersion achromatic objective
■ If available, a 20× or 25× achromatic objective is useful for examining centrifuged blood in capillary tubes (to detect motile trypanosomes and microfilariae).

Flatfield (plan) objectives
These popular objectives have additional lenses to correct for field curvature, i.e. they flatten the image across the field so that the entire field of view appears in focus at the same time.

Achromatic objectives are available as flatfield plan-achromats but are more expensive than the standard achromats.

Objectives for infinity corrected microscope systems
Most microscope objectives are made to work with microscopes having a standard 160 mm tubelength (160 mm is usually engraved on the objectives).

What are called infinity corrected objectives have recently been introduced by microscope manufacturers to meet the needs of specialist and research laboratories. Such objectives are computed for an 'infinite' optical tubelength and therefore allow for extra components to be easily inserted in the system. An accessory lens is fitted in the tube of the microscope so that a real image is formed in the focal plane of the eyepiece. Microscopes using infinity corrected systems are expensive and not needed for routine transmitted light microscopy.

Important: When ordering or needing to replace objectives for standard 160 mm tubelength microscopes, it is important to state that the objectives are for use with this tubelength of microscope. The figure 0.17 is often also engraved on objectives. This refers to the thickness in mm of cover glass with which the objective has been designed to work best.

Mechanical stage

A mechanical stage holds a slide in place and enables it to be examined in a controlled way. The specimen can be moved systematically up and down and across the stage, i.e. X and Y movements. The following type of mechanical stage is needed:

- Integral, smooth running mechanical stage.
- Preferably with vernier scales to enable specimens to be easily relocated.

Important: The type of mechanical stage that is supplied as an accessory and fitted to a microscope stage by one or two screws is not sufficiently reliable or robust for district laboratory work. It usually gives a less precise movement of the specimen and often requires repairing within a short period of time.

DIN standard for objectives

Most modern microscopes of 160 mm tubelength are fitted with DIN objectives. DIN is the abbreviation used to describe the German published standards relating to the measurement of objectives and other microscopical measurements. The DIN distance of an object to the shoulder of an objective is set at 45 mm. DIN objectives are longer than other objectives and should not therefore be interchanged with them. DIN objectives will only be parfocal with other DIN objectives.

Objectives found on older microscopes are usually engraved with their equivalent focal lengths, e.g. 16 mm for a 10× objective, 4 mm for a 40× objective, and 2 mm for a 100× objective.

Spring-loaded objectives

The high power objectives (40× and 100×) of modern microscopes are spring-loaded, i.e. the front mount of the objective will be pushed in rather than pushed through a specimen if such an objective is accidentally pressed against a specimen when focusing. Spring-loaded objectives help to protect a specimen and the front lens of an objective from being damaged.

Condenser and iris

The following type of condenser and fittings are recommended for routine transmitted light microscopy:

- Abbe type condenser with iris diaphragm.
- Facility to centre the condenser in its mount unless precentred by the manufacturer.
- Fitted with a filter holder of the swing-out type.

The importance of using the iris to increase or reduce the condenser aperture is described under *Use of a microscope*. If the lever which is used to open and close the iris is difficult to locate below the stage, it is recommended that the user lengthen the iris lever e.g. with a plastic sleeve (some microscope manufacturers do this).

Other condensers

Condenser with swing-out top lens (flip-top): Some microscopes are fitted with a condenser which has an upper lens which can be moved aside when using a very low power objective. This enables the light to fill the much larger field of view of the lower power objective. It is usually necessary also to lower the substage slightly. Such a condenser is not required for district laboratory work.

Achromatic-aplanatic condensers: These condensers are highly corrected for chromatic and spherical aberrations and are therefore expensive. They are not needed for routine transmitted light microscopy.

Focusing controls

The focusing mechanisms of the microscope must be:

- Smooth, particularly the fine focusing control.
- Reliable, robust, and not subject to drift.

Many modern microscopes have concentric coarse and fine focus knobs as shown in Plate 4.2.

Adjustable focus tension

This is shown in Plate 4.2. Turning the focus tension adjustment collar clockwise tightens the focus tension while turning the collar anti-clockwise loosens it. This allows the user to adjust the focus tension to suit their own preference. Care must be taken, however, not to loosen the focus tension too much otherwise the stage will drop downwards by itself and the specimen will drift out of focus.

Focus stop

Some microscopes are also fitted as standard with a focus stop mechanism operated by a lever located next to the left hand focusing control. The focus stop is used to prevent the stage from being moved upwards beyond a certain point (intended to protect the front lens of an objective from damage).

If a new microscope is received and it is not possible to focus a specimen because the focus stop is restricting the upward movement of the stage, the focus stop lever will need to be moved downwards to rest against the bar situated below the coarse focusing control. This will give unrestricted upward movement of the stage for focusing the specimen. When a microscope is used correctly a focus stop mechanism is not required.

Summary of the essential specifications of a microscope for district laboratory use

- Binocular microscope (160 mm tubelength), supplied with:
  - pair of 10× widefield eyepieces
  - if available, also pair of 7× eyepieces.
- Equipped with 10×, 40×, and 100× (oil) achromatic DIN objectives.
- Substage Abbe condenser, preferably pre-centred in mount, with iris and swing-out filter holder.
- Integral mechanical stage.
- Smooth and reliable coarse and fine focusing controls.
- Built-in illumination using a low wattage quartz halogen lamp, i.e. 6 V 10 W or 6 V 20 W.
- Electrical safety certification.
- Mirror unit.
- Supplied with non-drying immersion oil.

Tropical Health Technology Microscope

The Tropical Health Technology binocular microscope THT.BM shown in Plate 4.2 is suitable for district laboratory work. It is supplied with built-in 6 V 20 W halogen illumination, integral mechanical stage, achromatic 4×, 10×, 40×, and 100× objectives, 10× widefield high-eyepoint eyepieces and 7× eyepieces, precentred fitted Abbe condenser with iris and swing-out filter holder, mirror, 50 ml non-drying immersion oil, and colour plates to identify parasites, bacteria, and cells in specimens. It operates from 220–230 V 50 Hz AC mains electricity. The *Handy Mains 200 W* inverter as described in subunit 4.2 can be used to operate the microscope from a 12 V lead-acid battery.

The THT.BM microscope is available from Tropical Health Technology (see Appendix 11).

USE OF A MICROSCOPE

To achieve high quality microscopical reporting and prevent damage to the expensive optics and moving parts of a microscope, laboratory staff **must** be trained to use a microscope correctly and to handle it with care.

Using a microscope with built-in illumination

Position the microscope in a shaded part of the room on a secure bench or table that is free from vibration. Do not place it in front of a window where bright daylight will cause unwanted glare.

Use a seat of the correct height, i.e. one that will enable the microscope to be used with the back straight. Too high a seat will cause back and neck strain. If the seat is too high and difficult to adjust, raise the microscope to a convenient height by placing it on a block of wood.

Identifying the parts of the microscope

Use Plate 4.2 or the manufacturer's artwork to identify the essential parts of the microscope. The most important parts to identify are:

- Binocular head and its eyepieces.
- Revolving nosepiece (objective turret) with 10×, 40× and 100× objectives. On some microscopes a 4× objective may also be fitted.
- Mechanical stage with slide holder, spring arm, and movement controls.
- Abbe condenser with iris diaphragm and iris lever.

  Precentred condenser: A single screw will be seen which is used to remove the condenser should it ever become damaged and need repairing. When the condenser is not one that has been precentred, three centring screws will be seen.

- Swing-out filter holder with stop for holding it in place.
- Knob to focus the condenser i.e. move it up and down, positioned on left (not visible in Plate 4.2).
- Coarse and fine focusing controls on each side.
- Illuminator with lens (ground glass, light diffusing screen is located below lens).
- Lamp brightness control.
- Power ON/OFF switch.
- Mains cable socket, located at the back of the microscope.
- Fuse housing.

Setting up the microscope for routine use

The following instructions apply to microscopes fitted with an Abbe condenser and illumination system similar to that shown in Plate 4.2. For microscopes having special condensers and a more complex illumination e.g. illuminator with a field diaphragm, the manufacturer's instructions must be followed.

1 Turn the rotary lamp brightness control anti-clockwise to its lowest setting and then switch on the microscope.

2 Turn up the brightness control to about three quarters of its full power (final adjustment will be made at a later stage).

3 Carefully revolve the nosepiece until the 10× objective is located vertically above the stage. *Make sure there is no danger of the objective*

hitting the stage. If this appears likely, turn the coarse focusing control to increase the distance between the stage and objective (in modern microscopes the stage will move downwards whereas in older microscopes the objectives will move upwards).

4   Prepare a specimen slide such as a mounted stained thin blood film. A temporary mounted preparation can be made by adding a drop of oil to the lower third of the blood film and covering it with a cover glass. Make sure the underside of the slide is dry, clean, and free of stain marks.

5   Place the specimen slide, cover glass uppermost, on the front of the stage. Gently holding back the spring arm of the mechanical stage, push the slide back into the slide holder and release the arm slowly. The specimen will be held firmly.

Important: The spring arm and mechanisms of the mechanical stage can be easily damaged if the surface of the stage or underside of the slide is wet or has oil on it.

6   While looking from the side (not down the eyepieces), turn the coarse focusing control to bring the specimen close to the objective i.e. about 5 mm from the objective.

7   Looking down through the eyepieces, bring the specimen into focus by slowly turning the coarse focusing control in the opposite direction to increase the distance between the specimen and objective. The specimen will come into focus, first as a blurred image and then as a clear image.

Use the fine focusing control to obtain a sharp image (this will not be the best image because the condenser has yet to be focused and the illumination adjusted).

Correct use of a binocular head
The distance between the user's eyes (interpupillary distance) needs to match the distance between the eyepieces of the binocular head. If using the type of binocular head shown in Plate 4.2 (Seidentopf), pull the two bodies of the binocular upwards or downwards. If using a sliding type binocular head, slide the eyepieces nearer or further apart. The distance is correct when the two fields of view merge. If there are several users of the microscope, the interpupillary distance for each user can be recorded from the scale on the binocular head.

Adjust also for any difference in focusing between the eyes. First focus the specimen with the right eye through the fixed eyepiece and then without adjusting the focusing, adjust the left hand moveable eyepiece by turning the collar until the specimen is also in focus with this eyepiece.

8   Focus the condenser as follows:

–   Using the condenser focusing knob located on the left, raise the condenser to its topmost position.

–   Using the iris lever, open the iris fully. Check that the filter holder is located against its stop and not out of position and blocking the light.

–   Looking down the eyepieces and with the specimen in focus, *slowly* lower the condenser until the mottled image of the ground glass light diffusing screen (located below the lens of the illuminator) is seen in the background.

–   Slowly raise the condenser until the mottled image of the diffusing screen just disappears (this is usually about 1 mm below the condenser's topmost position). The condenser is now in focus and should be left in this position.

Note: Do not lower or raise the condenser when changing objectives and examining different specimens. The best images will be achieved by adjusting the lamp brightness control and using the iris lever to adjust the condenser aperture (explained later).

9   Check the centring of the condenser unless the microscope is fitted with a precentred condenser (if precentred there will be no centring screws, only a single screw holding the condenser in its mount). To check the centring of a condenser that is not precentred:

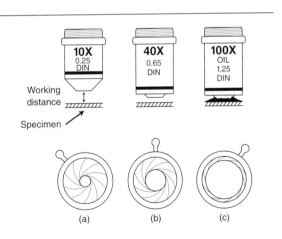

Fig. 4.3 Working distances of 10×, 40×, and 100× objectives and adjustment of condenser iris for each objective. (a) Iris about two thirds closed for 10× objective. (b) Iris open more for 40× objective. (c) Iris fully open for 100× objective. Note how closely the 40× and 100× objectives work to the slide.

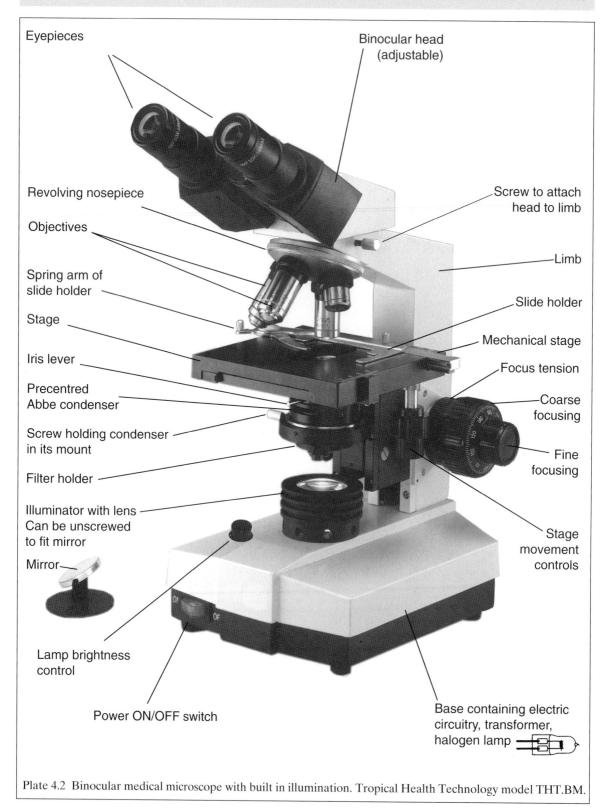

Eyepieces

Binocular head
(adjustable)

Screw to attach
head to limb

Revolving nosepiece

Limb

Objectives

Spring arm of
slide holder

Slide holder

Stage

Mechanical stage

Iris lever

Focus tension

Precentred
Abbe condenser

Coarse
focusing

Screw holding condenser
in its mount

Fine
focusing

Filter holder

Illuminator with lens
Can be unscrewed
to fit mirror

Stage
movement
controls

Mirror

Lamp brightness
control

Power ON/OFF switch

Base containing electric
circuitry, transformer,
halogen lamp

Plate 4.2 Binocular medical microscope with built in illumination. Tropical Health Technology model THT.BM.

– Remove the eyepieces and with the eyes positioned close to the eyepiece tubes, close the iris. Note whether the spot of light seen at the bottom of the eyepiece tubes is centrally located. If it is, the condenser is centred correctly and no adjustment is necessary.

– If the spot of light is off-centre, use the condenser centring screws to adjust the condenser in its mount until the spot of light is centrally placed.

– Replace the eyepieces.

Note: Once centred correctly, the condenser should remain centred unless it is transported when its centring should again be checked before use.

10 Looking down the eyepieces with the specimen in focus, obtain the best possible image by adjusting the condenser aperture and lamp brightness control. For the 10× objective, the condenser will need to be closed about two thirds to provide a good image. Adjust the lamp brightness control to a level which provides good illumination without glare.

Important: Use the lamp brightness control, not the iris to reduce the *intensity* of illumination. If the condenser aperture is closed too much there will be loss of detail (resolution) in the image.

If not sure how far to close the condenser aperture, remove the eyepieces and with the specimen in focus, look down the eyepiece tubes and slowly open and close the iris. The condenser aperture is closed by the correct amount when the edge of the iris just comes into view.

11 Examine the specimen with the 40× objective. Carefully revolve the nosepiece to bring the 40× objective into place. It will locate very close to the specimen. Providing the objectives are parfocal (in focus one with another), only slight focusing with the fine focusing control should be necessary to bring the specimen into sharp focus.

Open the condenser iris more (see Fig. 4.3) and increase the brightness control to obtain a bright clear image.

12 Examine the specimen with the 100× oil immersion objective. Revolve the nosepiece to move the 40× objective to one side and before bringing the 100× objective into position, place a drop of immersion oil on the specimen. Carefully locate the 100× objective. The lens of this objective should just dip into the drop of oil (providing the objectives are parfocal).

Use the fine focusing control to focus the specimen. Open the condenser iris fully and increase the illumination to give a bright clear image.

Non-drying immersion oil
Use a good quality non-drying synthetic immersion oil because this will not dry on a lens should the oil not be removed from the objective after use. *Never mix oils.* When changing oils, always remove completely the previous oil from an objective before using a new oil otherwise the image will appear blurred.

13 Before removing the specimen from under the oil immersion objective, revolve the nosepiece so that the objective moves to one side. Only then remove the slide from the slide holder.

Important: Moving the objective to one side will not alter its focusing. It will prevent what is the commonest way in which *very* expensive oil immersion objectives become damaged and need replacing. Scratching of the 100× objective lens can be easily seen by unscrewing the objective and examining the front lens of the objective with a magnifying lens. When used inverted, one of the eyepieces of the microscope can act as a magnifying lens (remove one of the eyepieces and turn it the other way up).

Note: To achieve high quality microscopy, prepare specimens correctly using standardized staining techniques and preparations of the correct thickness.

Important points when examining specimens

■ Before using a microscope, first clean the eyepieces, objectives, condenser lens, stage, and illuminator lens (explained more fully under *quality control, care and maintenance of the microscope*, see p. 120).

■ Use a cover glass when examining a specimen with the 10× or 40× objective. When using the 100× objective, allow the preparation to dry completely before placing oil on it.

■ *Focus continuously* to avoid organisms and structures in different planes being missed or misidentified.

■ Use the correct magnification of eyepiece and objective. Focus and scan first with a lower power before using a higher magnification.

Summary of how to use a microscope with built-in illumination

1 Position the microscope correctly and identify the essential parts.

2 Before switching on the microscope turn the lamp brilliance control to its lowest setting, then increase it to about three quarters of its power.

3 Bring the 10× objective into place.

4 Make sure the underside of the specimen slide and surface of the stage are completely dry and clean.

5 Place the specimen on the stage in the slide holder.

6 Focus the specimen with the 10× objective.

7 Focus the condenser (should be within 1 mm of its topmost position) and leave it in this position for all objectives.

8 If the microscope is not fitted with a precentred condenser, check the centring of the condenser.

9 *Examine the specimen with the 10× objective.*

Obtain the best image by:
− closing the iris about two thirds,
− adjusting the lamp brightness control to give good illumination with the minimum of glare.

10 Use the mechanical stage to examine the specimen systematically.

11 *Examine the specimen with the 40× objective.*

Obtain the best image by:
− opening the iris more,
− increasing the illumination.

12 *Examine the specimen with the 100× objective.* Move the 40× objective to the side, place a drop of oil on the specimen and bring the 100× objective into position. Obtain the best image by:
− opening the iris fully,
− increasing the illumination.

To prevent damage to the 100× objective lens, move the objective to one side before removing the specimen.

Difficulties in focusing

■ If the microscope is new and has a focus stop, check that this is not restricting the movement of the stage (see previous text *Focus stop*).

■ If using the 100× objective and no image can be focused, check that the oil has been added to the smear side of the slide.

■ If using the 100× objective and the image is not clear, check that sufficient oil has been added. The problem may also be due to a new type of oil being used without all the previous oil being cleaned from the slide and objective.

■ To assist in focusing with the 100× objective, prefocus the specimen first with the 10× objective (do not use the 40× objective unless the preparation is mounted and free of oil).

■ If the image cannot be focused with the 40× objective or is blurred, the objective lens probably has oil on it or has become contaminated from a wet preparation. Revolve the nosepiece and carefully clean the lens.

Note: To differentiate whether dirt seen in the image is from the objective or eyepiece, rotate one of the eyepieces. If the dirt also rotates it is the eyepiece that requires cleaning.

Using a microscope with a lamp and mirror

Whenever possible use a specially designed angled microscope lamp fitted with a halogen bulb, adjustable diaphragm, and lamp brightness control. Many microscope lamps are fitted with low voltage bulbs and therefore a transformer will be needed. Normally this will be supplied with the microscope lamp.

If no special microscope lamp is available, use an angled desk type lamp fitted with an ordinary tungsten opal 60 W bulb. Place a blue daylight filter in the filter holder below the condenser. To reduce the glare, stand in front of the bulb a piece of card with a 50 mm diameter hole cut in it for the light to pass through.

Set up the illumination and focus the condenser as follows:

1 Revolve the binocular head and position the microscope so that the mirror in the base is facing the lamp.

2 Place the front of the lamp about 200 mm away

from the microscope with the bulb directed towards the flat (plane) side of the mirror.

3 Turn on the lamp. If the lamp has a brilliance control, set it about three quarters of its power and if fitted with a diaphragm, open this about halfway.

4 Raise the condenser on the microscope to its topmost position and open the iris fully.

5 Looking down on the upper lens of the condenser, angle the flat side of the mirror to reflect light up through the condenser.

6 Using a specimen such as a mounted stained thin blood film, focus the specimen with the 10× objective (see previous text). Readjust the mirror to obtain the brightest light.

7 *Microscope lamp with diaphragm*
   - Adjust the lamp diaphragm until a hazy image of it appears in the background of the field of view.
   - Lower the condenser slightly until the image of the diaphragm becomes sharply focused. The condenser is now in focus and should be left in this position when using all three objectives.
   - If required, centre the lamp diaphragm.
   - Open the lamp diaphragm until the full field of view is illuminated.

   Lamp without a diaphragm
   - From the topmost position and with the iris fully open, slowly lower the condenser until an image of the lamp, e.g. lettering on the bulb, comes into view.
   - Slowly raise the condenser until the image of the lamp just disappears. The condenser is now in focus and should be left in this position when using all three objectives.

   Note: In practice, for most microscopes with an Abbe condenser, the correct position of the condenser will be within 1 mm of its topmost position which will coincide with the position at which the light is brightest.

8 If the condenser is not one that has been pre-centred by the manufacturer, check its centring (see previous text).

9 Obtain the best possible image by adjusting the condenser iris:
   - For the 10× objective the iris should be about two thirds closed. If the illumination is too bright and the lamp has no brightness

control, do *not* close further the condenser iris because this will result in loss of detail in the image. Use a ground glass filter in the filter holder to reduce the brightness.
   - For the 40× objective, open the condenser iris more.
   - For the 100× objective open the iris fully to obtain maximum illumination.

Using a microscope with daylight and a mirror
Ordinary daylight may be sufficient for some work with a monocular microscope but it is variable and difficult to control. Daylight is scarcely enough for oil immersion work and insufficient for a binocular microscope.

When using a monocular microscope with daylight, set up the illumination and focus the condenser as follows:

1 Revolve the head of the microscope and position the microscope with the mirror facing the window.

2 Raise the condenser to within 1 mm of its topmost position and open the iris.

3 Looking down on the upper lens of the condenser, angle the flat side of the mirror to reflect light up through the condenser.

   Caution: When using daylight, *never* attempt to reflect direct *sunlight* up through the microscope. This is both dangerous for the eyes and will provide unsuitable illumination. It is best to reflect light from a white sunlit wall or a white painted board outside the laboratory window.

4 Using a specimen such as a mounted stained thin blood film, focus the specimen with the 10× objective (see previous text). If required, readjust the angle of the mirror to obtain the brightest illumination.

5 If the condenser is not one that has been pre-centred by the manufacturer, check its centring (see previous text).

6 Obtain the best possible image by adjusting the condenser iris:
   - For the 10× objective, close the iris about two thirds.
   - For the 40× objective, open the iris more.
   - For the 100× objective, open the iris fully.

   Note: A monocular microscope is easier to use when it is fitted with a viewing aid (see previous text and Fig. 4.2).

QUALITY CONTROL, CARE AND MAINTENANCE OF A MICROSCOPE

Because of the importance of microscopy in patient care and the high cost of a microscope and its components, each district laboratory should monitor its microscopical work. The person in charge of the laboratory must ensure that:

■ Staff know how to use a microscope correctly and handle it with care. Clear instructions should be displayed close to the microscope.

■ A stock record card of the microscope is kept which gives the model, date and source of purchase, details of replacement parts, and maintenance schedule as recommended by the manufacturer. Essential components must be kept in stock, e.g. lamps and fuses.

■ Each day before use, the microscope is cleaned and its performance checked by a competent person using a specimen control slide (see following text). The daily quality control (QC) check of the microscope should be recorded and signed.

■ Any problem in the use of the microscope is reported immediately and remedied as soon as possible.

■ The microscope is securely stored at the end of the day's work.

Note: Microscopes are likely to be better cared for if responsibility for them is allocated to individual members of staff.[5]

During the visit of the district laboratory coordinator, the condition of each microscope should be checked, the daily quality control records inspected, stocks of essential components checked, and any microscopical reporting problems discussed.

Good microscopy practice

Daily cleaning and QC check before using the microscope

1 Using a clean cloth, wipe any dust and dirt from the stage and its controls, focusing knobs, and other surfaces of the microscope. Use a small soft brush to clean less accessible places, e.g. revolving nosepiece.

2 Using lens tissue or a separate piece of clean cotton cloth or cotton bud, clean the surface lens-es of the *dry* objectives (i.e. 4×, 10×, 20×, 40×), the upper lenses of the eyepieces, condenser lens, and illuminator lens. If required, dampen the cloth with clean water and a mild soap solution. Dry the lens with a dry cloth. Do *not* dismantle any lens.

Note: It is good practice to keep small pieces of cotton cloth laundered daily just for cleaning the microscope.

3 Carry out a quality control (QC) check to ensure the lenses are completely clean and the illumination system is correct. A specimen control slide such as a mounted stained blood film should be kept for the purpose of daily QC of the microscope. Record the QC checks i.e. for lenses and illumination.

Note: If an objective is not giving a clear image check whether it is completely clean. Remove it and examine the lens with a magnifying lens (e.g. an inverted eyepiece).

Care when using the microscope

– Do not force any mechanism, e.g. iris lever, focusing controls, or mechanical stage controls. Use these delicate mechanisms with care.

– Make sure the surface of the stage and the underside of the specimen are dry and clean before inserting the specimen in the slide holder.

Note: Whenever possible, cover wet preparations with cover glasses measuring 20 × 20 mm, not size 22 × 22 mm which make it easy for the fingers and stage of the microscope to become wet and contaminated.

– *Always* move the 100× objective to one side when inserting and removing specimens to prevent scratching of the front lens of the objective.

– Whenever possible use non-drying immersion oil. Avoid using thick yellow cedar wood oil.

– Do not mix immersion oils. When changing to a new oil, clean all the previous oil from the objective lens.

– Protect eyepieces that are not in use by placing them in a closed container.

At the end of the day's microscopy

1 Turn the lamp brightness control to its lowest setting, switch off the microscope, and remove the plug from the mains socket.

2 Using a piece of soft tissue or a soft piece of clean cotton cloth, wipe the immersion oil from the 100× objective and its surrounding mount.

Never use alcohol to clean off the oil because this will dissolve the cement holding the lens in its mount. If any oil is difficult to remove, use a cloth dampened with a *small* amount of xylene and immediately wipe the lens dry.

3 Do not leave an objective or eyepiece opening (port) empty. If the caps supplied with the microscope have been mislaid, prevent dirt from entering the opening by covering it with adhesive tape.

4 Decontaminate the stage of the microscope using a cloth dampened with 70% ethanol. Dry the surface.

5 Cover the microscope with its dust cover.

6 To prevent theft or unauthorized use, lock the microscope in a cupboard. Use two hands to carry the microscope (hold the limb and support the base).

In hot humid conditions: If the microscope is not to be used the next day, protect the lenses and other components from fungal growth by sealing the microscope in an airtight plastic bag with a container of dry (blue) self-indicating silica gel. About 100 g is adequate. The silica gel will remove moisture from the air inside the bag, providing a less humid environment. After use the silica gel will appear pink and require drying in an oven or in a container over a burner. When dry the silica gel will appear blue (active) again and should be stored immediately in an airtight container ready for reuse.

Do not place the microscope in a box with a lamp unless the box is sufficiently well ventilated otherwise heat from the lamp may damage the microscope.

Changing the lamp or a fuse

– Switch off the microscope and remove the plug from the mains socket.

– Follow the manufacturer's instructions for replacing a lamp or fuse.

Halogen lamp: Use a lamp of the correct voltage and wattage. If using a capsule type halogen lamp, use a long life lamp (see previous text). Hold the glass part of the lamp between a piece of tissue or cloth. Finger marking of the glass will reduce the life of the lamp. Always turn the lamp brightness control to its lowest setting before switching on the microscope. This will help to prolong the life of the lamp.

Fuse: Use a fuse of the correct rating. If the reason for the fuse blowing is not known ask a qualified electrician to check the electrical system.

Safety precautions when using a microscope with built-in illumination

■ Before purchasing and using a microscope, make sure it has a safety certificate (see previous text).

■ Use the microscope with the correct voltage supply. Read the manufacturer's literature.

■ Make sure the microscope is earthed via the mains plug. Use fuses of the correct rating in the mains plug and in the microscope fuse housing (read the manufacture's literature).

■ Always switch off and unplug the microscope from the mains:
  – at the end of the day's work.
  – when there is a storm with lightning.
  – when performing any cleaning and maintenance, e.g. changing a lamp, replacing a fuse, exchanging the illuminator in the base for a mirror unit.

■ Locate the microscope away from any source of water and out of direct sunlight.

■ Regularly check the electrical cable for signs of wear and loose connections in the mains plug.

■ If there is any electrical problem consult a qualified electrician.

Note: If operating the microscope from a 12 V lead-acid battery, follow the guidelines covering the *safe use of batteries* described in subunit 4.2.

SPECIAL FORMS OF MICROSCOPY

Most of the microscopy performed in district laboratory practice is routine transmitted light microscopy. Other forms of microscopy which may be used include:

■ Dark-field microscopy
■ Fluorescence microscopy
■ Micrometry (measurement)

Dark-field microscopy

This form of microscopy is used when maximum contrast is needed, e.g. to visualize transparent objects.

In dark-field (dark-ground) microscopy, a black patch stop below the condenser or a central blackout area in a special dark-field condenser prevents direct light from entering the objective and therefore the field of view is dark. Instead of passing through the centre of the condenser the light is reflected to

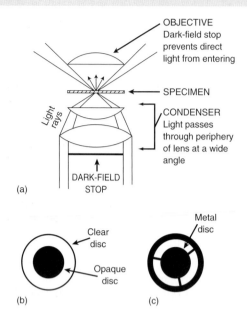

OBJECTIVE
Dark-field stop
prevents direct
light from entering

SPECIMEN

CONDENSER
Light passes
through periphery
of lens at a wide
angle

Light rays

DARK-FIELD
STOP

(a)

Clear
disc

Metal
disc

Opaque
disc

(b)   (c)

Fig. 4.4 (a) Principle of dark-field microscopy using a dark-field stop in the filter holder for the 10× and 40× objectives. (*Courtesy Dr W G Hartley*). (b) Dark-field stop made in the laboratory. (c) Manufactured metal dark-field stop.

pass through the outer edge of the condenser lens at a wide angle (see Fig. 4.4).

The specimen is illuminated by this wide angle of light, i.e. oblique light. Organisms and fine structures in the specimen which have a different refractive index to the fluid in which they are suspended, diffract or scatter the light and can be seen shining brightly against the dark background.

Unstained motile organisms such as the delicate treponemes of *Treponema pallidum*, and structures such as the sheath of pathogenic microfilariae, and the capsules of cryptococci, not normally seen by transmitted light microscopy, can be seen clearly using dark-field microscopy. Because these can be detected using the 10× and 40× objectives, an inexpensive dark-field stop can be used to obtain dark-field microscopy. A special dark-field condenser is required for use with the 100× objective (see later text).

Dark-field stop for the 10× and 40× objectives

A dark-field stop consists of a simple opaque disc, or stop, positioned in the filter holder below the condenser. The diameter of the opaque disc for use with the 40× objective is critical and must be correct. It is usually possible to use the same diameter of disc for the 10× objective as used with the 40× objective. Several manufacturers produce metal dark-field

stops to match their own microscopes. If however this useful accessory is not available, a dark-field stop can be made in the laboratory.

Making a dark-field stop for a microscope with built-in illumination

Providing the microscope has good illumination and the condenser has a swing-out filter holder, dark-field microscopy for use with the 10× and 40× objectives can be obtained using a dark-field stop made as follows:

1   Measure exactly in mm the internal diameter of the filter holder.

2   Make a disc of the diameter size of the filter holder from clear celluloid or other transparent rigid material, e.g. clear sheet as used in overhead projectors. Mark the centre of the disc with a small cross.

3   Using opaque card, cut out perfect discs (stops) of several different diameters to fit in the centre of the clear celluloid disc. Start with opaque discs of diameter 18 mm, 19 mm, 20 mm, and 21 mm. Mark the centre of each disc with a small cross.

    When testing each opaque disc for size, position it in the centre of the clear celluloid disc (matching the central crosses) using a small piece of plasticene or *Blutack*.

4   Turn the lamp brightness control to its maximum setting. Raise the condenser to its topmost position and open the iris fully.

5   Make a test specimen on a slide using a small amount of saliva taken hygienically from the side of the mouth (it should include a few epithelial cells). Cover the preparation with a cover glass. The slide and cover glass must be *clean* and the preparation not too thick.

6   Focus the specimen first with the 10× objective.

7   Place the dark-field stop in the filter holder and try each opaque disc until the best dark-field is seen with the 10× objective, i.e. dark background with the cells in the specimen brightly illuminated.

8   Focus the specimen with the 40× objective, and note the quality of the dark-field.

    If the field of view is not dark, use a larger size opaque disc. If dark but the cells are not brightly illuminated, decrease the disc size. Increase or decrease the diameter of the opaque disc by 1 mm each time until a size of disc is obtained that gives good dark-field with the 40× objective.

    Make a note of the diameters of the clear and opaque discs in case the original stop becomes damaged and needs replacing.

Using a dark-field stop with a microscope having built-in illumination

1   Prepare a *thin* wet unstained preparation on a slide and cover with a cover glass.

    Important: Do not use too dense a specimen and make sure the slide and cover glass are completely clean.

2   Locate the dark-field stop in the filter holder below the condenser.

3   Turn the brightness control to its maximum set-

ting, raise the condenser to its topmost position, and open fully the iris.

Note: A bright and correctly centred illumination is essential.

4 Focus and scan the specimen first with the 10× objective. Use the 40× objective to identify the organisms.

Value of dark-field microscopy

Dark-field microscopy is particularly useful for detecting:

- Motile *Treponema pallidum* in chancre fluid.
- Motile borreliae in blood.
- Motile leptospires in urine.
- Pathogenic microfilariae in blood. The sheath and nuclei can be clearly seen.
- Cryptococci in cerebrospinal fluid. The capsule surrounding the cells can be seen.
- Vibrios in specimens and cultures.

Using a special dark-field condenser

To obtain dark-field microscopy with the 100× objective, a special expensive oil immersion dark-field (dark-ground) condenser is needed. Also required is a funnel stop for inserting in the 100× objective (to reduce its NA), and a high intensity light source.

Instructions on how to use a dark-field condenser are usually supplied by the manufacturer. In district laboratory work it is rarely necessary to use a 100× objective to examine specimens by dark-field microscopy.

Fluorescence microscopy

In fluorescence microscopy, ultra-violet light which has a very short wavelength and is not visible to the eye (or just visible deep blue light) is used to illuminate organisms, cells, or particles which have been previously stained with fluorescing dyes called fluorochromes. These dyes are able to transform the invisible short wavelength ultra-violet light into longer wavelength visible light (or just-visible deep blue light into more visible yellow or orange light). The fluorescent stained organisms, cells, or particles can be seen glowing (fluorescing) against a dark background.

The effect produced by a fluorochrome depends on its excitation, i.e. short-wave radiation, and on the pH of the medium. Changes in pH can alter the emission wavelength. Bleaching, quenching, or oxygenation of the fluorochrome can reduce the intensity of the fluorescence.

Two types of fluorescence microscopy are used in medical laboratory work:

- Transmitted light fluorescence.

- Incident (reflected) light fluorescence, also called epifluorescence.

Transmitted light fluorescence

In transmitted light fluorescence, short wavelength light from a fluorescence lamp such as a mercury vapour or quartz halogen lamp passes through a primary, or excitation, filter which removes all the unwanted colours (wavelengths) of light and passes only those that are required. The transmission of this filter must match the emission peak of the fluorochrome being used.

The light is then brought to the specimen by a dark-field immersion condenser (a non-fluorescing immersion oil must be used). The fluorescence which is given off by the specimen passes through a secondary, or barrier, filter located between the objective and the eye which filters off all light other than the fluorescence wavelengths specific to the specimen.

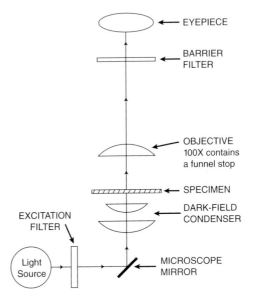

Fig. 4.5 Principle of transmitted light fluorescence.

Mercury vapour lamp

A mercury vapour lamp and its power supply are expensive and heavy and can be dangerous if not used correctly. A stable mains electricity supply is needed. The lamp requires about 20 minutes to warm up and if switched off it must cool before it is switched on again. Mercury vapour lamps are being increasingly replaced by quartz halogen lamps in new forms of fluorescence.

Incident light fluorescence

This simpler newer form of fluorescence involves illuminating the specimen from above (epifluorescence) using a dichroic mirror which is a special type of interference filter. It reflects selectively the shorter wavelength radiation and transmits the longer wavelength fluorescence, i.e. it is transparent to wavelengths above a given value and opaque to those below. The source of the shortwave radiation is usually a 100 W or 150 W halogen lamp.

Long wavelength fluorescence specific
to the specimen reaches the eye

EYEPIECE

BARRIER FILTER

Light Source

DICHROIC MIRROR
Reflects short wavelength excitation light on specimen. Transmits long wavelength fluorescence light.

EXCITATION FILTER

OBJECTIVE

SPECIMEN

Fig. 4.6 Principle of incident (reflected) light fluorescence.

The light passes through an excitation filter and is directed onto the dichroic mirror located above the specimen. This mirror reflects the short wavelength excitation light onto the specimen. The visible light from the reflected specimen passes back through the objective to the dichroic mirror which transmits the longer fluorescent wavelengths. A barrier filter ensures that only the fluorescence wavelengths specific for the specimen reach the eyepiece. No condenser is needed for incident fluorescence microscopy.

The development of incident fluorescence systems has lead to the availability of special 'fluorescence' objectives (containing an excitation filter, dichroic mirror, barrier filter) and halogen lamp units that can be used with most standard medical laboratory microscopes. An example is the low cost *FluoreslenS* system developed by Portable Medical Laboratories Inc (Appropriate Diagnostic Foundation), see Appendix 11. The *FluoreslenS* objective attaches to a standard microscope. It contains a fluorescence dichroic mirror, exciter filter and

barrier filter. When used with the fibre optic light source supplied (180 W halogen lamp), incident fluoresence microscopy can be performed to demonstrate AFB in sputum (see subunit 7.36 in Part 2) and a wide range of other fluorescence techniques. The system is shown below.

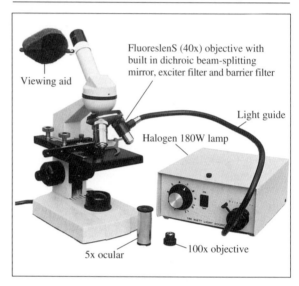

Incident fluorescence *FluoreslenS* system.
Courtesy of Portable Medical Laboratories.

Kawamoto acridine orange interference system

In the Kawamoto system, an interference filter specially designed for the flurochrome acridine orange is located in the filter holder of a substage condenser of a standard transmitted light microscope. The light source is a 100 W or 150 W halogen lamp. A barrier filter is inserted in the eyepiece(s).

Acridine orange (AO) fluoresces green (535 nm) when excited at wavelength 430 nm and red (650 nm) when excited at wavelength 492–495 nm. The Kawamoto narrow band pass interference filter is designed for the AO transmission peaks of 430 nm and 492–495 nm. The barrier filter used in the eyepiece has a cut-off wavelength of 515 nm.

Although the intensity of fluorescence emitted by the Kawamoto interference filter system is weaker than that produced by fluorescence microscopes, it has been found to be adequate for the detection of AO stained malaria parasites, trypanosomes, microfilariae, and bacteria. It provides a low cost method of obtaining fluorescence microscopy with acridine orange which is a particularly useful fluorochrome in both parasitology and bacteriology work.

Further information:
Readers should contact Professor Hiko Kawamoto, e-mail hiko@med.oita-u.ac.jp

Value of fluorescence microscopy
The following are the main applications of fluorescence microscopy:

- Examination of acridine orange stained specimens for the detection of malaria parasites, trypanosomes, microfilariae, *Trichomonas vaginalis*, *Entamoeba histolytica* (chromatoid bodies of cysts fluoresce), *Cryptosporidium* species, intracellular gonococci and meningococci, and the early detection of bacteria in blood cultures.

- Examination of auramine-phenol stained sputum and cerebrospinal fluid for acid fast bacilli (AFB).

- Immunodiagnosis by indirect and direct fluorescent antibody tests.

Micrometry

The measurement of objects using a calibrated eyepiece scale (micrometer) is called micrometry. The eyepiece scale requires calibration from a measured scale engraved on a glass slide, referred to as a stage graticule.

Required

- Eyepiece micrometer to fit into a 10× eyepiece or if available a special measuring 10× eyepiece. A suitable line scale for the eyepiece micrometer is one that is divided into 50 divisions.

- Stage graticule to calibrate the eyepiece scale. A suitable scale for the stage graticule is one that measures 2 mm in length with each large division measuring 0.1 mm (100 μm) and each small division measuring 0.01 mm (10 μm).

Availability of eyepiece micrometer and stage graticule

An eyepiece micrometer with a line scale having 100 divisions can be obtained from Pyser-SG1 (formerly Graticules Ltd), code No NE1 (see Appendix II). When ordering, the diameter of the graticule required must be stated, e.g. to fit an eyepiece of internal measurement (when top lens screwed off) 16 mm, 19 mm, or 21 mm.

A stage graticule measuring 2 mm in length with 0.1 mm and 0.01 mm divisions can be obtained from Pyser-SG1, code No. S22.

Alternatively, a calibrated measuring eyepiece may be available from a manufacturer for a specific microscope.

Calibrating an eyepiece micrometer using a stage graticule

The eyepiece micrometer will require calibration for each objective of the microscope at which measurements will be required. For convenience, a table can be prepared for each objective giving the measurements for 1 to 50 divisions of the eyepiece scale. The method of calibrating is as follows:

1 Unscrew the upper lens of a 10× eyepiece and insert the eyepiece micrometer disc with engraved side facing down. Alternatively, use a measuring eyepiece.

2 Place the stage graticule slide on the stage of the microscope and with the required objective in place, bring the scale into focus. Both the eyepiece scale and the calibration scale should be focused clearly. If required, unscrew slightly the top of the eyepiece lens to bring the eyepiece scale into sharp focus with the calibration scale of the stage graticule.

3 Adjust the field until the 0 line of the eyepiece scale aligns exactly with the 0 line of the calibration scale (see Fig. 4.7).

4 Look along the scales and note where a division of the eyepiece scale aligns *exactly* with a division of the calibration scale.

5 Measure the distance between the 0 point and where the alignment occurs. The measurements of the calibration scale are 0.1 mm to 2.0 mm. Each small subdivision measures 0.01 mm.

6 Count the number of divisions of the eyepiece scale covered between the 0 point and where the alignment occurs.

7 Calculate the measurement of 1 of the divisions of the eyepiece scale, in μm.

Example (as shown in Fig. 4.7)

Distance measured along stage graticule = 0.2 mm

Number of divisions of eyepiece scale = 27

1 division measures: $\dfrac{0.2}{27} = 0.0074$ mm

To convert mm to μm: $0.0074 \times 1000 = 7.4$ μm

8 Make tables giving the measurements for 1 to 50 eyepiece divisions.

Repeat the calibration and calculations for each objective at which measurements are required.

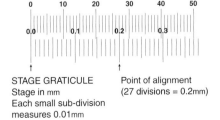

EYEPIECE MICROMETER
Scale showing 50 divisions of the 100 division scale

STAGE GRATICULE
Stage in mm
Each small sub-division
measures 0.01mm

Point of alignment
(27 divisions = 0.2mm)

Fig. 4.7 Calibration of an eyepiece micrometer scale using a stage graticule scale calibrated in mm. Example shows 27 divisions of the eyepiece micrometer aligning with 0.2 mm (200 μm) of the stage graticule. One division is therefore equal to 200 divided by 27 = 7.4 μm.

Measuring an object in a specimen, e.g. cyst

With the eyepiece micrometer scale and the cyst sharply focused, position the cyst along the scale and count the divisions covered. Refer to the previously prepared table for the objective being used to obtain the measurement for the number of divisions counted. This will give the size of the cyst in μm.

4.4 Equipment for purifying water

Water for laboratory use must be free from contaminants that could interfere with the performance of tests. The quality of water required is therefore dependent on the work carried out. In district laboratory work, water of an appropriate quality and quantity is required for:

- The preparation of:
  - stains and reagents used in staining techniques,
  - reagents used in clinical chemistry tests,
  - culture media and reagents used in microbiology,
  - reagents used in haematology and blood transfusion work.

- The rinsing of cleaned glassware, plastic-ware, syringes, lancets, and equipment components, e.g. cuvettes.

- Topping up of electrolyte in 12 V lead-acid batteries.

Depending on the requirements, available facilities, and quality of the laboratory's water supply (feed-water) the following methods can be used to obtain water of adequate purity and quantity:

- Distillation using a still.
- Filtration using a gravity filter and reusable ceramic filter of 0.9 μm porosity.
- Deionization (of filtered water) using mixed bed colour change deionizing resins.

Quality standards of purified water
The quality of purified water is graded according to the amount of biological matter, dissolved organic and inorganic material it contains. The *International Organization for Standardization* (ISO) specifies water quality as Grade 1, 2 or 3 (ISO 3696: 1987), the *British Standards Institute* has a simi-

lar grading (BS 3978: 1987), the *American Society for Testing and Materials* (ASTM) uses a Type 1, 2, 3 and 4 specification (ASTM D11 93–91) and the *National Committee for Clinical Laboratory Standards* (NCCLS) uses a Type 1, 11 and 111 specification (NCCLS 1988).

Water of ISO grade 3, ASTM Type 4, and NCCLS Type 111 produced by single distillation, deionization, or reverse osmosis, is recommended for the preparation of reagents and for laboratory analytical work. Such water should have an electrical conductivity at 25 °C of no more than 5 μS/cm.

Water suitable for use in district laboratories
Distilled or deionized water of ISO grade 3 (see previous text) is recommended for the analytical work carried out in district hospital laboratories but water of this purity may be difficult to obtain in laboratories with limited facilities. For most purposes, water with a conductivity of less than 20 μS/cm will be adequate.

In district hospitals where the pharmacy is distilling water for preparing intravenous solutions, it will usually be possible for the pharmacy also to supply the laboratory with distilled water.

In situations where neither the pharmacy nor the laboratory can operate a still, the most practical way for a hospital laboratory to obtain water of the quality it requires is by deionizing water that has been previously filtered.

For some staining procedures it may be possible to use filtered water without deionization providing control slides are used to ensure the staining reactions are correct. For some health centres therefore a gravity filter (0.9 μm porosity) may be all that is required if most of the work is microscopical and the water available for filtering is rainwater or water that is not heavily contaminated with salts.

Reagents for chemical tests and culture media will need to be prepared in the district hospital laboratory using distilled or deionized water and distributed, as required, to health centre laboratories.

Effectiveness of distillation, filtration, and deionization

	Distillation	Filtration (0.9 μm porosity)	Deionization
Dissolved ionized solids	E/G	P	E
Dissolved organics	G	P	P
Dissolved ionized gases	P	P	E
Particulates	E	E/G	P
Bacteria	E	E	P
Pyrogens	E	P	P

Note: Chart provides general guidelines.
E = Excellent, G = Good, P = Poor.

DISTILLATION

In the distillation process, impure water is boiled and the steam produced is condensed on a cold surface (condenser) to give chemically pure distilled water i.e. water from which non-volatile organic and inorganic materials are removed. Distillation does not remove dissolved ionized gases such as ammonia, carbon dioxide, and chlorine.

Distilled water should be clear, colourless and odourless. Providing the design of still ensures that the water contains only the condensed steam and the distillate is collected into a clean sterile container, the water will also be pyrogen-free.

Pyrogen: This is a substance, usually of bacterial origin, that can cause fever if transfused in an intravenous fluid.

A considerable volume of running water is required to operate a still (usually not less than 60 litre/hour to condense the steam) and the water feeding the still must not be heavily contaminated. Most stills are also operated from a heater of at least 3 kW consumption. A wide range of stills is available. The most expensive models are fully automatic (water-flow automatically set and maintained and on/off switch is automatic) and capable of producing highly purified water for research and specialist laboratory work, i.e. grade 1 and 2 water quality.

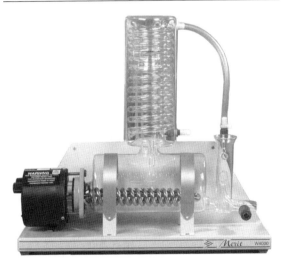

Plate 4.3 Merit water still. *Courtesy of Bibby Sterilin.*

The still shown in plate 4.3 is an example of a modern still capable of producing Grade 3 (ISO specification) quality water. The following specifications are based on this type of still.

Specifications of a still producing water suitable for district laboratories.

- Water is single distilled with an output of 4 litres/hour from a 3 kW heater.
- Distilled water has a conductivity of 3.0–4.0 μS/cm and resistivity of 0.25–0.35 megohm-cm.[a]
- Built-in safety thermostat.[b]
- Requires a running water supply of minimum flow 60 litres/hour (not heavily contaminated).
- Can be cleaned and descaled without being dismantled.

Recommended spares to keep in stock
Heater with built-in thermostat
Boiler
Condenser unit

NOTES

a　Conductivity is the measurement of a material's ability to conduct electric current. It is the reciprocal of resistance. Conductivity and resistivity measurements provide information on the quality of distilled and deionized water. The lower the conductance and higher the resistivity, the purer the water. Absolutely pure water has a conductivity of 0.055 micro Siemens/cm (μS/cm) and a resistivity of 18.3 megohms-cm (MΩ–cm)

b　A built-in thermostat is needed to protect a still and for safety reasons. It shuts off the power to the heater if the boiler runs dry. The thermostat resets automatically when the still has cooled.

Availability of *Merit Water Still*
The still shown in Plate 4.3 is the *Merit Water Still*, model W4000, manufactured by Bibby Sterilin Ltd (see Appendix II). It has the above specifications.
Recommended spares include a 3 kW heater (code A 6/6), boiler (W4000/B), and condenser unit (WC48/M2).

Use and care of a still

- Read carefully the manufacturer's instructions. Prepare a stock record card and written SOPs covering the use, cleaning, and care of the still.
- Ensure there is a sufficient supply of cool running water to feed the condenser.
- Do not allow the boiler to run dry.
- Collect the distilled water in a clean glass or plastic (not PVC) container previously rinsed with fresh distilled water.
- Avoid storing the distilled water for more than a few days. Keep the container capped.

- Regularly clean the still. If the water feeding the still is hard, the still will require frequent descaling as recommended by the manufacturer.

  Note: When buying a still, select one that can be cleaned without being dismantled, i.e. one in which the cleaning agent can be added to the boiler through a built-in funnel with a stopcock provided for drainage as shown in Plate 4.3.

- Do not use a still if any of the glass components appear cracked. Replace the damaged part.

FILTRATION

When using a gravity water filter fitted with a ceramic candle filter, 0.9 μm porosity, most bacteria, parasitic microorganisms, and suspended particles can be removed from the water but not dissolved salts.

Specifications of a gravity filter
The following specifications are based on the *Berkefeld* gravity filter shown in Fig. 4.8.

- 10 litres capacity with output of 40 litres/24 hour.[a]
- Fitted with two ceramic self-sterilizing *Sterasyl* candle filters of 0.9 μm porosity.[b]
- No external plumbing required.
- Easily cleaned and maintained (see later text).

Recommended spares to keep in stock: *Sterasyl* ceramic candle filters.

NOTES
a A reduction in output is an indication that the filters require cleaning.

b The *Sterasyl* ceramic filters fitted in the *Berkefeld* gravity filter contain fine particles of silver dispersed in their structure which prevent bacteria growing inside the filter.

Important: The use of *Sterasyl* filters that contain activated carbon, i.e. *Super Sterasyl* filters, is not recommended for laboratory use because some of the fine carbon particles can pass through the filter into the water. The carbon-containing *Super Sterasyl* filters are intended to improve the quality of the water when it is used for drinking.

Availability of *Berkefeld* filter
The 10 litre capacity polypropylene *Berkefeld* gravity filter model LP2, measures 590 mm high and is manufactured by Fairey Industrial Ceramics. (see Appendix II). It includes the polypropylene container with two *Sterasyl* candle filters and the required connections. Extra candle filters are available.

Use and maintenance of a gravity filter
If the water supply to the laboratory is heavily contaminated with particulate matter and there is no opportunity to use rainwater, leave the water to stand in a container overnight to allow the larger particles to sediment. Filter the upper layer of water. It is however preferable to use rainwater because this will contain less dissolved chemicals.

Harvesting rainwater
Collect the rain from as clean a surface as possible. If from a roof, clean the roof surface and the guttering to avoid dust, dead leaves and bird droppings being washed into the storage tank. Arrange the downspout so that the first water from each shower is diverted from the storage tank and allowed to run to waste.

Install a wire mesh screen over the top of the downspout and clean the screen regularly to prevent the collection of organic materials. Keep the storage tank covered. Seek also the advice of other people who harvest rainwater.

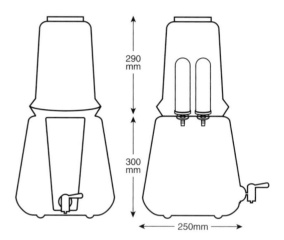

Fig. 4.8 *Berkefeld* polypropylene gravity water filter. *Left*: Front view. *Right*: Interior side view showing Sterasyl ceramic candles filters fitted.

Cleaning a gravity filter

The candle filters fitted in the *Berkefeld* gravity filter have a long-life (up to 1 year) providing they are cleaned regularly and handled with care to prevent cracking of the ceramic. The filters should be cleaned every week or more often if indicated. Filtering will slow down once the pores of the filter become clogged. To clean the ceramic filters:

1 Empty the upper and lower containers.

2 Carefully unscrew each filter.

3 Holding the screw-end of the filter, brush clean the filter using a stiff brush and clean water (brush away from the screw-end). DO NOT USE SOAP, DETERGENT, OR ANY CLEANING

FLUID because this will be soaked up by the filter making it unusable.

4 Clean the upper and lower containers and rinse the lower container with boiled filtered water.

5 Re-assemble the filters and discard the first 200–500 ml of filtered water. When the filters are new, follow the manufacturer's instructions.

DEIONIZATION

In deionization, impure water is passed through anion and cation exchange resins to produce ion-free water. Deionized water has a low electrical conductivity, near neutral pH and is free from water-soluble salts but is not pyrogen-free or sterile.

Impurities removed by deionization

Cations which may be present in the water such as calcium, magnesium, and sodium are exchanged by the cation resin which in turn releases hydrogen ions (H^+).

Anion impurities such as sulphate, bicarbonate, silica, nitrate, and chloride are exchanged by the anion resin which in turn releases hydroxyl (OH^-) ions. The hydrogen ions combine with the hydroxyl ions to give ion-free water (H_2O).

In district laboratories (without a still), water of the grade required for analytical work and making reagents can be obtained by deionizing water that has been previously filtered (see previous text). It is not practical or cost-effective to use deionizing resins without *first filtering* the water. The use of unfiltered water will lead to rapid contamination and exhaustion of the resins. The life of the resins can be maximized if soft filtered rainwater is used particularly in areas where the natural water is hard.

Low cost method of deionizing filtered water

Filtered water is most easily and economically deionized in district laboratories by passing water through a laboratory-made deionizer column using mixed bed colour change deionizer resin. This type of resin contains both cation and anion resins and an indicator that changes colour as the resin becomes exhausted.

A column of 150 g of resin, measuring approximately 45–50 mm in diameter and 135 mm long is contained in a polythene plastic tube suspended below the tap of a *Berkefeld* gravity filter. The filtered water trickles through the resin, is deionized, and passes through the small holes in the bottom of the tube into a collecting container as shown in Fig. 4.10.

Required

■ Plastic tube made from polythene tubing as shown in Fig. 4.9 to hold the deionizer resin.

When making the holes in the bottom of the tube, it is important to use a medium size sewing machine needle (size 90, not threaded) to ensure the deionized water passes through satisfactorily and the resin beads are fully retained.

■ Absorbent cotton wool pad to place on top of the resin column to prevent the water forming a channel through the resin.

■ Mixed bed colour change resin such as the *Purolite MB-400 QR/2048* high quality free-flowing, self-indicating resin mixture. As the resin exhausts its colour changes from light brown to red, from the top of the column downwards.

Conductivity readings of the deionized water are 0.1–1.0 µSm/cm. The reading rises to around 5.0 µS/cm when about 75% of the column appears red. When there remains only 20–25 mm of the active (light brown) resin in the bottom of the tube, the conductivity of the deionized water will rise to around 20 µS/cm. The resin should then be discarded.

Availability of Purolite MB-400 QR/2048 resin

The *Purolite MB-400 QR/2048* mixed bed self-indicating resin is manufactured by Purolite in 25 litre bags (18.3 kg), see Appendix 11. It can be obtained in packs of 1.8 kg (1 800 g), together with two free reusable plastic tubes and 12 cotton pads, from Developing Health Technology (see Appendix 11). This is sufficient to make 12 deionizing columns each containing approximately 150 g of resin.

Expected output figures

Based on using *Purolite MB-400 QR/2048* resin to deionize water filtered through a *Berkefeld* filter using the plastic tube method described, the following are the expected deionized water output figures for soft, medium, and hard water from 150 g of resin (one deionizing column):

Soft   (about 50 mg/t.d.s): 55–65 litres
Medium (about 200 mg/t.d.s): 15–17 litres
Hard   (about 300 mg/t.d.s): 11–12 litres

Note: t.d.s = total dissolved solids

Method of use

1 Fill the deionizer plastic tube to the 135 mm mark with deionizer resin (see Fig. 4.9). Tap the tube on the bench to pack down the resin.

2 Place a cotton wool pad on top of the resin column.

3 Suspend the tube under the tap of the gravity water filter (see Fig. 4.10). The end of the tap should be centrally located above the resin column and sufficiently inside the tube to prevent any non-deionized water trickling down the outside of the tube.

4 Place a plastic water collecting container on a stool or crate below the deionizer tube. Insert a

plastic funnel in the neck of the bottle to collect the deionized water.

5   *Slowly* turn on the tap of the water filter to obtain a trickle of water.

Important: For satisfactory deionization the water must pass through the resin column *slowly* and *evenly*. It will take about 1 hour to obtain 4–5 litres of distilled water.

If the water is allowed to pass through the column rapidly it will form a channel through or down the side of the resin instead of passing evenly through the entire resin bed. Uneven passage of the water will be indicated by the resin chaning colour unevenly down one side of the column. If this is noticed unhook the tube from the tap and turn it the other way round.

6   When about 75% of the resin column appears red, check the conductivity reading of the deionized water using an appropriate meter such as the Hanna *Pure Water Test* meter (see later text).

When a meter is not available, discard the resin when there remains only about 20 mm of light brown resin in the bottom of the tube. At this point the conductivity of the water will be reading around 20 μSm/cm. Do not discard the plastic tube, this can be reused.

Maintenance of the deionizer resin

The laboratory-made deionizer plastic column method of deionizing water allows laboratory staff to prepare pure water when it is needed and in the amounts required at a much lower cost than using a commercially produced resin cartridge unit (see following text). To maximize the life of the resin the following are important:

– Keep the deionizer tube out of sunlight to avoid inactivating the indicator.

– When not in use, remove the deionizer tube and store it in a dark place. This will protect the indicator and also minimize contamination of the resin column. When first used after storage, discard the water passing through the column for the first 5 minutes.

– Keep unused resin in an *opaque, sealed, airtight* plastic bag or tin.

Safety precautions

Deionizer resin can cause irritation if it is allowed to enter the eye or skin. It is therefore advizable to wear plastic gloves and protective eye goggles when filling the plastic tube. The resin beads are insoluble in

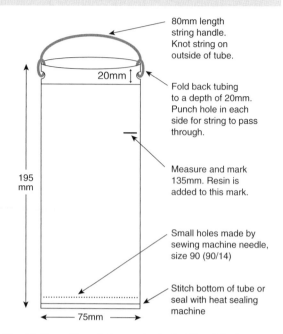

Fig. 4.9 Reusable polythene tube for holding deionizer resin.

water. Store the resin below 50 °C away from nitric acid and strong oxidizers.

Use of commercially produced resin cartridges

Commercially produced cartridges containing mixed bed colour change resins are available from several suppliers. Most units are designed for use with mains running tap water which provides the pressure needed to force the water *up* through the resin column. They are not designed for gravity use, e.g. using filtered water.

Resin cartridges are not recommended for use in district laboratories in tropical countries because of their high cost. The resin column rapidly becomes contaminated well before all the resin is exhausted.

Measuring the conductivity of deionized water

Collect some of the deionized water in a beaker and measure its conductivity using an inexpensive hand-held *Pure Water Test* meter such as that manufactured by Hanna Instruments, which measures over the range 0.1 to 99.9 μS/cm with a readability of 0.1 μS/cm. It is shown in Fig. 4.11.

A reading of below 5.0 μS/cm indicates that the deionized water is of Grade 3 standard (see previous text). If the reading is greater than 20 μS/cm, the water is not suitable for analytical work. Such a reading indicates that the deionizer resin is exhausted and requires replacing.

If when using a Hanna meter, no figures appear but a small ε symbol appears in the right hand corner of the display window, the conductivity of the

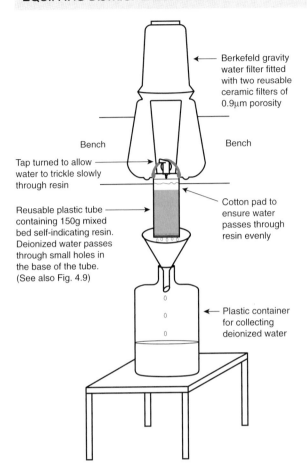

Berkefeld gravity water filter fitted with two reusable ceramic filters of 0.9μm porosity

Bench

Bench

Tap turned to allow water to trickle slowly through resin

Cotton pad to ensure water passes through resin evenly

Reusable plastic tube containing 150g mixed bed self-indicating resin. Deionized water passes through small holes in the base of the tube. (See also Fig. 4.9)

Plastic container for collecting deionized water

Fig. 4.10 Low cost practical method of obtaining pure water in district laboratories. The water is first filtered and then deionized using a laboratory-made deionizer column.

water is greater than 99.9 μS/cm, i.e. beyond the reading range of the meter.

Availability of the Hanna *Pure Water Test* meter
The Hanna *Pure Water Test* hand-held meter measuring 0.1 to 99.9 μS/cm complete with batteries is available from Hanna Instruments (see Appendix II). The meter is operated from four 1.4 V batteries (small flat batteries, similar to those found in digital watches).

4.5 Equipment for weighing

To make essential reagents, stains, and culture media a balance is required that weighs accurately and precisely within the range and readability (sensitivity) required.

Balances manufactured for medical laboratory use include:

■ Mechanical balances,
■ Electronic (microprocessor controlled) balances.

Mechanical balances: These balances include the single pan, trip, and torsion types. They do not require mains electricity or battery power and are currently less expensive than microprocessor controlled balances of similar readability. Mechanical balances are less widely available than electronic balances.

Electronic balances: A wide range of top-loading and analytical electronic balances is available. Electronic

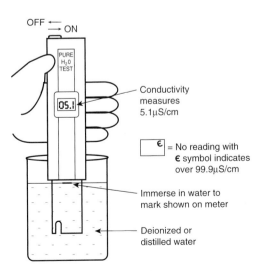

OFF ← ON

PURE H₂0 TEST

Conductivity measures 5.1μS/cm

ϵ = No reading with ϵ symbol indicates over 99.9μS/cm

Immerse in water to mark shown on meter

Deionized or distilled water

Fig. 4.11 Hanna Pure Water Test Meter.

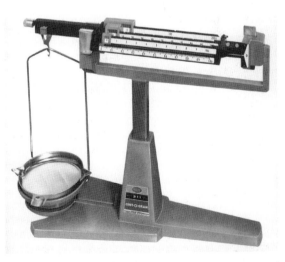

Plate 4.4 Ohaus 311 mechanical beam balance, readability of 0.01 g and capacity of 311 g, suitable for district hospital laboratories.

balances are single pan balances that use an electromagnetic force instead of weights. They are operated from mains electricity and often also from battery power. They weigh rapidly and usually have built-in taring which allows the weight of the weighing vessel to be 'zeroed'. Many models incorporate applications for industry and education and therefore have menus which provide multiple application modes and multiple weighing units (not required for district laboratory work).

In tropical countries with high relative humidity, electronic balances tend to have a reduced working life. Electric storms can also interfere with the performance of an electronic balance, necessitating its recalibration.

BALANCES FOR USE IN DISTRICT LABORATORIES

Mechanical balances with a readability of 0.01 g. The Ohaus model 311 balance is recommended for district hospital laboratories. It is available from Ohaus Corporation (see Appendix 11). A similar lower costing mechanical balance called the AQ3115 is available from Adam Equipment (see Appendix 11).

Specifications of the Ohaus 311 balance

- Mechanical beam balance, i.e. no separate weights are required.
- Readability of 0.01 g.
- Capacity of 311 g.[a]
- Easy to use with magnetic damping.[b]
- Zero adjustment.
- Stainless steel removable pan.
- Robust and can be easily maintained by the user. Does not require electricity or batteries.

NOTES

a   The weights are divided between four beams:
1st beam: 0 to 1 g with 0.01 g divisions, 2nd beam: 0 to 10 g with 1 g divisions, 3rd beam: 0 to 100 g with 10 g divisions, 4th beam: 0 to 200 g with 100 g divisions.
b   Magnetic damping lowers the time required to reach an accurate reading by minimizing the time it takes for the pointer to come to rest.

Electronic balances with readability of 0.01 g
For district hospital laboratories an electronic balance without multiple application modes, having a readability of 0.01 g and operating from both battery and mains power, is suitable. An example of such a balance at an affordable price is the *AQT 200 Compact balance* shown in Plate 4.5. It is available from Adam Equipment (see Appendix 11).

Specifications of the AQT 200 Compact balance

- Capacity of 200 g with readability of 0.01 g and repeatability of 0.02 g.
- Easy to use with large clear LCD.
- Operates from mains electricity using AC adaptor (supplied) or from 6 AA batteries (not supplied).
- Low battery indicator and auto shut-off to conserve battery life.
- Autocalibration using keypad (200 g calibration weight should be ordered separately).
- Built-in spirit level and height adjustable feet.
- 3 seconds stabilization time.
- Windshield draught excluder provided.
- Operating temperature, 0–40 °C.
- Weighs 1.2 Kg.
- Measures 195 wide × 240 deep × 70 mm high with 130 mm platform diameter.
- Provided with clearly written *User Manual*.

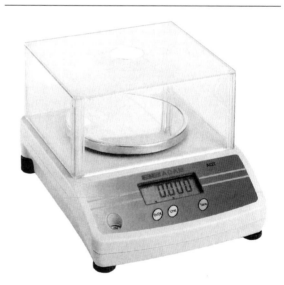

Plate 4.5 AQT 200 Compact electronic balance, showing windshield draught excluder in position.
Courtesy of Adam Equipment.

Other Ohaus mechanical balances
In addition to the balances described, the Ohaus Corporation and Adam Equipment also supply other beam and trip balances of varying capacity and readability (0.1 g and 1 g).

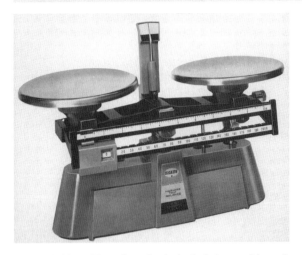

Plate 4.6 Ohaus Havard mechanical trip balance with readability of 0.1 g and capacity of 2 000 g.

The balance shown in Plate 4.6 is the Ohaus Havard trip balance model 1415. It has a capacity of 2 000 g and readability of 0.1 g. It is useful for weighing chemicals and culture media in large amounts and when required, for balancing centrifuge buckets.

USE AND CARE OF BALANCES

A balance is a delicate instrument that requires practical instruction in its correct use. The following apply when using a balance:

- Read carefully the manufacturer's instructions. Prepare a stock record card and written SOPs covering the use, cleaning, and care of the balance.

- Always handle a balance with care.

- Position the balance on a firm bench away from vibration, draughts, and direct sunlight. Electronic balances require protection against magnetism and static electricity. Make sure the balance is level, adjusting if necessary the screws on which it stands. A spirit level or plumb line is often provided to assist in levelling the instrument.

- Before starting to weigh, zero the balance as directed by the manufacturer. If using a beam balance, check the positioning of the beam.

- Weigh chemicals at room temperature in a weighing scoop (if provided) or small beaker (avoid using plastic containers when using an electronic balance). NEVER weigh chemicals directly on a balance pan. Place the weighing vessel in the centre of the pan.

- When adding or removing a chemical, remove the container to avoid spilling any chemical on the balance pan.

- When using an analytical double pan balance, bring the pans to rest before adding or removing a chemical.

- If using a box of weights, *always* use the forceps provided to add or remove weights. Protect the weights from dust, moisture, and fungal growth.

- After completing the weighing, return the balance to zero weight. Use a small brush to wipe away any chemical which may have been spilt.

- In humid climates, place a suitable desiccant such as reusable self-indicating silica gel inside the case of an analytical balance.

- Keep a small notebook by the balance in which to make the necessary weighing calculations and to record the date of preparation of reagents.

- Keep the balance and surrounding area clean. When using a mechanical balance do not let dirt accumulate near the pivots and bearings. Use a fine brush or an air syringe to remove dust particles. Keep the balance covered when it is not in use.

- Do not use an electronic balance when there is an electrical storm.

- When using an electronic balance, check the calibration frequently as instructed by the manufacturer. Remove the balance pan when moving the balance.

Checking the accuracy of a balance

The accuracy of a balance should be checked regularly as recommended by the manufacturer. If the balance is of the analytical double pan type, the knife edges should be checked periodically. When at rest the pans should not leave the stirrups. If separate weights are used, have the accuracy of these checked from time to time. When using an electronic balance, use a calibration weight as recommended by the manufacturer.

4.6 Equipment for pipetting and dispensing

Highly infectious pathogens can be found in specimens sent to the laboratory for testing; and harmful and corrosive chemicals are frequently used to analyze samples. For these reasons mouth-pipetting is banned in medical laboratories (see also subunit 3.2).

Changing to safe methods of pipetting and dispensing can be achieved simply and economically and often improves the quality of analytical work.

Factors that need to be considered when selecting manual and automated devices for pipetting and dispensing specimens and reagents include:

- level of accuracy and precision required,
- how well the device performs,
- whether the device will need to be autoclaved,
- ease of use,
- workload,
- whether the user will be able to maintain and calibrate the device,
- cost of the device, consumables, replacement parts,
- availability.

Most district laboratories will probably find that they need to use several different devices for the collection of capillary blood, measuring venous blood, serum, urine, and other body fluids. A safe method of aspirating blood in ESR tests is described in subunit 4.12.

Capillary and micropipette fillers

Bulb capillary filler

An inexpensive small bulb aspirator as shown in Fig. 4.12 is suitable for use with calibrated capillaries, particularly when measuring and dispensing blood and serum. It is available from Developing Health Technology (DHT), see Appendix 11. The bulb has a hole which is left uncovered when the blood or serum is being drawn into the capillary. The hole is covered with the finger when expelling and rinsing the sample from the capillary. Calibrated capillaries measuring 10–200 µl are available from DHT and other suppliers.

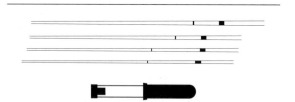

Fig. 4.12 Bulb capillary filler for use with calibrated capillaries for measuring 10µl to 200 µl specimen volumes.

Capillary and micropipette filler

This thumb wheel aspirator is a safe alternative to using a mouth-piece and rubber tubing when collecting blood samples. It is particularly useful because it can be used with both calibrated capillaries and micropipettes such as white shell-back 20 µl and 50 µl micropipettes.

The device is easily controlled using a thumb wheel and the angle at which the capillary or micropipette is held can be adjusted. It is shown in Fig. 4.13 and is available from DHT.

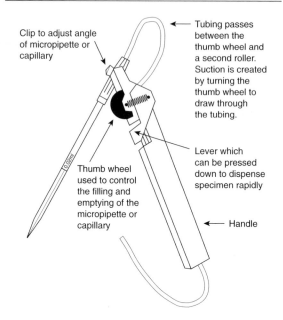

Clip to adjust angle of micropipette or capillary

Tubing passes between the thumb wheel and a second roller. Suction is created by turning the thumb wheel to draw through the tubing.

Thumb wheel used to control the filling and emptying of the micropipette or capillary

Lever which can be pressed down to dispense specimen rapidly

Handle

Fig. 4.13 Combined capillary and micropipette filler.

Pipettors

Pipettors are automated hand-held single or multichannel liquid handling devices. They include fixed and variable volume pipettors that are operated manually or electronically. Depending on their principle of operation, they are described as air displacement pipettors or positive displacement pipettors.

Air displacement and positive displacement pipettors

Pipettors operate by means of a piston (plunger) with liquids being transferred and dispensed by displacement.

When there is a layer of air separating the piston from the liquid, the term air displacement pipettor is used. To dispel the last drop of liquid from the pipettor, the plunger needs to be fully depressed, i.e. the fluid is expelled in two stages.

When the piston is in direct contact with the liquid the pipettor is referred to as a direct, or positive, displacement pipettor and special glass or plastic capillaries are used instead of plastic tips.

Both air and positive displacement pipettors are manufactured to high standards of accuracy and precision. The use of positive displacement pipettors is recommended when measuring particularly viscous fluids and when high levels of accuracy and reproducibility are required. For routine district laboratory work air displacement pipettors are adequate and generally more available. The *Volac UNI* range of pipettors are economically priced easy to use pipettors with good accuracy and reproducibility. They are available from Poulten and Graf (see Appendix 11).

Fixed volume pipettors

A fixed volume pipettor as shown in Fig. 4.14, measures a single volume of liquid. It is more convenient and less complicated to use than a variable volume pipettor and costs less.

Volac UNI range of fixed volume pipettors
The range includes the following capacities:

10 μl, code R770/B
20 μl, code R770/D
50 μl, code R770/H   } Require yellow *Volac*
100 μl, code R770/N   micropipettor tips, code
200 μl, code R770/Q   } D590*

250 μl, code R770/R   } Require blue *Volac*
500 μl, code R770/U   micropipettor tips, code
1000 μl, code R770/Y   } D592*

*Tips are supplied in bulk packs of 1000 (non-sterile), boxed in packs of 100 (non-sterile), or boxed in packs of 100 (sterile). Specify when ordering.

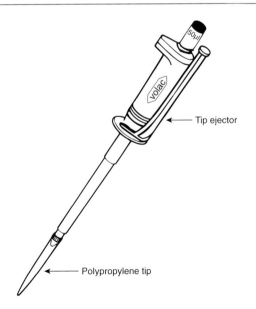

Fig. 4.14 Fixed volume *Volac pipettor* with built-in tip ejector.

Variable volume pipettors

A variable volume pipettor is calibrated to measure and dispense μl volumes continuously over a set range, usually digitally although electronic devices are also available. Changing from one volume to another requires great care. A thorough knowledge is required of μl measurements and for some pipettors, also how vernier scales work. Variable volume pipettors are expensive (almost twice the price of fixed volume pipettors).

Volac UNI range of variable volume pipettors
The range includes the following:

20–100 μl, code R780/B
40–200 μl, code R780/C
200–1000 μl, code R780/E
1000–5000 μl, code R780/F
2000–10 000 μl, code R/780/G

Tips: Yellow *Volac* tips, code D590 are used for pipettors of capacity up to 200 μl, blue *Volac* tips, code D592 for 100–1000 μl, white long *Volac* tips, code D893 for 1000 to 5000 μl and blue long *Volac* tips, code D894 for 2000–10 000 μl.

Note: Always use the tips recommended by the manufacturer for a particular pipettor.

How to use an air displacement pipettor
Pipetting aqueous solutions using normal forward pipetting:
– Fill and empty the tip twice with the liquid. Press the plunger to the first stop.
– With the pipettor held *vertically* and the tip 1–2 mm below the surface of the liquid, release the plunger smoothly and slowly to aspirate the fluid.
– To dispense, touch the tip at an angle against the side of the receiving vessel, press to the first stop, wait a few seconds, then press the plunger to the second stop to expel all the fluid.

Pipetting plasma, high viscosity fluids and very small volumes, using reverse pipetting:
– Fill and empty the tip twice with the liquid. Press the plunger to the second stop.
– With the pipettor held vertically and the tip 1–2 mm below the surface of the liquid, release the plunger slowly and smoothly to fill the tip. Wipe the outside of the tip.
– With the tip against the side of the receiving vessel, press the plunger to the first stop to dispense the required volume. *Do not* press to the second stop (the liquid remaining in the tip should be discarded).

Diluting whole blood using repetitive pipetting.
– Fill and empty the tip twice with the blood. Press the plunger to the first stop.
– With the pipettor held vertically and the tip well below the surface of the blood, release the plunger smoothly and slowly to aspirate the blood.
– Remove the pipettor and wipe carefully the

outside of the tip. Dip the tip into the diluent well below the surface. Press the plunger slowly and smoothly several times to fill and empty the tip until all the blood is expelled. Depress the plunger to the second stop to empty the tip completely.

Important
- Always read carefully the manufacturer's instruction regarding the use and care of a pipettor.
- When not in use, always store a pipettor upright in a stand. Never leave a pipettor on its side with tip attached containing fluid.
- Keep the pipettor clean, particularly the nozzle.
- Every few months, depending on usage, arrange for the pipettor to be checked for accuracy and precision. Re-calibration of a pipettor requires the use of an analytical balance of readability 0.0001 g (not normally found in a district laboratory) and specialist training.
- Do not use a tip unless it forms a complete seal with the pipettor.

Reuse of plastic tips
Most manufacturers of pipettors will not recommend the reuse of plastic tips. In some situations, however, tips may need to be decontaminated, washed, and reused. Most plastic tips are made from polypropylene and are therefore durable. To reuse, the tips *must* be well cleaned to remove all traces of protein and disinfectant, rinsed well, and dried completely. Only reuse a tip when it fits the pipettor perfectly.

Specimen measuring syringes

When measuring specimens such as urine, a polypropylene (autoclavable) *Exacta-Med* syringe can be used. These low cost syringes with tip extenders, clear blue markings, and a barrel with a narrow black silicon seal make it easy to measure volumes with sufficient accuracy. The following syringes are suitable:

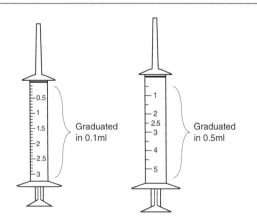

Fig. 4.15 3 ml and 5 ml polypropylene measuring syringes.

- 3.0 ml syringe which is graduated in 0.1 ml divisions.
- 5 ml syringe which is graduated in 0.5 ml divisions.

Measuring syringes are available from DHT (see Appendix 11).

Graduated plastic bulb pipettes
Graduated plastic bulb pipettes (*Pastettes*) can also be used for measuring body fluids such as urine in most basic clinical chemistry tests performed in district laboratories. The following *Pastettes* are useful:

- 1 ml *Pastette* graduated at 0.5 ml and 1 ml.
- 3 ml *Pastette* graduated from 0.5–3.0 ml in 0.5 ml divisions.

Ungraduated *Pastettes* of varying length are also available and are useful for transferring serum and other fluids from tubes and specimen containers. *Pastettes* are manufactured from polyethylene and cannot therefore be heat sterilized. They can however be decontaminated using a suitable disinfectant such as diluted bleach, washed, dried, and reused several times for work not requiring a sterile pipette. *Pastettes* are available from DHT (see Appendix 11).

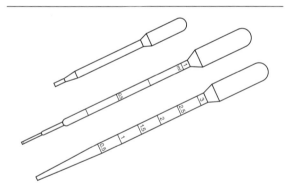

Fig. 4.16 Examples of useful graduated and non-graduated plastic (polyethylene) bulb pipettes (*Pastettes*).

Glass Pasteur Pipettes

These are needed when a sterile Pasteur pipette is required. Glass Pasteur pipettes can be made in the laboratory or bought ready-made. *Volac* glass Pasteur pipettes are recommended because they are made with a slightly heavier wall thickness to reduce breakages in use and in transit. They are available in sizes 150 mm, 230 mm, 270 mm, 310 mm and 350 mm, plain or plugged or sterilized, 250/box with two PVC teats, from Poulten and Graf (see Appendix 11).

Devices for use with pipettes

Effective, easy to control devices that can be used to draw up and dispense fluid from pipettes include:

■ Low cost DHT pipette fillers

■ *Pi-pump 2500* pipette filler

Bulbs with valves: A range of large bulb devices fitted with valves are available for the controlled filling and emptying of pipettes. Some of these are complex and tiring to use and also expensive.

DHT pipette fillers

These popular devices are inexpensive and easy to handle, giving excellent control of fluid levels. The pipette holding part of the device is made of a soft thermoplastic material. All sizes of pipette are easily inserted and held firmly. Three models are available from DHT:

– DHT pipette filler DPF.002 for use with pipettes up to 2 ml.

– DHT pipette filler DPF.005 for use with 5 ml pipettes.

– DHT pipette filler DPF.010 for use with 10 ml pipettes.

A DHT pipette filler is shown in Fig. 4.17.

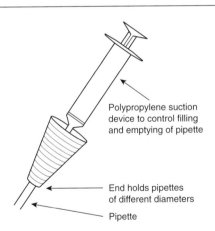

Fig. 4.17 Low cost controlled pipette filler that can be used with pipettes of different diameters.

Pi-pump 2500 pipette filler

This polypropylene thumb-wheel device made by Hecht is lightweight and very easy to operate. It gives excellent control of the level of fluid both when aspirating and dispensing. All the fluid can be dispensed by depressing the side lever or dispensed in measured volumes using the thumb-wheel as shown in Fig. 4.18.

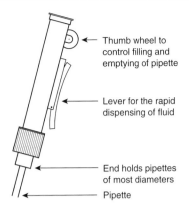

Fig. 4.18 *Pi-pump 2500* for use with pipettes of 1 ml to 10 ml.

The end of the green 10 ml *Pi-pump* is flexible and tapered, enabling it to be used with most pipettes up to 10 ml, including 1 ml and 2 ml pipettes (it is not necessary to purchase the smaller volume *Pi-pump*). The Pi-pump 2500 is available from DHT.

Similar designs of pipette filler: Other pipette fillers with a similar design to the green 10 ml *Pi-pump 2500* e.g. referred to as *Fast Release Pipette Fillers* are available but lack the special tapered anti-slip end of the *Pi-pump* made by Hecht.

Caution: When inserting a pipette into the end of a pipette filling device, always hold the *upper end*, not the middle or lower tapered end of the pipette. Serious injuries to the hand or wrist can occur when a long glass pipette is held lower down and snaps when it is being pushed into a device.

Reagent dispensers

Automatic bottle top or handheld devices are widely available for the rapid repetitive pipetting and dispensing of reagents. Some dispensers are very expensive. An inexpensive method of dispensing reagents is to use manual reagent syringe dispensers.

DHT manual syringe reagent dispensers

Reagent is aspirated by a polypropylene syringe having clear markings and narrow black silicone seal. It is fitted with a two-way valve. Fluid is drawn to the graduation mark each time by the user. The tubing can be left in the reagent and the syringe left attached to the tubing. In between use the syringe can be held in a small bottle or other container positioned next to the reagent bottle (see Fig. 4.19).

Such a system for dispensing reagents is not only safe for the user but also minimizes the contamination of reagents which can occur when pipettes

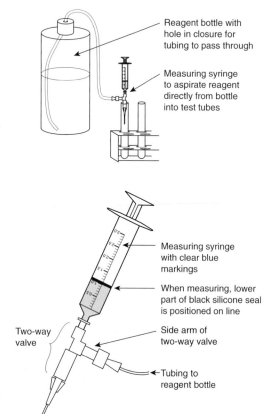

Reagent bottle with hole in closure for tubing to pass through

Measuring syringe to aspirate reagent directly from bottle into test tubes

Measuring syringe with clear blue markings

When measuring, lower part of black silicone seal is positioned on line

Two-way valve

Side arm of two-way valve

Tubing to reagent bottle

Dispensing probe

Fig. 4.19 DHT inexpensive manual syringe dispensing system. *Upper*: Complete system with reagent bottle, tubing and syringe (2.5 ml or 5.0 ml) with two-way valve. *Lower*: Measuring syringe with two-way valve suitable for measuring volumes up to 2.5 ml.

are used, keeps reagents capped when in use, and prevents the inaccuracy in liquid handling which can occur when pipettes are used and reagent is not wiped from the outside of a pipette but dispensed with the measured volume.

The DHT syringe reagent dispensing system is supplied complete with measuring syringe, two-way valve, tubing, 500 ml plastic reagent bottle and separate top with hole in it.

Principle of displacement

When changing from using pipettes to other devices for liquid handling which are based on displacement (e.g. syringe systems, dispensers, dilutors), it is important to understand the principle of displacement.

When using a syringe device, dispenser, or dilutor, the fluid is measured by displacement. Such a system requires priming before use, i.e. filling and emptying to remove air from the system. It is not usually possible to remove *every* air bubble and this does not matter providing the air bubble is *not*

dispensed with the fluid but remains in the end of the syringe tubing or dispensing arm.

Depending on the volume required, the following DHT syringe reagent dispensers are available:

- For volumes from 0.5 ml to 2.5 ml, use the 2.5 ml syringe dispenser graduated in 0.1 ml divisions.

- For volumes 3.0 ml, 3.5 ml, 4.0 ml, 4.5 ml and 5 ml, use the 5 ml syringe dispenser graduated in 0.5 ml divisions.

  Note: DHT manual syringe dispensers are not available for measuring volumes between 3.0 and 5 ml that require 0.1 ml graduations.

Labmax bottle top dispenser

One of the less expensive bottle top dispensers which is easy to use and maintain and has auto-calibration is the *Labmax* bottle top dispenser manufactured by Labnet International Inc. (see Appendix 11). Model D5370–5 dispenses 1–5 ml in 0.1 ml increments.

The *Labmax* bottle dispenser has a glass cylinder housed in polypropylene. The piston mechanism does not use fluid lubricant. A reagent guard valve prevents accidental discharge of reagent when the dispenser is not in use. Reagent is syphoned back into the bottle. A unique closed circuit air purging system allows air and bubbles to be eliminated without loss of reagent. The graduations are easy to read. The dispenser is supplied with a range of adaptors to fit commonly used reagent bottles.

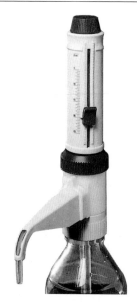

Plate 4.7 *Labmax* bottle top dispenser. *Courtesy of Labnet International Inc.*

4.7 Centrifuges

A centrifuge sediments particles (cells, bacteria, casts, parasites) suspended in fluid by exerting a force greater than that of gravity. The greater the outward pull due to rotation, i.e. centrifugal force, the more rapid and effective is the sedimentation. Heavy particles sediment first followed by lighter particles.

Centrifugal force increases with the speed of rotation, i.e. revolutions of the rotor per minute (rpm) and the radius of rotation. The actual sedimentation achieved at a given speed depends therefore on the radius of the centrifuge. Most techniques requiring a centrifugation stage will usually specify the required relative centrifugal force (RCF) expressed in gravities (g). For example, an RCF of 2 000 xg refers to a force 2 000 times the force of gravity. Most centrifuge manufacturers specify both the maximum RCF (separating capacity) and rpm of which a centrifuge is capable.

Calculating the RCF

The RCF can be calculated providing the rpm and the radius (in mm) of the centrifuge are known. The radius is measured from the centre of the centrifuge shaft to the tip of the centrifuge tube. The RCF can be calculated using a normogram or from the following formula:

$$RCF (g) = 1.118 \times radius (mm) \times rpm^2 \times 10^{-6}$$

In district laboratory work the following centrifuges are required:

- General purpose bench centrifuge
- Microhaematocrit centrifuge

GENERAL PURPOSE CENTRIFUGE

Specifications of a general purpose centrifuge for district laboratories

- Designed for centrifuging clinical samples, i.e. sealed centrifuging chamber with no ventilation holes in the base of the chamber.
- Microprocessor controlled digital display or electronic analogue dial controlled.[a]
- Fixed angle 4 to 12-place (depending on workload) rotor that can accommodate capped conical tubes of capacity 15 ml.[b]
- Brushless drive induction motor or brushed drive motor with spare carbon brushes supplied.

- Variable speed with maximum RCF of not less than 1000 g
- Fitted with a timer.
- Has a safe lid interlock (prevents the lid from opening before the rotor has stopped) and an easy to use mechanical lid release mechanism to recover samples should there be a power failure.[c]
- Easy to balance and preferably fitted with an imbalance detector that stops the centrifuge should the rotor be loaded incorrectly.
- Strong impact-resistant body and lid that will prevent debris from being projected into the laboratory should the rotor head crack and break up.

NOTES

a   Many manufacturers are replacing analogue dial operated centrifuges with microprocessor digital display models that can be operated with greater efficiency and accuracy. However, some microprocessor controlled centrifuges are very expensive and complex to use, offering the user a wide range of programmable functions. Such models are needed for specialist laboratory work. For district laboratories, a microprocessor controlled centrifuge with essential easy to use functions is recommended or an analogue centrifuge fitted with safety lid interlock.

b   Most small bench centrifuges have a fixed angle rotor for greater efficiency and performance. They are easier to obtain and less expensive than equivalent swing-out rotor models. A swing-out rotor centrifuge with sealed holders (buckets) is recommended for use in specialist microbiology laboratories.

Note: Not all bench top centrifuges can accommodate capped 15 ml capacity conical tubes (122–125 mm in length). Some can only take round bottomed tubes up to 100 mm in length, i.e. uncapped tubes which are less safe to use.

c   Not all centrifuges sold as having a lid interlock prevent the user from opening the centrifuge before the rotor has stopped. Centrifuges bearing the CE mark (sold in Europe) are fitted with a safe lid interlock. Some lid lock devices simply stop the motor, allowing the user to open the lid before the rotor has stopped spinning which can result in the release of infectious aerosols into the laboratory. Purchasers should check with the manufacturer on the type of lid lock and also the mechanism for releasing the lid in the event of a power failure.

A general purpose centrifuge is needed:

- To sediment cells, bacteria, and parasites in body fluids for microscopical examination, e.g. blood, urine, cerebrospinal fluid.

- To obtain serum, wash red cells, and perform emergency compatibility testing (crossmatching).
- To perform parasite concentration techniques.
- To obtain serum or plasma for antibody testing and clinical chemistry tests.

Microhaematocrit centrifuge

A microhaematocrit centrifuge is needed:

- To diagnose and monitor anaemia when a reliable measurement of haemoglobin is not possible.
- To measure PCV to calculate mean cell haemoglobin concentration (MCHC) in the investigation of iron deficiency and other forms of anaemia.
- To perform microhaematocrit concentration techniques to detect motile trypanosomes and microfilariae.

Note: The specifications and use of microhaematocrit centrifuges can be found in subunit 8.5 in Part 2 of *District Laboratory Practice in Tropical Countries*.

Variable speed analogue bench centrifuge

The 6-place analogue fixed angle rotor centrifuge shown in Plate 4.8 is manufactured by Nickel-Electro (model NE 020GT/1), see Appendix 11. It is suitable for use in small district laboratories because it is robust, has a variable speed control (500–3500 rpm) with maximum RCF of 1300 g, and is fitted with an electronic timer (0–30 minutes). A push button starts and stops the centrifuge.

The NE 020GT/1 centrifuge has a brushed drive motor (100 W rating, 230 V 50 Hz) and is fitted with a safety lid interlock which prevents the centrifuge from being opened before the rotor stops. Warning indicator lights are fitted for rotation and lid unlock. A special tool is provided to unlock the lid manually should a power failure occur. Tubes up to 15 ml capacity including capped tubes can be used. The centrifuge measures 340 mm wide × 290 mm deep × 225 mm high (lid closed) and weighs 15 kg.

Operating the NE 020GT/1 centrifuge from a 12 V lead-acid battery

Because the NE 020GT/1 is a variable speed brushed drive motor centrifuge with a 100 Watt rating, it is possible to use the *Handy Mains Inverter* described in subunit 4.2 to power the centrifuge

from a 12 V lead-acid battery. The workload *must not* require frequent or prolonged use of the centrifuge because this will lead to excessive discharging of the battery. The safety guidelines described in subunit 4.2 regarding the use and care of a 12 V lead-acid battery should be followed.

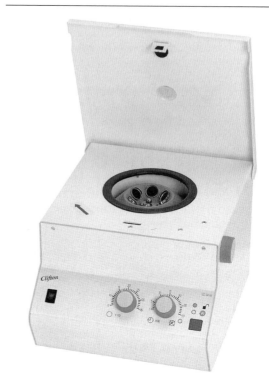

Plate 4.8 Nickel-Electro variable speed analogue 6-place interlock lid centrifuge. *Courtesy of Nickel-Electro.*

Variable speed Hermle microprocessor controlled bench centrifuge

The Hermle Z 200 A microprocessor controlled, variable speed, 12-place angle rotor centrifuge is recommended for district hospital laboratories. It is shown in Plate 4.9. The rotor is designed to take tubes up to 133 mm in length, i.e. conical capped tubes. It has a maximum RCF of 4 185 g (6 000 rpm) which the user controls by turning a knob. A small knob is also used to operate the timer which can be set in 0.5 minute intervals up to 30 minutes. Being microprocessor controlled, both the selected speed and time of centrifuging are digitally displayed (see Plate 4.9). If required, both the speed and time can be altered during a run or the centrifuge stopped before the set time.

The Hermle Z 200 A has an automatic braking system, a safe lid interlock, and an imbalance detector which automatically stops the centrifuge if the rotor is not balanced. Should there be a power failure, the lid can be manually opened by pulling a cord located in a recess in the side of the centrifuge.

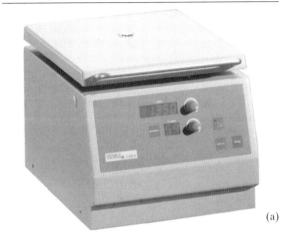

(a)

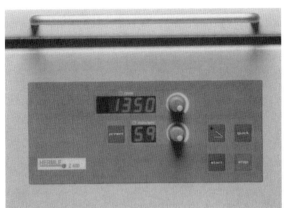

(b)

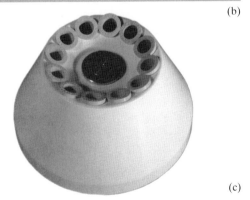

(c)

Plate 4.9 (a) Hermle Z 200 A, variable speed microprocessor controlled bench centrifuge.
(b) Control panel of Hermle Z 200 A centrifuge, showing speed control knob and display (upper), timer knob and display (lower), lid open indicator, start and stop knobs.
(c) Fixed angle 12 × 15 ml rotor of Hermle Z 200 A centrifuge. *Courtesy Hermle Labortechnik.*

The centrifuge can withstand a ±10% voltage fluctuation. Should a voltage fluctuation be greater than the built in ±10% tolerance, a voltage error code will be displayed in the speed control window and the centrifuge will stop. The Z 200 A centrifuge is fitted with a brushed drive, direct current, 100 W motor. It can only be operated from a mains electricity supply.

Availability of the Hermle Z 200 A centrifuge
The Z 200 A centrifuge is manufactured by Hermle Labortechnik (see Appendix 11). Complete with 12 × 15 ml rotor, the Z 200 A centrifuge measures 280 wide × 260 high × 370 deep mm and weighs 13 Kg. A separate angle rotor with inserts that take 6 Universals is available for the Z 200 A. When ordering, the voltage required must be stated.

Spare carbon brushes (part 940.204) should also be purchased for the Z 200 A centrifuge with a request for instructions on how to change the brushes. Instructions for changing the brushes are given in the *Service Manual*. Only a *User Manual* is normally provided with the centrifuge. Servicing departments should obtain a copy of the Hermle Z 200 A centrifuge *Service Manual*.

Other Hermle centrifuges

Hermle also supplies a brushless drive microprocessor controlled centrifuge with swing out rotor and sealed tube buckets (Z 300) with similar controls to the Z 200 A, but with a larger body. It measures 355 × 330 × 475 mm and weighs 27 Kg. The swing out rotor with sealed buckets is shown in Plate 4.10. A rotor that can take two microtitration plates is also available for use with the Z 300 centrifuge.

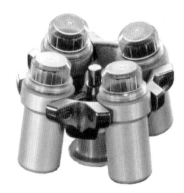

Plate 4.10 Swing out rotor with sealed buckets as used with the Hermle Z 300 microprocessor controlled centrifuge. *Courtesy of Lab Plant Ltd.*

Hand-operated centrifuges

Hand-operated centrifuges are dangerous both because of the injury that can be caused as the uncased buckets rotate and the serious risk of infection from aerosol dispersion.

In some countries the sale and use of hand-operated centrifuges has been banned. If the use of such a centrifuge is unavoidable it is important to locate the centrifuge in a safe place and use only capped plastic tubes.

USE AND CARE OF CENTRIFUGES

Although most modern centrifuges are fitted with an imbalance detector and lid interlock, it is important for laboratory workers to know how to use a centrifuge correctly to prevent it becoming damaged and breakages occurring. Also, many centrifuges in current use in district laboratories may not be fitted with the latest safety features.

Correct use and care of a centrifuge
- Place the centrifuge on a firm level bench out of direct sunlight, towards the back of the bench. Leave a clear area of 30 cm around the centrifuge (safety recommendation).
- Read the manufacturer's instructions. Prepare a stock record card and written SOPs covering the use, cleaning, and maintenance of the centrifuge.

Tubes and containers to use in a centrifuge
- Whenever possible use plastic tubes made from polystyrene or autoclavable copolymer or polypropylene. *Do not use thin-walled* glass tubes or vials that are sold as 'disposable' because they will break easily even when applying a low RCF.
- If using glass tubes, use round-bottomed tubes as these are less easily broken than conical tubes. Always examine tubes and other containers for cracks or chips before using them in a centrifuge.
- When using a swing-out rotor centrifuge, make sure the tubes are not too long otherwise they will be broken when the buckets swing out to their horizontal position.
- Cap tubes or containers (unless using sealed tube holders) and *do not* overfill them, particularly when using a fixed angle rotor centrifuge. Leave a gap of at least 20 mm from the top of the fluid to the rim of the tube or container.
- Do not insert a cotton wool plug or other loose fitting bung in a tube because this will be forced down into the fluid during centrifugation.

Balancing a centrifuge
- Check that the buckets or tube holders are correctly positioned in the centrifuge and that if required, each bucket contains its cushion (correctly located).

- Make sure that the contents on each side of the centrifuge are balanced. Read carefully the manufacturer's instructions particularly when using multi-tube carriers. Providing the same type and thickness of tube or container are used and the centrifuge is of the 'self-balancing' type, it is usually sufficient to balance the fluid contents of opposite buckets or tube holders by eye.

  If the centrifuge is not 'self-balancing', use a simple trip balance to check the weights (see subunit 4.5). If required, add water or a weak disinfectant solution to a bucket (using a wash-bottle) to balance the weights.

Note: Some centrifuges are fitted with an imbalance detector. This will stop a centrifuge from operating if it is not balanced. Imbalance can cause breakages and also wear out the bearings of a centrifuge which may lead to serious spin-off accidents.

Using a centrifuge
- Do not centrifuge at a higher speed or for a longer period than is necessary. This is important because many new models of centrifuge are capable of operating at very high speeds.
- When using an analogue type centrifuge, make sure that the speed control of the centrifuge is set at zero before starting the centrifuge and always increase the speed slowly. Immediately return the speed control to zero if there is any indication of imbalance or breakage.
- If using a centrifuge that can be fitted with both swing out and fixed angle rotors, do not operate the centrifuge at a higher speed than that recommended for the rotor being used (microprocessor controlled centrifuges have built-in rotor recognition to avoid rotors being used at incorrect speeds).
- If using a centrifuge that is not fitted with a lid interlock, or automatic brake, do not attempt to stop the rotor by hand because this can release aerosols, cause injury and will also damage the bearings of the centrifuge.
- *Never* open the centrifuge until the motor has stopped and the rotor has stopped spinning, otherwise infectious aerosols may be sprayed into the laboratory.
- Turn off a centrifuge and remove the plug from the wall socket at the end of each day's work and when there is an electrical storm.

Procedure if a breakage occurs: It is usually obvious from the noise that a glass tube or vial has broken or a bucket has failed. When a breakage occurs great clouds of aerosols may be dispersed. To reduce the risk of infection:

– Switch off the centrifuge but do not open it immediately. Allow at least 30 minutes for the droplets to settle.

– Wearing protective rubber gloves, remove and decontaminate the bucket and debris by autoclaving or boiling. Use forceps to dispose of the glass safely.

– Clean the centrifuge rotor and bowl with a suitable disinfectant.

Maintenance of a centrifuge

Most centrifuges become damaged and accidents occur because the buckets or rotor head have corroded or the buckets have not been placed correctly in the rotor. The following is essential preventive maintenance for centrifuges:

■ Clean the centrifuge and tube holders weekly or more often if indicated. Do not use corrosive cleaning fluids, particularly alkaline solutions. If centrifuging corrosive or alkaline samples in metal buckets, e.g. samples containing sodium hydroxide or saline solutions, make sure the buckets are rinsed and cleaned regularly.

■ At least every 3 months check the metal parts of the centrifuge for corrosion damage and cracks.

■ Examine regularly the electrical flex for signs of wear and check the plug for loose connections.

■ If the centrifuge is fitted with a brushed drive motor, the carbon brushes will require replacing periodically as instructed by the manufacturer. The motor will not run when the brushes have worn down. Prior sparking of the motor may occur.

Note: Always purchase spare carbon brushes with a brushed drive motor centrifuge and ask the manufacturer for instructions on how to change the brushes if these are not given in the *User Manual*. If it is difficult to change the brushes request the help of a qualified electrician.

4.8 Laboratory autoclave

In an autoclave, pressure is used to produce high temperature steam to achieve sterilization. The temperature of saturated steam at atmospheric pressure is approximately 100 °C. When water is boiled at an increasing pressure the temperature at which it boils and of the steam it forms, rises, i.e. temperature increases with pressure. At a pressure of 1.1 bar (15 lb/in^2, or 15 psi), the temperature of the saturated steam rises to 121 °C. Autoclaving at 121 °C for 15–20 minutes is required for sterilization. Both the temperature and holding time must be correct.

SI unit for pressure: Most pressure gauges on autoclaves are calibrated in pounds per square inch (lb/in^2, or psi) or in bars. The SI unit for pressure force is the pascal (Pa). In SI units, 1 psi is equivalent to 6.9 k Pa and 15 psi to 104 k Pa. Using bars, 1.1 bar is equivalent to 104 kPa or 15 psi.

Temperature

To obtain the correct temperature for sterilization *all* the air must first be removed from the autoclave. A mixture of hot air and steam will not sterilize. It has been estimated that if about 50% of air remains in the autoclave the temperature will only be 112 °C and heat penetration will be poor.

It must also be remembered that at high altitudes, atmospheric pressure is reduced and therefore the pressure required to achieve 121 °C will need to be increased. At 2 100 m (7 000 feet) a pressure of 18.5 psi is required to raise the temperature to 121 °C. The pressure should be raised 0.5 psi for every 300 m (1 000 feet) of altitude. Alternatively, a lower temperature and longer sterilizing time can be used (see later text).

Timing

Before commencing timing, sufficient time must first be allowed for the saturated steam to permeate the entire load and for heat transfer to occur. The heat-up time will depend on the type of autoclave and items being sterilized.

To prevent accidents and injury it is important to allow sufficient time after sterilization for the pressure to return to zero and for the load to cool. If the steam discharge tap is opened before the pressure gauge is reading zero, any fluid in the load will boil and bottles may explode. Several hours may be required for agar to cool to 80 °C for safe handling.

Other sterilizing cycles

Autoclaving at 121 °C for 15–20 minutes is recommended for most laboratory applications. Autoclaves used for sterilizing instruments and packs used in operating theatres, often referred to as clinical autoclaves, are usually designed to sterilize at 134 °C for 10 minutes or 126 °C for 11 minutes. Autoclaves operating at 121 °C are sometimes referred to as culture media autoclaves.

In district laboratories an autoclave is used for:

■ Sterilizing reusable syringes, specimen containers, tubes, pipettes, petri dishes, and other articles of equipment and laboratory- ware that need to be sterile before use and can withstand autoclaving. Items made from glass, metal, and plastic such as nylon, copolymer, or polypropylene can be autoclaved.

■ Sterilizing culture media and swabs for use in microbiology work. Most agar and liquid culture media can be autoclaved. Steaming at 100 °C in an autoclave with the lid left loose is used to sterilize media containing ingredients that could be decomposed or inactivated at temperatures over 100 °C.

■ Decontaminating specimens and other infectious waste prior to disposal (see subunit 3.4).

AUTOCLAVES FOR USE IN DISTRICT LABORATORIES

District hospital laboratories should be equipped with a reliable autoclave of adequate capacity. Small health centre laboratories will require an autoclave mainly for decontaminating specimens and infectious waste. For this purpose a less expensive pressure cooker is suitable.

Important: Staff *must* be adequately trained in the use of an autoclave or pressure cooker.

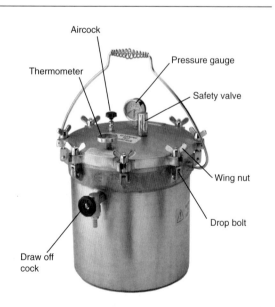

Plate 4.11 Dixon non-electric autoclave of 14 litre capacity, model ST 18, operating at 121 °C using an external heat source such as an electric hot plate, gas burner, or primus stove. *Courtesy of Dixon Surgical Instruments.*

Specifications of an autoclave for district hospital laboratories

● Capable of operating a 121 °C sterilizing cycle.

● Capacity of 14 to 30 litres, depending on workload.

● No plumbing in of the autoclave is required.

● Where mains electricity is unavailable, restricted, or intermittent, the autoclave should be capable of being used with an external heat source such as a hot plate, gas burner, or primus (kerosene) stove.

● Fitted with a thermometer and pressure gauge.

● Easy and safe to use with approved lid locking and pressure release safety valve.

● Supplied with metal tray or wire mesh basket.

● Thermostatically controlled and fitted with an automatic electric cut-out to prevent the autoclave from boiling dry (electric models).

● Supplied with clear operating and maintenance instructions.

Accessories and spares

– Gas burner or primus stove for a non-electric autoclave
– Metal stand if using gas or a primus stove
– Lid seal gasket
– Pressure release safety valve
– Spare washers for valves
– Timer
– TST (Time, Steam, Temperature) control indicator strips (121 °C for 15 minutes).

Dixon autoclaves

A robust aluminium constructed autoclave of 14 litre capacity with the above specifications, and capable of operating from an electric hot plate, gas burner, or primus stove, is the model ST18 shown in Plate 4.11. It is manufactured by and available from Dixon Surgical Instruments (see Appendix 11). The internal chamber measures 280 mm diameter × 230 mm deep. An electric thermostatically controlled 15 litre capacity, i.e. ST 19T is also available.

Dixon also manufactures 30 litre capacity, 121 °C operating autoclaves in stainless steel (280 mm diameter × 490 mm deep). The thermostatically controlled electric model ST 3028, is shown in Plate 4.12. It is fitted with a 2 kW heater and automatic

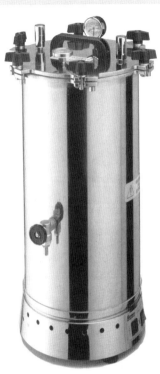

Plate 4.12 Dixon electric 2 kW heater autoclave of 30 litre capacity, model ST 3028, operating at 121 °C with temperature control and automatic cut-out. *Courtesy of Dixon Surgical Instruments.*

cut-out. The code for the gas/kerosene model is ST 3028G.

Further information on autoclaves: Details of more complex electric laboratory autoclaves, i.e. downward displacement autoclaves, can be found in the 8th edition *Microbiological Methods* (see Recommended Reading).

Prestige microprocessor controlled autoclave with automatic cycle

Microprocessor controlled electric autoclaves are widely available but expensive compared with manually operated models. Prestige Medical manufacture portable small capacity microprocessor controlled electronic autoclaves at affordable prices.

The *Prestige Classic* autoclave model 210024, as shown in Plate 4.13, has an automatic 121 °C/22 minute sterilizing cycle and important safety features. The chamber has a capacity of 12 litres, diameter of 210 mm, and height of 328 mm. The maximum load weight is 4 kg. The power consumption is 1500 W (50–60 Hz). It is supplied

with a large basket and wire support and clearly written *User Manual*.

Prestige electronic autoclaves have a mechanical interlock system which prevents the lid from being removed whilst pressure remains in the chamber. A gasket offset device prevents pressure build up if the lid is not correctly fitted. Electronic detectors turn off the power if there is insufficient water in the chamber for the safe operation of the autoclave. A one step operation starts the automatic cycle. A buzzer sounds when the sterilizing cycle is complete.

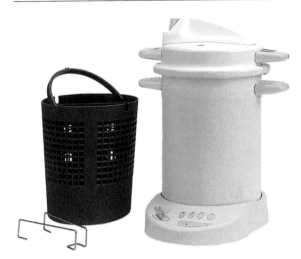

Plate 4.13 Electronic 12 litre Prestige *Classic* autoclave model 210024 with automatic 121 °C, 22 minute sterilizing cycle. *Courtesy of Prestige Medical.*

USE AND CARE OF AUTOCLAVES

The correct use of an autoclave is essential to protect against injury and to ensure sterilization. Always follow carefully the manufacturer's instructions and recommendations. Locate the autoclave in a safe place, particularly if using a primus stove or gas burner to heat the autoclave. Do not mix loads, i.e. autoclave infectious material separate from non-infectious articles. Always use the correct volume of water in the autoclave each time it is used (it must not be allowed to boil dry).

Decontamination of specimens and infectious waste

Place the articles for decontamination in wide, shallow, leak proof, solid bottomed containers, not more than 200 mm deep. Do not cover the containers.

When decontaminating infectious material in

plastic bags, do not over-pack the bags. Leave them unsealed with their tops folded back.

Sterilizing culture media

Place bottles and tubes of culture media in wire or polypropylene baskets. Limit the amount of culture medium in bottles to 500 ml. Leave the caps loose (tighten after autoclaving).

Always sterilize a medium at the correct temperature and for the correct length of time as instructed in the method of preparation. Under-autoclaving can result in an unsterile medium whereas over-autoclaving can cause precipitation, lowering of pH, or the destruction of essential components in a medium.

Sterilizing laboratory-ware

After cleaning, prepare reusable items for sterilization as follows:

Syringes: Wrap polypropylene, nylon, or glass syringes, barrel alongside plunger, in a clean cloth and close with adhesive tape or tie with a cloth strip.

Lancets and scalpel blades: Wrap stainless steel reusable lancets and scalpel blades individually in clean pieces of non-shiny porous paper (can be reused) and place in a small tin or other autoclavable container. Sterilize with the lid open (close after autoclaving).

Pipettes: Plug glass or polypropylene pipettes with non-absorbent cotton wool and wrap individually in non-shiny porous paper (X-ray wrapping paper is suitable) or place in a metal or polypropylene canister (leave the top off during autoclaving).

Specimen containers, tubes, petri dishes, and other laboratory-ware: Place polypropylene and heat resistant glass containers, tubes, and other items in wire baskets or other suitable open sided holders. When loading make sure the caps of the containers and tubes are loosened (tighten after autoclaving).

Using a manually operated autoclave with thermometer and pressure gauge

1 Add the correct amount of water to the autoclave as directed in the manufacturer's *User Manual*.

2 When loading the autoclave, leave sufficient space between articles for the steam to circulate freely. Do not allow articles to touch the sides of the chamber or stand in the water. Use a tray or wire stand in the bottom of the chamber.

3 Place a control TST (Time, Steam, Temperature) indicator strip in the centre of the load where steam penetration is likely to be slowest (see later text, *Control of an autoclave*).

4 Secure the lid of the autoclave as instructed by the manufacturer.

5 Open the aircock (air outlet) and close the draw-off cock (see Plate 4.11).

6 Heat the autoclave. If using an electric autoclave, switch on the power to maximum setting. If using a model without a built-in heater, apply heat from an electric hot plate, gas burner, or primus stove. When the water begins to boil, air and steam will be expelled through the aircock.

7 Allow the correct length of time for all the air to be expelled as instructed by the manufacturer.

Checking whether all the air has been expelled
It is possible to check whether all the air has been removed from an autoclave by connecting one end of a length of tubing to the air outlet and immersing the other end in a container of water. All the air has been expelled when no more bubbles can be seen emerging from the tubing into the water.

8 Close the aircock (air outlet). This will cause the pressure to rise and with it the temperature of the saturated steam.

9 When the required pressure has been reached (15 psi) as shown on the pressure gauge, and the excess steam begins to be released from the safety valve, reduce the heat and begin timing using a timer. The heat should be sufficient to maintain the required pressure for the duration of the sterilizing time.

Depending on altitude, set the timer as follows:

Altitude metres (m)	Time minutes
0	15 (121 °C)
500	20 (120 °C)
1 000	25 (119 °C)
1 500	30 (118 °C)
2 000	35 (117 °C)
2 500	40 (116 °C)

10 At the end of the sterilizing time, turn off the heat and allow the autoclave to cool naturally. This will usually take several hours particularly for agar culture media to cool sufficiently for safe handling.

11 When the thermometer reads below 80 °C and the pressure gauge registers zero, slowly open the draw-off cock to vent the autoclave. Open the aircock and wait for a few minutes before opening the lid.

Important: To avoid fluids boiling and injuries from burns or exploding bottles, NEVER open the draw-off cock or aircock, or attempt to open the lid of an autoclave until the temperature has fallen to below 80 °C and the PRESSURE READS ZERO.

Some models of electric autoclave are fitted with a safety device that prevents opening when the autoclave is still under pressure or thermal lock.

12 Open the lid of the autoclave as instructed by the manufacturer and carefully unload it.

Caution: Wear full face and hand protection when opening and unpacking an autoclave, particularly when it contains bottled fluids which may still be over 100 °C even when the temperature inside the autoclave is below 80 °C. On contact with air at room temperature the bottle may explode. If possible, leave the autoclave to cool overnight before opening it.

13 Check the TST control strip to ensure sterilization has been satisfactory (see later text).

Using a steam sterilizer (pressure cooker)

The following instructions apply when using a steam sterilizer (pressure cooker):

1 Prepare the articles for sterilizing as described previously.

2 Add the correct amount of water to the sterilizer as instructed in the manufacturer's *User Manual*. Use distilled or deionized water or if unavailable, use filtered rain water.

3 Load the sterilizer. Do not pack it too tightly or allow the articles to stand in the water or touch the sides of the chamber. Use the tray provided.

4 Place a control TST strip in the centre of the load (see *Control of an autoclave*).

5 Check that the lid gasket is correctly located and close the sterilizer as instructed by the manufacturer.

6 Press the lever of the pressure valve downwards.

7 Make sure the small metal pin in the safety valve is pushed down.

8 Apply heat to the sterilizer using an electric hot plate, gas burner, or primus stove.

9 When steam can be seen emerging *strongly* from the pressure valve, time 5 minutes. During this time air will be expelled with the steam.

10 After 5 minutes, reduce the heat until steam can still be clearly heard escaping from the pressure valve.

11 Begin timing 15 minutes. Make sure sufficient heat is applied to ensure the steam continues to emerge from the pressure valve.

Note: Most steam sterilizers are designed to operate at 121 °C for 15 minutes at 2 500 m and at 125 °C at sea level, therefore use 15 minutes up to 2 500 m. Between 2 500 m and 7 000 m, use 30 minutes.

12 At the end of the sterilization time, turn off the heat and *leave the sterilizer and its contents to cool.*

13 Lift the lever of the pressure valve and wait 15 minutes.

Important: Do not open the sterilizer until it has cooled and been fully vented.

14 Open the sterilizer and unload it. Examine the TST strip to ensure sterilization has been satisfactory.

Caution: Wear full face and hand protection when opening and unpacking the sterilizer.

Control of an autoclave

An autoclave thermometer, depending on its location, gives an indication of the temperature of the steam in the chamber or in the drain of an autoclave, not in the load. Ideally, therefore, all autoclaves should be tested with a thermocouple to find the time it takes to bring the load to 121 °C. The thermocouple leads should be placed in the centre of the load where heat penetration is slowest and the thermocouple connected to a recorder to produce a graph of the time/temperature conditions during the sterilizing cycle.

When a thermocouple and recorder are not available, an indication of the effectiveness of a sterilizing cycle can be obtained by incorporating in the load a chemical indicator that monitors time, steam, and temperature, such as an TST control strip.

Use of TST control strips

TST (Time, Steam, Temperature) control strips for use in autoclaves and pressure cookers incorporate a yellow chemical indicator in a circular area on the end of each strip. The control strip should be placed in the load where heat penetration is likely to be slowest (usually in the centre). Only when the conditions for sterilization have been met, i.e. correct heat/time ratio in saturated steam, will the yellow colour of the indicator dot change to a purple-blue colour, matching the purple-blue of the comparison dot shown on the strip. The change is abrupt and distinctive, avoiding any misinterpretation of the result.

The Albert Browne TST sterilizer control strips must be stored in the dark because direct sunlight will cause deterioration of the chemical indicator. In conditions of high relative humidity, unused strips should be sealed in an airtight plastic bag. Providing they are stored correctly, the strips have a 3 year shelf-life from date of manufacture.

Availability: TST control strips both for testing autoclaves operating at 121 °C and at higher temperatures are available in packs of 100 from the Browne Group (see Appendix 11). Code 2342, 121 °C/15 mins and also from Prestige Medical, code 219276 (121 °C/15 mins).

Other methods of monitoring the performance of autoclaves
Browne's indicator tubes: These contain a chemical that changes from red to green when the required temperature has been reached for the correct length of time. They cost about the same as the Browne's TST control strips but only monitor time and temperature. Also, being made of glass they are less safe to use than the TST strips.

Adhesive sterilization tape: This is not a reliable way of testing whether a sterilizing cycle has been effective. The heat/moisture sensitive ink which forms the bands on the tape and changes to a dark colour after autoclaving, does not record accurately the conditions during the sterilizing cycle. The tape is useful in showing when an article has been autoclaved.

Care and maintenance of autoclaves

- Read and follow carefully the manufacturer's instructions. Prepare a stock record card and written SOPs covering the use, care, and maintenance of the autoclave (see end of subunit 4.1).

- Hold in stock a spare lid gasket, safety valve, and spare valve washers (seals).

- Clean the inside of the autoclave after use and also around the valve and stopcocks. Make sure the vent is not blocked. Do not use a corrosive cleaning chemical.

- Check regularly for signs of wear and damage. Examine particularly whether:
  - the lid seal gasket is flexible and unperished and is not allowing steam to escape from the lid.
  - the flex is undamaged.
  - the pressure gauge is in working order and reading zero at atmospheric pressure.
  - the safety valve is free moving and in working order (read carefully the *User Manual* on how to check and clean the safety valve).
  - the aircock and draw-off cock are undamaged and working correctly with no leakage from seals.

- Do not use an autoclave if it is defective. Obtain the help of a qualified engineer to repair a defective autoclave and test it before reuse.

- Use a time, steam, and temperature control to check the performance of an autoclave (see previous text).

4.9 Incubator, water bath, heat block

Incubation at controlled temperatures is required for bacteriological cultures and some blood transfusion, serological, haematology and clinical chemistry tests. For bacteriological cultures, an incubator is required whereas for the other tests a dry heat block is recommended or a water bath.

INCUBATOR

Microorganisms require incubation at the temperature and in the humidity and gaseous atmosphere most suited to their metabolism.

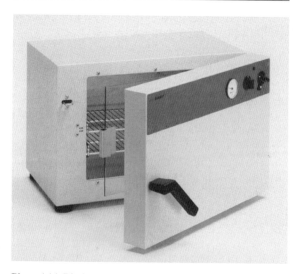

Plate 4.14 Binder 28 litre incubator with inner door and temperature display. *Courtesy of WTB Binder.*

Binder B28 incubator

The incubator shown in Plate 4.14 is the WTB Binder 28 litre, hydraulic thermostat controlled, natural convection incubator with analogue temperature display and overheat protection. It is fitted with an internal glass door. The inside of the incubator measures 280 mm high × 400 mm wide × 250 mm deep. Its operating range is 30 to 70 °C with ±1 °C accuracy. It has a power rating of 250 W and weighs 18 Kg.

Availability

The WTB Binder B28 litre incubator is manufactured by and available from WTB Binder GmbH (see Appendix II).

Specifications of an electric incubator for district microbiological laboratories

- Natural convection model with overheat protection, i.e. over temperature cut-out.[a]
- Capable of operating at 35 °C ± 2 °C with hydraulic thermostat temperature control or microprocessor controlled.[b]
- Fitted with a temperature display to provide a continuous readout of temperature or supplied with a thermometer for insertion through the vent hole in the roof of the incubator.
- Capacity suited to the workload. An incubator of 28 litre capacity as shown in Plate 4.14 will be adequate for most district laboratories.
- Non-tip adjustable shelves.
- Corrosion resistant durable outer case.
- Easy to clean and maintain and supplied with adequate *User Manual.*

NOTES

a   A natural convection incubator is recommended in preference to a fan air circulation model because a fan can cause the drying out of cultures.

b   While microprocessor controlled incubators provide a more sensitive control of temperature compared with hydraulic thermostatically operated incubators, most electronic models are more expensive to buy, service, and repair.

Note: Some manufacturers fit an inner glass door that enables cultural reactions to be viewed with the minimum of heat loss (see Plate 4.14).

Cultura M mains and battery low cost small incubator

The inexpensive *Cultura M* mains and battery operated incubator is suitable for use in district laboratories where the microbiology workload is small with only a few specimens requiring culturing or where there is a need for portability. Because the incubator has an operating temperature range of 25–45 °C, it can also be used for incubating water samples. It is lightweight, weighing just over 1 kg and measures

internally, 220 mm wide × 150 mm deep × 120 mm high (externally 310 × 155 × 168 mm). The *Cultura M* incubator can be used in either the horizontal or vertical position (see Plate 4.15). When used in the vertical position, a simple candle jar can be fitted inside the incubator.

The *Cultura M* incubator is constructed from white ABS plastic. It has a base shelf and transparent styrolux door. It is thermostatically controlled by a temperature regulator. Accuracy is ±1 °C. A thermometer is supplied.

Two models are available:

- *Cultura M* AC mains 220 V (or 110 V) only model.
- *Cultura M* AC mains and 12 V DC battery model. It is supplied with two separate leads. When using the incubator with a 12 V lead-acid battery, the battery lead with crocodile clips is used. When using the incubator with mains electricity, the lead with built-in converter is used (when ordering, state the voltage required (220 V or 110 V).

Availability

The *Cultura M* incubators are available from the manufacturer Almedica (see Appendix II). The *Cultura M* mains AC and 12 V DC model complete with thermometer, battery leads and AC mains lead with built-in converter has an order code 70702. The electric only model 220 V has an order code 70700, and the 110 V model, 70701.

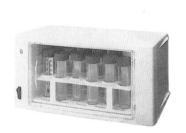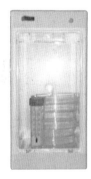

Plate 4.15 Mains and battery operated small portable Almedica *Cultura M* incubator with temperature range 25–45 °C (thermometer supplied). Can be used horizontally, *(left)* or vertically *(right)*.

Use and care of an incubator

■   Read carefully the manufacturer's instructions. Prepare a stock record card and written SOPs covering the use, care, and maintenance of the incubator (see end of subunit 4.1).

- Make sure the incubator is positioned on a level surface and that none of the ventilation openings are obstructed. Check that the flex is lying safely.

- If the incubator does not have a temperature display, insert a thermometer in the vent hole through the roof of the incubator. Adjust the thermostat dial until the thermometer shows the correct reading, i.e. 35 °C for the routine incubation of bacteriological cultures.

- Before incubating cultures and tests and following overnight culturing of microorganisms, check the temperature.

- Clean the incubator regularly, making sure it is first disconnected from its power supply.

- Every 3–6 months (depending on the age and condition of the incubator), check the incubator and flex for signs of wear.

- At the time of purchase, it is advisable to buy a spare thermostat and thermometer if these are of a special type and not available locally.

WATER BATH

In district laboratories a water bath is required to incubate bottles of culture media, liquids in flasks or other large containers, and when incubating samples in test tube racks. When only a few samples in tubes require incubating, it is more convenient and less expensive to use a dry heat block (see later text).

Specifications of a water bath for district laboratories
- Unstirred with hydraulic thermostat or electronic temperature control.[a]
- Operating over a temperature range from ambient to 60 °C or above, with safety cut-out.
- Having a 4 litre capacity.[b]
- Fitted with a thermometer.
- Supplied with a lid.[c]

NOTES
a Electronic temperature controlled water baths provide a more sensitive control of temperature but they are more expensive. Hydraulic thermostat controlled water baths having a 0.25-0.5 °C sensitivity are suitable for district laboratory work. Stirred water baths cost more than unstirred models. They are not required for district laboratory work.

b Water baths require filling with distilled water, or if

unavailable, with boiled or filtered rain water. It is therefore best to select the lowest capacity of bath that will handle the workload. A 4 litre capacity bath will usually be adequate (see Plate 4.16).

c A plastic or stainless steel lid, preferably gabled, is required to prevent heat loss from the bath and particles from entering.

Clifton NE1-4 unstirred analogue water bath
The water bath shown in Plate 4.16 is the Nickel-Electro *Clifton* unstirred, hydraulic thermostat, 4 litre capacity bath, model NE1-4. The inside of the bath measures 300 mm long × 150 mm wide × 150 mm deep (externally, 332 × 185 × 290 mm). It has a 500 W heater and is fitted with a safety cut-out. The sheathed immersion heater is located in the base of the bath under a perforated sheath. The sensitivity of the bath is ±0.25 °C, with a temperature range ambient +5 °C–100 °C. There is an illuminated on/off switch and 'heater-on' indicator. The power consumption of the heater is 400 W. The NE1-4/GLI-4/TC-1 Clifton bath is supplied with fitted angle thermometer and white plastic gabled lid.

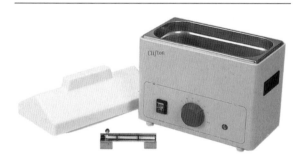

Plate 4.16 Nickel-Electro 4 litre capacity unstirred Clifton water bath with thermometer (fits to side of bath) and plastic gabled lid. *Courtesy of Nickel-Electro.*

Use and care of a water bath
- Read the manufacturer's instructions. Prepare a stock record card and written SOPs covering the use, care, and maintenance of the water bath (see end of subunit 4.1).

- Fill the bath and *maintain its level* with distilled water or if unavailable with boiled water, preferably boiled filtered rain water. This is necessary to minimize salts depositing on the heater.

- To minimize the growth of microorganisms in the water, add a bactericidal agent to the water such as merthiolate (thiomersal) at a dilution of 1 in 1 000.

- Before incubating samples, check that the temperature of the water is correct.

- Ensure that the level of the water is above the level of whatever is being incubated.

- Use the lid to prevent loss of heat from the bath and to minimize particles from entering the water. When removing the lid after incubation, take care to avoid any water entering uncapped tubes. Whenever possible, use capped tubes.

- Clean the water bath regularly, taking care not to damage the heating unit. If there is a build up of scale on the heater and sides of the bath, this can be removed by using the juice of a lemon or filling the bath with 10% w/v citric acid and leaving it until the deposit has dissolved.

- Unplug the bath from the wall socket when not using it, when there is an electric storm, and when cleaning the bath and carrying out any maintenance work.

- Every 3–6 months, check the bath for corrosion, the flex for wear, and the plug for any loose connections.

Heat block

In district laboratories where the workload is small and an incubator is not required because no bacteriological culture work is performed, a heat block is recommended for incubating samples in test tubes.

Compared with a water bath, a heat block (dry bath incubator) is less expensive to run, requires very little maintenance, and because water is not used, there is no risk of moisture entering tubes and interfering with reactions. It is usually less expensive to buy than a water bath.

Note: When used with a solid undrilled aluminium block (provided upon request by most manufacturers), a heat block can function as a small hot plate. However, unlike a hot plate it is not possible to increase or decrease the temperature rapidly.

Cole-Parmer analogue heat block
The heat block shown in Plate 4.17 is the electric analogue double block dry block heater model 36401–03 (240 V) supplied by Cole-Parmer (see Appendix 11). It has a maximum temperature of 130 °C and is fitted with dual bimetallic thermostats (high and low), which make it easy to control the temperature. The temperature stability is ±0.75 °C. Power consumption is 180W.

Specifications of a heat block for district laboratories
- Heat block that holds one or two blocks of the required hole diameters and preferably alphanumerically labelled for ease of identification. More than one block will be required if different diameters of tubes are being used.[a]
- Analogue thermostatic temperature control that provides stability of the block temperature at ±0.5 °C or ±0.75 °C.[b]
- Supplied with a thermometer which fits the thermometer-drilled hole in the block (may need to be ordered separately).

NOTES
a   To ensure good heat transfer and the correct incubating temperature of samples, the size of hole in the block must be correct for the diameter of tube used.
b   Digital heat blocks are also available that are microprocessor controlled, providing temperature stability as low as ±0.1 °C. These models, however, are considerably more expensive than the analogue thermostatically controlled heat blocks.

A range of aluminium heating blocks is available covering tubes of external diameters of 6, 10, 13, 16, 20 and 25 mm. A combination block holds three 25 mm tubes, five 13 mm tubes and six 6 mm tubes (code C–36400–56). This block and a block holding twenty 10 mm tubes are shown in Plate 4.17. A solid block is also available (code C–36400–60). Single size hole blocks are alphanumerically labelled (letters and numbers identify the holes). A Celsius scale spirit thermometer is required to set the temperature. This needs ordering separately. Each block has a hole for insertion of a thermometer.

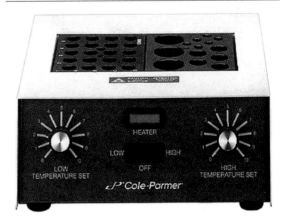

Plate 4.17 Cole-Parmer analogue two block heater with dual thermostats fitted with a combination block and labelled single tube size block. *Courtesy of Cole-Parmer.*

Use and care of a heat block

■ Keep a thermometer in the heat block and check that the temperature is correct before using the block. Allow time for the heat block to heat up before using a thermometer to set the thermostat at the temperature required.

■ Use the correct size of diameter tube in the block, i.e. one that fits the hole exactly.

■ Clean the block regularly as recommended by the manufacturer. Never use caustic cleaning materials. If required, an aluminium block can be autoclaved.

■ Disconnect the heat block from the electricity supply by removing the wall plug at the end of each day's work and before cleaning the unit.

4.10 Colorimeter

In district laboratories a colorimeter is used to measure haemoglobin and other substances in body fluids which can alter in concentration in disease and during treatment.

Colorimetry

A colorimeter is used to measure the concentration of a substance in a patient's sample by comparing the amount of light it absorbs with that absorbed by a standard preparation that contains a known amount of the substance being tested. A coloured solution of the substance being measured or a coloured derivative of it is produced. Coloured solutions absorb light at given wavelengths in the visible spectrum.

Visible light spectrum

Wavelengths between 400 nm and 700 nm form the visible light band of the electromagnetic spectrum, referred to as the visible light spectrum. Wavelengths of about 700 nm are seen by the eye as red colours while those of progressively shorter wavelengths give rise in turn to the colours orange, yellow, green, blue and finally violet which is produced by short wavelengths of 400 nm.

Wavelengths greater than 700 nm are known as infrared or heatwaves and cannot be seen by the eye while vibrations with wavelengths of less than 400 nm are known as ultraviolet (UV) light and these also cannot be seen by the eye.

Beer-Lambert law

Most colorimetric analytical tests are based on the Beer-Lambert law which states that under the correct conditions the absorbance of a solution when measured at the appropriate wavelength is directly proportional to its concentration and the length of the lightpath through the solution. Using a standard, this law can be applied to measuring the concentration of a substance in an unknown (test) solution by using the formula:

Concentration of test =

$$\frac{\text{Absorbance (A) of test}}{\text{Absorbance (A) of standard}} \times \text{Concentration of standard}$$

Terminology: Formerly the amount of light absorbed by a coloured solution, i.e. absorbance, was referred to as optical density, or OD.

In colorimetric tests, the lightpath is kept constant by using optically matched cuvettes usually of 10 mm lightpath distance or tubes of known lightpath distance. In selecting the correct band of wavelengths to use, both the maximum absorbance and selectivity of the wavelengths for a particular substance need to be considered.

For the Beer-Lambert law to hold true, both the solution being tested and the instrument used to measure the absorbance must meet certain requirements.

Solution requirements: The solution must be the same throughout (homogeneous) and the molecules of which it is composed must not associate or dissociate at the time absorbance is being measured. The substance being measured in the solution should not react with the solvent.

Reagent blanks must be used to correct for any absorption of light by solvents. A reagent blank solution contains all the reagents and chemicals used in the chemical development of the colour but lacks the substance being assayed. Alternatively, a reagent blank may contain all components except a vital reagent.

Instrument requirements: The instrument used in colorimetric tests must show satisfactory accuracy, sensitivity, reproducibility and linearity at the different wavelengths used.

The cuvettes used in the instrument must be optically matched, free from scratches, clean, and of the correct lightpath distance. A 10 mm lightpath cuvette is recommended for the clinical chemistry tests included in this publication.

Note: To determine whether a test method and the colorimeter used to measure a particular substance obey the Beer-Lambert law, it is essential to prepare what is called a calibration graph (see later text).

INSTRUMENTS USED TO READ ABSORBANCE

Absorbance can be measured using a:

■ Colorimeter (filter absorption spectrometer, or filter photometer).
■ Spectrophotometer (absorption spectrometer).

The main differences between a colorimeter and a spectrophotometer are as follows:

Colorimeter

When using a colorimeter, absorbance can be measured only within certain wavelength ranges with filters being used to obtain the required wavelength range.

Most colorimeters are supplied with colour filters that correspond to the Ilford Spectrum filters No. 600–609 which cover the wavelength ranges within the visible light spectrum, 400–700 nm. These filters have a wavelength band width of 40 nm and are suitable for most of the colorimetric test methods performed in district laboratories.

Interference filters

Most filter photometers and some colorimeters are supplied with, or make available as optional accessories, narrow band interference filters (typically 10 nm band width). These are more expensive and sensitive than colour filters and because they are available for reading at wavelengths beyond the visible spectrum (providing the instrument is fitted with a suitable lamp), they can increase the range of tests performed and the number of commercially available test kits that can be used.

Spectrophotometer

When using a spectrophotometer, absorbance can be measured at specific wavelengths. A diffraction grating, prism, or other device is used to disperse white light into a continuous spectrum, enabling wavelengths of monochromatic (one colour) light to be selected.

A spectrophotometer is mainly used when tests require reading at specific wavelengths, e.g. to reduce interference from unwanted chromogens. Compared with a colorimeter, a spectrophotometer is considerably more expensive, usually less rugged, and requires greater technical skill and a stable electricity supply for its reliable performance. Its use is not required for most district laboratory work.

Specifications of a colorimeter for district laboratories

● Preferably operating from both AC mains electricity and rechargeable battery.
● Preferably digital readout of absorbance.
● Wavelength range: 400–700 nm using 40 nm band width colour filters.
● Whenever possible, the colour filters should be glass mounted in a sealed unit inside the colorimeter to avoid them being mislaid or finger marked, fading in bright light, or being damaged from fungal growth.
● Can be used with easily obtainable 10 mm lightpath cuvettes.
● Preferably fitted with a cuvette chamber that holds two cuvettes.
● Capable of reading small sample volumes, to enable semi-micro methods to be used to reduce the cost of tests.
● Easy to use, clean and maintain.

Note: Laboratories carrying out a wide range of clinical chemistry tests using test kits may need to consider using a colorimeter fitted with interference filters and capable of providing readouts in both absorbance and concentration units.

Biochrom C0 7000 tropicalised colorimeter

A colorimeter with the above specifications is the digital readout C0 7000 *Colourwave Medical Colorimeter* shown in Plate 4.18. It is manufactured by Biochrom Ltd (see Appendix 11). The C0 7000 colorimeter operates from both mains electricity and internal rechargeable battery that is recharged from the adapter supplied. All ten filters (400–700 nm) are supplied with the colorimeter (see following text). They are glass sealed and mounted on a special filter wheel housed inside the colorimeter. A filter window shows which filter is in place (see Plate 4.18).

Fluid volumes as low as 1.6 ml can be read in the C0 7000 colorimeter. It is designed for use with 10 mm lightpath cuvettes or tubes of 10, 12, and 16 mm diameter using the adaptors supplied. The colorimeter has been tropicalised for use in hot and humid environments. The filters are encased in glass to protect them from fungal attack. The PCB is coated to preserve it from damage by heat up to 45 °C and from humidity. The CO 7000 measures 180 × 150 × 60 mm and weighs 0.6 kg. There is a drain hole at the bottom of the cuvette compartment so that spills of fluids drain harmlessly through the instrument.

Availability
The C0 7000 colorimeter is available from Biochrom Ltd (see Appendix II) It is supplied with 10 built in tropicalised filters (400–700 nm), starter pack of 10 plastic cuvettes, mains adapter, internal NiMH rechargeable battery, and fitted tungsten lamp (3V 1W). Spare lamps are available, code 80–3000–55.

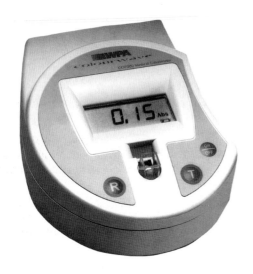

Plate 4.18 WPA Biochrom. *Colourwave C0 7000 Colorimeter. Courtesy of Biochrom Ltd.*

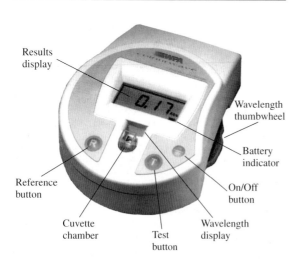

Plate 4.19 Controls of the *Colourwave C0 7000 Colorimeter. Courtesy of Biochrom Ltd.*

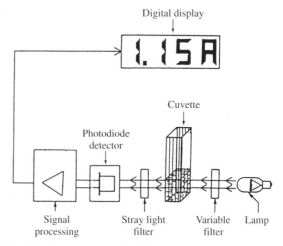

Fig. 4.20 Optical path of C0 7000 colorimeter.

USE AND CARE OF A COLORIMETER

- Read carefully the *User Manual.* Prepare a stock record card and written SOPs covering the use, care, and maintenance of the colorimeter.

- Use the correct type of cuvette or tube in the colorimeter as recommended by the manufacturer. Make sure that the cuvette (or tube) is clean and its optical surfaces are dry and free from finger marks and scratches.

- Bring the filter into place before switching on the colorimeter. Before use, allow sufficient time for the colorimeter to stabilize as instructed in the *User Manual.*

- Before reading the absorbance of a solution, check that it is clear, there are no air bubbles in it, and that it is at room temperature to avoid condensation forming on the outside of the cuvette or tube. Clean the outside of the cuvette with tissue to remove any marks from the optical surfaces.

- Calibrate the colorimeter for each test method (see later text).

- If a spillage occurs, immediately clean the colorimeter using water and detergent if required. Do not use organic solvents.

- To prolong the life of the lamp, switch off the colorimeter after use. At the end of the day's work disconnect it from the mains socket and cover the instrument with its protective dust cover.

- When needing to replace the lamp, usually indicated by difficulty in zeroing the instrument or no reading in the display, use a lamp of the correct specifications as detailed in the *User Manual.*

Always keep spare lamps in stock. Replace the lamp as instructed by the manufacturer. Take care not to finger mark the glass bulb.

Use of a colorimeter, based on the C0 7000 instrument

The essential components of a typical digital colorimeter such as the C0 7000 are shown in Fig. 4.20 and Plate 4.19.

Method of use

1 Place the colorimeter on a solid surface that is free from mechanical vibration. Do not place the instrument in direct sunlight or on the same bench as a centrifuge.

2 Ensure that the colorimeter is connected correctly to its adapter which plugs into the mains electricity supply. Alternatively, use the inbuilt battery, ensuring that there is sufficient battery charge. This will be indicated by a small battery symbol on the display. When there is only 1 bar of the symbol showing, the colorimeter needs to be charged (a full battery charge will take 8–12 hours. When fully charged the battery will last approximately 1 month).

3 Turn the filter thumbwheel until the required filter is shown in the wavelength display. The filter to use will usually be stated in the test method. The filters supplied can be used to cover the following ranges of wavelengths:

Wavelength Required	Filter to use
400–419 nm	400 nm
420–449 nm	440 nm
450–479 nm	470 nm
480–509 nm	490 nm
510–539 nm	520 nm
540–569 nm	550 nm
570–589 nm	580 nm
590–634 nm	590 nm
635–689 nm	680 nm
690–700 nm	700 nm

4 Turn on the colorimeter by pressing the on/off button. The display will show all digits and then revert to 0.00 Abs with the battery indicator showing full or partial charge. The green *Power Indicator* lamp will come on. Allow at least 2 minutes for the instrument to stabilize.

5 Transfer at least 1.6 ml of the reagent blank solution or distilled water (as specified in the test method) to a plastic or glass cuvette of 10 mm lightpath distance (macro or semimacro cuvettes can be used).

Important: Do not finger mark the clear optical surfaces of the cuvette and avoid air bubbles

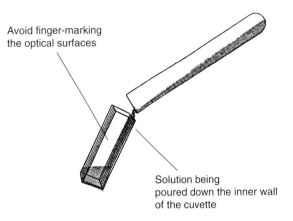

Avoid finger-marking the optical surfaces

Solution being poured down the inner wall of the cuvette

Fig. 4.21 How to transfer a solution from a tube to a cuvette, avoiding air bubbles.

forming when transferring the solution to the cuvette see Fig. 4.21. If reusing a plastic cuvette, make sure it is completely clean and its optical sides are scratch free.

6 Insert the blank solution in the cuvette chamber, making sure the clear optical surfaces of the cuvette are dry and facing *front-to-back* in the cuvette chamber.

7 Press button R once to reset the display to read zero. This is known as referencing.

8 Transfer at least 1.6 ml of the sample solution (standard, control, or patient's) to another cuvette. Remove the blank solution and insert the sample solution.

9 Press the test button T to give the absorbance reading for the sample.

10 Calculate the concentration of the control and test samples as instructed in the test method.

Calculation factor given in test kit methods
Where a test kit method provides a factor to calculate test results, this is based on reading the test at the wavelength specified. The factor will be different when using a colorimeter because of the 40 nm band width of the filter. To obtain the correct factor, when using a colorimeter, calibrate the test method (see following text).

Calibrating a colorimeter

As previously mentioned, when introducing a new test method it is necessary to establish whether the absorbance of the substance being measured increases in a linear way with its concentration. From the calibration graph, test results can be obtained.

Calibration of a test method involves:

- Preparing and testing a series of dilutions of the substance being assayed, i.e. standards, as described in the test methods in the clinical chemistry section (see *Calibration* text). For the calibration of most tests, five standards are used.

- From the absorbance readings obtained for the standards, prepare a calibration graph by plotting the absorbance of each standard against its concentration and examining whether a straight line (linear) calibration is produced. The preparation and use of a calibration graph is described as follows:

Method of preparing a calibration graph

1 Take a sheet of graph paper and rule the vertical axis and the horizontal axis. Mark the vertical axis *Absorbance*. Mark the horizontal axis *Concentration* and give the units of measurement (see Fig. 4.22).

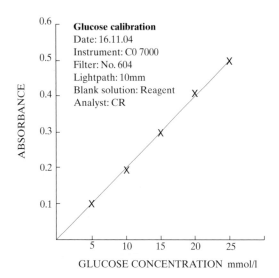

Fig. 4.22 Example of a calibration graph used to calibrate a glucose test method.

2 Depending on the range of concentrations and absorbance readings, divide each axis into the most suitable units for easiest reading. Use as much of the graph paper as possible.

3 Test each standard following the specified method. Plot the absorbance of each standard solution against its concentration, marking each point with a small neat cross (see Fig. 4.22).

4 Join each cross, making sure that the line passes through the point of origin in the bottom left hand corner (equivalent to the reagent blank).

5 Write in the top right-hand corner of the graph:
- date
- instrument used
- filter or wavelength at which the absorbances were measured
- lightpath distance of the cuvette (usually 10 mm)
- blank solution used to zero the instrument, i.e. water or a reagent blank solution
- initials of analyst (person who performed the calibration).

Linear calibration: If the line obviously looks as though it should be a straight line but one or two points are slightly off the line, this usually indicates inaccurate pipetting. A line of 'best fit' can be drawn if only one or two points are off the line. If a line of 'best fit' cannot be drawn, the calibration must be repeated.

    If only one point is off the line this should be disregarded and a straight line drawn through the origin and all the other points. Ideally the line passing through zero should be at an angle of 45°. If this is not so and the angle is too steep or too flat, repeat the readings using the filter or wavelength near to maximum absorption.

    If a straight line can be drawn through the points plotted as shown in Fig. 4.23, then absorbance is directly proportional to concentration. The Beer-Lambert law applies and its formula can be used (see following text).

Non-linear calibration: When the calibration is non-linear, the points will follow a curve, not a straight line. The curved line should be drawn smoothly and pass through the point of origin as shown in Fig. 4.24.

    When the graph is non-linear, the Beer-Lambert law and its formula cannot be applied (see following text).

Note: An analytical method where the Beer-Lambert law applies will have better performance characteristics than a method where the law cannot be applied.

Using a calibration graph to obtain test results

The procedures for determining the concentration of test and control samples depend on whether the calibration is linear or non-linear.

Using a linear calibration graph

When the calibration graph is linear, the following formula can be used to calculate the concentration of unknown samples:

Concentration of test (CT) =

$$\frac{\text{Absorbance of test (AT)}}{\text{Absorbance of standard (AS)}} \times \frac{\text{Concentration of}}{\text{standard (CS)}}$$

or in the abbreviated form:

$$CT = \frac{AT}{AS} \times CS$$

Alternatively, a table covering the appropriate range of values can be prepared from the calibration graph. Results can be read from the table providing the reading of the standard (put through with each batch of tests) agrees with the table and the control result is correct.

Note: If the reading of the test solution is beyond the limits of the graph or the range of the instrument, the final coloured solution can be diluted with an appropriate diluent and the absorbance of the diluted fluid read. The result is multiplied by the dilution factor. It is however better practice to dilute the specimen and repeat the test.

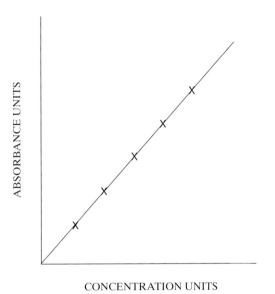

Fig. 4.23 Linear calibration showing a straight line joining the points plotted.

Using a non-linear calibration graph

When a test method produces a non-linear calibration, the values of the test and control samples must be read from the calibration graph. The formula based on the Beer-Lambert law *cannot* be used. A table covering the appropriate range of values can be prepared from the calibration graph.

The reading of the standard must be checked to make sure it agrees with the calibration graph and the control result must be correct.

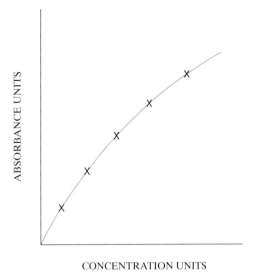

Fig. 4.24 Non-linear calibration showing a curved line joining the points plotted.

Need for control and standard with each batch of tests

A quality control sample must be carried through at the time of calibration and with each batch of tests. Only if the control sample gives the correct result can a calibration graph be used to determine patients' samples.

Control sample

A control sample contains a known amount of the substance being assayed. It is carried through every stage of the procedure in exactly the same way as patients' samples. It is the best indication that a method, reagents, and instrument are functioning satisfactorily.

When determining the concentration of unknown samples, the instrument, the method, and the reagents must be the same as those used for the standard solutions.

At least one of the standards used to prepare the calibration graph should be included in each batch of tests carried through. The amount of analyte in this standard solution should be carefully chosen to give the best performance possible. Best performance is required at concentrations where clinical decisions are made.

Note: The reagent blank must be treated in exactly the same way as the standards.

4.11 Mixers

Mixers that may be required in district laboratories, depending on the type of work performed and workload, include:

- Roller mixer, particularly for mixing blood specimens and control samples.

- Rotator (orbital mixer) for the controlled mixing of agglutination tests such as the RPR test.

- Vortex mixer for the safe mixing and emulsifying of samples particularly in microbiology and clinical chemistry laboratories and for dissolving substances in the preparation of reagents.

- Combined magnetic stirrer and hot plate, mainly used in the preparation of culture media and reagents, and when needing to heat liquids.

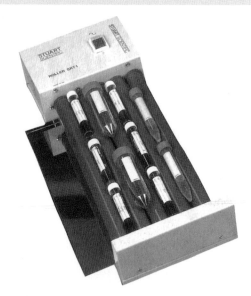

Plate 4.20 SRTI Stuart five-roller mixer that rotates and tilts specimens. *Courtesy of Bibby Sterilin.*

ROLLER MIXER

A roller mixer, rather than a revolving disc type of mixer (rotary mixer), is preferred for mixing blood and other specimens because it is easier to use, provides gentle but thorough mixing of specimens, can mix specimens in a variety of containers including Universals, and can be easily decontaminated and cleaned.

Specifications of a roller mixer for district laboratory work
- Five roller capacity.

- Provides rotary and tilt mixing of specimens.

- Fixed speed (33 rpm or 40 rpm).

- Easy to decontaminate and clean.

Stuart roller mixer
An example of a roller mixer with the above specifications is the SRTI 5 roller mixer shown in Plate 4.20. It is manufactured by Bibby Sterilin (see Appendix 11).

The roller mixer weighs 5 kg and measures 500 mm long × 200 mm wide by 90 mm high. To accommodate large diameter bottles one or more of the rollers can be removed.

ROTATOR (ORBITAL MIXER)

A rotator with the following specifications is required for mixing RPR agglutination tests used in the investigation of syphilis. Such a rotator is also useful for other slide or tile agglutination tests performed in microbiology, haematology, and blood transfusion laboratories.

Specifications of a rotator for RPR and other slide agglutination tests
- Operating at a speed of 100 rpm.

- Rotating in a 15–20 mm diameter orbit.

- Preferably with timer (RPR tests require 8 minutes rotation).

- Supplied with a lid to prevent drying of samples.

Immutrep battery and mains rotator
A rotator with the above specifications is the *Immutrep Rotator* shown in Plate 4.21. It is available from Developing Health Technology (see Appendix 11).

The rotator has a fixed speed of 100 rpm and an orbiting diameter of 15–20 mm. It is supplied with a lid. The platform can accommodate two agglutination plates. The *Immutrep Rotator* is supplied with 8 × 1.5 V rechargeable batteries and also with a mains adaptor making it possible to power the rotator from mains electricity or from batteries.

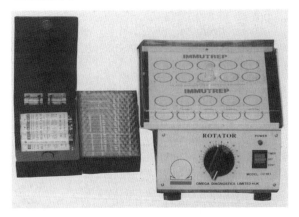

Plate 4.21 Rotator that can be operated from mains electricity or batteries, rechargeable from the mains or from solar power pack *(left)*. *Courtesy of Omega Diagnostics Ltd.*

The batteries can also be recharged from a solar panel (available as an accessory). A 12 V input is also fitted to the rotator to enable it to be powered from a 12 V lead-acid battery (leads not supplied). It has a built-in timer. After rotating for 8 minutes at 100 rpm, the rotator stops automatically.

VORTEX MIXER

When needing to mix and emulsify cultures and specimens, a vortex mixer provides a safe way of doing this, reducing the risk of infection from aerosols providing the mixer is used correctly.

Specifications of a vortex mixer for use in district laboratories
- Variable speed control.
- Preferably providing vortex mixing and gentle shaking.
- Provided with a range of easily interchangeable heads enabling samples to be mixed in tubes, flasks, beakers, and microtitration plates.
- Option for unattended use for longer continuous mixing of samples.
- Heads must be made of chemically-resistant treated material that will not absorb fluids and can be easily decontaminated and cleaned should a spillage occur.
- Stable base that holds the mixer securely on the bench and prevents it vibrating during use.

Vortex Genie 2 variable speed mixer
A variable speed, combined vortex mixer and shaker with the above specifications is the *Vortex Genie 2* shown in Plate 4.22. It is manufactured by Scientific Industries (see Appendix II). The standard unit is supplied with two heads: a 76 mm diameter black rubber platform head for vortexing or shaking liquids in flasks, beakers, single or multiple tubes, and a black rigid cup head for use with single tubes.

Two separate accessory packs are available for use with the *Vortex Genie 2*:

- H301 which is the *Multiple Sample Head Starter Set*. This includes a 152 mm diameter platform head with two inserts, one for taking 60 microtubes (5–10.5 mm in diameter) and the other for holding a microtitration plate (96 wells).

- H302 which is the *Large Sample Head Set* for beakers, flasks, and large tubes. It includes a recessed platform, elastic bands, and inserts for tubes of 10–37 mm diameter.

The *Vortex Genie 2* weighs 4.8 Kg, has a power consumption of 60 W, and measures 156 mm long × 121 mm deep × 165 mm high. When ordering, the voltage required must be stated.

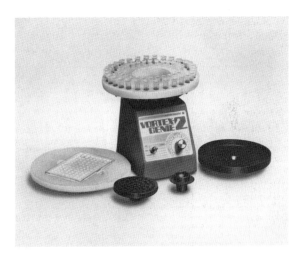

Plate 4.22 *Vortex Genie 2* variable speed mixer with accessories. *Courtesy of Scientific Industries.*

MAGNETIC STIRRER MIXER AND HOT PLATE
This is a useful piece of equipment because it combines a magnetic stirrer and hot plate in a single unit. Each function can be used independently.

Clifton analogue magnetic stirrer hot plate

Plate 4.23 shows the Clifton MSH.1 magnetic stirrer hot plate manufactured by Nickel-Electro (see Appendix II). The magnetic stirrer has a maximum speed range 100–1500 rpm with electronic speed control. The hot plate has a rapid warm-up and is manufactured from solid aluminium which cannot crack and chip like a glass ceramic plate. The hot plate is controlled by an energy regulator. It measures 140 mm in diameter.

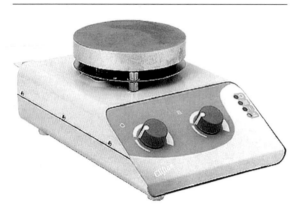

Plate 4.23 Clifton MSH.1 analogue magnetic stirrer hot plate. *Courtesy of Nickel-Electro.*

The MSH.1 magnetic stirrer hot plate has a power consumption of 425 W (hot plate 400 W). Its overall dimensions are 315 × 240 × 172 mm. It is supplied with two PTFE followers (spinbar magnets), one 20 mm long and the other 40 mm. The motor is fitted with one shot over-temperature/over-current safety device. The magnetic stirrer is capable of stirring up to 5 litre volumes. The unit weighs 5.1 kg. When ordering, the voltage required must be stated.

USE AND CARE OF MIXERS

- Read the manufacturer's *User Manual*. Prepare a stock record card and written SOPs covering the use, care, and maintenance of the mixer (see end of subunit 4.1).

- A practical demonstration must be given when training staff how to use a vortex mixer. Do not allow students to use the equipment without supervision.

- Make sure the containers used on a roller mixer have leakproof caps.

- Should a spillage occur, immediately clean the mixer as recommended by the manufacturer.

- Take special care when using a stirring hot plate. Use it in a safe place, well away from flammable chemicals. Turn it off immediately after use. If the unit has a ceramic plate, take care not to crack, scratch, or chip the ceramic. If damaged, the equipment must *not* be used. This risk can be avoided by purchasing a magnetic stirrer hot plate which has an aluminium plate (see previous text).

Expected heat and chemical resistance of plastics commonly used to make laboratory plastic-ware

	LDPE	HDPE	PP	PMP	PS	PVC	PC	PTFE
Translucent	Yes	Yes	Yes	Clear	Clear	Varies	Clear	No
Heat								
Autoclavable, 121 °C, 15–20 min	No	15 min	Yes	Yes	No	No	Yes	Yes
Hot air oven sterilization	No	No	No	No	No	No	No	Yes
Chemicals								
Acetic acid	●	●	●	●	●	●	●	●
Acetone	●	●	●	●	X	X	X	●
Ammonium hydroxide, 28% w/v	●	●	●	●	●	●	X	●
Benzoic acid, saturated	●	●	●	●	●	●	●	●
Boric acid	●	●	●	●	●	●	●	●

	LDPE	HDPE	PP	PMP	PS	PVC	PC	PTFE
Butyl alcohol	●	●	●	●	●	●	●	●
Calcium hydroxide	●	●	●	●	●	●	X	●
Calcium hypochlorite	●	●	●	●	●	●	X	●
Carbon tetrachloride	X	●	●	●	X	X	X	●
Chloroform	X	●	●	X	X	X	X	●
Citric acid	●	●	●	●	●	●	●	●
Cresol	X	●	●	X	X	X	X	●
Diethyl ether, see *Notes*	X	X	X	X	X	X	X	●
Ethyl acetate	●	●	●	●	X	X	X	●
Ethyl alcohol	●	●	●	●	●	●	●	●
Ethylene glycol	●	●	●	●	●	●	●	●
Formaldehyde (aqueous)	●	●	●	●	●	●	●	●
Glycerol (glycerine)	●	●	●	●	●	●	●	●
Hydrochloric acid, 35% v/v	●	●	●	●	●	●	●	●
Hydrogen peroxide	●	●	●	●	X	●	●	●
Methyl alcohol	●	●	●	●	●	●	●	●
Nitric acid, 10% v/v	●	●	●	●	●	●	●	●
Nitric acid, 70% v/v	X	●	X	●	X	X	X	●
Phenol	●	●	●	●	●	●	●	●
Phosphoric acid, concentrated	●	●	●	●	●	●	●	●
Potassium hydroxide, concentrated	●	●	●	●	●	●	X	●
Potassium permangate	●	●	●	●	●	●	●	●
Salicylic acid, saturated	●	●	●	●	●	●	●	●
Silver nitrate	●	●	●	●	●	●	●	●
Sodium hydroxide, concentrated	●	●	●	●	●	●	X	●
Sodium hypochlorite, 0.5% w/v	●	●	●	●	●	●	X	●
Sulphuric acid, dilute	●	●	●	●	●	●	●	●
Sulphuric acid, concentrated	X	●	●	●	X	X	X	●
Toluene	X	X	X	X	X	X	X	●
Trichloroacetic acid	●	●	●	●	●	●	●	●
Trichloroethylene	X	X	X	X	X	X	X	●
Urea	●	●	●	●	●	●	X	●
Xylene	●	●	X	X	X	X	X	●

Key: ● = Resistant at 20 °C. X = Appreciable reaction, not recommended.
Abbreviations: LDPE = Low density polyethylene, HDPE = High density polyethylene (more rigid and less permeable than LDPE), PP = Polypropylene, PMP = Polymethylpentene (TPX), PS = Polystyrene, PVC = Polyvinyl chloride, PC = Polycarbonate, PTFE = Polytetrafluoroethylene.
Notes: Tubes made from polypropylene (PP) copolymer or polycarbonate (PC) can be used with the formol ether concentration technique. The reactions of copolymer are similar to those of polypropylene. Products made from PS and PMP are brittle at ambient temperature and may crack or break if dropped.

4.12 General laboratory-ware for district laboratories

Besides the main items of equipment described in subunits 4.3–4.11, district laboratories depending on the tests they perform, will also require many of the items included in this subunit.

The quantity of each item required will depend on the work of the laboratory, frequency of ordering, source(s) of supply, prices and available finance.

ITEM	SPECIFICATION AND ORDERING INFORMATION

PLASTIC-WARE

Information on the resistance of different plastics to chemicals and heat can be found on pages 160–161. Although many of the items listed under PLASTIC-WARE are also manufactured in glass, plastic-ware is recommended because it is break-resistant and therefore safer to use, easier to transport, and more economical because of its durability.

Beakers
Polypropylene beakers suitable for general use, e.g. *Tri-pour* graduated type. Suggested capacities: 50 ml, 100 ml, 250 ml, 1 000 ml. Order by description and capacity.

Cylinders
Polypropylene, with clear graduations. Suggested capacities: 50 ml, 250 ml, 500 ml. Order by description and capacity.

Cuvettes
Polystyrene, 10 mm lightpath, 40 mm height. Order by description. Usual quantity: 100 cuvettes per pack.

Volumetric flasks
Preferably clear PMP or TPX with stopper. Suggested capacities: 100 ml, 250 ml, 500 ml, 1 000 ml (mainly needed for making standards). Order by description and capacity.
Note: Glass volumetric flasks are generally less expensive but not as durable.

Funnels
Polypropylene, preferably ribbed for rapid filtering. Suggested sizes: diameter 35–40 mm, 60–70 mm, 90–100 mm, 140–150 mm. Order by description and diameter size.
Note: Larger size plastic funnels can usually be obtained inexpensively from a local store or market.

Measuring jug
Polypropylene, 1 litre (1 000 ml) capacity, graduated tall jug (saves buying an expensive 1 litre cylinder). Order by description.

Strainer (sieve)
Small plastic strainer, approximately 65 mm top diameter (needed for faecal concentration technique). Obtain locally (nylon plastic tea strainer is suitable).

Water storage container
Polyethylene 5 litre container with handle and removable tap.

GLASSWARE

Microscope slides
Size 76 × 26 mm, prewashed with *ground polished edges* and twin-frosted end (one end frosted both sides) for easy labelling using a lead pencil. Order by size and description. Usual pack: 50 or 100 slides per box.

Cover glasses
Preferably size 20 × 20 mm, No. $1\frac{1}{2}$ thickness (stronger for reuse). Usual pack: 100 cover glasses per box.
Note: Size 22 × 22 mm can also be used but when covering wet preparations this leaves very little space on each side of the cover glass, resulting in the underside of the slide and fingers becoming easily contaminated.

Counting chamber
See Haemocytometer under *WBC counting equipment*.

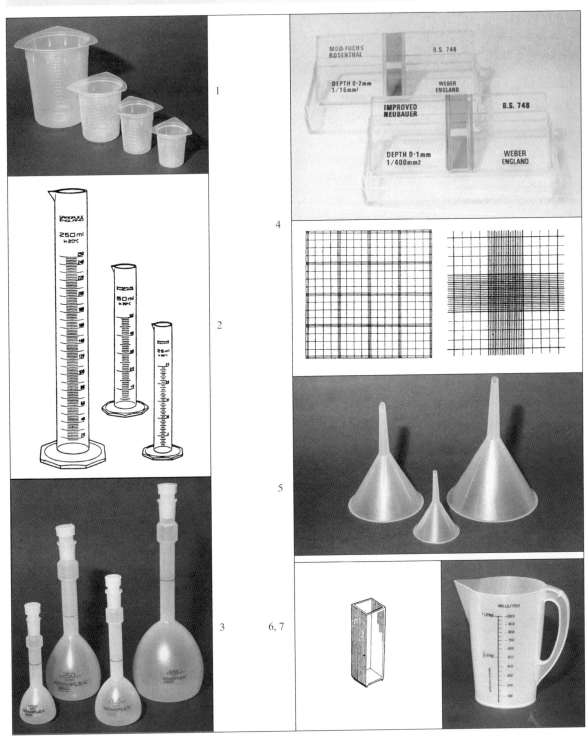

1 Tripour beakers. 2 Cylinders. 3 Plastic volumetric flasks. 4 Fuchs Rosenthal chamber and ruling *(left)*, improved Neubauer chamber and ruling *(right)*. 5 Ribbed funnels. 6 *Left:* Polystyrene 10 mm cuvette. 7 *Right:* Tall plastic measuring jug.

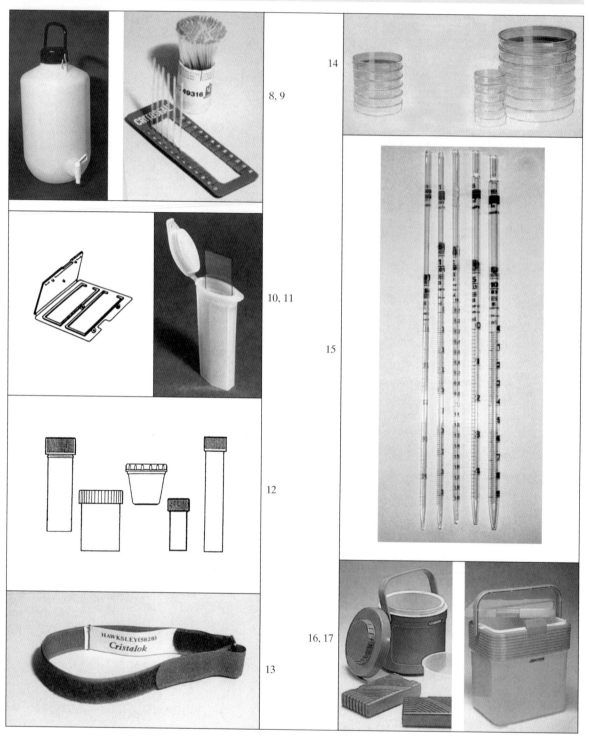

8 Polyethylene water container.   9 Haematocrit tubes and sealant.   10 Slide mailer for 2 slides.   11 Leakproof slide mailer for 4 slides.   12 Specimen containers.   13 Tourniquet with velcro ends.   14 Petri dishes (glass and plastic).   15 Graduated pipettes. 16 Insulated flask.   17 Cool box for transporting specimens.

Petri dishes (reusable)	Standard size (*Pyrex*): Lid diameter 80 mm (base 74 mm), or lid 100 mm (base 94 mm). Usual pack: 10 dishes. *Note*: Autoclavable plastic dishes made from PMP are available (*Nalgene*) but considerably more expensive than *Pyrex* glass dishes. Usual pack: 10 dishes.
Graduated pipettes	Class B accuracy, type 3 graduated pipettes are suitable. Suggested capacities: 0.2 ml, 0.5 ml, 1 ml, 2 ml, 5 ml, 10 ml. *Types*: refer to graduations. *Type 1* reads zero at top, capacity at shoulder. *Type 2* reads capacity at top, zero at outlet. *Type 3* reads zero at top, capacity at outlet. *Type 4* reads zero at top, capacity at outlet with blowing-out of last drop. *Plastic pipettes*: For some forms of work, plastic pipettes are suitable but not as easy to clean as glass pipettes. Pipettes made from polypropylene are more chemically resistant and durable than those made from polystyrene (see plastic resistance chart at the end of this subunit).
Pastettes	See *Plastic bulb pipettes*, described in subunit 4.6.
Westergren pipettes	See *ESR equipment*.
Micro-pipettes	Clear glass or white shellback (Sahli type). Available: 20 μl (0.02 ml), 50 μl (0.05 ml), 100 μl (0.1 ml). Used mainly for collecting capillary blood (see also subunit 4.6). *Note*: These pipettes are of the containing type, i.e. pipette needs to be rinsed in diluent to ensure none of the sample remains in the pipette.
Calibrated capillaries	Calibrated for a single volume with a line marked on the capillary. Available: 20 μl (0.02 ml), 50 μl (0.05 ml), 100 μl (0.1 ml), 200 μl (0.2 ml). Used mainly for collecting capillary blood (see also subunit 4.6). Usual pack: 200 or 250 capillaries per box.
Haematocrit capillaries	– *Plain* (without heparin): 75 mm long, for use with anticoagulated blood, e.g. EDTA blood. Usual pack: 100, 200, or 250 capillary tubes per box. – *Heparinized*: 75 mm long, for the direct collection of capillary blood, e.g. when measuring PCV. Usual pack: 100, 200, or 250 capillary tubes per box.
Pipette fillers	See subunit 4.6, *Equipment for pipetting and dispensing*.

SPECIMEN CONTAINERS (REUSABLE)

All containers must have leak-proof caps, preferably screw caps that do not require a liner. For reuse, order containers without a label (most labelled containers use water-insoluble adhesive labels which are difficult to remove). Purchase *water soluble* adhesive labels (see *Stationery*).

Urine container	Glass, 20–30 ml capacity wide-neck Universal is suitable. *Note*: If it is not necessary to autoclave the container (specimen is not for culture), a polystyrene plastic container can be used. A polypropylene Universal, although more durable and autoclavable, is not recommended because it is not possible to see whether the specimen is clear or cloudy.
Faecal container	Preferably polypropylene, 25–30 ml capacity, wide-neck container. *Note*: Whenever possible use a disposable container for faeces.
Sputum container	Preferably polypropylene, 60–120 ml capacity, wide-neck container. *Note*: Whenever possible use a disposable container for sputum.
Blood containers (reusable)	– *Venous clotted blood container* Glass, 10 ml capacity, flat bottomed vial (tube) about 16 × 100 mm with plastic cap that does not require a liner. *Note*: Do not use a plastic container. A glass container is required for good blood clotting and clot retraction. – *EDTA anticoagulated blood container* Polystyrene or glass container of 2.5 ml capacity preferably with pink cap (add EDTA anticoagulant in the laboratory).

– *Serum or plasma container*
Polypropylene plastic container of 5 ml capacity, preferably with white screw cap.

– *ESR container.* See *ESR equipment.*

– *Fluoride-oxalate container*
Polystyrene or glass container of 2.0 ml or 2.5 ml capacity, preferably with yellow cap (add fluoride-oxalate in the laboratory).

TRANSPORTING SPECIMENS

Slide mailer Leakproof reusable polythene box, suitable for the safe transport of up to four microscopical slide preparations (76 × 26 mm slides).

Cool box or flask Well insulated box or cool bag supplied with freezer packs or if transporting very few specimens, a wide neck, shatter resistant, plastic bodied *Thermos* flask. Usually locally available.

Note: Information on insulated containers for transporting blood and specimens that require careful temperature control can be obtained from WHO Expanded Programme for Immunization (EPI), World Health Organization EPI Unit, 1211 Geneva, 27-Switzerland.

BLOOD COLLECTION ITEMS

Tourniquet Elasticated arm band with velcro ends is suitable. Alternatively, about 360 mm of *soft* flexible latex rubber tubing.

Sphygmomanometer (Pressure cuff) Anaeroid sphygmomanometer with pressure dial, rubber tubing, bulb, and velcro ends. Needed for checking the blood pressure of blood donors.

Spencer Wells forceps Needed to clamp tubing when collecting blood from donors. Stainless steel Spencer Wells forceps about 125 mm long is suitable.

Syringes (reusable) Polypropylene or nylon with Luer end. Suggested capacities: 2.5 ml, 5 ml, 10 ml.

Needles Long length hypodermic, with polypropylene or metal hub. For collecting venous blood from adults, order 19 g (gauge) about 35 mm long. For children, order 23 g, about 25 mm long. Usual pack: 100 needles per box.

Lancets (prickers) Preferably stainless steel with long point (*Steriseal* type). Usual pack: 200 lancets per box.

Blood donor bags See *Collection of blood from donors*, described in subunit 9.2 Part 2 of *District Laboratory Practice in Tropical Countries.*

Blood collection card Whatman card with filter paper circles for collecting blood samples (spots) for use mainly in surveys. Each blood spot measures 16 mm in diameter and requires 100 µl of blood. Using a $\frac{1}{8}$ punch, about 1.3 µl of serum is obtained after lyzing the dried blood spot.

REAGENT AND MEDIA CONTAINERS

Use glass or good quality plastic bottles that have a leak-proof screw-cap that does not require a liner. For culture media, use glass containers that can be autoclaved.

Brown or other opaque container Needed for light sensitive reagents and stains. Obtainable in glass or plastic. Useful capacities: 250 ml, 500 ml, 1 litre, 2.5 litre.

Clear or translucent container Glass or good quality plastic. Useful capacities: 60–100 ml, 250 ml, 500 ml, 1 litre.

Dropper bottle – *Translucent polythene*: 15 ml container with dropper plug and cap. Suitable for physiological saline (when making faecal preparations), and dispensing immersion oil.

– *Amber polythene*: 15 ml container with dropper plug and cap. Suitable for iodine (when making faecal preparations).

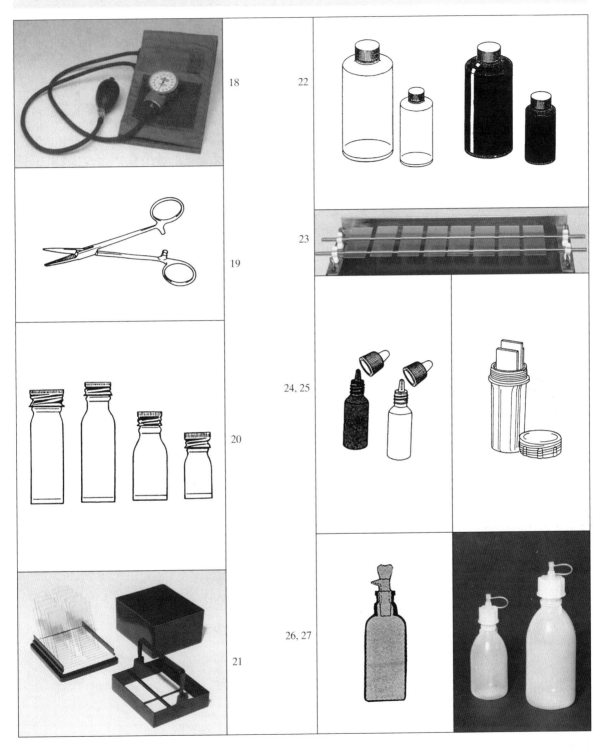

18 Pressure cuff. 19 Spencer Wells forceps. 20 Universal, McCartney, and bijoux bottles. 21 Slide staining trough. 22 Clear and amber reagent containers. 23 Slide staining rods. 24 Saline and iodine droppers. 25 Coplin container. 26 TK staining bottle. 27 Spout staining containers.

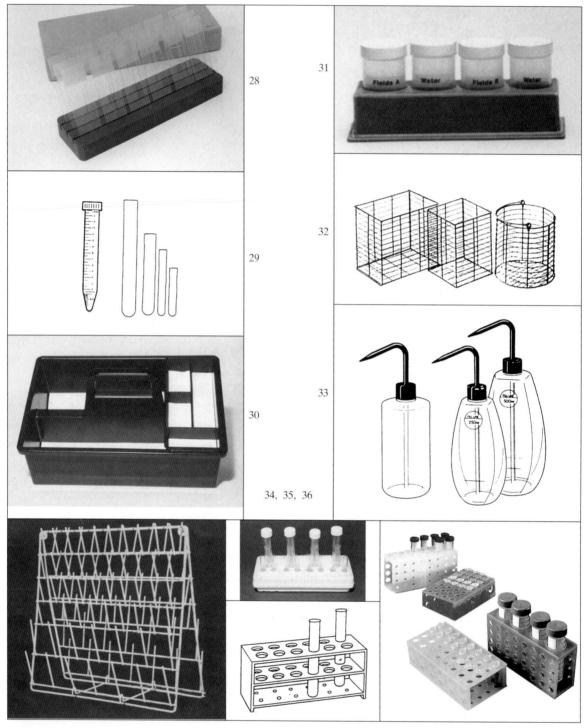

28 Slide draining rack.   29 Centrifuge and round base tubes.   30 Collecting tray.   31 Malaria rack.   32 Storage and autoclave baskets.   33 Wash bottles.   34 Drying rack.   35 Plastic crossmatch rack *(upper)*, test-tube rack *(lower)*.   36 Polypropylene 4-way combi-racks. Single rack has 4 sizes of hole to accommodate different sizes of tubes: 32 × 8 mm holes for 0.5 ml microtubes, 32 × 12 mm holes for 1.5 ml and 2 ml microtubes, 12 × 17 mm holes for 15 ml tubes, and 4 × 30 mm holes for Universals. The racks can also be joined together. Produced in green, blue, orange, yellow or neutral. Made by Scientific Specialities Inc (available from DHT, Alpha Labs and Radleys).

Bijou bottle	For use mainly in microbiology. Glass, with aluminium cap and rubber liner that can be autoclaved. Order extra caps and liners.
Universal or McCartney bottle	For use mainly in microbiology. *McCartney*: glass, 28 ml capacity with narrow neck, aluminium screw cap and rubber liner. *Universal*: glass, 25 ml capacity with wide neck, aluminium screw cap and rubber liner. Order extra caps and liners.

STAINING EQUIPMENT (MANUAL TECHNIQUES)

Staining rods	Stainless steel adjustable length rods in holders with levelling screws, for fitting across sink.
Coplin jar	Screw cap cylindrical polypropylene container with grooves for holding up to 10 slide preparations (back to back).
Slide staining trough	Black acetyl trough with rack for holding up to 25 slide preparations and lid which has a holder for draining slides. Useful for batch staining.
Malaria staining containers	Polypropylene, 100 ml capacity wide-neck containers for Fields' staining of thick blood films (dip technique).
Stain dispensing container	– *TK type*: Amber glass, 100 ml capacity with groove in stopper. Can be closed when not in use. – *Spout-type*: Translucent polythene bottle with pouring spout which can be closed when not in use. Useful capacities: 100 ml, 250 ml.
Wash bottle	Polythene, with dispenser tube. Useful capacities: 250 ml, 500 ml. *Solvent venting wash bottles*: The caps of these wash bottles are fitted with a valve which vents volatile solvent vapour, eliminating solvent drip. Useful when wash bottles are used with volatile reagents, e.g. alcoholic reagents.

TUBES

Centrifuge tubes	Conical tubes, 10–15 ml capacity, preferably graduated and made from break-resistant autoclavable copolymer or polypropylene. Order with caps for the safe centrifuging of specimens. *Note*: Most small bench centrifuges can only accommodate capped tubes up to 100–110 mm in length, i.e. of 10 ml or 12 ml capacity. The Hermle Z200A centrifuge is an exception in that it can accommodate longer length 15 ml capacity conical tubes (see subunit 4.7). Copolymer tubes can be used in the formol ether faecal concentration test.
Round base tubes	Good quality reusable glass tubes (not disposable glass) of the following sizes are needed for routine haematology, blood transfusion, serology, and clinical chemistry tests: 9.5 × 63 mm, 12 × 75 mm, 13 × 100 mm, 16 × 150 mm. *Note*: For crossmatching, 9.5 × 65 mm glass tubes are recommended instead of precipitin tubes because they can be easily washed and reused.
Flat base tubes	Glass, 10 ml capacity capped vials (for clotted venous blood). See *Specimen containers*.

RACKS AND TRAYS

Order racks and trays that can be disinfected (bleach solution) and easily cleaned, such as nylon coated wire or racks made from aluminium, polypropylene, ABS, or other plastic.

Tube racks	– To hold 12 or more tubes, 75 mm long × 10–13 mm diameter. – To hold 12 or more tubes, 100 mm long × 11–13 mm diameter. – To hold 12 or more tubes, 125–150 mm long × 15–20 mm diameter. Order by diameter size and length of tube to put in rack and by number of holes required. Racks holding several sizes of tubes are available.

Crossmatch rack	Preferably for crossmatching up to 4 units of blood with places for patient's clotted blood sample, donor's red cell suspension tubes, and crossmatch tubes.
EDTA or ESR rack	To hold 12 or more EDTA or ESR containers up to 5 ml capacity, 15–18 mm diameter.
Universal rack	To hold Universal or McCartney bottles, 25 mm diameter.
Bijou rack	To hold 12 or more bijou bottles.
Slide draining rack	Block (PVC or other plastic) with angled slots to hold 12 or more slides upright for smears to dry after staining.
Drying rack	Peg rack for draining washed glassware and plasticware, preferably two sided and free standing with panels measuring about 500 × 420 mm (polythene coated wire is suitable). Alternatively, wooden pegs in a wall hanging board made locally.
Baskets	For microbiology work, square or round wire baskets (zinc plated, stainless steel or polypropylene), required for autoclaving culture media and specimens.
Trays	Required to hold sputum, faecal and other specimen containers safely, i.e. contain any spillages. Usually locally available (plastic trays are suitable).
Collecting tray	Light weight partitioned container with handle. Needed for ward collection of specimens from patients. Plastic 'tool box' type container is suitable. Usually locally available.
Slide box	Plastic or wooden box with lid and slots to take up to 50 or more slides. Needed for storing control and teaching slide preparations.

BURNERS

Bunsen burner	Portable butane gas burner such as locally available *International Camping Gaz*. Microbiology laboratories with a gas supply should try to obtain a burner with a protective tube, e.g. *Bactiburner*, to avoid particles being dispersed when flame sterilizing wire loops. The *Bactiburner* is available for use with calor, propane or butane gas.
Spirit burner	Metal spirit burner with wick and screw cap. Order spare length of wick.
Tripod and gauze	Metal tripod and stainless steel gauze having ceramic centre.

ESR EQUIPMENT (WESTERGREN METHOD)

ESR kit: A kit consisting of all the items needed to perform ESR tests safely is available from Developing Health Technology (DHT). Kit consists of safe 6-place Westergren stand, glass Westergren pipettes, reusable ESR containers with roll of 1 000 water-soluble adhesive labels, anticoagulant hand dispenser, rack, and 1 hour mechanical timer/ringer. Items are also available individually.

ESR stand	Stand holding 6 or more Westergren pipettes that can be easily disinfected and cleaned. Supplied with spirit level and pipette suction devices (pipette fillers) to avoid dangerous mouth-pipetting.
ESR pipettes	Reusable Westergren glass pipettes.
ESR blood containers	Reusable polystyrene or glass containers of 2.5 ml capacity for holding 0.5 ml anticoagulant and 2 ml of blood, preferably with mauve cap. Purchase empty and unlabelled. In the laboratory, add sodium citrate and label. (Use *water-soluble* adhesive labels).
60 minute timer	See *Timers*.

WHITE BLOOD CELL (WBC) MANUAL COUNTING EQUIPMENT

WBC kit: A kit consisting of all the items needed to perform manual total WBC counts is available from Developing Health Technology (DHT). Kit consists of bright line Improved Neubauer haemocytometer, hand tally counter, hand syringe dispenser to measure diluting fluid, 50 µl calibrated capillaries, reusable WBC dilution containers, and rack. Also available individually.

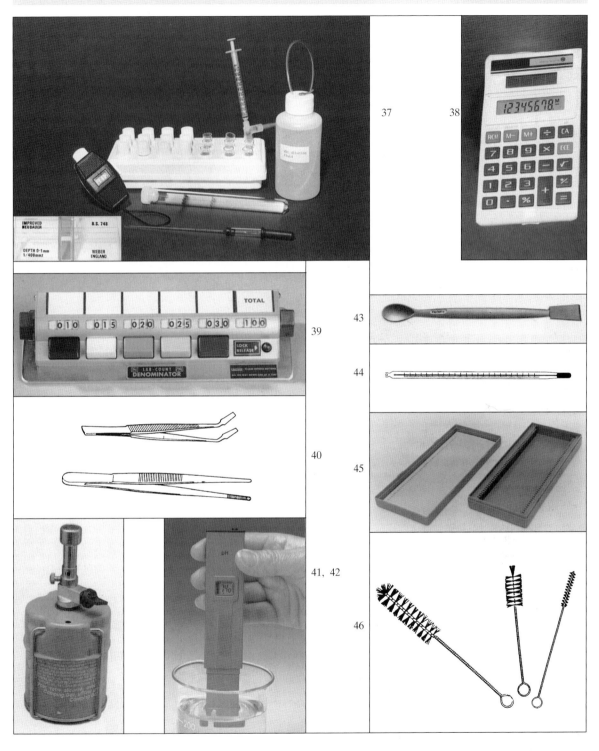

37 DHT kit for counting WBC. 38 Solar powered battery calculator. 39 Mechanical WBC differential counter. 40 Laboratory forceps. 41 Labogaz burner. 42 Hanna battery pH meter. 43 Spatula with spoon. 44 Spirit thermometer. 45 Slide box. 46 Cleaning brushes.

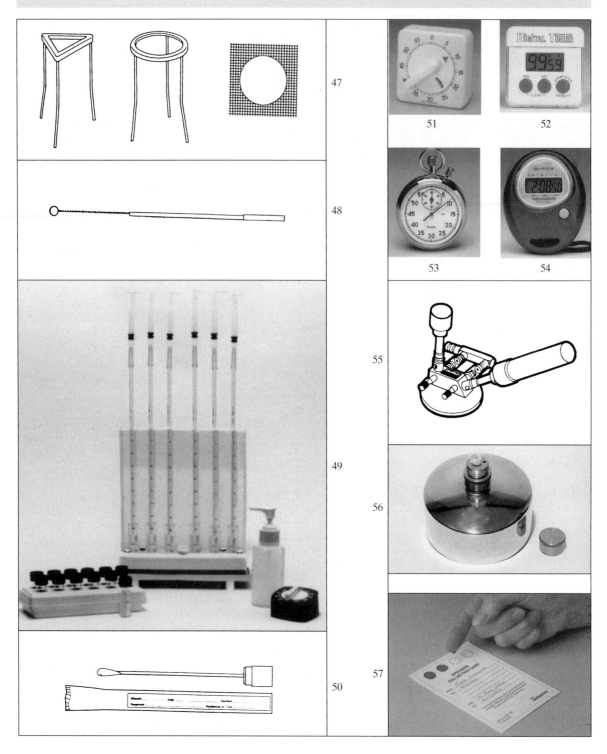

47 Metal tripods and gauze.   48 Wire loop in holder.   49 DHT safe ESR kit.   50 Transport swab.   51 Mechanical timer.
52 Digital battery timer.   53 Mechanical stop-watch.   54 Digital battery stop-watch.   55 *Bactiburner*.   56 Metal spirit burner with screw cap.   57 Blood collection filter paper card.

Improved Neubauer haemocytometer

Needed for counting white blood cells and platelets. Order bright clear line (metallized surface), double grid Improved Neubauer ruled haemocytometer (counting chamber). It is usually supplied with two cover glasses. Order extra haemocytometer cover glasses.

Note: Less expensive chambers are available without bright line rulings. These are *not* recommended because the non-bright line rulings make it difficult to perform cell counts accurately. Low cost bright line haemocytometers are available from DHT.

Fuchs Rosenthal haemocytometer

For counting cells in cerebrospinal fluid (csf). Order bright line, double grid Fuchs Rosenthal ruled haemocytometer. It is usually supplied with two cover glasses. Order extra cover glasses (same as used for Improved Neubauer chamber).

Note: This chamber is recommended for counting white cells in csf because it has a depth of 0.2 mm (twice the depth of an Improved Neubauer ruled chamber).

Hand tally counter

Plastic or metal cased, mechanical hand counter, mainly for counting white cells and platelets.

Differential cell counter

Mechanical 5-unit differential counter with totalizer for performing white blood cell differential counts (available from DHT).

TIMERS (MECHANICAL)

Note: Mechanical timers do not require batteries for their operation.

60 minute timer

1–60 minute mechanical interval timer with ringer is needed for timing staining techniques, clinical chemistry tests, and ESR tests. Often available locally (cooking timer).

Stop-watch

A 60 minute stop-watch with a seconds hand is required, mainly for timing coagulation tests and for some clinical chemistry tests.

Note: Chrome metal body stop watches with jewelled lever movement are considerably more expensive than electronic digital stop-watches. When purchasing a digital model, ensure that the type of battery required can be obtained locally.

THERMOMETER, FORCEPS, SPATULA, WIRE LOOP

Thermometer

General purpose, −10 to 110 °C, red spirit thermometer (or if unavailable, mercury) with 1 °C subdivisions.

Note: A spirit thermometer is recommended in preference to a mercury thermometer because the spirit in the bulb is not toxic like mercury and will not therefore become a hazard should the thermometer break. Also, red spirit thermometers are easier to read.

Forceps

Stainless steel straight forceps about 125 mm long with blunt tips and a block end (referred to as dissecting forceps).

Note: Spencer Wells forceps is listed under *Blood Collection items*.

Spatula

Preferably stainless steel about 140 mm long with a scoop at one end and narrow bent blade at the other. If not available, a polypropylene flat blade spatula about 100 mm long is suitable (less expensive than the scoop/blade stainless steel spatula).

Wire loop (reusable)

Nickel-chromium wire loop of diameter 2 mm, holding 1/500 ml and no longer than 60 mm in length. Order as a complete loop with handle. Alternatively, purchase ready-made 1/500 ml nickel-chromium wire loops and wire loop holder with screw-chuck head.

PH EQUIPMENT

pH meter

Low cost, robust, electronic, hand held water-proof meter, having a range of pH 0.1–14.0 and resolution of pH 0.1 with automatic calibration and temperature compensation, e.g. *Hanna pH 3 meter* operated by 4 × 1.4 V batteries which give approximately 700 h working life. Has a built-in low battery warning. Order also pH 7 buffer.

Note: This type of pH meter has a protected glass electrode which if correctly used should last 3–5 years. The electrode cannot be replaced. Between use the electrode should be immersed in pH 7 buffer (*not* distilled or deionized water).

pH papers

These are suitable for use in small district laboratories where the accurate measurement of pH is not required, e.g. checking the pH of buffered water used in staining techniques. *Useful papers*: Whatman range (10 books per box, each book having 20 leaves) pH 1.0–11.0 in steps of 1.0, pH 5.2 to 6.7 in steps of 0.5, and pH 6.8 to 8.3 in steps of 0.5. Also needed is neutral litmus paper that turns red when a reaction is acid and blue when alkaline.

CLEANING EQUIPMENT

Discard containers

Plastic containers (purchase locally) for soaking items prior to washing:

- Bucket(s) for infected glassware, plasticware, and reusable specimen containers.
- Long container for pipettes.
- Container for slides.
- Small container for cover glasses.

Washing containers

General purpose domestic plastic washing-up bowls (purchase locally).

Brushes

Nylon or bristle head brushes of various sizes:
- Large size, 70–90 mm diameter head.
- Small size, 40–50 mm diameter head.
- Test tube brush with diameter head of about 12 mm.
- Nail brush.

Rubber gloves

Domestic type, reusable rubber gloves (purchase locally) to protect hands when washing glassware and plasticware.

Detergent

Detergent soap (purchase locally).

Disinfectant

See subunit 3.4.

Hand soap

Preferably medicated hand soap or if unavailable, simple non-perfumed hand soap.

DRESSINGS

Cotton wool

Absorbent type (sold as a roll).

Cellulose wadding

To make small swabs for cleansing the skin prior to blood collection (sold as a roll). Less expensive than cotton wool.

Elastoplast tape

About 20 mm wide, to tape dressings and to tape around the neck of specimen containers to ensure a complete seal (when transporting or mailing specimens).

Elastoplast dressings

Small circular elastoplasts suitable for covering needle puncture wounds following the collection of venous blood.

Scissors

Stainless steel scissors for cutting cloth, tape and dressings.

Note: A second pair of scissors is useful for other general purposes, e.g. cutting paper.

STATIONERY, MARKERS, AND CALCULATOR

Labels for specimens

Preferably self-adhesive (water soluble adhesive) or if unavailable dry glue labels or roll of gummed paper.

Note: 1 000-label rolls of water-soluble self-adhesive labels for sticking on specimen containers are available from DHT (see Appendix II). EDTA labels have pink red print and show blood level. ESR labels have mauve print and show blood level. Other specimen labels are printed in black.

Labels for reagent containers	Preferably self-adhesive labels, suitable for labelling reagent containers.
Hazard labels	To identify hazardous chemicals (see subunit 3.5) such as those that are flammable, oxidizing, toxic, harmful, corrosive, explosive.
Filter paper	Whatman grade 1 filter paper is suitable. Sold as 100 papers per box. Useful sizes: 70 mm, 125 mm, 185 mm diameter.
Record books	Ruled exercise books (preferably large hard-back books) for recording patient data and test results (purchase locally). Separate books are needed for:

– Blood tests
– Urine tests
– Faecal tests
– Blood donation book
– Blood grouping and crossmatching
– Microbiology microscopy and serology
– Microbiology culture and sensitivity.

Graph paper	A4 size pad, ruled 1, 5, and 10 mm squares. Usual pack: 50 sheets per pad. Needed to prepare calibration graphs.
Marker pen	*Waterproof*, black ink felt tip marker(s) of medium tip for the permanent labelling of containers.
Diamond marker pen	For writing on glass. Durable, clear writing diamond pen, preferably with a wooden handle (avoid retractable point pens).
Chinagraph (grease) pencils	Black grease (wax) pencils, preferably of the peel back *Blaisdell* type to avoid the need to use a pencil sharpener which tends to break the lead.
Black lead pencils	Needed for labelling the frosted end of glass slides. Order pencils with a medium or soft lead. Purchase also a pencil sharpener.
Sellotape	Polypropylene, 25 mm wide is suitable.
Ruler	Plastic or wood, 30 cm (12 inch) long.
Pens	Non-leaking blue or black biro(s) and red biro(s).
Elastic bands	Box of assorted sizes.
Paper clips	About 30 mm in length (sold in boxes).
Calculator	Basic, easy to use solar charged battery calculator with clear digital display, e.g. Sharp solar calculator, EL 334.

SWABS

Applicator sticks	Wooden applicator sticks to make cotton wool swabs for collecting specimens. Usual quantity: 500 or more sticks per box.
Ready-made swabs	Sterile cotton wool swab in sterile tube. Usual quantity: 100 tubed swabs per box.
Transport swabs	Tube or plastic bag containing sterile Amies transport medium with sterile cotton wool swab inserted in cap of tube. Usual quantity: 100 transport medium swabs per box.

Availability: If not available locally, most of the items described in this subunit can be obtained economically from Developing Health Technology (see Appendix II). DHT has no minimum order value and makes items available in quantities appropriate for district laboratories.

Note: Azlon is now part of Bibby Sterilin (see Appendix 11)

REFERENCES

1 Guidelines on equipment donations. *Contact*, October, 1994, pp. 11–14.

2 *Principles of management of health laboratories.* World Health Organization, Alexandria, 1993. WHO Regional Publications, Eastern Mediterranean Series, No. 3.

3 *Basic malaria microscopy. Part 1 Learner's Guide.* World Health Organization, Geneva, 1991.

4 **Payne D.** A lens too far? *Transactions of the Royal Society of Tropical Medicine and Hygiene*, 1993, 87, p496. Correspondence.

5 **Opoku-Okrah et al**. Improving microscope quality is a good investment for under-resourced laboratories. *Transaction, Royal Society Tropical Medicine and Hygiene*, 2000, 94, p. 582.

RECOMMENDED READING

Johns WL, El-Nageh MM. *Selection of Basic Laboratory Equipment for Laboratories with Limited Resources.* WHO Eastern Mediterranean Series, No 17, 2000. Available from WHO, PO Box 7608, Nasr City, Cairo, Egypt.

Manual of Basic Techniques for a Health Laboratory, World Health Organization, Geneva, 2nd edition, 2003.

Maintenance and repair of laboratory, diagnostic and imaging, and hospital equipment. WHO, Geneva, 1994. Obtainable from Distribution and Sales, WHO, 1211 Geneva, 27, Switzerland.

Skeet M. and Fear D. Care and safe use of hospital equipment. VSO 1995. Obtainable from VSO Books, Voluntary Service Overseas, 317 Putney Bridge Road, London SW15 2PN, UK.

El-Nageh MM et al. *Basics of Quality Assurance for Intermediate and Peripheral Laboratories.* WHO Eastern Mediterranean Series, No 2, 2002. Available from WHO, PO Box 7608, Nasr City, Cairo, Egypt.

Guidelines for Health Care Equipment Donations, WHO, Geneva, March 2000, WHO/ARA/97.3.

Colling C et al. *Microbiological Methods*, 8th edition, 2004. Arnold-Hodder Headline.

Resources for Appropriate Healthcare Technologies for the Developing World
website www.iee.org/OnComms/pn/healthtech/aht.cfm

WHO Essential Healthcare Technology
website www.who.int/eht

Health Exchange: Special issue on Appropriate Healthcare Technology for the Developing World, Nov 2004. Available from IHE/RedR, 1 Great George St, London SW1P 3AA, UK. E-mail: info@ihe.org.uk website www.ihe.org.uk/pub.htm

Chapter 5 Parasitological Tests

ACKNOWLEDGEMENT
for
Colour Plates

Acknowledgement and gratitude are expressed to all those who kindly supplied transparencies and artwork to illustrate the Parasitology Chapter. Special thanks are due to:

Mr Anthony Moody for supplying transparencies for Plates 5.5c, 5.6 *right*, 5.12 *right*, 5.14, 5.15, 5.17, 5.26, 5.34, 5.41, 5.61 and 5.67 *right*.

Mr John Williams for supplying transparencies for Plates 5.5a, 5.5b, 5.50 *left*, 5.52, and 5.57.

Professor Wallace Peters for supplying artwork for Plates 5.36, 5.50 *right*, 5.51 and 5.53 *left*.

Dr Richard W Ashford for supplying the transparency for Plate 5.20.

Professor H Zaiman for permission to reproduce Plate 5.38 *left*.

Dr KE Mott and the World Health Organization for the use of Plate 5.42 *right*.

Bernhard-Nocht Institut für Schiffs und Tropentrankheiten for the use of Plate 5.42 *left*.

Africa Health and CDC for permission to reproduce Plate 5.70.

Wolfe Medical Publications for permission to reproduce Plate 5.56.

Tropical Doctor and Drs BOL Dukes and J Anderson for permission to reproduce Plate 5.60.

Professor Tom Oriehel for supplying artwork for Plate 5.58d

Orchid Biomedical Systems for supplying artwork for Plates 5.47 and 5.48.

Binax Inc. for supplying artwork for Plates 5.49 and 5.59.

WB Saunders Company and Dr W Jann Brown for permission to reproduce Plate 5.24.

5

Parasitological tests

5.1 Parasitology in district laboratories and quality assurance of tests

The investigation of parasitic infections forms a major part of district laboratory practice. Depending on the parasitic diseases found locally and their importance, the following investigations are among those performed in district laboratories:

Tests

■ Examination of faecal specimens   *Subunit*
for intestinal parasites: 5.3–5.5

Entamoeba histolytica	*Enterobius vermicularis*
Giardia lamblia	*Stronglyoides stercoralis*
Balantidium coli	*Trichuris trichiura*
Cryptosporidium (HIV related)	*Schistosoma* species
Isospora belli (HIV related)	*Taenia* species
Cyclospora (HIV related)	*Opisthorchis* species
Ascaris lumbricoides	*Fasciolopsis buski*
Ancylostoma duodenale	*Fasciola hepatica*
Necator americanus	*Capillaria* species

                 Subunit

■ Testing urine for schistosome eggs.   5.6
■ Testing blood for malaria parasites.   5.7
■ Testing blood and c.s.f. for trypanosomes
(African trypanosomiasis).   5.8
■ Investigation of Chagas' disease.   5.9
■ Examination of specimens
for *Leishmania* parasites.   5.10
■ Testing blood for microfilariae   5.11
■ Skin snips for *Onchocerca* microfilariae.   5.12
■ Testing sputum for *Paragonimus eggs.*   5.13
■ Less frequently needed parasitology
tests to investigate: 5.14
    – Amoebic liver abscess
    – Amoebic meningoencephalitis
    – Toxoplasmosis

    – Hydatid disease
    – Trichinosis
    – Dracunculiasis

QUALITY ASSURANCE OF PARASITOLOGY TESTS

The importance of quality assurance and standard operating procedures (SOPs) are explained in sub-unit 2.4. The following apply to the quality assurance of the pre-analytical, analytical, and post-analytic stages of parasitology investigations.

Pre-analytical stage

This involves:

– Selecting parasitology tests appropriately.
– Collecting, transporting and storing specimens correctly.
– Ensuring the request form is completed correctly.
– Checking the specimen and request form when they reach the laboratory.

Appropriate selection of parasitology tests

The clinical and/or public health reasons for requesting a parasitology test must be clear. Laboratory staff and those requesting tests should know the approximate cost of each test (see subunit 2.2), the information provided by the test and the limitations of the test procedure. Most microscopical parasitology tests are diagnostic but how well a test detects a particular parasite depends on the species of parasite, degree and stage of infection, type of specimen, sensitivity of the technique used and experience of the microscopist. The detection of parasites can also be influenced by medication given to or taken by the patient before the specimen is collected.

Correct collection and transport of specimens

The following are important:

● Use specimen containers that are leak-proof, clean, dry, and free from traces of antiseptics and disinfectants.

● If an anticoagulated blood specimen is required, use a suitable anticoagulant, e.g. sodium citrate for microfilariae and EDTA (sequestrene) for malaria parasites and trypanosomes. Mix the blood well but gently with the anticoagulant.

Use of EDTA: The blood must be examined within 1 hour of collection to avoid morphological changes in the appearance of parasites and the exflagellation of *Plasmodium* gametocytes.

- Protect specimens from direct sunlight and heat. Thick blood films require special protection from dust, flies, and ants. In conditions of high humidity, an incubator or portable dryer may be needed to prevent distortion of the parasites which can occur when thick-blood films are left to dry slowly.

- Ensure specimens arrive in the laboratory as soon as is feasible after they are collected. Some specimens must be delivered to the laboratory for rapid examination, for example:

  - a dysenteric faecal specimen or rectal scrape for the detection of motile *E. histolytica* trophozoites.

  - cerebrospinal fluid for the detection of motile trypanosomes.

  - discharge specimen for the detection of motile *T. vaginalis*.

Such specimens require examination within 15–20 minutes after collection. In general, all other specimens unless a result is required urgently, should reach the laboratory within 1 hour of collection to avoid loss or distortion of parasites.

- When needing to transport specimens to a specialist parasitology laboratory, use a suitable fixature or preservative (see end of this subunit).

- Label the specimen carefully with the patient's name and identification number, and also the date and time of collection.

Request form

A correctly completed request form must accompany all specimens. An example of a suitable format is described in subunit 2.2. For parasitology investigations, it is important to provide adequate clinical information and details of any drugs given to or taken by the patient before the specimen was collected. This information is particularly relevant when examining blood for malaria parasites. For epidemiological purposes, the patient's village or locality should also be written on the request form.

Checking the specimen and request form

As well as checking that the specimen is clearly labelled and is accompanied by the correct request form it is important to check that the container is not leaking, that the specimen is suitable for the test being requested and has been delivered to the laboratory within the time specified for the particular investigation. Appropriate action should be taken if a test result is required urgently or there are clear problems in identification or collection.

Analytical stage

This involves:

- Making sure the parasitology test method is valid and appropriate.

- Preparing a clearly written SOP for each test (see subunit 2.4).

- Controlling stains and reagents.

- Ensuring slides, cover glasses and other glassware and plasticware are clean.

- Knowing how to use equipment correctly, particularly a microscope.

- Following appropriate health and safety measures.

Quality control (QC) of parasitology test methods

- Use the most suitable method for detecting and identifying a particular parasite and follow exactly the technique as detailed in the SOP. For some parasites and situations it may be appropriate to use a concentration technique, for example:

  - to detect the eggs of intestinal parasites that are excreted only intermittently or in small numbers, e.g. *Taenia* or *Schistosoma* species.

  - to detect microfilariae in blood.

  - to diagnose a serious disease such as African trypanosomiasis when trypanosomes are not found by direct techniques.

- For microscopical examinations, make preparations of the correct thickness, e.g. thick blood films, and faecal suspensions. Whenever possible, standardize the amount of specimen used. For faecal preparations, ensure the specimen is well emulsified in the saline or iodine.

- Wipe the back of slides clean after staining.

- Standardize the number of microscope fields or amount of preparation examined before reporting 'no parasite detected'. Ensure any additional relevant information is included in the report, e.g. presence of large numbers of pus cells in faecal preparations, marked eosinophilia in blood films, or the presence of malarial pigment in white cells.

- Use visual aids and standard control slides of parasites (prepared in the laboratory) to improve the accuracy and reproducibility of microscopical reporting and reduce inter-reader variability. Control slides are also needed as reference material when training newly qualified staff.

Note: The preservation of parasites and preparation of 'permanent' slide preparations are described at the end of this subunit.

- Ensure staff are well trained and the work of trainees and newly qualified personnel is supervized adequately. When a new test method is introduced, an SOP must be prepared and the procedure adequately demonstrated, controlled, and reviewed by the technologist in charge.

Controlling stains and reagents

This involves standardizing the concentrations of working stains and staining times (may require changing for different batches of stain). Newly prepared stains must be checked before use and monitored during use. Stains and reagents must be stored correctly and where indicated checked regularly for contamination. The following control measures apply to the stains and reagents commonly used in parasitology tests.

Physiological saline: This is used mainly to make wet faecal preparations.

- Prepare the reagent using distilled water, deionized water, or boiled filtered water.
- Dispense the saline preferably from a small dropper bottle (which can be closed when not in use) to avoid contaminating the reagent. Renew frequently to ensure the saline is isotonic and has not become concentrated due to evaporation. The use of non-isotonic saline can affect the motility and morphology of parasites.
- Check daily for contamination (particularly for flagellates or ciliates) by examining a drop of the reagent on a slide using the 10× and 40× objectives with condenser iris closed sufficiently to give good contrast.

Dobell's iodine: This is used mainly to identify cysts in faecal preparations.

- Keep the reagent in a dark brown dropper bottle or if this is not possible, cover the outside of the container with opaque paper or tinfoil.
- Check the performance of the reagent by using it to stain the glycogen inclusions of *I. buetschlii* cysts.

Methanol (methyl alcohol): Absolute methanol is required as a fixative for thin blood films and as a constituent of Giemsa and other alcohol-based

Romanowsky stains.

- Use a good quality methanol. Technical grade methanol (lower priced) is suitable for making reagents such as 70% v/v alcohol and acid alcohol but because it contains traces of water it is unsuitable as a fixative for blood films or for making Romanowsky stains.
- Avoid moisture from the atmosphere entering the methanol. Make sure the cap of the stock bottle is tight. For routine use, transfer a small quantity from the stock bottle to a *dry* dispensing bottle (that can be closed in between use).

Buffered reagents: Buffered water and buffered saline are used in parasitology techniques.

- Prepare a buffered reagent carefully, weighing accurately the dry chemicals and checking the pH. Alternatively, use buffer tablets.
- Store buffered reagents at 2–8 °C in tightly stoppered (preferably plastic) bottles. When in use, avoid leaving the reagents in sunlight (encourages the growth of algae). Check for contamination (cloudiness) at regular intervals.

Giemsa stain: This is used mainly for staining malaria parasites, trypanosomes, leishmanial parasites, and microfilariae.

- Use a reliable and if possible a ready-made standardized stain (e.g. BDH/Merck).
- Store the stock stain in a dark bottle and take precautions to avoid moisture entering the stain. For routine use, transfer a small quantity of the stock stain to a dry dispensing bottle (that can be closed in between use).
- Check the quality of all new batches of Giemsa (especially if not using a ready-made stain) by using it to stain malaria parasites. If available, use a species that shows Schüffner's dots (*P. vivax* or *P. ovale*). For control purposes, thick and thin blood films can be prepared from fresh blood, dried, folded individually in paper, sealed in a plastic bag, and stored in a freezer at −20 °C.

Note: If using Leishman stain, control this in the same way as described for Giemsa stain.

Field's stain: This is used for staining malaria parasites and is also useful for staining leishmanial parasites, trypanosomes, microfilariae, and *Giardia* flagellates.

- Prepare the stains from Fields' stain powders A and B, using hot distilled water or heated boiled filtered water (70–100 °C). Filter the stains.
- Check the quality of the stains by staining thick

films containing malaria parasites.

Note: Although Fields' stains A and B are stable and the same staining solutions can be used many times (with regular filtering) for staining thick films, to promote standardization and for safety reasons, it is better to change the stains frequently (see subunit 5.7).

Slides and cover glasses

It is important to make sure glass microscope slides and cover glasses are completely clean. After use, soak slides and cover glasses in separate containers (in a suitable disinfectant) to avoid damaging the fragile cover glasses. Rinse well in clean water and dry between clean cotton cloths. If available buy thicker (No 1 ½) cover glasses as these will last longer.

Plastic cover glasses: Although plastic cover glasses are available, they are more difficult to clean. Most scratch easily and some disinfectants can damage the plastic.

Controlling microscopy

- Train staff how to use and maintain a microscope correctly as described in subunit 4.3. It is particularly important to clean frequently the lenses of the eyepieces and objectives. The 40× objective can become easily contaminated when examining wet preparations.

- Use an appropriate intensity of light for each objective and obtain adequate contrast by adjusting the condenser iris diaphragm for the type of specimen and objective being used (see subunit 4.3).
  When contrast is insufficient, parasites will be missed in unstained preparations, particularly trypanosomes in csf, *T. vaginalis* in discharges, motile *E. histolytica*, *Giardia* trophozoites, and protozoal cysts and oocysts in faecal preparations.
  When light is insufficient for use with an oil immersion objective, e.g. use of daylight with a binocular microscope, it will be particularly difficult to identify malaria parasites in thick blood films.

- Focus continuously to detect parasites and identify morphological features.

- Examine preparations first with a low power objective to detect larger parasites, eosinophilia or other white cell abnormalities in blood films, and to identify areas of the correct thickness and, or, staining to examine with a higher magnification.

- Use both the 10× and 40× objectives to examine faecal preparations to avoid missing small parasites, e.g. *I. belli* cysts, small fluke eggs, or cysts of *Giardia*.

- Examine specimens for a sufficient length of time

to avoid false negative reports and to ensure mixed infections are not missed, e.g. mixed *Plasmodium* infections.

Control of centrifuging

The force and the length of time of centrifugation are important when sedimenting parasites, e.g. when performing the formol ether (or ethyl acetate) concentration technique to sediment faecal parasites. If incorrectly centrifuged, faecal debris may also be sedimented with the parasites. Centrifuging at too great a force can destroy trypanosomes or cause the loss of a sheath from a pathogenic microfilaria species. Details of how to use and maintain a centrifuge can be found in subunit 4.7.

Health and safety in parasitology work

All specimens sent to the laboratory for parasitology investigations may contain highly infectious organisms and *must be handled and examined with care* following the guidelines contained in subunit 3.3, *Microbial hazards.*

Fingers can become easily contaminated when preparing wet preparations and blood smears, therefore protective gloves should be worn. Staff must wash their hands thoroughly before attending patients, when leaving the laboratory and before eating and drinking. Other personal safety measures are described in subunit 3.2. Specimens must be disposed of safely as described in subunit 3.4.

Stock alcoholic stains, methanol and particularly diethyl ether are fire hazards and must not be used near an open flame (see also subunits 3.5 and 3.7).

Post-analytical stage

Quality assurance of this stage includes:

- Reporting and verifying parasitology test results.

- Taking appropriate action(s) when a result has serious implications for the care or treatment of a patient or is of public health importance.

- Interpreting test results correctly.

The following are important:

- Standardize the reporting of results, particularly for microscopical tests. The method of reporting must be clearly written in the SOP.

  Where appropriate, a test should be reported semi-quantitatively, e.g. malaria parasites in blood films, or eggs in faeces. The specimen examined must be stated and also if a concentration technique has been used.

- Write reports clearly and neatly using standardized forms that can be inserted in a patient's notes (not results 'charted' by nursing staff, see subunit 2.2).

- Ensure that any abbreviation or plus sign scheme used in the report is clearly understood by those receiving the report.

- Include in the report any information that could assist in interpreting a result or lead to a better understanding or treatment of a patient's condition. Laboratory staff should understand the meaning of test results.

- Check all reports before they are issued. The technologist in charge should also verify any unusual or unexpected result.

- Communicate immediately any serious result to the medical officer caring for the patient, e.g. finding of trypanosomes in blood or csf, or a heavy falciparum parasitaemia in a young child with anaemia.

- Keep written dated records of all parasitology investigations performed in the laboratory.

PRESERVATION OF PARASITES AND PREPARATION OF PERMANENT MOUNTS

The preservation of parasites and preparation of permanent mounts of parasites in specimens are required:

- For the control of microscopical parasitology tests and for training purposes.

- When specimens are sent to peripheral laboratories as part of an external parasitology quality assessment programme.

- When specimens need to be sent to a Reference Laboratory for parasite identification.

- When specimens are collected in the field, for example during epidemiological surveys.

Permanent mounts

Stained dry specimens

Malaria parasites, trypanosomes, microfilariae, leishmania amastigotes and other parasites in stained smears are best preserved by using a plastic polymer mountant such as *DPX*, *HystoMount* or *Permount*. Place a drop of mountant on the dry, oil-free film or smear, cover with a cover glass, and leave to air-dry. When dry peel off the excess mountant. Such preparations can be kept for several years with good preservation of parasite morphology and little fading of the stain, loss of transparency, or shrinkage of the mountant.

Wet specimens

A temporary preparation of a wet mounted specimen can be made by simply sealing around the cover glass with one of the plastic polymer mountants mentioned above. To make a permanent mount of a faecal specimen containing eggs and cysts, it is necessary to make the mount from faeces that have been mixed with Bayer's preservative (see following text) or from the sediment obtained following formol ether concentration of the faeces (see subunit 5.4). The simplest method of making a permanent mount is to use the double cover glass technique:

1 Place a drop of Bayer preserved faeces or formol ether faecal sediment on a 22×22 mm square cover glass. Cover with a smaller size cover glass, e.g. a round 19 mm diameter or 18×18 mm square cover glass.

2 Using absorbent tissue remove the excess fluid from around the small cover glass.

3 Place a drop of *DPX*, *HystoMount*, *Permount* or similar plastic polymer mountant on a microscope slide.

4 Lower the slide, drop downwards, on top of the cover glass preparation and turn the preparation over (larger cover glass will be uppermost). The mountant should fill the area around the small cover glass, sealing in the specimen.

5 Allow the preparation to air-dry overnight. To ensure complete sealing, the preparation can be ringed with clear nail varnish.

Preservatives and fixatives for faecal parasites

For teaching purposes and external QA programmes it is useful to be able to preserve parasites in faecal specimens, particularly eggs and cysts. To preserve and identify *E. histolytica* trophozoites, special fixatives and staining procedures are required.

Preservation of eggs and cysts using Bayer's solution

Bayer's solution is recommended because it preserves well the morphology of faecal eggs and cysts. It is a modified formalin solution containing copper chloride, glacial acetic acid, and formalin. The stock solution is stable indefinitely at room temperature. Bayer-preserved faeces can be examined unstained in direct preparations (sampling from the sediment) or examined after concentration by the formol ether technique.

Bayer's solution is used as follows:

1 Prepare a working solution by diluting Bayer's

stock solution (Reagent No 10) 1 in 10, e.g. use 1 ml stock solution and 9 ml of distilled or filtered water.

2 Emulsify about 1 g of faeces in 3-4 ml of Bayer's working solution. Use a leak-proof screw cap container.

Note: If the chemicals to make Bayer's solution are not available, 10% v/v formol saline can be used, but this will not preserve faecal cysts and eggs as well as Bayer's solution nor for as long a period.

Fixation of faeces for *E. histolytica* trophozoites
Routinely, *E. histolytica* trophozoites are usually identified in dysenteric specimens by their motility and ingested red cells. Only occasionally is it necessary to fix and stain faeces for *E. histolytica*. The choice of fixative depends on the staining method used. SAF (sodium acetate, acetic acid, formaldehyde) fixative is commonly used when an iron haematoxylin staining method is used and PVA (polyvinyl alcohol) or absolute methanol when using a trichrome staining method. Details of these fixatives and staining procedures can be found in the WHO *Training Manual, on Diagnosis of Intestinal Parasites* (WHO/CTD/SIP/98.2), 1998, and other publications covering parasitology methods.

Preservation of schistosome eggs in urine
S. haematobium eggs can be preserved in urine by adding 1 ml of 1% v/v domestic bleach solution to every 10 ml of urine. The specimen can be examined after centrifugation, gravity sedimentation, or by the Nuclepore filtration technique. The bleach also prevents the precipitation of phosphates.

Note: When preserved with bleach, the urine is unsuitable for chemical testing, e.g. for the detection of protein or blood. Also, it will not be possible to detect red cells microscopically in bleach preserved urine because the red cells are lyzed by the chemical.

Preservation of worms
When required specimens can be fixed and preserved as follows:

1 Wearing protective gloves and eyeshields, make up the fixative solution as follows:

95% v/v ethanol . . . . .50 ml
Distilled or boiled water . . . . .45 ml
Formaldehyde solution, concentrated . . . . .10 ml
Glacial acetic acid .5 ml

Caution: Formaldehyde and glacial acetic acid have an irritating vapour, therefore ensure the laboratory is well ventilated. The 95% ethanol solution is flammable, therefore keep it well away from any open flame.

2 Transfer the fixative solution to a beaker and heat to 60–65 °C.

3 If the specimen is a fluke or tapeworm segment, flatten it between two slides held loosely together with an elastic band.

4 Place the specimen in the fixative and stir gently for a few minutes. Leave the specimen in the fixative overnight.

5 Transfer the specimen to a container of 5% v/v glycerine in 70% v/v ethanol. Transport or store the specimen in this solution.

5.2 Features and classification of parasites of medical importance

In diagnosing parasitic infections and participating in the control of parasitic diseases, laboratory personnel need to understand the relevant features of parasites of medical importance, particularly those that are found in their area.

Parasitism
A parasite is an organism that is entirely dependent on another organism, referred to as its host, for all or part of its life cycle and metabolic requirements. Parasitism is therefore a relationship in which a parasite benefits and the host provides the benefit. The degree of dependence of a parasite on its host varies. An obligatory parasite is one that must always live in contact with its host. The term free-living describes the non-parasitic stages of existence which are lived independently of a host, e.g. hookworms have active free-living stages in the soil.

Terms used to describe parasite hosts
Definitive host: This is the host in which sexual reproduction takes place or in which the most highly developed form of a parasite occurs. When the most mature form is not obvious, the definitive host is the mammalian host.

Intermediate host: This is the host which alternates with the definitive host and in which the larval or asexual stages of a parasite are found. Some parasites require two intermediate hosts in which to complete their life cycle.

Reservoir host: This is an animal host serving as a source from which other animals can become infected. Epidemiologically, reservoir hosts are important in the control of parasitic diseases. They can maintain a nucleus of infection in an area.

Zoonosis
This term is used to describe an animal infection that is naturally transmissible to humans either directly or indirectly via a vector.* Examples of parasitic diseases that are zoonoses include: leishmaniasis, South American trypanosomiasis, rhodesiense trypanosomiasis, japonicum schistosomiasis, trichinosis, fascioliasis, hydatid disease, and cryptosporidiosis.

* A vector is an agent, usually an insect, that transmits an infection from one human host to another. The term mechanical vector is used to describe a vector which assists in the transfer of parasitic forms between hosts but is not essential in the life cycle of a parasite, e.g. a fly that transfers amoebic cysts from infected faeces to food that is eaten by humans.

PRACTICAL CLASSIFICATION OF PARASITES OF MEDICAL IMPORTANCE

The following is a basic generally accepted practical classification of the medically important parasitic protozoa and helminths.

PROTOZOA
Single-celled organisms
Multiply in human host

Amoebae
Entamoeba histolytica
Acanthamoeba species
Naegleria species

Flagellates
Giardia lamblia
Trichomonas vaginalis
Trypanosoma species
Leishmania species

Ciliates
Balantidium coli

Coccidia
Blood and tissue coccidia:
Plasmodium species
Toxoplasma gondii

Intestinal coccidia:
Isospora belli
Cryptosporidium parvum
Cyclospora cayetanensis

Microsporidia
Encephalitozoon species
Enterocytozoon species

Note: Other species are likely to emerge in association with HIV.

HELMINTHS
Multicellular worms
Do not normally multiply in human host

Trematodes (Flukes)
Schistosoma species

Paragonimus species
Fasciolopsis buski
Fasciola hepatica
Opisthorchis (Clonorchis) sinensis
Opisthorchis viverrini

Lesser medical importance:

Metagonimus yokagawai
Heterophyes heterophyes
Dicrocoelium dendriticum

Cestodes (Tapeworms)
Taenia species
Echinococcus granulosus (larvae)
Diphyllobothrium latum
Vampirolepis nana (less important)

Nematodes (Roundworms)
Intestinal nematodes:

Ascaris lumbricoides (large roundworm)
Enterobius vermicularis (threadworm)
Trichuris trichiura (whipworm)
Strongyloides stercoralis
Ancylostoma duodenale (hookworm)
Necator americanus (hookworm)

Filarial and other tissue nematodes:

Wuchereria bancrofti
Brugia species
Loa loa
Onchocerca volvulus
Drancunculus medinensis (Guinea worm)
Trichinella species

PROTOZOA

Amoebae
Amoebae consist of a shapeless mass of moving cytoplasm which is divided into granular endoplasm and clear ectoplasm. They move by pushing out the ectoplasm to form pseudopodia (false feet) into which the endoplasm then flows. Amoebae reproduce asexually by simply dividing into two (binary fission).

E. histolytica lives in the intestine as a trophozoite, i.e. vegetative stage of protozoa showing motility and the ability to grow, feed, and reproduce. It produces resistant cysts by which it is transmitted.

Flagellates
Flagellates possess at some stage of their life cycle one or more long hair-like flagella for locomotion. They reproduce asexually by binary fission.

G. lamblia is an intestinal flagellate that is bilaterally symmetrical having two nuclei, two axonemes, and four pairs of flagella. Motile trophozoites can be found in faeces and also cysts by which *G. lamblia* is transmitted.

Trypanosoma and *Leishmania* species possess a prominent kinetoplast (mass of mitochondrial DNA) and are transmitted by insects. *Trypanosoma* species live in the blood and tissues. *Leishmania* species live intracellularly in macrophages.

Ciliates
Ciliate trophozoites are covered with short hairs (cilia) by which they move. They reproduce asexually by binary fission and sexually by conjugation. Ciliates possess two dissimilar nuclei (macronucleus and micronucleus) and a large contractile vacuole. They form cysts by which they are transmitted.

Coccidia
Coccidia are intracellular parasites that reproduce asexually by a process called schizogony (merogony) and sexually by sporogony.

Plasmodium species (malaria parasites), normally found in the liver and red cells, are transmitted by anopheline mosquitoes. *T. gondii* and the intestinal coccidia are transmitted by the ingestion of oocysts. (*T. gondii* can also be transmitted congenitally). Intestinal coccidia are particularly important as pathogens in immunosuppressed or immunodeficient persons, e.g. those infected with HIV.

Microsopiridia
Microsopridia are obligate intracellular spore-forming microorganisms, normally pathogenic in fish, insects, and other invertebrates and mammals. In humans they have been reported as pathogens in those infected with HIV. In host cells, there are successive cycles of schizogony (merogony) followed by sporogony from which many spores are produced.

HELMINTHS

Flukes
Flukes are unsegmented mostly flat leaf-like worms (schistosomes are an exception) without a body cavity. They vary in size from 1 mm (*H. heterophyes*) to 70 mm (*F. buski*) in length. They have oral and ventral suckers (attachment organs). The digestive system consists of a mouth and an oesophagus which divides to form two intestinal caeca (branched in some species). There is no anus but an excretory system composed of excretory cells called flame cells, collecting tubules, and an excretory pore. There is a simple nervous system.

Parasitic flukes of medical importance belong to the subclass Digenea. Two generations are required to complete their life cycle. There is an asexual generation in which multiplication occurs (in sporocyst or redia stage), and a sexual generation which produces eggs. In humans only the adults are found.

With the exception of schistosomes, flukes are hermaphroditic (male and female reproduction organs in the same individual) and produce eggs that are operculated (with lids). To develop, the eggs must reach water. Snails serve as the first or only intermediate host. Most flukes parasitize a wide range of animals.

Adult flukes of *Schistosoma* species live in the blood venules around the gut or bladder. Hypersensitivity reactions to the eggs cause tissue damage. *Paragonimus* flukes parasitize the lungs. *F. hepatica*, *O. sinensis*, *O. viverrini* and *D. dendriticum* live in the biliary tract, and *F. buski*, *H. heterophyes*, and *M. yokagawai* parasitize the small intestine.

Tapeworms
The body of a tapeworm is segmented and tapelike. It consists of a head (scolex) and many proglottids (segments). There is no body cavity. The scolex has suckers and in some species also hooks that attach the tapeworm to its host. There is no mouth or digestive system. A tapeworm obtains its nutrients through its body surface. There is a simple excretory system similar to that in flukes.

Tapeworms are hermaphroditic. Proglottids are formed from behind the head. Newly formed proglottids are small and immature. Mature proglottids contain fully developed reproductive organs (several testes, bilobed ovary, and a uterus which may be coiled or consist of a central stem with side branches). Proglottids that contain eggs are called gravid segments. In most species the eggs are released when a gravid segment becomes detached and ruptures.

With the exception of *E. granulosus*, tapeworms that parasitize humans live in the small intestine often growing to great lengths. Only the larval stages of *E. granulosus* (non-human tapeworm) are found in humans.

Nematodes
Nematodes are cylindrical worms. They have a body cavity and a cuticle (skin) which may be smooth, spined, or ridged. The adults of some species are very long, e.g. *D. medinensis*, measuring 1 metre or more. The mouth is surrounded by lips, or papillae. In some species, e.g. hookworms, the lips open into a buccal cavity which has cutting or tooth-like plates. The digestive system is a simple tube which ends in an anus. There is an excretory system and a nervous system.

Sexes are separate with the male worms being smaller than the females. Females are either viviparous (produce larvae) or oviparous (lay eggs). The discharged eggs may hatch directly into infective larvae or they may require special conditions in which to hatch and up to three developmental stages before becoming infective larvae. Each stage involves a shedding of the old cuticle (moulting).

For most nematodes of medical importance, humans are the only or most significant hosts. Most of the medically important intestinal nematodes are geohelminths, i.e. soil-transmitted (spread by faecal contamination of the soil). A person becomes infected by swallowing infective eggs (*A. lumbricoides*, *T. trichiura*, *E. vermicularis*) or by infective larvae penetrating the skin (hookworms, *S. stercoralis*). Before becoming adults in their human host the larvae of hookworms, *A. lumbricoides*, and *S. stercoralis* migrate through the heart and lungs for about 10 days during which time the larvae grow and develop.

The infective larvae of filarial nematodes are transmitted through the bite of an insect vector. *T. spiralis* is transmitted by ingestion of larvae in infected tissue and *D. medinensis* by ingestion of an infected intermediate host (*Cyclops*).

LIFE CYCLES OF PARASITES

In preventing the spread of parasitic diseases and in selecting and evaluating control interventions, it is important to know the life cycles of parasites, the hosts and vectors, and the human and environmental factors that are involved. Life cycles also provide information on the tissues infected and the parasitic forms that can be found in specimens from patients.

Direct life cycle

When a parasite requires only one species of host in which to complete its development it is said to have a direct life cycle. Important parasites in humans that have a direct life cycle include:

E. histolytica	*S. stercoralis*
G. lamblia	*T. trichiura*
A. lumbricoides	*A. duodenale*
E. vermicularis	*N. americanus*

Indirect life cycle

When two or more species of hosts are required, the life cycle is referred to as indirect. Examples of parasites that have an indirect life cycle include:

Plasmodium species　　O. volvulus
Trypanosoma species　　P. westermani
Leishmania species　　Schistosoma species
W. bancrofti　　　　　　Taenia species
B. malayi　　　　　　　F. buski
L. loa　　　　　　　　　D. latum

Note: Life cycles of the medically important parasites are described in the subsequent subunits of this chapter.

Transmission of parasites

Transmission routes of the medically important parasites are summarized in Chart 5.1. In tropical and developing countries the following are among the factors that contribute to the spread and increase in incidence of parasitic infections:

- Inadequate sanitation and unhygienic living conditions leading to faecal contamination of the environment.

- Lack of health education.

- Insufficient water and contaminated water supplies.

- Failure to control vectors due to ineffective interventions, insecticide resistance, lack of resources, and suspension of surveillance and control measures (e.g. during war and conflict).

- Poverty, malnutrition and for some parasites, increased susceptibility due to co-existing HIV infection.

- Development schemes introducing opportunities for vector breeding and infection of the workforce, e.g. poorly designed irrigation schemes and dam projects.

- Failure of drugs to treat parasitic infections effectively.

- Climatic factors.

- Population migrations causing poor health, loss of natural immunity, exposure to new infections, and people being forced to live and work closer to vector habitats and reservoir hosts, often in overcrowded conditions, e.g. refugee camps.

Further information: Readers are referred to, *Short textbook of public health medicine for the tropics*, *Public health – an action guide to improving health in developing countries*, and *Medical entomology*. For availability, see Recommended Reading.

PARASITIC DISEASE

Not all parasitic infections cause disease of clinical significance. Both parasitic and host factors are involved.

Parasitic factors include:
- strain of parasite and adaptation to a human host.
- number of parasites (parasite load).
- site(s) occupied in the body.
- metabolic processes of the parasite, particularly the nature of any waste products or toxins produced by the parasite during its growth and reproduction.

Host factors include:
- genetic factors.
- age and level of natural immunity.
- intensity and frequency of infection.
- immune responses to the infection.
- presence of co-existing disease or condition which reduces natural immune responses, e.g. pregnancy, or infection with HIV.
- whether there is undernutrition or malnutrition.
- life style and work of the person infected.

Examples: A light infection with an intestinal parasite which has little reproductive potential in a well nourished individual is likely to be of little or no consequence. An infection, however, with malaria parasites (which have a high reproductive potential) in a pregnant woman or non-immune child can be serious or even life-threatening.

Mortality rates and disease burden

The following table taken from the *2004 World Health Report* provides estimates (2002 figures) of the number of deaths caused by major parasitic diseases and their disease burden using disability-adjusted life years (DALYs), that is the number of healthy years of life lost due to premature death and disability.*

	Deaths (thousands)		Disease burden (DALYs)* (thousands)		
	Male	Female	Total	Male	Female
Malaria	607	665	46 485	22 243	24 242
African trypanosomiasis	31	17	1 525	966	559
Chagas' disease	8	7	667	343	324
Schistosomiasis	10	5	1 701	1 020	681
Leishmaniasis	30	21	2 089	1 249	840
Lymphatic filariasis	0	0	5 777	4 413	1 364
Onchocerciasis	0	0	484	280	204
Ascariasis	1	2	1 817	910	907
Trichuriasis	2	1	1 007	519	488
Hookworm disease	2	1	58	31	27

*Further information on how DALYs are calculated and used to make decisions and set priorities in health care can be found in the *2004 World Health Report* (Explanatory Notes) and in *Short Textbook of Public Health Medicine for the Tropics* (see Recommended Reading)

Recent advances: Sequencing of the genomes of parasites that cause major tropical diseases by the UNICEF/UNDP/World Bank/WHO Programme for Research and Training on Tropical Diseases (TDR), is expected in the future to lead to the development of new diagnostics, drugs, and vaccines to diagnose, treat, and control important parasitic diseases.[1]

Table 5.1 Parasites found in different specimens

Specimen	Parasite	Form
FAECES	E. histolytica	cyst, trophozoite
	G. lamblia	cyst, trophozoite
	T. hominis	trophozoite
	B. coli	cyst, trophozoite
	I. belli	oocyst
	C. parvum	oocyst
	C. cayetanensis	oocyst
	Microsporidia	spores
	T. solium	egg, segment
	T. saginata	egg, segment
	V. nana	egg
	D. latum	egg[a]
	D. caninum	egg capsule[a]
	O. sinensis	egg
	O. felineus	egg
	H. heterophyes	egg
	M. yokagawai	egg
	F. hepatica	egg
	F. gigantica	egg
	F. buski	egg[b]
	Dicrocoelium	egg
	G. hominis	egg
	Schistosoma spp	egg
	A. lumbricoides	egg, worm
	E. vermicularis	worm[c]
	S. stercoralis	larva
	T. trichiura	egg
	A. duodenale	egg
	N. americanus	egg
	Trichostrongylus	egg
	Capillaria spp	egg
	Paragonimus spp	egg[d]
BLOOD	Plasmodium spp	trophozoite schizont[e], gametocyte
	Trypanosoma spp	trypomastigote
	W. bancrofti	microfilaria
	B. malayi	microfilaria
	L. loa	microfilaria
	Mansonella spp	microfilaria
URINE	S. haematobium	egg[c]
	S. mansoni	egg[f]
	T. vaginalis	trophozoite
	W. bancrofti	microfilaria[f]
	O. volvulus	microfilaria[f]

Specimen	Parasite	Form
VAGINAL DISCHARGE	T. vaginalis	trophozoite
SPUTUM	Paragonimus spp	egg[g]
CSF	Trypanosoma spp	trypomastigote
	Naegleria	trophozoite
BONE MARROW	L. donovani	amastigote
	L. infantum	amastigote
LYMPH GLAND ASPIRATE	Trypanosoma spp	trypomastigote
	L. donovani	amastigote
	L. infantum	amastigote
	T. gondii	trophozoite
LIVER ASPIRATE	E. histolytica	trophozoite
	L. donovani	amastigote
	L. infantum	amastigote
SPLEEN ASPIRATE	L. donovani	amastigote
	L. infantum	amastigote
SKIN	Leishmania spp	amastigote
	O. volvulus	microfilaria
	D. medinensis	larva (ulcer fluid)
	E. vermicularis	egg (perianal skin)
MUSCLE	Trichinella	larva
RECTAL SCRAPING	E. histolytica	trophozoite
	Schistosoma spp	egg
DUODENAL ASPIRATE	G. lamblia	trophozoite
	C. sinensis	egg
	F. hepatica	egg
	S. stercoralis	larva

Notes
a   Sometimes segments are found in faeces.
b   Occasionally flukes are found in faeces.
c   Sometimes the egg is seen in faeces.
d   Eggs are more commonly found in sputum.
e   Schizonts of *P. falciparum* are rarely seen in blood films.
f   Not often found in urine.
g   Occasionally flukes are found in sputum.

PARASITES ASSOCIATED WITH HIV

An increasing number of parasites are being associated with human immunodeficiency virus (HIV) infection and AIDS. They include:

– *Cryptosporidum*, *I. belli*, and *Cyclospora*, causing enteritis with secretory diarrhoea (see subunit 5.4.4).

– *Microsporidia*, causing diarrhoea with wasting, eye disease, and disseminated disease (see subunit 5.4.4).

- *Blastocystis hominis,* causing severe enteritis (see subunit 5.4.1).
- *P. falciparum,* with HIV immunosuppression increasing parasitaemia and worsening malaria in pregnancy (see subunit 9.7).
- *Leishmania* species, with HIV coinfection causing reactivation of latent infections, rapid progression of disease and disseminated disease (see subunit 5.10).
- *T. gondii,* causing cerebral toxoplasmosis (see subunit 5.14.3).

- *Acanthamoeba* species, causing ulceration of the skin and infections in other tissues (see subunit 5.14.2).
- *T. cruzi,* causing meninogoencephalitis, myocarditis and reactivation of latent infections (see subunit 5.9).

Note: *Pneumocystis jiroveci* (formerly *Pneumocystis carinii*) which can cause life-threatening pneumonia in HIV infected persons is described in subunit 7.18.52 in Part 2.

Chart 5.1 Distribution and transmission of parasites of medical importance

Parasite Distribution	Definitive host	Intermediate host	Transmission	Disease
PROTOZA				
Entamoeba histolytica Worldwide[a]	Human	–	Cysts ingested	Amoebic dysentery Amoebic liver abscess
Giardia lamblia Worldwide[a]	Human	–	Cysts ingested	Giardiasis Malabsorption Diarrhoea
Trichomonas vaginalis Worldwide	Human	–	Flagellates sexually transmitted	Trichomoniasis (vaginitis and urethritis)
Balantidium coli Worldwide	Pig Human	–	Cysts ingested	Balantidial dysentery
Trypanosoma cruzi Central and South America	Armadillo, oppossum, cat, dog, Human	Triatomine bug	Trypomastigotes in bug faeces enter through bite wound	Chagas' disease South American trypanosomiasis
Trypanosoma b. rhodesiense, Sub-Saharan Africa	Game animals Human	Tsetse fly	Trypomastigotes transmitted by insect bite	African trypanosomiasis (Sleeping sickness)
Trypanosoma b. gambiense Sub-Saharan Africa	Human Pig	Tsetse fly	As above	As above
Leishmania donovani, L. infantum See subunit 5.10	Rodent, dog, wolf, fox Human	Sandfly	Promastigotes transmitted by insect bite	Visceral leishmaniasis Co-infection with HIV
L. major, L. tropica, L. peruviana, L. mexicana, L. aethioopica, L. braziliensis, L. panamensis, L. guyanensis See subunit 5.10	Dog, rodent, sloth, hydrax, anteater Human	Sandfly	Promastigotes transmitted by insect bite	Cutaneous leishmaniasis Mucocutaneous leishmaniasis
Plasmodium falciparum Tropics, Sub-tropics	Anopheline mosquito	Human	Sporozoites transmitted by insect bite	Malignant tertian malaria Cerebral malaria
Plasmodium malariae Tropics, Sub-tropics	As above	As above	As above	Quartan malaria
Plasmodium vivax Tropics, Sub-tropics	As above	As above	As above	Benign tertian malaria

Parasite Distribution	Definitive host	Intermediate host	Transmission	Disease
Plasmodium ovale W. Africa, E. Africa, Asia, S. America	As above	As above	As above	Ovale tertian malaria
Isospora belli Worldwide	Human	–	Oocysts ingested	Isosporiasis Diarrhoea[b] Malabsorption
Cryptosporidium species Worldwide	Domestic animals, livestock, wildlife Human	–	Oocysts ingested	Cryptosporidiosis Diarrhoea[b] Malabsorption
Cyclospora cayetanensis Worldwide	Human (? animals)	–	Oocysts ingested	Persistent diarrhoea[b]
Toxoplasma gondii Worldwide	Cat, lynx	Herbivores, pig, bird, rodent. Human	Oocysts ingested in cat faeces. Tissue cysts ingested in undercooked meat. Transplacental transmission	Toxoplasmosis Cerebral toxoplasmosis[b] Congenital toxoplasmosis
Microsporidia Worldwide	Human and animal hosts depending on species	–	Spores ingested	Diarrhoea, nephritis, neurological disorders, conjunctivitis, disseminated disease[b]
FLUKES				
Opisthorchis sinensis China, Korea, Vietnam, Japan	Human. Dog, cat, pig, mouse, camel	1st: snail 2nd: fish	Metacercariae ingested in fish	Clonorchiasis, cholangitis, pancreatitis, cholangiocarcinoma
Opisthorchis viverrini Thailand, Laos	Civet cat Human	1st: snail 2nd: fish	Metacercariae ingested in fish	Opisthorchiasis, cholangitis, cholangiocarcinoma, liver cancer
Fasciola hepatica Worldwide	Sheep, cattle Human	Snail	Metacercariae ingested on water plants	Fascioliasis
Fasciolopsis buski Far East	Human Pig	Snail	Metacercariae ingested on water plants	Fasciolopsiasis
Metagonimus yokagawai Mainly Far East	Human Cat, dog, rat, pig	1st: Snail 2nd: Fish	Metacercariae ingested in fish	Metagonimiasis
Paragonimus westermani Far East, Indonesia, Malaysia, India	Human Carnivores	1st: Snail 2nd: Crab, crayfish	Metacercariae ingested in crab or crayfish	Paragonimiasis
Other Paragonimus spp Far East, Africa, India, Central/South America	Carnivores Human	As above	As above	As above
Schistosoma haematobium Africa, Middle East	Human Baboon	Snail	Cercariae penetrate skin	Urinary schistosomiasis
Schistosoma mansoni Africa, South America, Caribbean	Human Rodent Baboon	Snail	Cercariae penetrate skin	Intestinal schistosomiasis
Schistosoma mekongi Cambodia, Laos	Human Dog	Snail	Cercariae penetrate skin	Intestinal schistosomiasis

Parasite Distribution	Definitive host	Intermediate host	Transmission	Disease
Schistosoma japonicum China, Philippines, Indonesia	Cat, dog, rat, pig, buffalo, cattle, sheep, goat Human	Snail	Cercariae penetrate skin	Intestinal schistosomiasis

TAPEWORMS

Parasite Distribution	Definitive host	Intermediate host	Transmission	Disease
Taenia solium Worldwide	Human	Pig	Cysticerci ingested in pork Eggs ingested	Taeniasis Cysticercosis
Taenia saginata Worldwide	Human	Cattle	Cysticerci ingested in beef	Taeniasis
Echinococcus granulosus Worldwide	Dog, wolf, fox, hyaena, jackal	Sheep, cattle, goat, camel Human is accidental host	Eggs ingested	Echinococcosis Hydatid cyst
Vampirolepis nana Formerly *Hymenolepis nana* Worldwide	Mainly human	–	Eggs ingested	Hymenolepiasis
Diphyllobothrium latum Mainly temperate great lake areas	Human Dog, cat, seal, bear, fox	1st: Crustacean 2nd: Fish	Plerocercoids ingested in fish	Diphyllobothriasis
Spirometra species Far East, Central Africa	Carnivores	1st: *Cyclops* 2nd: Reptiles, small mammals, game animals Human	Procercoids ingested in *Cyclops*. Plerocercoids in frog tissue applied to sores and wounds	Sparganosis

NEMATODES

Parasite Distribution	Definitive host	Intermediate host	Transmission	Disease
Ascaris lumbricoides[a] Worldwide	Human	–	Eggs ingested	Ascariasis. Intestinal blockage. Pneumonitis (larvae)
Toxocara canis Worldwide	Dog	–	Eggs ingested	Visceral larva migrans
Enterobius vermicularis Worldwide	Human	–	Eggs ingested	Enterobiasis (pinworm, threadworm infection)
Strongyloides stercoralis Worldwide[a]	Human	–	Larvae penetrate skin. Also auto-infection	Strongyloidiasis Malabsorption
Stronglyoides füelleborni Tropical Africa, Papua New Guinea	Primates Human	–	Eggs ingested	Swollen belly syndrome in infants
Trichuris trichiura Worldwide[a]	Human	–	Eggs ingested	Trichuriasis (whipworm infection)
Ancylostoma duodenale Tropics Sub-tropics	Human	–	Larvae penetrate skin Drinking contaminated water	Hookworm disease Anaemia
Necator americanus As above	Human	–	Larvae penetrate skin	As above
Animal hookworms Worldwide	Dog, cat	–	Larvae penetrate skin	Cutaneous larva migrans

Wuchereria bancrofti Tropical Africa, India, SE Asia, Pacific Is., Central and South America	Human	Mosquito	Larvae transmitted by insect bite	Lymphatic filariasis (bancroftian)
Brugia species SE Asia, Far East, SW India, Indonesia	Human Monkey, cat	Mosquito	Larvae transmitted by insect bite	Lymphatic filariasis (brugian)
Loa loa West/Central Africa (rain forests)	Human	Tabanid fly *(Chrysops)*	Larvae transmitted by insect bite	Loiasis (Calabar swelling)
Onchocerca volvulus West/Central Africa, Central America, Middle East	Human	Blackfly	Larvae transmitted by insect bite	Onchocerciasis (River blindness, 'Sowda')
Dracunculus medinensis Sub-Saharan Africa, India, Arabian peninsula	Human	*Cyclops*	Larvae ingested in crustacean	Dracunculiasis (Guinea worm disease)
Trichinella spiralis Africa, Asia, S. America	Pig, bushpig, wild carnivores, rat Human	Same individual as definitive host	Larvae ingested in meat from wild pig or carnivore	Trichinosis

Notes:
a   Commonest in tropics and subtropics.
b   Severe infection can occur in immunosuppressed or immunodeficient persons, e.g. those with AIDS.

5.3 Direct examination of faeces and concentration techniques

This subunit includes:

- The clinical and public health reasons for examining faecal specimens for parasites.
- Collection of faecal specimens for parasitic examination.
- Direct examination of faeces for intestinal parasites.
- Faecal concentration techniques.

Reasons for examining faecal specimens for parasites

In district laboratories the examination of faecal specimens for parasites is requested:

- To identify the parasitic causes of blood and mucus in faeces and differentiate amoebic dysentery from bacterial dysentery.
- To identify intestinal parasitic infections that re-

quire treatment, i.e. those associated with serious illhealth, persistent diarrhoea, weight loss, intestinal malabsorption and the impairment of development and nutrition in children.

Also, to identify chronic significant infections that if not treated can lead to serious complications developing later in life, e.g. intestinal schistosomiasis leading to portal hypertension, or chronic *O. viverrini* infection leading to cancer of the bile duct.

- To detect serious hookworm infection in patients with severe iron deficiency anaemia, especially in a pregnant woman or child.

Heavy worm infections
Although hookworms and most other nematodes, flukes and tapeworms do not multiply in humans, moderate and heavy infections can occur when a person becomes infected with a heavy parasite load and reinfected frequently. Symptoms in children tend to be more severe and may occur with lower worm loads, particularly when there is undernutrition or co-existing illhealth.

- To assist in the surveillance and control of local parasitic infections caused by geohelminths (soil transmitted nematodes), and helminths transmitted by the ingestion of infected meat, freshwater fish, crabs, or shell-fish.

Importance of infection rates
In the control and management of parasitic helminth infections, it is important to know prevalence rates (proportion of those infected with a parasite at any one time), ages, and groups of those infected. When prevalence of infection is low, the mean worm burden is usually low and heavy infections are rare, whereas with high prevalence rates (e.g. over 50%) the worm burden increases and with it the severity of infection. A knowledge of prevalence rates of geohelminths provides information on the degree of faecal contamination of the environment.

Collection of faecal specimen for parasitic examination

For clinical purposes, a fresh faecal specimen is required. It should be uncontaminated with urine and collected into a suitable size, clean, dry, leak-proof container. The container need not be sterile but must be free of all traces of antiseptics and disinfectants (also a bedpan if this is first used to collect a specimen from an inpatient). A large teaspoon amount of faeces is adequate or about 10 ml of a fluid specimen. Several specimens collected on alternate days may be required to detect parasites that are excreted intermittently, e.g. *Giardia*.

Unsuitable containers: Avoid using containers made from leaves, paper, or cardboard (including matchboxes) because these will not be leakproof, may not be clean, and can result in the faecal contamination of hands and surfaces. If no leakproof container is available, a non-leakproof container can be used providing the specimen is first sealed in a plastic bag. This, however, is not recommended for the routine collection of faeces because the plastic bag is difficult to label and can be a hazard to laboratory staff.

Important: Dysenteric and watery specimens must reach the laboratory as soon as possible after being passed (within 15 minutes) otherwise motile parasites such as *E. histolytica* and *G. lamblia* trophozoites may not be detected. Other specimens should reach the laboratory within 1 hour of being collected. Specimens must be labelled correctly and accompanied by a correctly completed request form (see subunit 5.1).

Public health faecal specimens. The Public Health Laboratory should provide the district laboratory with containers and detailed instructions on the method of collecting specimens. The collection technique will depend on the parasite being investigated, the method that will be used to examine the faeces, and whether any fixative or preservative is required.

Caution: Faecal specimens, like other specimens received in the laboratory, must be handled with care to avoid acquiring infection from infectious parasites, bacteria, or viruses. Faeces may contain:

– infective forms of parasites such as *S. stercoralis*, *E. vermicularis*, *T. solium*, *G. lamblia*, *E. histolytica*, or *C. parvum*.

– bacteria such as *V. cholerae*, *Shigella* or *Salmonella* species.

– viruses including hepatitis viruses, HIV, and rotaviruses.

DIRECT EXAMINATION OF FAECES FOR PARASITES

Routinely faecal specimens are examined in district laboratories by direct technique. This involves:

■ Reporting the appearance of the specimen and identifying any parasitic worms or tapeworm segments.

■ Examining the specimen microscopically for:
  – motile parasites such as the larvae of *S. stercoralis* and trophozoites of *E. histolytica*, *G. lamblia*, and more rarely, *B. coli*,
  – helminth eggs,
  – cysts and oocysts of intestinal protozoa.

Need for faecal concentration techniques

The direct examination of faeces is essential to detect motile parasites and is usually adequate to detect significant helminth infections. Important exceptions are *Schistosoma* species because only a few eggs are usually produced even in moderate and severe infections, therefore a concentration technique should be performed when intestinal schistosomiasis is suspected and no eggs are found by direct examination.

Concentration techniques may also be required:

– To detect *Strongyloides* larvae, the eggs of *Taenia*, cysts of *G. lamblia*, and to make it easier to detect small parasites, e.g. small fluke eggs, or the oocysts of intestinal coccidia prior to staining.

– To check whether treatment has been successful.

– To quantify intestinal parasites.

Note: The techniques used to concentrate and quantify faecal parasites are described at the end of this subunit.

Reporting the appearance of faecal specimens
Report the following:

● Colour of the specimen.
● Consistency, i.e. whether formed, semiformed, unformed, watery.
● Presence of blood, mucus, and, or, pus. If blood is present note whether this is mixed in the faeces. If only on the surface this indicates rectal or anal bleeding.
● Whether the specimen contains worms, e.g. *A. lumbricoides* (large roundworm), *E. vermicularis* (threadworm) or tapeworm segments, e.g. *T. solium*, *T. saginata*.

Blood and mucus in faeces

Blood and mucus may be found in faeces from patients with amoebic dysentery, intestinal schistosomiasis, invasive balantidiasis (rare infection), and in severe *T. trichiura* infections. Other non-parasitic conditions in which blood and mucus may be found include bacillary dysentery, *Campylobacter* enteritis, ulcerative colitis, intestinal tumour, and haemorrhoids.

Presence of pus

This can be found when there is inflammation of the intestinal tract. Many pus cells can be found in faecal specimens from patients with bacillary dysentery. They can also be found in amoebic dysentery but are less numerous.

Pale coloured specimens

Pale coloured and frothy specimens (containing fat) can be found in giardiasis and other infections associated with intestinal malabsorption. Pale coloured faeces (lacking stercobilinogen) are also excreted by patients with obstructive jaundice.

Microscopical examination of faecal specimens

Examine immediately those specimens containing blood and mucus and those that are unformed because these may contain motile trophozoites of *E. histolytica* or *G. lamblia*.

Examination of dysenteric and unformed specimens

1 Using a wire loop or piece of stick, place a small amount of specimen, to include blood and mucus on one end of a slide. Without adding saline, cover with a cover glass and using a tissue, press gently on the cover glass to make a thin preparation.

2 Place a drop of eosin reagent (Reagent No. 23) on the other end of the slide. Mix a small amount of the specimen with the eosin and cover with a cover glass.

Value of eosin: Eosin does not stain living trophozoites but provides a pink background which can make them easier to see.

3 Examine immediately the preparations microscopically, first using the 10× objective with the condenser iris *closed sufficiently* to give good contrast. Use the 40× objective to identify motile trophozoites, e.g. *E. histolytica* amoebae (see subunit 5.4.1) or *G. lamblia* flagellates (see 5.4.1).

Note: The eggs of *Schistosoma* species and *T. trichiura*, and the trophozoites of *B. coli* can also result in specimens containing blood and mucus.

Examination of semi-formed and formed faeces

1 Place a drop of fresh physiological saline (Reagent No 50) on one end of a slide and a drop of iodine (Reagent No 38) on the other end.

To avoid contaminating the fingers and stage of the microscope, do not use too large a drop of saline or iodine.

2 Using a wire loop or piece of stick, mix a small amount of specimen, about 2 mg, (matchstick head amount) with the saline and a similar amount with the iodine. Make smooth *thin* preparations. Cover each preparation with a cover glass.

Important: Sample from different areas in and on the specimen or preferably mix the faeces before sampling to distribute evenly any parasites in the specimen. Do not use too much specimen otherwise the preparations will be too thick, making it difficult to detect and identify parasites.

3 Examine systematically the entire saline preparation for larvae, ciliates, helminth eggs, cysts, and oocysts. Use the 10× objective with the condenser iris *closed sufficiently* to give good contrast.

Use the 40× objective to assist in the detection and identification of eggs, cysts, and oocysts. Always examine several microscope fields with this objective before reporting 'No parasites found'.

4 Use the iodine preparation to assist in the identification of cysts (see following text).

5 Report the number of larvae and each species of egg found in the entire saline preparation as follows:

Scanty . . . . 1–3 per preparation
Few . . . . 4–10 per preparation
Moderate number . . . . 11–20 per preparation
Many . . . . 21–40 per preparation
Very many . . . . over 40 per preparation

Note: Plate 5.1 shows the relative sizes of helminth eggs and a *Strongyloides* larva in a saline preparation as seen in a microscope field viewed with the 10× objective and 10× widefield eyepiece. Plate 5.2 shows the relative sizes of protozoan trophozoites, cysts, and oocysts in saline and iodine when viewed with the 40× objective and 10× eyepiece.

Identification of larvae: In a fresh faecal specimen, *S. stercoralis* is the only larva that will be found. It can be easily detected in a saline preparation by its motility and large size. It is described in subunit 5.5. If the specimen is not fresh, *S. stercoralis* will require differentiation from hookworm larvae (see subunit 5.5).

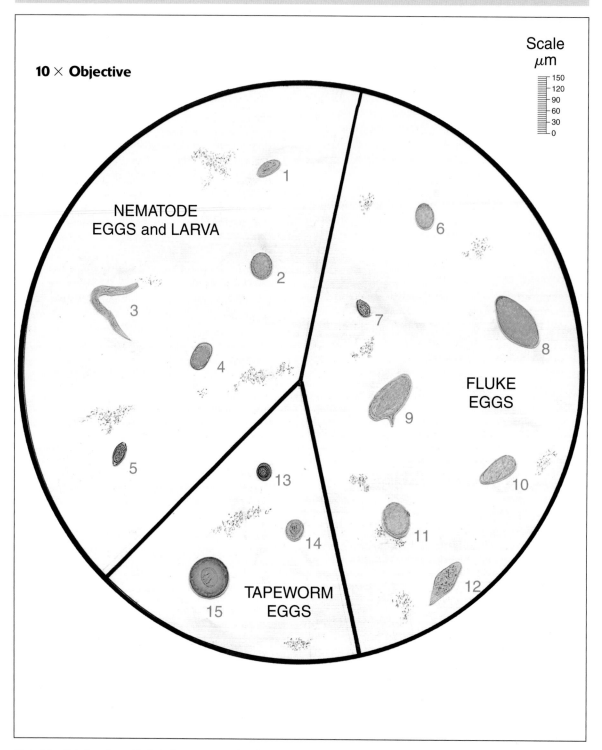

Plate 5.1   Relative sizes of helminth eggs as seen in microscope field using the 10× objective (with 10× eye-pieces). Eggs are as seen in a saline preparation.

1. *E.vermicularis*,   2. *A.lumbricoides*,   3. *S.stercoralis* larva (motile),   4. Hookworm,   5. *T.trichiura*,   6. *D.latum*,   7. *O.sinensis*, 8. *Fasciola* sp,   9. *S.mansoni*,   10. *Paragonimus* sp,   11. *S.japonicum*,   12. *S.intercalatum*,   13. *Taenia* sp,   14. *V.nana*,   15. *H.dimunuta*.

Note: Helminth eggs found in faeces are described in subunit 5.5 and also shown on p. 428.

Identification of helminth eggs: Eggs are recognized by their:

- size,
- colour (colourless, pale yellow, brown),
- morphological features.

Note: Some helminths also have a limited geographical distribution.

The relative sizes and colour of the eggs of the common nematodes, flukes, and tapeworms are shown in Plate 5.1. Each species is described and illustrated in subunit 5.5 and also on p. 428.

Identification of intestinal flagellates: The trophozoite of *G. lamblia* and its differentiation from non-pathogenic flagellates that can be found in faeces is described in subunit 5.4.

Identification of ciliates: *B. coli* is the only ciliate found in human faeces (rare infection). The trophozoite and cyst are described and illustrated in subunit 5.4.

Identification of cysts and oocysts: In saline and eosin preparations, protozoan cysts and oocysts can be recognized as refractile bodies (shine brightly when focused). Cysts can be identified by their shape, size, nuclei, and inclusions as seen in an iodine preparation (see Plate 5.2 on p. 197).

Iodine stains nuclei and glycogen but not chromatoid bodies. Burrows stain or Sargeaunt's stain can be used to stain chromatoid bodies (see subunit 5.4).

The cysts of *E. histolytica/E. dispar* and those of *G. lamblia* and their differentiation from non-pathogenic or other species are described in subunit 5.4.

The identification of the oocysts of the coccidia, *I. belli*, *C. parvum*, and *C. cayetanensis* are also described in subunit 5.4.

Faecal leukocytes: The presence of polymorphonuclear neutrophils (pus cells) in faeces is mainly associated with inflammatory diarrhoea caused by bacteria.

Non-parasitic structures found in faeces: Care must be taken not to report as parasites those structures that can be normally found in faeces such as muscle fibres, vegetable fibres, starch cells (stain blue-black with iodine), pollen grains, fatty acid crystals, soaps, spores, yeasts, and hairs (see Plate 5.3).

Large numbers of fat globules may be seen in faeces when there is malabsorption. Charcot Leyden crystals (breakdown products of eosinophils) can sometimes be seen in faeces (also in sputum) in parasitic infections. They appear as slender crystals with pointed ends, about 30–40 μm in length as shown in Plate 5.3.

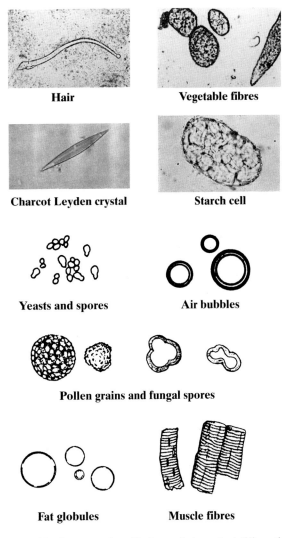

Hair   Vegetable fibres

Charcot Leyden crystal   Starch cell

Yeasts and spores   Air bubbles

Pollen grains and fungal spores

Fat globules   Muscle fibres

Plate 5.3   Structures found in faeces that required differentiation from parasites.

FAECAL CONCENTRATION TECHNIQUES

The need for faecal concentration techniques has been discussed at the beginning of this subunit. The following techniques are commonly used to concentrate faecal parasites in district laboratories:

- Sedimentation techniques in which parasites are sedimented by gravity or centrifugal force, e.g. formol ether concentration method which is the most frequently used technique because it concentrates a wide range of parasites with minimum damage to their morphology.

- Floatation (also spelt flotation) techniques in which parasites are concentrated by being floated in solutions of high specific gravity, i.e. solutions that are denser than the parasites being concentrated. Examples include the zinc sulphate method and saturated sodium chloride method.

Unlike the formol ether sedimentation technique, a single floatation technique cannot be used to concentrate a wide range of parasites because of differences in the densities of parasites and the damage that can be caused by floatation fluids to some parasites.

For certain parasites and situations (see later text), floatation techniques are recommended and can be easily performed in the field with the minimum of equipment, providing adequate health and safety measures are taken.

Choice of concentration technique
The method to use will depend on:

- why the technique is being performed, the species of parasite requiring concentration, and how well its morphology is retained by a particular technique.

- the number of specimens to be examined and time available.

- the location, e.g. field or laboratory situation and equipment available.

- experience of staff performing the technique.

- health and safety considerations.

The techniques that are recommended for the different parasites are shown in Chart 5.3.

Formol ether concentration technique
This is recommended for use in district laboratories because it is rapid and can be used to concentrate a wide range of faecal parasites from fresh or preserved faeces. Eggs that do not concentrate well by this technique are those of *Fasciola* species and *Vampirolepis nana* but concentration of these parasites is not usually required. Risk of laboratory acquired infection from faecal pathogens is minimized because organisms are killed by the formalin solution. The technique, however, requires the use of highly flammable ether or less flammable ethyl acetate (see following text). When concentrating the oocysts of coccidia, an additional centrifugation stage is required.

Formalin-acetone concentration: A technique using acetone instead of ether has been descirbed by Parija *et al. Tropical Doctor*, 2003, 33, pp. 163–163

Commercially available devices, e.g. *Parasep* and *Evergreen* faecal parasite concentrator kits eliminate the tube and filter process, so reducing the risk of aerosol contamination.

Principle
In the Ridley modified method, faeces are emulsified in formol water, the suspension is strained to

Chart 5.3 Faecal concentration techniques and their application

Parasite	Formol ether	Sat. NaCl[a]	Zn SO$_4$[b]
CYSTS			
G. lamblia	●	–	●
E. histolytica/ E. dispar	●	–	●
OOCYSTS			
I. belli	●[c]	–	–
C. parvum	●[c]	–	–
C. cayetanensis	●[c]	–	–
EGGS			
A. lumbricoides	●	●	–
Hookworm	●	●	–
T. trichiura	●	–	●
Schistosoma sp	●[d]	–	–
Taenia sp	●	–	–
Opisthorchis sp	●	–	●
LARVAE			
Strongyloides	●[e]	–	–

NOTES
a   Saturated sodium chloride, specific gravity 1.200.
b   Zinc sulphate, 33% v/v, specific gravity 1.180.
c   Use formol ether oocyst concentration technique.
d   Formol detergent gravity technique is also suitable (see sub-unit 5.5).
e   Water emergence technique in which larvae remain motile is also recommended (see subunit 5.5).

remove large faecal particles, ether or ethyl acetate is added, and the mixed suspension is centrifuged. Cysts, oocysts, eggs, and larvae are fixed and sedimented and the faecal debris is separated in a layer between the ether and the formol water. Faecal fat is dissolved in the ether.

Required

- Formol water, 10% v/v.*

*Prepare by mixing 50 ml of strong formaldehyde solution with 450 ml of distilled or filtered rain water.

- Diethyl ether or ethyl acetate.*

*Diethyl ether is a highly flammable and volatile chemical and therefore its replacement by a less flammable chemical such as ethyl acetate or acetone is recommended by some workers. When using ethyl acetate, greater care needs to be taken when discarding the faecal debris layer to prevent remixing with the sediment. Insoluble particles of ethyl acetate may form under the cover glass. In some countries ethyl acetate is difficult to obtain. It has an unpleasant odour.

- Sieve (strainer) with small holes, preferably 400–450 μm in size.*

*The small inexpensive nylon tea or coffee strainer available in most countries is suitable (can be used many times and does not corrode like metal sieves).

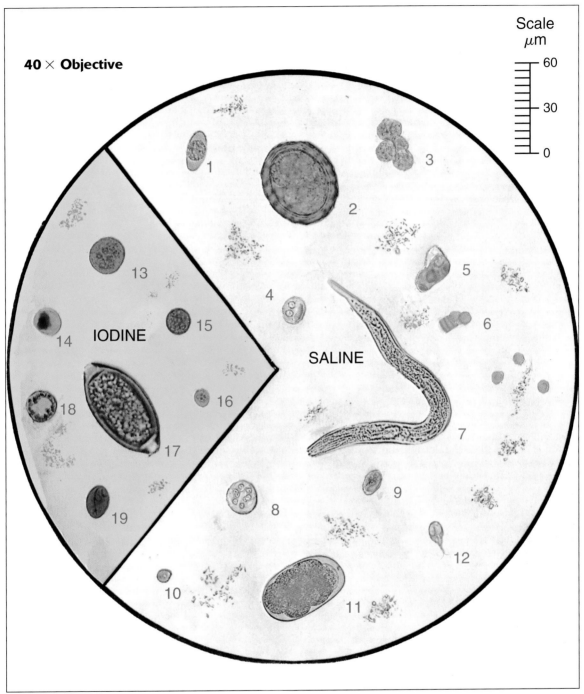

Plate 5.2 Relative sizes of trophozoites and cysts of intestinal protozoa, common nematode eggs and larva of *Strongyloides* as seen in microscope field using the 40× objective (with 10× eyepieces).

1. *I.belli* oocyst, 2. *A lumbricoides* egg, 3. Leucocytes, 4. *E.histolytica/E.dispar* cyst, 5. *E.histolytica* trophozoite (motile), 6. Red cells, 7. *S.stercoralis* larva (motile), 8. *E.coli* cyst (mature), 9. *G.lamblia* cyst, 10. *C.mesnili* cyst, 11. Hookworm egg, 12. *G.lamblia* trophozoite (motile).

Iodine preparation: 13. *E.coli* cyst, 14. *I.buetschlii* cyst, 15. *E.histolytica/E.dispar* cyst, 16. *V.nana* cyst, 17. *T.trichiura* egg, 18. *Blastocystis hominis*, 19. *G.lamblia* cyst.

Note: Trophozoites, cysts and oocysts found in faeces are described in subunit 5.4.

Method

1　Using a rod or stick, emulsify an estimated 1 g (pea-size) of faeces in about 4 ml of 10% formol water contained in a screw-cap bottle or tube.

Note: Include in the sample, faeces from the surface and several places in the specimen.

2　Add a further 3–4 ml of 10% v/v formol water, cap the bottle, and mix well by shaking.

3　Sieve the emulsified faeces, collecting the sieved suspension in a beaker.

4　Transfer the suspension to a conical (centrifuge) tube made of strong glass, copolymer, or polypropylene. Add 3–4 ml of diethyl ether or ethyl acetate.

Caution: Ether is highly flammable and ethyl acetate is flammable, therefore use well away from an open flame, e.g. flame from the burner of a gas refrigerator, Bunsen burner, or spirit lamp. Ether vapour is anaesthetic, therefore make sure the laboratory is well-ventilated.

5　Stopper* the tube and mix for 1 minute. If using a Vortex mixer, leave the tube unstoppered and mix for about 15 seconds (it is best to use a boiling tube).

* Do not use a rubber bung or a cap with a rubber liner because ether attacks rubber.

6　With a tissue or piece of cloth wrapped around the top of the tube, loosen the stopper (considerable pressure will have built up inside the tube).

7　Centrifuge immediately at 750–1 000 g (approx. 3000 rpm) for 1 minute.

After centrifuging, the parasites will have sedimented to the bottom of the tube and the faecal debris will have collected in a layer between the ether and formol water as shown in Fig. 5.1.

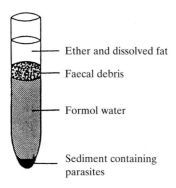

Ether and dissolved fat

Faecal debris

Formol water

Sediment containing parasites

Fig. 5.1　Formal ether sedimentation concentration technique, after centrifugation.

8　Using a stick or the stem of a plastic bulb pipette, loosen the layer of faecal debris from the side of the tube and *invert* the tube to discard the ether, faecal debris, and formol water. The sediment will remain.

9　Return the tube to its upright position and allow the fluid from the side of the tube to drain to the bottom. Tap the bottom of the tube to resuspend and mix the sediment. Transfer the sediment to a slide, and cover with a cover glass.

10　Examine the preparation microscopically using the 10× objective with the condenser iris *closed sufficiently* to give good contrast. Use the 40× objective to examine small cysts and eggs. To assist in the identification of cysts, run a small drop of iodine under the cover glass (see subunit 5.4).

Although the motility of *Strongyloides* larvae will not be seen, the non-motile larvae can be easily recognized.

11　If required, count the number of each species of egg in the entire preparation. This will give the approximate number per gram of faeces.

Formol ether oocyst concentration technique[2]

Follow steps 1 to 6 of the above method. Continue as follows:

7　Centrifuge immediately at *low* speed, i.e. RCF 300–400 g (about 1 000 rpm) for 1 minute.

8　Using a plastic bulb pipette or Pasteur pipette, carefully remove the entire column of fluid below the faecal debris and ether and transfer this to another centrifuge tube.

9　Add formol water to make the volume up to 10–15 ml. Centrifuge at RCF 750–1 000 g (about 3 000 rpm) for 5–10 minutes.

10　Remove the supernatant. Tap the bottom of the tube to resuspend and mix the sediment. Transfer the sediment to a slide and examine for oocysts using the 40× objective.

Note: Cryptosporidium and *Cyclospora* oocysts are best identified in a modified Ziehl-Neelsen stained smear as described in subunit 5.4 (with experience *Cyclospora* oocysts can be identified in unstained preparations). *I. belli* oocysts can be easily identified in an unstained wet preparation (see subunit 5.4). The modified formol ether method is recommended in preference to Sheather's sucrose floatation technique for concentrating *Cryptosporidium* because recovery and subsequent staining of the oocysts are better after the formol ether method.

Zinc sulphate floatation technique

As shown in Chart 5.3, the zinc sulphate technique is recommended for concentrating the cysts of *G. lamblia* and *E. histolytica/E. dispar*, and the eggs of *T. trichiura* and *Opisthorchis* species.

Other nematode eggs are concentrated less well. The technique is not suitable for concentrating eggs or cysts in fatty faeces. Adequate safety precautions should be taken because faecal pathogens are not killed by zinc sulphate.

Principle

A zinc sulphate solution is used which has a specific gravity (relative density) of 1.180–1.200. Faeces are emulsified in the solution and the suspension is left undisturbed for the eggs and cysts to float to the surface. They are collected on a cover glass.

Required

– Zinc sulphate solution, 33% w/v Reagent No 69, specific gravity, 1.180–1.200.

> Use a hydrometer to check that the specific gravity of the solution is correct. Adjust with distilled water or more chemical if required.

– Test tube (without a lip) of about 15 ml capacity which has a completely smooth rim.

– Strainer (nylon coffee or tea strainer is suitable).

Method

1 Fill the tube about one quarter full with the zinc sulphate solution. Add an estimated 1 gram of faeces (or 2 ml if a fluid specimen). Using a rod or stick, emulsify the specimen in the solution.

2 Fill the tube with the zinc sulphate solution, and mix well. Strain the faecal suspension to remove large faecal particles.

3 Return the suspension to the tube. Stand the tube in a completely vertical position in a rack.

4 Using a plastic bulb pipette or Pasteur pipette, add further solution to ensure the tube is filled to the brim.

5 Carefully place a completely clean (grease-free) cover glass on top of the tube. Avoid trapping any air bubbles.

6 Leave undisturbed for 30–45 minutes to give time for the cysts and eggs to float.

> Note: Do not leave longer because the cysts can become distorted and the eggs will begin to sink.

7 Carefully lift the cover glass from the tube by a straight pull upwards. Place the cover glass face downwards on a slide.

Caution: Avoid contaminating the fingers. Mature *E. histolytica* and *G. lamblia* cysts are infective when passed in the faeces.

8 Examine microscopically the entire preparation using the 10× objective with the condenser iris closed sufficiently to give good contrast. Use the 40× objective, and run a drop of iodine under the cover glass, to identify the cysts (see subunit 5.4).

9 Count the number of *T. trichiura* eggs to give the approximate number per gram of faeces.

Note: Parasites can also be recovered from the surface of the floatation fluid after centrifuging. If however, a centrifuge is available, the safer formol ether technique is recommended for concentrating eggs and infective cysts from faecal specimens.

Saturated sodium chloride floatation technique

The saturated sodium chloride technique is a useful and inexpensive method of concentrating hookworm or *Ascaris* eggs, e.g. in field surveys.

Preparation of saturated sodium chloride solution

Stir sodium chloride (e.g. table salt) into hot clean distilled or boiled filtered water until no more can be dissolved. Add a few more grams of the salt so that a layer of the undissolved salt remains in the bottom of the stock container. Mix well and leave the undissolved salt to sediment. When cool, filter some of the solution and use a hydrometer to check that the specific gravity is 1.200.

Immediately before use, filter the amount of solution required from the stock bottle and recheck the specific gravity.

Method

The technique is the same as that described for the zinc sulphate floatation technique except that a saturated solution of sodium chloride is used and a flat bottomed vial (50 mm tall and 20 mm wide) is used instead of a tube. A glass slide is used to recover the eggs instead of a cover glass. Eggs can be recovered after about 20 minutes.

Stoll's technique for counting helminth eggs

1 Weigh 3 g of faeces in a screw-cap container. Add 42 ml of water* to give a 1 in 15 dilution of the faeces. If the faeces is a formed specimen, use sodium hydroxide 0.1 mol/l (N/10) solution instead of water.

> *Formol water:* The use of formol water as used in the formol ether concentration technique is recommended as this will kill faecal pathogens, making the technique safer.

2 Using a rod, break up the faeces and mix it with the water. Cap the container and shake hard to complete the mixing.

3 Without delay, using a wide bore Pasteur pipette (previously marked to measure the required volume), remove 0.15 ml of the suspension and transfer this to a slide.

Cover with a long cover glass or if unavailable with two square cover glasses side by side.

4 Examine systematically the entire preparation, using the 10× objective with the condenser iris reduced to give good contrast. Include in the count any eggs lying outside the edges of the cover glass because these are also contained in the 0.15 ml sample.

5 Multiply the number of eggs counted by 100 to give the number of eggs per gram of faeces.

Note: If the faeces is not a formed specimen, the following additional calculation is necessary to give the number of eggs per gram of faeces:

Fluid specimen . . . . multiply by 5
Unformed watery specimen . . . . multiply by 4
Unformed soft specimen . . . . multiply by 3
Semiformed specimen . . . . multiply by 2

5.4 Identification of faecal protozoan trophozoites, cysts and oocysts

This subunit describes the following intestinal protozoa:

1 *E. histolytica* and its differentiation from non-pathogenic amoebae.
2 *G. lamblia* and its differentiation from non-pathogenic flagellates.
3 *B. coli.*
4 Intestinal coccidia: *I. belli, Cryptosporidium* species, *C. cayetanensis.*

Briefly described:
Blastocystis hominis
Microsporidia

Note: The laboratory diagnosis of amoebic liver abscess is described in subunit 5.14.1.

1   *Entamoeba histolytica*

E. histolytica is endemic in many parts of tropical and subtropical Africa, Asia, Mexico, South America, and China. Distribution is related more to inadequate environmental sanitation and poor personal hygiene than to climate. It is transmitted by the faecal-oral route with infective cysts being ingested in food, water, or from hands contaminated with faeces, *E. histolytica* has a direct life cycle as shown in Fig. 5.2.

Differentiation of invasive *E. histolytica* from non-invasive *E. dispar*

Formerly a pathogenic invasive strain and a non-pathogenic strain of *E. histolytica* were thought to exist. Using isoenzyme-electrophoretic techniques, these two 'strains' have now been recognized as separate species.[3,4] *Entamoeba histolytica* is the invasive pathogenic species and *Entamoeba dispar* (originally described by Brumpt in 1925) has been designated the non-invasive non-pathogenic species. The two species are morphologically identical. Trophozoites containing ingested red cells can be identified as *E. histolytica* but the cysts of *E. histolytica* and *E. dispar* cannot be differentiated microscopically and should therefore be reported as *E. histolytica/E. dispar. E. histolytica* causes amoebic dysentery and amoebic liver abscess.

Note: *E. histolytica* can be differentiated from *E. dispar* using molecular techniques.[5] An ELISA is available from Techlab Inc. which uses monoclonal antibody to detect specific *E. histolytica* lectin (adhesin) in faeces. Details of the assay (*E. HISTOLYTICA, T5017*), prices and distributors can be obtained from Techlab Inc. (see Appendix 11).

Amoebic dysentery
Amoebic dysentery occurs when *E. histolytica* trophozoites invade the wall of the large intestine and multiply in the submucosa, forming large flask-shaped ulcers. The amoebae ingest red cells from damaged capillaries. Compared with bacillary dysentery, the onset of amoebic dysentery is less acute, lasts longer, and there is usually no significant fever. Without treatment dysenteric attacks may recur for several years.

Amoebic liver abscess
Occasionally *E. histolytica* amoebae are carried to the liver in the portal circulation and form abscesses, usually in the right lobe. Amoebic liver abscesses are more common in adults than in children with a higher frequency in men (3 to 1 rate). There is pain and tenderness over the liver, wasting, and fever with chills and night sweats. Patients with large or multiple abscesses may become jaundiced and anaemic. There is usually a raised white cell count with neutrophilia and a significantly raised ESR.

The centre of the abscess contains a viscous pink-brown or grey-yellow fluid consisting of digested liver tissue. It is referred to as 'pus' but contains very few pus cells. As *part of treatment* (not diagnosis) the fluid may be aspirated and sent to the laboratory to examine for trophozoites. Amoebic liver abscess can be diagnosed serologically as described in subunit 5.14.1.

Prevention and control of *E. histolytica* infection

- Preventing faecal contamination of the environment by using latrines and protecting water supplies from faecal contamination.

- Handwashing after defaecation and before eating.

- Covering food and water to prevent contamination from flies which can act as cyst carriers.

- Not eating green salads or other uncooked foods which may contain cysts, usually as a result of fertilization with untreated human faeces.

- Boiling drinking water (*E. histolytica* cysts are killed at 55 °C).

- Health education, particularly of food handlers, and also in schools and community health centres.

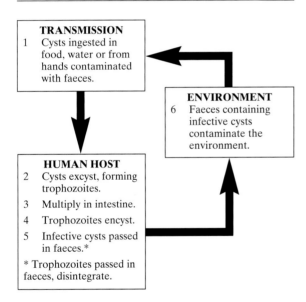

| TRANSMISSION |
| 1 Cysts ingested in food, water or from hands contaminated with faeces. |

| ENVIRONMENT |
| 6 Faeces containing infective cysts contaminate the environment. |

| HUMAN HOST |
| 2 Cysts excyst, forming trophozoites. |
| 3 Multiply in intestine. |
| 4 Trophozoites encyst. |
| 5 Infective cysts passed in faeces.* |
| * Trophozoites passed in faeces, disintegrate. |

Fig 5.2   Transmission and life cycle of *Entamoeba histolytica, Giardia lamblia, Balantidium coli.*

LABORATORY DIAGNOSIS

The laboratory diagnosis of amoebic dysentery is by finding *E. histolytica* trophozoites in a *fresh* (still warm) dysenteric faecal specimen or rectal scrape. Specimens must be examined without delay, otherwise identification of the trophozoites becomes impossible because the amoebae lose their motility, extrude food vacuoles containing red cells, and round up.

Examination of a dysenteric specimen for *E. histolytica* trophozoites

1   Using a wire loop or piece of stick, place a small amount of blood and mucus on one end of a slide. Without adding saline, cover with a cover glass and using a tissue, press gently on the cover glass to make a thin preparation.

2   Place a drop of eosin reagent (Reagent No. 23) on the other end of the slide. Mix a small amount of the specimen with the eosin and cover with a cover glass.

    Value of eosin: Eosin does not stain living amoebae but provides a pink background which can make the motile amoebae easier to detect.

3   Examine immediately the preparations microscopically, first using the 10× objective with the condenser iris *closed sufficiently* to give good contrast. Use the 40× objective to identify motile *E. histolytica* trophozoites.

Trophozoite of *E. histolytica*

- Average size is about 25 × 20 μm (see Plate 5.2 in subunit 5.3).

- Shows active amoeboid movement (directional) in fresh warm specimen.

- In dysenteric specimens, the amoebae contain ingested red cells. This is diagnostic of *E. histolytica.*

- Single nucleus is present which has a central karyosome (not always visible).

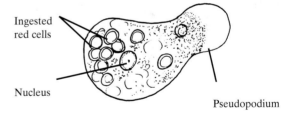

Ingested red cells

Nucleus

Pseudopodium

Fig. 5.3   Morphology of *E.histolytica* trophozoite.

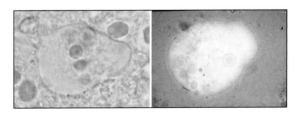

Plate 5.4   *Left: E.histolytica* trophozoite in dysenteric faecal specimen. Note the ingested red cells (diagnostic feature). *Right: E.histolytica* trophozoite containing red cells as seen in an eosin preparation. See also Plate 5.2 (p. 197).

Cysts of E. histolytica/E. dispar

With the recognition that *E. histolytica* is morphologically identical but genetically distinct from *E. dispar* (see previous text), cysts, formerly reported as *E. histolytica* should now be reported as *E. histolytica/ E. dispar.*

Cysts of *E. histolytica/E. dispar*

- Round, measuring 10–15 µm.
- Contain, 1, 2 or 4 nuclei with a central karyosome (special staining techniques are required to show details of nuclear structure).
- Chromatoid bodies (aggregations of ribosomes) can be seen particularly in immature cysts. They do not stain with iodine but can be stained with Burrow's stain or Sargeaunt's stain (see following text).

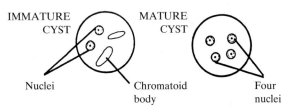

Fig. 5.4. Morphology of immature and mature *E.hisolytica /E.dispar* cysts.

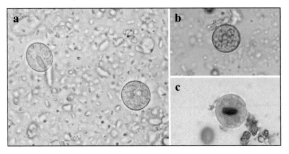

Plate 5.5 *E.histolytica/E.dispar* cysts showing chromatoid bodies. **a** Immature single nucleus cyst in saline, **b** Iodine stained mature 4 nuclei cyst, **c** Burrow stained chromatoid body in cyst. See also Plate 5.2 on p. 197.

Staining of chromatoid bodies
The simplest technique is to make a saline suspension of faeces in a small tube, add 2 or 3 drops of Burrow's stain (Reagent No 15) or Sargeaunt's stain (Reagent No 55) and mix. Leave the suspension overnight or at least 6 hours. Examine microscopically for stained chromatoid bars (blue if using Burrow's stain, green if using Sargeaunt's stain).

If facilities for fluorescence microscopy are available, acridine orange can be used to demonstrate chromatoid bars in *E. histolytica/E. dispar* cysts.

Differentiation of cysts of non-pathogenic species of amoebae that can be found in faeces

The commonest seen cysts that require differentiation from *E. hystolytica/E. dispar* are *Entamoeba hartmanni* (similar in appearance but smaller than *E. histolytica/E. dispar*, measuring 7–9 µm), *Entamoeba coli*, *Iodamoeba buetschlii*, *Endolimax nana*. The differentiating features of these cysts are summarized in Chart 5.2 and the appearances of the cysts in saline and iodine preparations are shown in Plate 5.2 on p. 197.

Chart 5.2 Differentiation of small cysts that can be found in faeces

Species	Size	Nuclei	Chromatoid body	Glycogen inclusion
CYSTS OF AMOEBAE				
Entamoeba histolytica/ E. dispar	10–15 µm	1–4	Present (immature cyst)	Diffuse
Entamoeba hartmanni	7–9 µm	1–4	Present (immature cyst)	Diffuse
Entamoeba coli	15–30 µm	1–8	Rare Needle-like	Diffuse
Iodamoeba buetschlii	9–15 µm	1	–	Compact mass
Endolimax nana	7–9 µm	4 Hole-like	–	–

Note: Refer also to Plate 5.2 on p. 197.

Blastocystis hominis

This anaerobic intestinal protozoan can be found in faeces and is sometimes confused with cysts. It is usually non-pathogenic but may cause acute enteritis in persons with immunodeficiency (being increasingly reported from persons with HIV).

Appearance: *B. hominis* is round and about the size of an *E. coli* cyst but shows great variation in size. It has peripheral cytoplasm, a central vacuole but no nucleus. It can be recognized from the granules which form a ring around the periphery. The granules stain with iodine (see Plate 5.2 on p. 197).

---

2 Giardia lamblia*

---

* Also called *Giardia intestinalis* and *Giardia duodenalis.*

G. lamblia has a worldwide distribution and is particularly common in the tropics and subtropics, in areas where water supplies and the environment become faecally contaminated. In endemic areas, young children are more frequently infected than adults, particularly those that are malnourished.

G. lamblia is transmitted by the faecal-oral route. G. lamblia has a direct life cycle (see Fig. 5.2). Infection with G. lamblia is called giardiasis.

Giardiasis
Although many infections, particularly in adults are without symptoms, G. lamblia can cause abdominal pain, severe diarrhoea, flatulence, vomiting, weight loss, malabsorption with lactose intolerance, and in children, impairment of growth. Symptoms can be severe particularly in children under 3 years of age, and in the undernourished. Those with reduced immune responses, gastrointestinal disorders or intestinal bacterial infections, tend to be more susceptible to *Giardia* infection.

Prevention and control of *G. lamblia* infection
Giardiasis may be reduced by improving environmental sanitation and personal hygiene to prevent food, water, and hands becoming contaminated with faeces containing cysts.

The cysts are not killed in food or water stored at 4–6 °C. Like the cysts of *E. histolytica*, those of *Giardia* are resistant to the concentrations of chlorine normally used for the treatment of domestic water supplies.

LABORATORY DIAGNOSIS

Faecal specimens containing G. lamblia may have an offensive odour and are pale coloured, fatty and float in water. The preparation of faecal specimens for microscopical examination is described under *Direct examination of faecal specimens* in subunit 5.3.

The laboratory diagnosis of giardiasis is by:

- Finding G. lamblia trophozoites in *fresh* diarrhoeic specimens particularly in mucus. They are often difficult to detect because they attach themselves to the wall of the intestine.

  Several specimens collected at different times may need to be examined. A Giemsa or Field's stained faecal smear should be examined if giardiasis is suspected but no trophozoites are detected in a wet faecal preparation, and also to confirm the identity of the flagellates.

- Finding G. lamblia cysts in more formed specimens. The cysts are excreted irregularly. Often large number may be present for a few days followed by fewer numbers for a week or more. Several specimens may need to be examined and a concentration technique used.

Concentration of Giardia cysts
G. lamblia cysts can be concentrated using the Ridley modified formol ether centrifuge technique in which formol water is used (see subunit 5.3).[3] Alternatively, the cysts can be concentrated using a zinc sulphate floatation technique as detailed in subunit 5.3. A drop of Sargeaunt's stain (Reagent No 55) can be added to the preparation to make detection of the cysts easier.

Note: In giardiasis, the number of trophozoites or cysts present in faecal specimens cannot be taken as an indication of the severity of infection.

Duodenal aspirates: Occasionally giardiasis can be diagnosed by detecting *G. lamblia* trophozoites in duodenal contents, but this should only be considered when giardiasis is clinically suspected and no parasites are detected after examining several faecal specimens. The use of *Enterotest* (string test) is not recommended for the collection of duodenal specimens because of the very high cost of the test.

Trophozoite of G. lamblia

- Small pear-shaped flagellate with a rapid tumbling and spinning motility, often likened to a falling leaf.

- Measures 12–15 × 5–9 μm (see Plate 5.2 to compare size of G. lamblia with other intestinal protozoa).

- Has a large concave sucking disc on the ventral surface (attaches trophozoite to the intestinal mucosa).

- It has four pairs of flagella, two axonemes, and two nuclei which stain well (Giemsa or Field's technique).

- A single or two curved median bodies are present (function unknown).

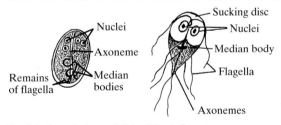

Fig. 5.5 Morphology of *G.lamblia*. *Left*: cyst. *Right*: trophozoite.

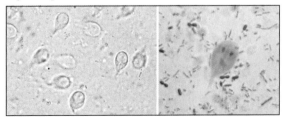

Plate 5.6 *Left*: *G.lamblia* trophozoites in saline preparation, *Right*: Field's stained *G.lamblia* trophozoite as seen with 100× objective. See also Plate 5.2 on p. 197.

Cyst of G. lamblia

- Small and oval measuring 8–12 × about 6 μm.

- Internal structures include four nuclei grouped at one end (sometimes difficult to see), axonemes, median bodies, and remains of flagella. These structures can be seen in unstained preparations but are more clearly defined in an iodine preparation.

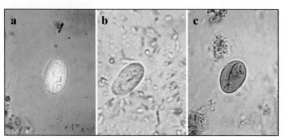

Plate 5.7   Cysts of *G.lamblia* **a** In eosin preparation, **b** In saline preparation, **c** In iodine preparation. See also Plate 5.2.

Differentiation of G. lamblia from non-pathogenic flagellates that can be found in faeces

Intestinal non-pathogenic flagellates that require differentiation from *G. lamblia* include:

- *Chilomastix mesnili*

- *Pentatrichomonas hominis* (formerly *Trichomonas hominis*)

- *Enteromonas hominis*

- *Retortamonas intestinalis*

Trophozoites of the above mentioned flagellates can be easily differentiated from *G. lamblia* by their shape and movement (in a fresh specimen) and because they have only one nucleus (and fewer flagella).

The only other small protozoan trophozoite that has two nuclei is the flagellate, *Dientamoeba fragilis* but this organism, although related to the genus *Trichomonas*, has no flagella or median bodies and looks like a small (9–15 μm) amoeba (it was formerly grouped with the amoebae). Cysts are produced by *C. mesnili*, *E. hominis*, and *R. intestinalis*. They can be easily differentiated from those of *G. lamblia* because they are smaller (under 8 μm) and do not have the same characteristic appearance of *G. lamblia* (do not contain remains of flagella). The cysts of *E. hominis* are oval in shape and have four nuclei (but not grouped to one end). *C. mesnili* cysts

are lemon-shaped. The cysts of *R. intestinalis* are pear-shaped.

Diagnosis of giardiasis using an antigen test
Several tests are commercially available for detecting *Giardia* specific antigen in faecal specimens using a monoclonal antibody reagent. The antigen is stable and can be detected in fresh faeces (not those treated with PVA or MIF fixatives). The presence of antigen indicates active infection. It is produced as *G. lamblia* multiplies in the intestine.

Giardia-Strip is a rapid, simple to perform immunochromatographic strip test developed by Coris BioConcept to detect the membrane antigens of *G. lamblia* cysts in unconcentrated fresh faeces. The test takes 15 minutes to perform. Positive results are indicated by clearly visible pink-red lines. *Giardia-Strip* is both a chronic and acute-phase screening test. It has been correlated with enzyme immunoassay and microscopy methods, giving an accuracy of 92.9%, sensitivity of 91.6%, and specificity of 93.5%. The strips require storage at between 4–37 °C in a dry environment. Each kit contains 25 strips and buffer solution to dilute the faeces. Once opened the strips have a shelf-life of 15 weeks. Details of distributors and prices can be obtained from Coris BioConcept (see Appendix 11). Information on the principle of the test, method, and performance characteristics can be found on the company's website www.corisbio.com.

---

3   *Balantidium coli*

B. coli is an uncommon parasite of humans. It commonly infects pigs and has a worldwide distribution. Human infections have been reported mainly from Central and South America, Papua New Guinea, the Philippines and other tropical areas among those who keep pigs and use pig faeces as fertilizer.

   B. coli is transmitted by the ingestion of infective cysts in food or water or from hands contaminated with pig faeces. *B. coli* has a direct life cycle similar to that of *E. histolytica* and *G. lamblia* except a pig, not a human is the natural host. *B. coli* causes balantidial dysentery. It is the only ciliate that can parasitize humans.

Balantidial dysentery
Infection with *B. coli* can be asymptomatic. Balantidial dysentery occurs when the ciliates invade the wall of the large intestine, causing inflammation and ulceration with blood and mucus being passed in the faeces. Intestinal perforation is a serious complication of balantidiasis.

Prevention and control of balantidiasis
In pig rearing areas, infection with *B. coli* can be avoided by not eating food which is likely to be contaminated with pig faeces, protecting water supplies from faecal contamination, and improving personal hygiene.

   B. coli cysts are infective as soon as they are excreted in the faeces. They are rapidly killed by drying but in moist conditions they can remain infective for several weeks.

LABORATORY DIAGNOSIS

Balantidial dysentery is diagnosed by finding the motile trophozoites of *B. coli* in a *fresh* dysenteric faecal specimen, examined in the same way as described for amoebic dysentery. In chronic infections, *B. coli* cysts can be found in formed or semi-formed faeces.

Trophozoite of B. coli

- Large, easily seen oval shaped ciliate with a rapid revolving motility, measuring 50–200 × 40-70 μm.
- With careful focusing, the beating cilia can be seen particularly in the region of the funnel-shaped cytostome.
- Often contains ingested red cells.
- A large macronucleus may be seen. A very small micronucleus lies close to the macronucleus but this can only be seen in stained preparations.
- One of two contractile vacuoles may be visible.

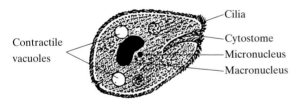

Fig. 5.6   Morphology of *B.coli* trophozoite.

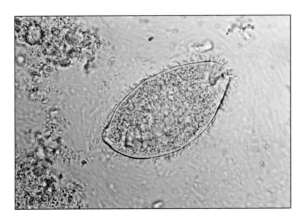

Plate 5.8   *B.coli* trophozoite in saline preparation.

Cyst of B. coli

- Large, round, thick walled, measuring 50–60 μm in diameter.
- Cilia (inside wall) can sometimes be seen in younger cysts.
- Macronucleus stains well with iodine.

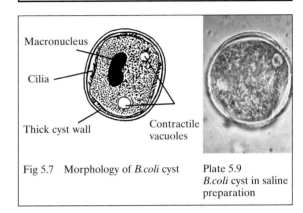

Fig 5.7   Morphology of *B.coli* cyst   Plate 5.9
                                               B.coli cyst in saline
                                               preparation

4   Human intestinal coccidia:
Isospora belli, Cryptosporidium parvum, Cyclospora cayetanensis

I. belli, C. parvum and *C. cayetanensis* are thought to have a worldwide distribution. *C. parvum* is particularly prevalent in tropical countries.

Other *Cryptosporidium* species: Increasingly, other *Cryptosporidium* species are being reported as causing human infections, including *C. hominis* (formerly *C. parvum* genotype 1) which is morphologically indistinguishable from *C. parvum*, and of lesser importance, *C. meleagridis, C. canis,* and *C. felis*.

I. belli, Cryptosporium, and *C. cayetanensis* are transmitted by the faecal-oral route with infective oocysts being ingested. The oocysts of *I. belli* and *C. cayetanensis* are not infective when passed in faeces. They require several days in the environment in which to mature. The oocysts of *Cryptosporidium* are infective when excreted in the faeces.
Water-borne outbreaks of *C. parvum* and *C. cayetanensis* have been reported from tropical countries and elsewhere. *Cryptosporidium* oocysts are particularly resistant to disinfectants, including chlorine at concentrations normally used to treat drinking water supplies. *Cryptosporidium* infection rates are higher in the warm wet season, and lower in the drier cool months.

The life cycle of *I. belli*, *Cryptosporidium* and *C. cayetanensis* is typical of sporozoa, i.e. there is an asexual reproductive stage (schizogony) and a sexual development cycle (sporogony), as summarized in Fig. 5.8. They complete their life cycle in a single host. *C. parvum* infects a wide range of domestic animals and wildlife.

I. belli, *C. parvum* (*C. hominis* and other species) and *C. cayetanensis* are being increasingly reported as causes of enteritis and as opportunistic pathogens in immunocompromised persons.

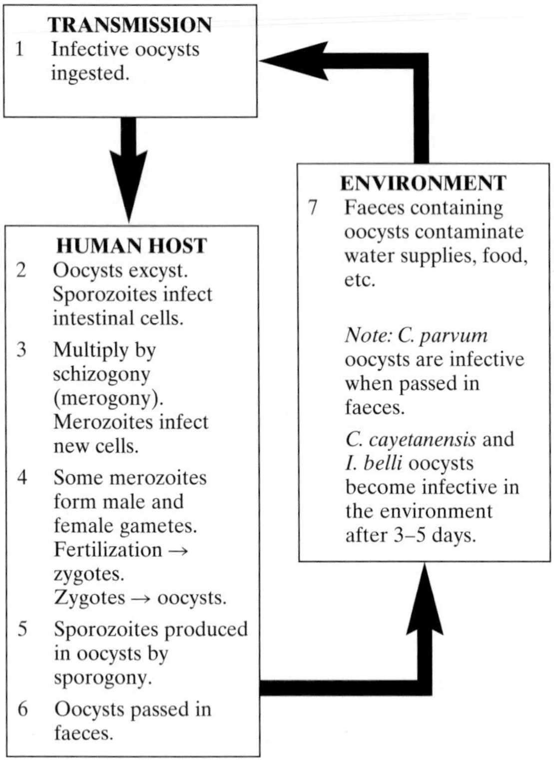

```
┌─────────────────────────────┐
│  TRANSMISSION               │
│  1  Infective oocysts       │
│     ingested.               │
└─────────────────────────────┘

┌─────────────────────────────┐      ┌──────────────────────────┐
│  HUMAN HOST                 │      │  ENVIRONMENT             │
│  2  Oocysts excyst.         │      │  7  Faeces containing    │
│     Sporozoites infect      │      │     oocysts contaminate  │
│     intestinal cells.       │      │     water supplies, food,│
│                             │      │     etc.                 │
│  3  Multiply by             │      │                          │
│     schizogony              │      │  Note: C. parvum         │
│     (merogony).             │      │  oocysts are infective   │
│     Merozoites infect       │      │  when passed in          │
│     new cells.              │      │  faeces.                 │
│                             │      │                          │
│  4  Some merozoites         │      │  C. cayetanensis and     │
│     form male and           │      │  I. belli oocysts        │
│     female gametes.         │      │  become infective in     │
│     Fertilization →         │      │  the environment         │
│     zygotes.                │      │  after 3–5 days.         │
│     Zygotes → oocysts.      │      └──────────────────────────┘
│                             │
│  5  Sporozoites produced    │
│     in oocysts by           │
│     sporogony.              │
│                             │
│  6  Oocysts passed in       │
│     faeces.                 │
└─────────────────────────────┘
```

Fig 5.8 Transmission and life cycle of intestinal coccidia: *Cryptosprodium parvum*, *Isospora belli*, and *Cyclospora cayetanensis*.

Intestinal coccidiosis
I. belli infection is rarely serious and can be asymptomatic but severe diarrhoeal disease can occur in AIDS patients.

C. parvum is widely spread in the environment. It has been reported as an important cause of diarrhoeal disease in young children and toddlers in developing countries. In persons with depressed immune responses, particularly those with AIDS, infection with *Cryptosporidium* can cause acute and often fatal diarrhoeal disease and also respiratory disease. Autoinfection can occur with infective oocysts sporulating in the intestine. Disseminated disease may occur. Person to person transmission is common and animal hosts are also important sources of human infections.

C. caytanenis has been described as a cause of prolonged diarrhoea in tropical countries and elsewhere. It can cause severe prolonged diarrhoea in those infected with HIV.

LABORATORY DIAGNOSIS

Diarrhoeal disease caused by *I. belli*, *C. parvum* and *C. cayetanenis* is diagnosed by finding oocysts in faecal specimens. Specimens are usually watery and often have an offensive smell. Pus cells are not found.

I. belli

Oocysts of *I. belli* can usually be identified in direct wet preparations, prepared and examined as described in subunit 5.3. If required the oocysts can be concentrated by the formol ether oocyst concentration technique (see subunit 5.3). The oocysts can be easily missed if the illumination of the microscope is too bright.

Cryptosporidium and *C. cayetanensis*

Oocysts of *Cryptosporidium* and *C. cayetanensis* can be detected in wet preparations but they are more easily identified in smears stained by the modified Ziehl-Neelsen (Zn) method following concentration by the formol ether oocyst concentration technique as described at the end of subunit 5.3.

Modified Ziehl-Neelsen (Zn) method for *Cryptosporidium* and *C. cayetanensis*

Reagents
– Carbol fuchsin stain*   No. 17
– Malachite green stain*   No. 41

　*Same as used in the Zn technique for staining AFB in sputum

– Acid alcohol 1% v/v

　This can be made by diluting 3% acid alcohol (Reagent No. 3) as used in the Zn technique for staining AFB, i.e. add 30 ml of the 3% acid alcohol to 60 ml of distilled or deionized water and mix.

1　Prepare a smear from the sediment obtained by the formol ether oocyst concentration technique (see end of subunit 5.3). Air-dry the smear. Fix the smear with methanol for 2–3 minutes.

2　Stain with *unheated* carbol fuchsin for 15 minutes. Wash off the stain with water.

3 Decolorize with 1% acid alcohol for 10–15 seconds. Wash off with water.

4 Counterstain with 0.5% malachite green (or methylene blue) for 30 seconds. Wash off with water and stand the slide in a draining rack for the smear to dry.

5 Examine the smear microscopically for oocysts, using a low power magnification to detect the oocysts and the oil immersion objective to identify them.

Oocysts of Isospora belli

In unstained wet preparation:

● Oval, measuring 20–33 × 10–19 μm.

● Usually contains a granular zygote as shown in Plate 5.10 (right).

● Occasionally more mature sporulated oocysts can be found (particularly if the specimen is not fresh), containing two sporocysts (each with four sporozoites) as shown in Plate 5.10 (left).

Note: Iodine does not stain oocysts. In a modified Zn stained smear, there is an overall red-pink staining of the oocysts.

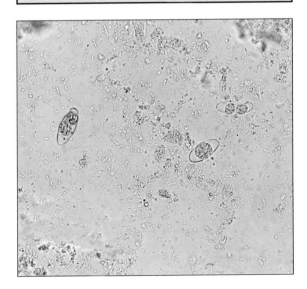

Plate 5.10   *I.belli* oocysts in saline preparation. *Right*: Oocyst containing granular zygote. *Left*: Oocyst containing two sporocysts.

Oocysts of Cryptosporidium

In unstained direct wet faecal preparations the small oocysts of *Cryptosporidium* are difficult to differentiate from yeasts and other small spherical structures found in faeces. Examination of a modified Zn stained smear is required, or if there are facilities for fluorescence microscopy, an auramine phenol staining technique can be used to demonstrate *Cryposporidum* oocysts.

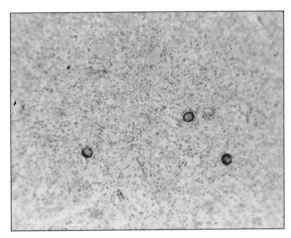

Plate 5.11   Pink-red stained *Cryptosporidium* oocysts in modified Ziehl-Neelsen stained faecal smear.

Oocysts of Cryptosporidium

In modified Zn stained smear:

● Small, round to oval, pink red stained bodies measuring 4–6 μm, as shown in Plate 5.11.

   Note: Older oocysts stain palely.

● Some oocysts may contain a single deeply stained red dot.

Note: Yeasts and faecal debris often stain pale red but these structures can usually be distinguished from cryptosporidia. Some bacterial spores are also acid fast but most of these are too small to cause confusion.

***Crypto-strip* test to detect *Cryptosporidium parvum* oocysts**
Crypto-strip is a rapid, simple to perform immunochromatographic strip test developed by Coris BioConcept to detect the membrane antigens of *C. parvum* oocysts in fresh diluted faeces. The test takes 10 minutes to perform. It is a highly specific acute phase screening test, capable of detecting 50–100 oocysts in 100 μl of faeces. Each kit contains 25 strips and buffer solution used to dilute the faeces. The strips require storage between 4–37 °C in a dry environment. Once opened, the strips have a shelf-life of 15 weeks. Details of local distributors and prices can be obtained from Coris BioConcept (see Appendix 11). Information on the principle and performance of the test can be found on the company's website www.corisbio.com.

Oocysts of Cyclospora cayetanensis
In unstained direct wet preparations, *C. cayetanensis* oocysts appear as spherical bodies with a central refractile morula-like structure (often with a greenish tinge) as shown in Plate 5.12 (right).

Oocysts of *C. cayetanensis*
In modified Zn stained smear:

- Round, irregularly stained bodies, measuring 8–10 μm in diameter (larger than *Cryptosporidium*).
- Oocysts often contain red staining granules.
- Some oocysts may appear as unstained glassy wrinkled spheres.

Note: C. cayetanensis does not stain with iodine. The oocyst wall auto-fluoresces blue when exposed to ultra violet light at wavelength 365 nm.

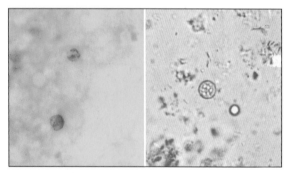

Plate 5.12   *Left*: *Cyclospora* oocysts in Ziehl-Neelsen stained faecal smear. *Right*: *Cyclospora* oocysts in unstained preparation showing morula-like centre.

Microsporidia
Microsporidia are small, obligate intracellular protozoan parasites. In host cells the parasites develop and multiply (merogony), producing large numbers of infective spores (sporogony). Microsporidia infect a wide range of vertebrates, and invertebrates. Microsporidia are being increasingly reported as pathogens in patients with late HIV disease.

Microsporidia in AIDS patients
Microsporidia species most frequently reported in association with AIDS are *Enterocytozoon bieneusi*, *Encephalitozoon intestinalis* and *Encephalitozoon hellem*. Intestinal microsporidiosis is the commonest infection, caused mainly by *E. bieneusi*. It produces persistent diarrhoea with wasting. *E. intestinalis* infects the intestine, gall bladder, liver, kidney. *E. hellem* is associated with infection of the cornea and conjunctiva, causing kerato-conjunctivitis. Other species have been reported as causing disseminated infections. Infection is probably by spores being ingested, inhaled, or inoculated (eye). The spores are highly resistant in the environment.

LABORATORY DIAGNOSIS

Several staining techniques have been developed to detect the spores of microsporidia in faeces, including a modified trichrome technique (for laboratories able to obtain the required reagents) and a modified Fields technique which uses reagents more likely to be available in district laboratories.

Modified Fields technique for staining microsporida spores in faeces[6]
The examination of fresh formalin treated faeces is recommended*

*Formalin inhibits the growth of fungal spores (which may be mistaken for microsporidia spores) and also makes the sample microbiologically safe.

It is *essential* to include a positive control smear.

Method

1   Mix 1 volume of unformed or fluid faeces with 3 volumes of 10% formalin solution (Reagent No 29).

2   Place 2 drops (about 20μl) of the faeces-formalin suspension on a slide and make a smear using a wooden applicator stick. Allow to air-dry. Fix the smear with absolute methanol for 2 minutes and allow to air-dry.

3   Cover the patient's smear and positive control smear with 0.5ml diluted Fields stain B*.

* Mix 1ml Fields stain B (Reagent No 26) with 4 ml pH 7.2 buffered saline (Reagent No 49).

4   *Immediately* add an equal volume of Fields stain A (Reagent No 25) and mix with the diluted Fields stain B. Leave to stain for 3 minutes at room temperature.

5   Gently wash off the stain with clean tap water.

6   Counterstain with 0.25% malachite green * for 2 minutes. Rinse off the stain with clean tap water and allow the smears to air-dry.

* Dissolve 0.5 g malachite green in 200 ml distilled or deionised water.

7   Examine the smears microscopically using the 100× oil immersion objective.

Results: Microsporidia spores are oval in shape and stain grey-blue often with an unstained central or polar area. The spores are *very small* (some just larger than bacteria)* and may be seen in clumps.

* Spores of microsporida reported to infect humans measure from 1.0–1.6 × 0.9 μm to 4.0–4.5 × 2.0–2.5μm.

5.5 Identification of helminth eggs and larvae found in faeces

This subunit describes the following helminths that can be found in faeces:

Nematodes: 1 *Ascaris lumbricoides*
(Round worms) 2 *Trichuris trichiura*
             3 Hookworms:
                Ancylostoma duodenale
                Necator americanus
             4 *Strongyloides stercoralis*

Briefly described: *Trichostrongylus* species, *Ternidens diminutus*, *Oesophagostum* species, *Capillaria philippinensis*, *Strongyloides füelleborni*

Trematodes: 5 *Schistosoma* species:
(Flukes)   *S. mansoni, S. intercalatum,*
                S. japonicum, S. mekongi
             6 *Opisthorchis* (*Clonorchis*) *sinensis*
             7 *Opisthorchis viverrini*
             8 *Fasciola* species:
                F. hepatica, F. gigantica
             9 *Fasciolopsis buski*

Briefly described: *Heterophyes heterophyes, Metagonimus yokagawai, Opisthorchis felineus, Dicrocoelium dentriticum, Gastrodiscoides hominis, Echinostoma* species

Cestodes: 10 *Taenia* species:
(Tapeworms)   *T. solium, T. saginata*
            11 *Diphyllobothrium latum*
            12 *Vampirolepis nana*

Briefly described: *Hymenolepis diminuta, Dipylidium caninum*

Recovered from perianal specimens:

            13 *Enterobius vermicularis*

1   *Ascaris lumbricoides**

* Also known as the large intestinal roundworm.

A. lumbricoides has a worldwide distribution. It is particularly common in the tropics and subtropics in places where environmental sanitation is inadequate and untreated human faeces are used as fertilizer (night-soil). In 2002, WHO estimated that there were 1450 million persons infected with *A. lumbricoides* and annually 60 000 dying from ascariasis.[7]

A. lumbricoides is spread by faecal pollution of the environment. A person becomes infected by ingesting infective eggs in contaminated food or from hands that have become faecally contaminated.

The mature worms live free in the intestine. Fertilized female worms produce many eggs per day. The eggs can remain viable in soil and dust for several years. These factors contribute to the widespread and often heavy *Ascaris* infections which can be found especially among children of 3–8 years whose fingers become contaminated while playing on open ground. The worms can live 1–2 years in their host.

The direct life cycle of *A. lumbricoides* is summarized in Fig. 5.9. Eggs passed in the faeces are non-embryonated. They require about 30–40 days in the environment (or less in higher temperatures) in which to mature to the infective stage. The larva does not hatch until the egg is ingested.

A. lumbricoides causes ascariasis (roundworm infection). In young children, heavy infections cause or contribute significantly to malnutrition.

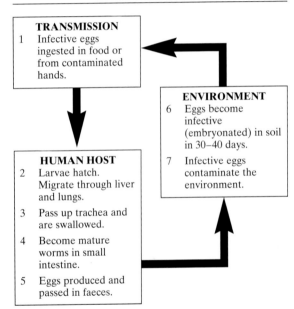

Fig 5.9   Transmission and life cycle of *Ascaris lumbricoides*.

Ascariasis
During their migration, *Ascaris* larvae can cause inflamma-tory and hypersensitive reactions including pneumonia-like symptoms, attacks of coughing, and bronchial asthma. Eosinophilia is common and there is often urticaria. Signs of toxaemia may develop and very occasionally neurological disorders.

Developing and mature worms in the intestine frequently cause abdominal pain, nausea, diarrhoea and vomiting. Intestinal muscle may become damaged and absorption impaired. *A. lumbricoides* infection in children is known to affect gastrointestinal function. Protein digestion or absorption is impaired, the absorption of fat decreases, and lactase activity in the small intestine is reduced. Infected children are often vitamin-A deficient and have low serum albumin levels. Frequent exposure to infection may result in impairment of physical and intellectual development. *Ascaris* worms are large and in heavy infections, especially in children, worm masses can cause obstruction or perforation of the intestine and occasionally obstruction of the bile duct and pancreatic duct. Other complications include liver abscesses and appendicitis caused by migrating worms. Worms can pass though the anus or be vomited.

Measures to prevent and control ascariasis

- Preventing soil becoming faecally polluted by:
  - Using latrines and avoiding the use of untreated human faeces as fertilizer.
  - Treating infected individuals as part of a control programme, especially children.
- Preventing infection by:
  - Washing hands before eating.
  - Avoiding eating uncooked vegetables, green salads and fruits which may be contaminated with faeces containing *Ascaris* eggs.

LABORATORY DIAGNOSIS

■ Finding *A. lumbricoides* eggs in faeces. Concentration techniques are rarely required. The method of preparing and examining specimens is described in subunit 5.3.

■ Identifying *A. lumbricoides* worms expelled through the anus or mouth.

A. lumbricoides worms

Freshly expelled *Ascaris* worms are pinkish in colour with an appearance similar to earthworms. They measure 12–35 cm in length and taper at both ends. The tail of the male is curved and has small rod-like projections (spicules). There is a small mouth surrounded by three lips.

Caution: Always use forceps to handle *Ascaris* worms because they can cause asthma and other allergic reactions. If storing *Ascaris* eggs in formol saline, e.g. for teaching purposes, first treat the faecal deposit with hot (70–80 °C) formol saline. This will prevent the eggs from developing to an infective stage.

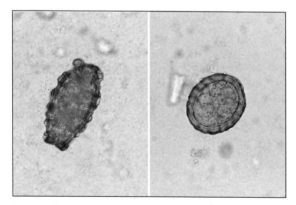

Plate 5.13 *Left*: Infertile egg of *A.lumbricoides*. *Right*: Fertile egg of *A.lumbricoides*. See also Plates 5.1 and 5.2.

Eggs of A. lumbricoides

Usually fertilized eggs are found in faeces but occasionally infertile eggs are produced by unfertilized female worms.

FERTILIZED EGG

- Yellow-brown, oval or round, measuring 50–70 μm long by 30–50 μm wide.
- Shell is often covered by an uneven albuminous coat (mammilated).
- Contains a central granular mass which is the unsegmented fertilized ovum.

Decorticated egg: This term is used to describe an egg that has no albuminous coat. A decorticated egg has a smooth shell and appears pale yellow or colourless.

INFERTILE EGG

- It is darker in colour and has a thinner wall and more granular albuminous covering.
- More elongated than a fertilized egg, measuring about 90×45 μm.
- Contains a central mass of large granules.

---

2   *Trichuris trichiura**
* Also known as whipworm.

T. trichiura is found worldwide but is more common in moist warm climates in areas where faecal contamination of the environment occurs. It is rarely found in arid areas and at high altitudes. WHO estimates (2002) that globally there are 1050 million persons infected with *T. trichiura*.[7]

Infection is by ingesting infective eggs in contaminated food or from contaminated fingers. Children are more often infected than adults, due to playing on faecally contaminated ground. The direct life cycle of *T. trichiura* is summarized in Fig. 5.10. Many eggs are produced. They remain infective for several months in moist warm soil but they are unable to withstand drying.

T. trichiura causes trichuriasis (whipworm infection). Symptomatic infections are mainly in children.

Trichuriasis

Light infections produce few symptoms. In young children, severe infections can cause chronic diarrhoea, intestinal ulceration with blood and mucus being passed in the faeces, iron deficiency anaemia, failure to develop at the normal rate, weight loss, and prolapse of the rectum. Massive infections can be fatal. Eosinophilia is common. Severe trichuriasis is thought to increase the risk of disease with *Entamoeba histolytica* and pathogenic enterobacteria such as *Shigella* species. Migrating worms occasionally cause appendicitis.

Measures to prevent and control trichuriasis are the same as those described for *A. lumbricoides* (see subunit 5.5.2).

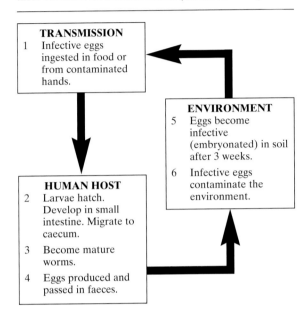

TRANSMISSION
1 Infective eggs ingested in food or from contaminated hands.

ENVIRONMENT
5 Eggs become infective (embryonated) in soil after 3 weeks.
6 Infective eggs contaminate the environment.

HUMAN HOST
2 Larvae hatch. Develop in small intestine. Migrate to caecum.
3 Become mature worms.
4 Eggs produced and passed in faeces.

Fig 5.10   Transmission and life cycle of *Trichuris trichiura*.

LABORATORY DIAGNOSIS

The laboratory diagnosis of *T. trichiura* infection is by finding *T. trichiura* eggs in faeces. Concentration techniques are rarely required to detect significant infections. The method of preparing and examining specimens is described in subunit 5.3.

Note: Heavy infections can be diagnosed clinically by examining the rectum for worms using a proctoscope.

Egg of *T. trichiura*
- It is yellow-brown and measures about 50 × 25 μm.
- Has a characteristic barrel shape with a colourless protruding mucoid plug at each end.
- Contains a central granular mass which is the unsegmented ovum.

Capillaria philippinensis
C. philippinensis is a very small whipworm which is normally parasitic in fish-eating birds but can infect

humans causing capillariasis. As its name suggests it is found in the Philippine Islands where it is fairly widely distributed in northern Luzon. It is also found in Thailand.

C. philippinensis is transmitted by the ingestion of infective embryonated eggs in raw, undercooked, or pickled fish. The larvae develop into mature worms in the small intestine. Immature eggs are passed in the faeces. Occasionally infective larvae develop in the intestine and cause autoinfection.

Laboratory diagnosis
This is by finding the eggs in faeces. They can be few and therefore if infection is suspected and the eggs are not found in direct preparations, a concentration technique should be used, such as the formol ether concentration method described in subunit 5.3.

Egg of *C. philippinensis*
Features used to identify the egg and differentiate it from *T. trichiura* are as follows:
- Smaller than *T. trichiura*, measuring about 45 × 21 μm.
- It is yellow-brown but less elliptical in shape than *T. trichiura*.
- The plugs (one at each end of the egg) are smaller and do not protrude like those of *T. trichiura*.

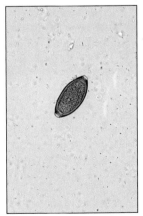
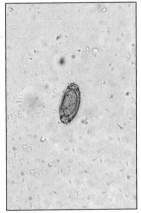

Plate 5.14 Egg of *T.trichiura*. See also Plates 5.1 and 5.2.
Plate 5.15 Egg of *C.philippinensis*.

Capillariasis
Early and mild infections cause abdominal pain, intestinal 'gurgling', and chronic watery diarrhoea. Heavy infections can lead to muscle wasting and oedema caused by loss of protein and severe malabsorption of fats and sugars. Plasma potassium, sodium, and calcium are reduced.

3   Hookworms

Hookworm infection is caused by:

– *Necator americanus*
– *Ancylostoma duodenale*

Hookworms are widespread in the tropics and sub-tropics. In 2002, WHO estimated that there were 1300 million persons infected with hookworms and 65 000 deaths annually from hookworm disease.[7]

N. americanus is more commonly found in the Far East, South Asia, Pacific Islands, tropical Africa, Central and South America.

A. duodenale is found in the Middle East, in countries around the Mediterranean, north China and north India, but it can also be found with *N. americanus* in west Africa, South-East Asia, the Pacific Islands and South America.

Hookworm infection is spread by faecal pollution of the soil. Infection occurs when infective filariform larvae penetrate the skin, especially when a person is walking barefoot on infected ground. *A. duodenale* can also be transmitted by ingesting infective larvae.

The direct life cycle of hookworms is summarized in Fig. 5.11. *A. duodenale* larvae can delay their development into adult worms for several months until conditions favour transmission. The mature worms live in the small intestine (1–10 years). They become attached to the wall of the small intestine by sucking part of the mucosa into their mouth-parts. The mouth of *A. duodenale* is large and has teeth-like structures whereas that of *N. americanus* has cutting plates. Hookworms suck blood from their host but much of the blood passes through the worm undigested. Some of the iron in the undigested red cells is reabsorbed by the host.

The worms, particularly *A. duodenale*, move around in the intestine in search of new sites from which to suck blood. The abandoned sites continue to bleed for some time. About twice as many eggs are produced by *A. duodenale* than from *N. americanus*. Eggs are normally excreted in the faeces 4–7 weeks after infection.

The first stage larva that hatches from the egg is called a rhabditiform larva. It feeds, and in warm well-oxygenated soil, develops into the infective filariform larva. The infective non-feeding larvae can remain viable in damp warm soil for up to 2 years.

Hookworm infection and hookworm anaemia
The first sign of hookworm infection is frequently a skin reaction at the site of larval penetration. This is known as 'ground itch' and is usually more intense in those previously infected. During migration of the larvae, mild respiratory symptoms may develop and also an eosinophilia.

Adult hookworms cause chronic blood loss. It has been estimated that a single *A. duodenale* worm ingests about 150 μl (0.15 ml) of blood per day and a *N. americanus* worm about 30 μl (0.03 ml). The test for occult blood in faeces is positive.

Iron deficiency anaemia: This usually develops with heavy prolonged infection, especially with *A. duodenale*. It may be severe and even fatal especially in those with inadequate iron stores and a low iron intake. Infected pregnant women are also at risk of becoming anaemic due to their increased need for iron. Loss of protein can lead to oedema.

Measures to prevent and control hookworm infection

● Preventing soil from becoming infected by improving environmental sanitation, particularly by the use of latrines and health education.

● Preventing infective larvae penetrating the feet by wearing adequate protective footware. Open sandals are not effective barriers to infection.

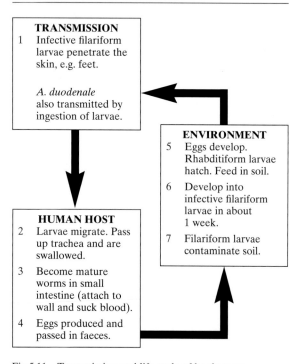

Fig 5.11   Transmission and life cycle of hookworms: *Ancylostoma duodenale* and *Nectar americanus*.

LABORATORY DIAGNOSIS

The laboratory diagnosis of hookworm infection is by finding hookworm eggs in faeces. Morphologically, the eggs of *A. duodenale* and *N. americanus* cannot be differentiated. The direct examination of faeces as described in subunit 5.3 is usually adequate to detect the eggs. If required the eggs can be concentrated by the formol ether concentration technique or the saturated salt floatation technique (see subunit 5.3).

Note: Hookworm infection is usually accompanied by a blood eosinophilia.

Egg of hookworm (N. americanus or A. duodenale)

In faecal specimens less than 12 hours old, a hookworm egg has the following appearance:

- It is colourless with a thin shell which appears microscopically as a black line around the ovum.
- Oval in shape, measuring about 65×40 μm.
- Contains an ovum which appears segmented (usually 4–8 cell stage).

Note: If the specimen is more than 12 hours old, a larva may be seen inside the egg. If the faeces is more than 24 hours old, the larva may hatch and must then be differentiated from a *Strongyloides* larva (see subunit 5.5.4).

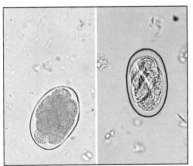
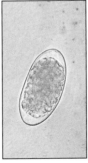
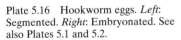

Plate 5.16   Hookworm eggs. *Left:* Segmented. *Right:* Embryonated. See also Plates 5.1 and 5.2.

Plate 5.17   Egg of *Trichostrongylus.*

Eggs that can be mistaken for hookworm eggs

Hookworm eggs need to be distinguished from the eggs of *Trichostrongylus* species, *Ternidens deminutus*, *Oesophagostum* species, and *Strongyloides füelleborni* (nematodes normally parasitic in animals which can infect humans). A brief description of these parasites can be found after the egg descriptions except *S. füelleborni* which is described after *Strongyloides stercoralis* (see 5.5.4).

Egg of Trichostrongylus

Compared with a hookworm egg, the egg of *Trichostrongylus* is:

- Longer and thinner than a hookworm egg, measuring 85–115 μm in length.
- More pointed at one or both ends as shown in Plate 5.17.
- Usually appears more segmented.

Egg of Ternidens deminutus

The egg of *Ternidens deminutus* has a similar structure to a hookworm egg but is much larger, measuring about 85 μm in length and contains more cells.

Egg of S. füelleborni

It often contains a larva. When at the non-embryonated segmented stage, it closely resembles a hookworm egg except that it is smaller, measuring about 50×35 μm (see end of 5.5.4).

Egg of Oesophagostum species

It is about the same size as that of a hookworm but is passed in the faeces in an advanced stage of development.

Trichostrongylus species

Trichostrongylus nematodes, occasionally referred to as pseudo-hookworms, are mainly parasites of ruminants, equines, and rodents but several species can infect humans.

Infections have been reported from parts of Africa, Egypt, Indonesia, Iran, Iraq, South-East Asia, India, Japan, and Chile.

A person becomes infected by ingesting third stage larvae in contaminated food or drink. The adult worms live in the small intestine with the head penetrating the mucosal wall. The head is without cutting teeth or plates. Eggs are produced which are passed in the faeces. They require differentiation from hookworm eggs (see previous text).

Like hookworms, *Trichostrongylus* worms also suck blood from their host. The clinical features of trichostrongyliasis, however, are less severe than those of hookworm infection and treatment is different.

Ternidens deminutus

T. deminutus is a nematode which resembles a hookworm. It is normally parasitic in monkeys and baboons but can infect humans, where infections have been reported mostly from South Africa and East Africa.

Transmission is probably by ingestion of third stage larvae. The worms are found in the large intestine. Like hookworms, *T. deminutus* worms also suck blood from their host and anaemia may develop in heavy infections. *T. deminutus* eggs can be found in faeces and require differentiation from hookworm eggs (see previous text).

Oesophagostum species

Human infections with *Oesophagostum* species have a high prevalence in West and East Africa. An infection rate of 30% has been reported from Togo and Ghana. Eggs resembling those of hookworm (see previous text) are passed in the faeces. In the soil the eggs hatch and the larvae develop into infective stages.

Infection is by the ingestion of infective larvae. The larvae develop in the large intestine where they form nodules and abscesses. When mature the worms leave the nodules and become attached to the intestinal wall.

4   *Strongyloides stercoralis**

* Also known as the dwarf threadworm.

S. stercoralis has a world-wide distribution. It is endemic in many tropical and subtropical countries including those of Africa, Asia and South America, particularly in humid areas.

Infection with *S. stercoralis* can occur:

– By infective filariform larvae penetrating the skin.

– By autoinfection (self-infection) with rhabditiform (first stage) larvae developing into infective filariform larvae in the intestine or on perianal skin followed by penetration of the intestinal wall or perianal skin. Autoinfection enables untreated infections to persist for many years.

The direct life cycle of *S. stercoralis* is summarized in Fig. 5.12. Unlike other soil-transmitted helminths, *S. stercoralis* can reproduce in the soil (warm moist conditions). Adult worms which live in the small intestine are females and eggs are produced parthenogenetically from which rhabditiform larvae hatch. Larvae, not eggs are therefore excreted in the faeces. In the soil the larvae develop within a week into free-living male and female worms. The females produce a further generation of rhabditiform larvae. These develop into infective filariform larvae. The free-living cycle in the soil can be repeated several times. The infected filariform larvae require a human host in which to become mature worms.

Strongyloidiasis

When penetrating the skin, *S. stercoralis* larvae can cause an itchy dermatitis and rash. During migration of the larvae, allergic and respiratory symptoms may occur. Most infections are without serious symptoms. Heavy infections (especially common in children) can cause dysentery, malabsorption, steatorrhoea, and dehydration with electrolyte disturbance. Abdominal pain is common and occasionally finger clubbing. There is usually an eosinophilia.

Hyperinfection: Autoinfection with *S. stercoralis* can become overwhelming and sometimes fatal when the body's normal immune responses are reduced, e.g. by drugs, steroids, malnutrition, pregnancy or puerperium, or when other diseases are present which cause immunosuppression. In such infections, larvae can be found in most tissues and serous cavities of the body. Ulcerative enterocolitis can occur with dysentery or rec-

tal bleeding. It is therefore important to check for strongyloidiasis in those at risk of developing disseminated hyperinfection. Little evidence exists for hyperinfection occurring in persons co-infected with HIV.

Prevention and control of *Strongyloides* infection are as described for hookworm infection.

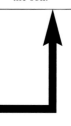

TRANSMISSION
1   Infective filariform larvae penetrate skin, e.g. feet. Autoinfection also occurs.

ENVIRONMENT
6   In soil larvae become free-living worms. Produce more rhabditiform larvae.*
* Free-living cycle can be repeated several times.
7   Become infective filariform larvae in the soil.

HUMAN HOST
2   Larvae migrate. Pass up trachea and are swallowed.
3   Become mature worms in small intestine.
4   Eggs laid. Hatch rhabditiform larvae in intestine.
5   Rhabditiform larvae:
– passed in faeces, or
– become filariform larvae in intestine, causing autoinfection.

Fig 5.12   Transmission and life cycle of *Strongyloides stercoralis.*

LABORATORY DIAGNOSIS

The laboratory diagnosis of *S. stercoralis* infection is by finding motile *S. stercoralis* larvae in fresh faeces. The larvae can also be found in duodenal aspirates, but this method of diagnosis is not usually necessary. In disseminated infections, larvae can be found in most body fluids. Because *S. stercoralis* larvae tend to be excreted intermittently and their numbers can be few, the following technique should be used if infection is suspected and the larvae are not detected by direct examination.

Water emergence technique for detecting *Strongyloides* larvae in faeces

A *fresh* (not more than 2 hours old) formed or semiformed faecal specimen is required. The method is as follows:

1 Using a piece of stick, make a central deep depression in the specimen. Fill the depression with warm water (not over 37 °C).

2 Incubate the specimen in a 35–37 °C incubator or on a warm part of the bench for 1½–3 hours during which time the larvae will migrate out of the faeces into the warm water.

3 Using a plastic bulb pipette or Pasteur pipette, transfer some of the water to a slide and cover with a cover glass. Alternatively, transfer all the water to a conical tube, centrifuge, and transfer the sediment to a slide.

4 Examine the preparation microscopically for motile larvae using the 10× objective with the condenser iris *closed sufficiently* to give good contrast.

Note: S. stercoralis larvae are also well concentrated by the formol ether technique described in subunit 5.3.

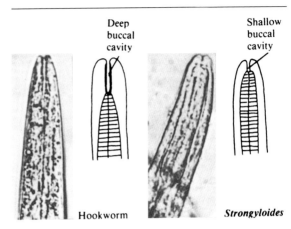

Plate 5.19   *Left*: Deep buccal cavity of hookworm. *Right*: Shallow buccal cavity of *S.stercoralis*.

Strongyloides füelleborni

S. füelleborni is a natural parasite of monkeys and dogs but it can also infect humans. The subspecies *S. füelleborni füelleborni* is found in tropical Africa, and the subspecies *S. füelleborni kellyi* is found in Papua New Guinea. Young children and infants, including babies as young as 2 months old, have been reported as being infected.

In Papua New Guinea, *S. füelleborni* infections are associated with an acute and often fatal infantile disease known as 'swollen belly illness'. Further information can be found in the paper of Ashford *et al.*[8] *S. füelleborni* infection can be diagnosed by finding eggs in fresh faeces. Many eggs may be present and typically appear embryonated. Often the eggs are mistakenly reported as those of hookworm. Other laboratory findings include a very low serum protein level, moderate eosinophilia, and sometimes anaemia.

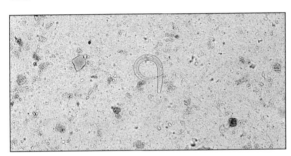

Plate 5.18   Larva of *S.stercoralis* as seen with 10× objective. See also Plates 5.1 and 5.2.

Rhabditiform larvae of S. stercoralis

● It is actively motile.*

  *Following formol ether concentration, the larvae are immobilized.

● It is large, measuring 200–250 μm × 16 μm, and unsheathed.

● Shows a typical rhabditiform large bulbed oesophagus.

● It can be distinguished from a hookworm larva (sometimes seen in faeces more than 24 h old) by its shorter buccal cavity (mouth cavity) as shown in Plate 5.19.

Note: The buccal cavity can be more easily seen by running a drop of Dobell's iodine under the cover glass to immobilize the larva, and using the 40× objective to examine the depth of the buccal cavity.

Egg of S. füelleborni

● It is colourless, oval in shape and measures about 50 × 35 μm, i.e. smaller than hookworm eggs which they can resemble.

● May contain a partially developed larva.

Important: If there is a delay in examining the faeces, the larva will hatch.

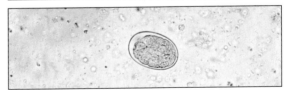

Plate 5.20   Egg of *S.füelleborni*.

5   Intestinal *Schistosoma* species

Eggs of the following species can be found in faeces:

- Widespread species:
  Schistosoma mansoni
  Schistosoma japonicum

- Less widespread species:
  Schistosoma intercalatum
  Schistosoma mekongi and related species,
  S. malayensis

Animal schistosomes may occasionally infect humans.
S. mattheei is the most significant species.

Note: S. *haematobium* causes urinary schistosomiasis.
It is described in subunit 5.6.

Distribution
An estimated 200 million people in 74 countries
have schistosomiasis (includes *S. haematobium* infections) with it is thought 200 000 persons dying
annually from the disease.[9, 10] Infection rates are
highest among children.

S. mansoni is endemic in 52 countries. It is widespread in many African countries, Madagascar, and
parts of the Middle East, South America (especially
Brazil), and the West Indies. *S. mansoni* occurs with
S. haematobium in 41 countries of Africa and the
eastern Mediterranean. Water development projects
for water conservation, irrigation, and hydroelectric
power have contributed to the spread of *S. mansoni*
and changes in its distribution.

S. japonicum is widely distributed in mainland
China, parts of the Philippines, and western
Indonesia.

S. mekongi is found in Lao People's Democratic
Republic, Cambodia and Thailand in the Mekong
River Basin. Prevalence rates are estimated at
15–50% with children (up to 15 y) being more commonly infected. A schistosome similar to *S. mekongi*
called *S. malayensis* (recently recognized) is found in
the foothills and mountainous regions of Malaysia.

S. intercalatum has a high infectivity rate but is
limited in its distribution mainly to West and Central
Africa, i.e. Zaire, Gabon, and Cameroon. Infections
have also been reported from the Republic of Sao
Tome (island off West Africa).

Natural hybrids of *S. haematobium* and *S. intercalatum* occur
in Cameroon.

Transmission and life cycle
Schistosoma species are transmitted by cercariae
penetrating the skin when a person is bathing, washing clothes, fishing, or engaged in agricultural work
or other activity involving contact with water that has
been faecally contaminated and contains the snail
hosts of the parasites. In its snail host the parasite
multiplies and develops to its infective cercarial stage.

Hosts
Humans are the most significant definitive hosts of *S. mansoni*
and *S. intercalatum*. Intermediate hosts of *S. mansoni* are
aquatic snails, (*Biomphalaria* species for *S. mansoni* and
Bulinus species for *S. intercalatum*). They are found on vegetation in ponds, streams, rivers, lakes, dams, irrigation channels and rice paddies. *S. japonicum* infects a wide range of
animals including water-buffaloes, dogs, cats, cattle, pigs,
sheep, goats, and wild rodents. Dogs are important reservoir
hosts in the transmission of *S. mekongi*. The snails that serve
as intermediate hosts for *S. japonicum* (*Oncomelania* species)
and *S. mekongi* (*Neotricula* species) are amphibious (water
and land snails). They live mainly on vegetation along river
banks and in rice paddies. Development and reproduction in
the snail takes 3–5 weeks.

The indirect life cycle of *Schistosoma* species is
summarized in Fig. 5.13. Following infection, the cercariae develop into schistosomula which migrate via
the lungs to the liver. In the portal venous system,
the schistosomula become mature flukes and pair.
The paired flukes migrate to the mesenteric veins
which drain the large intestine. The venules of the
rectum and lower large intestine are the main sites
involved. The female flukes lay eggs in the capillary
venules. Some of the eggs penetrate through into
the lumen of the intestine and are excreted in the
faeces. Other eggs become lodged in the tissues.
Infection to egg-laying normally takes 4–8 weeks. In
their human host, schistosomes live for up to 5
years, sometimes longer.

Intestinal schistosomiasis
S. mansoni, *S. japonicum*, *S. mekongi*, and *S. intercalatum* cause intestinal schistosomiasis. Damage to
the liver and intestinal tract and the complications
arising from chronic infection are caused by a
cellular reaction to the eggs in the tissues. By
acquiring host antigens, the flukes are protected
from host immune reactions.

S. mansoni schistosomiasis
There may be irritation and a skin rash at the site of cercarial
penetration ('swimmer's itch'). The majority of *S. mansoni*
eggs penetrate through the intestinal wall and are excreted in
the faeces sometimes with blood and mucus (estimated egg
output is 100–300 eggs/day). Host reaction to eggs lodged in
the intestinal mucosa leads to the formation of granulomata,
ulceration, and thickening of the bowel wall. Large granulomata cause colonic and rectal polyps.

A proportion of the eggs reach the liver through the portal vein. In the liver, reaction to the eggs may eventually cause thickening of the portal vessels known as claypipe-stem fibrosis. Prolonged heavy infection can lead to a marked enlargement of the liver with fibrosis, portal hypertension, and ascites. The spleen may also become enlarged. Death from haematemesis can occur from ruptured oesophageal varices.

Salmonella infections in patients with *S. mansoni* tend to become chronic and prolonged. Hepatitis B infections have been reported as more common and prolonged in *S. mansoni* infected persons, particularly those with hepatosplenic schistosomiasis.

S. japonicum and S. mekongi schistosomiasis
About 2–60 days after infection a severe immune reaction to the products of young flukes and eggs may occur. It is known as Katayama reaction and takes the form of an acute illness with fever, muscular and abdominal pain, spleen enlargement, urticaria, and eosinophilia. Although this can also occur with other schostosome infections, it is more common with *S. japonicum*.

The clinical features and pathology of *S. japonicum* infection are similar to, but often more severe, than those of *S. mansoni* infection. The egg output of *S. japonicum* is higher (about 500–3 500 eggs/day). Enlargement of the liver and spleen is common in all age groups. Cerebral schistosomiasis and the depositing of eggs in other parts of the body also occur more frequently with *S. japonicum* infections.

S. intercalatum schistosomiasis
The commonest clinical symptoms are dysentery and lower abdominal pain. *S. intercalatum* eggs trapped in the tissues appear to cause less host immune reaction and damage than the eggs of other schistosomes. Highest prevalence and intensity of infection occur in those aged 5–14 years.

Measures to prevent and control schistosomiasis
- Avoiding contact with water known to contain cercariae by:
  - Providing safe water supplies in villages.
  - Constructing footbridges across infested rivers and streams.
  - Providing safe recreational bathing sites, especially for children.

- Preventing water becoming contaminated with eggs by:
  - Health education and providing sanitation facilities.
  - Treating infected persons.
  - Protecting water supplies from faecal pollution by animal reservoir hosts (*S. japonicum*).

- Minimizing the risk of infection from new water conservation and irrigation schemes and hydroelectric developments by:
  - Treating workers when necessary.
  - Siting settlements away from canals, drains, and irrigation channels and providing latrines and sufficient safe water for domestic use.
  - Lining canals with cement and keeping them free from silt and vegetation in which snails can breed.
  - Filling in formerly used irrigation ditches with clean soil to bury snail hosts.
  - Varying the water levels in the system.

- Destroying snail intermediate hosts, mainly by:
  - Using molluscicides where this is affordable and feasible, and will not harm important animal and plant life.

TRANSMISSION
1. Cercariae penetrate skin when person in contact with contaminated water.

HUMAN HOST*
2. Cercariae → schistosomula. Migrate through lungs and liver.
3. Become mature flukes in portal venous system. Flukes pair.
4. Migrate to veins of lower large intestine (*S. haematobium* to veins of bladder).
5. Eggs laid in venules. Burrow through into intestine (eggs of *S. haematobium* into bladder).
6. Eggs passed in faeces. (*S. haematobium* in urine).

  * *S. japonicum* also infects animals.

FRESH WATER
7. Eggs reach water. Miracidia hatch.
Snail host
8. Miracidia penetrate snail. Become sporocysts and multiply (2 generations). Sporocysts → cercariae.
9. Cercariae leave snail. (*S. japonicum* attaches to water vegetation).

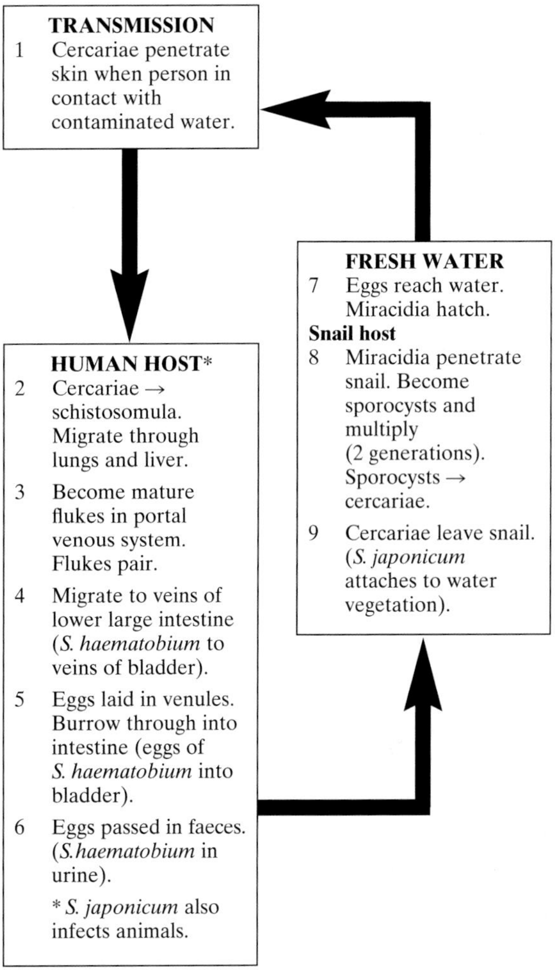

Fig 5.13   Transmission and life cycle of *Schistosoma* species.

- Removing vegetation from locally used water places, draining swamps, and other measures to eradicate snail habitats.
- Taking environmental measures to prevent seasonal flooding which results in an increase in snail numbers and transmission.

- Treating water supplies by:
  - Using a chlorine disinfectant where possible.
  - Storing water for 48 hours to allow time for any cercariae to die.
  - Using filter systems at water inputs to prevent cercariae from entering.

Further information: Readers are referred to the paper of Crompton *et al*[11], the WHO Report *Prevention and control of schistosomiasis and soil-transmitted helminthiasis*[7], and the WHO website www.who.int/health-topics/schisto.

LABORATORY DIAGNOSIS

The laboratory diagnosis of intestinal schistosomias is by:

■ Finding schistosome eggs in faeces by direct examination or more commonly by using a concentration technique. The specimen will often contain blood and mucus.

■ Examining a rectal biopsy for eggs when they cannot be found in faeces, especially after a patient has been partially treated.

Other findings

– There may be a blood eosinophilia and a raised erythrocyte sedimentation rate (ESR). Patients are often also anaemic.

– In patients with hepatic disease, serum total protein is raised due to raised globulin, serum albumin is often low, and serum alkaline phosphatase and aspartate aminotransferase (AST) activities are usually raised.

Examination of faeces for schistosome eggs

The preparation and examination of faeces by direct technique and the semi-quantitative reporting of egg numbers are described in subunit 5.3. Knowing the approximate number of eggs gives an indication of the intensity of infection. When eggs are not found in direct preparations a concentration method should be performed, such as the formol ether technique as described in subunit 5.3, or if a centrifuge is not available by the formol detergent gravity technique (see *Field survey techniques*). Even in moderate to severe symptomatic infections (particularly those of *S. mansoni* and *S. intercalatum*) a concentration technique may be required to detect the eggs.

Schistosoma species that can be found in faeces

Depending on geographical area, eggs of the following *Schistosoma* species can be found in faeces:

S. mansoni (Africa, S. America, Caribbean, Middle East).
S. intercalatum (West and Central Africa).
S. japonicum (China, Philippines, Indonesia).
S. mekongi (Lao PDR, Cambodia, Thailand).

Very occasionally, the eggs of *S. mattheei* (animal schistosome) are detected. *S. mattheei* is mainly found in parts of South Africa, Zaire and Zimbabwe.
Natural hybrids of *S. haematobium* and *S. mattheei* occur.

Egg of *S. mansoni*

● It is pale yellow-brown, large, and oval, measuring about 150 × 60 μm.

● Has a characteristic side (lateral) spine.

Note: Sometimes the spine may appear terminal like that of an *S. haematobium* egg but if the egg is rolled over by pressing gently on the cover glass the spine will be seen to be lateral.

● Contains a fully developed miracidium.

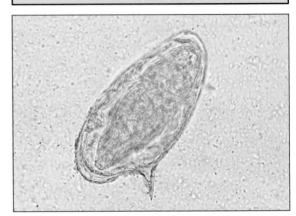

Plate 5.21   Egg of *S.mansoni* with lateral spine.

Egg of *S. japonicum*

● It is colourless or pale yellow-brown, large and round to oval, measuring about 90 × 65 μm.

● A very small hook-like spine (rudimentary spine) can sometimes be seen projecting from the egg wall but often it is hidden by faecal debris and red cells.

● Contains a fully developed miracidium.

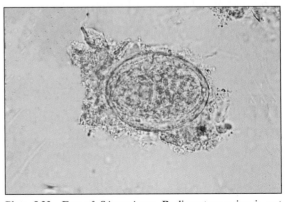

Plate 5.23   Egg of *S.japonicum*. Rudimentary spine is not visible. See also Plate 5.1 on p. 194..

Egg of S. mekongi

- It is similar to but smaller and rounder than the egg of *S. japonicum*, measuring about 56 × 66 μm.
- Has a small knob-like spine similar to the egg of *S. japonicum*.

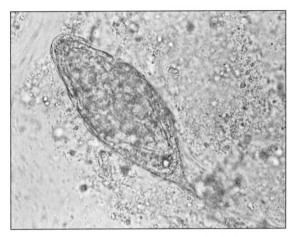

Plate 5.22   Egg of *S.intercalatum* with terminal spine.

Egg of S. intercalatum

- It is pale yellow-brown, large, and elongate, measuring about 180 × 60 μm.
- Has a characteristic long spine at one end (terminal spine) which may appear bent.

  Note: Because of its terminal spine, the egg of *S. intercalatum* can resemble that of *S. haematobium* but unlike *S. haematobium* the egg of *S. intercalatum* is usually found in faeces, not in urine and it is also larger.

- Contains a fully developed miracidium.
- Unlike other terminally-spined schistosome eggs, the egg of *S. intercalatum* is usually acid fast (Ziehl-Neelsen staining).

S. mattheei (animal schistosome)
This species is a natural parasite of cattle, sheep, goats, zebras, and antelopes. It has been reported as infecting up to 30% of persons in parts of South Africa. It also occurs in Zimbabwe and Zaire.

The eggs of *S. mattheei* are usually found in those already infected with *S. haematobium* or *S. mansoni*. It is thought hybridization occurs between *S. mattheei* and *S. haematobium*. Infection with *S. mattheei* is rarely serious.

Eggs of S. mattheei
The eggs are usually excreted in faeces. They have a terminal spine and therefore require differentiating from those of

S. haematobium and *S. intercalatum*.

The egg of *S. mattheei* is larger than the egg of *S. haematobium*, measuring about 220 × 60 μm. The terminal spine is not as long as that of *S. intercalatum*. Unlike *S. intercalatum*, the shell of *S. mattheei* is not acid fast (Ziehl-Neelsen staining).

Examination of a rectal biopsy for schistosome eggs

When schistosome eggs cannot be found in faeces they can sometimes be found in a rectal biopsy. The eggs are often non-viable and calcified.

A biopsy is examined as follows:

1 Immediately after removal, place the tissue in physiological saline and soak it for 30–60 min.

2 Transfer the tissue to a slide and cover with a cover glass. With care, press on the cover glass to spread out the tissue and make a sufficiently thin preparation.

3 Examine the entire preparation microscopically for eggs using the 10× objective with the condenser iris *closed sufficiently* to give good contrast. Constant focusing is necessary to detect the eggs.

   Note: if the preparation is too thick to examine, add a drop of lactophenol solution (Reagent No 40) and wait a few minutes for the tissue to clear sufficiently.

4 Identify the eggs and estimate the number of uncalcified eggs in the biopsy and the proportion that are calcified (black). Uncalcified and calcified eggs of *S. mansoni* in tissue are shown in Plate 5.24.

Schistosome eggs found in rectal biopsies: A rectal biopsy, depending on geographical area, may contain the eggs of *S. mansoni*, *S. intercalatum*, *S. japonicum*, *S. mekongi*, and occasionally the eggs of *S. haematobium* (described in subunit 5.6).

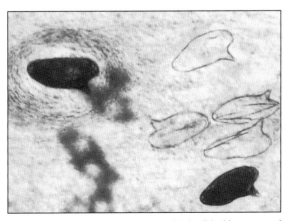

Plate 5.24   Uncalcified and calcified (black) eggs of *S.mansoni* in rectal biopsy.

FIELD SURVEY TECHNIQUES

In assessing the effectiveness of schistosomiasis control strategies, the district laboratory may be requested to participate in surveys to estimate prevalence and intensity of infection in the community.

Kato-Katz technique

In recent years several modified Kato techniques have been developed for the semi-concentration and semiquantitative estimation of schistosome eggs in faeces. Such techniques have been shown to be of value in schistosomiasis epidemiology and control work.

In the Kato-Katz technique faeces are pressed through a mesh screen to remove large particles. A portion of the sieved sample is then transferred to the hole of a template on a slide. After filling the hole, the template is removed and the remaining sample (approx. 10 mg, 20 mg, or 50 mg depending on size of template) is covered with a piece of cellophane soaked in glycerol (glycerine). The glycerol 'clears' the faecal material from around the eggs. The eggs are then counted and the number calculated per gram (g) of faeces.

Note: Further information on the Kato-Katz technique can be found in the WHO publication *Manual of basic techniques for a health laboratory*, 2nd edition, WHO, Geneva.

Compared with other field techniques for detecting and quantifying schistosome eggs in faeces, the Kato-Katz technique is less sensitive, is unsuitable for fluid or hard specimens, can alter the morphological appearances of eggs, and the technique is less safe and hygienic. Alternative field techniques have been suggested such as the sodium hydroxide digest technique, details of which can be found in the paper of Marshall et al.,[12] the Stoll helminth egg counting technique (see subunit 5.3), and the formol detergent gravity technique described in the following text.

Formol detergent field technique for concentrating and quantifying schistosome eggs

This technique is reproducible, inexpensive, simple, safe and hygienic to perform (formalin kills faecal pathogens) and gives good preservation of schistosome eggs. It is more sensitive than the Kato-Katz technique because more faeces is used. With simple modification, the technique can also be used to detect other faecal parasites.

The following are required:
- Formol detergent solution. Reagent No. 28
- Universal container with a conical base and measuring spoon (*Sterilin* type).
- Sieve (strainer) with small holes (preferably 400–450 µm in size). The small nylon tea strainer available in most countries is suitable.

The method is as follows:

1 Dispense about 10 ml of the formol detergent solution into a Universal container.

2 Using the spoon attached to the cap of the container, transfer a *level* spoonful of faeces to the container (approx. 300 mg when using a *Sterilin* spoon), and mix *well* in the solution to break up the faeces. Tighten the cap and shake for about 30 seconds.

3 Sieve the emulsified faeces, collecting the sieved suspension in a beaker. Return the sieved suspension to the conical based Universal container.

4 Stand the container upright in a rack for 1 hour (do not centrifuge).

5 Using a plastic bulb pipette or a Pasteur pipette, remove and discard the supernatant fluid, taking care not to disturb the sediment (containing schistosome eggs) which has formed in the base of the container.

6 Add about 10 ml of 10% formol detergent solution, and mix well for a minimum of 30 sec.

Leave to sediment for a further 1 hour. Further 'clearing' of the faecal debris will take place.

Note: The schistosome eggs are fixed and will not overclear or become distorted.

7 Using a plastic bulb pipette or Pasteur pipette, remove and discard the supernatant fluid, taking care not to remove the fine sediment that has collected in the conical base of the container.

8 Transfer the *entire* sediment to a slide and cover with a 22 × 40 mm cover glass or if unavailable with two smaller square cover glasses.

9 Systematically examine the *entire* sediment microscopically for schistosome eggs using the 10× objective with the condenser iris *closed sufficiently* to give good contrast.

Count the number of eggs and multiply the number counted by 3 to give the approximate number per gram (g) of faeces.

Interpretation of schistosome egg counts
The definition of a heavy infection is area-specific and may vary from 100/800 eggs per gram of faeces.

Modified technique to detect other parasitic eggs, oocysts, and larvae:

Perform the method as far as step 4. Instead of removing the supernatant fluid, *add* a further 10 ml, shake well, and leave the suspension to sediment overnight. Continue as described in steps 7–9, reporting the numbers of each species of helminth egg seen.

Serological diagnosis of schistosomiasis

Serum antibody tests have a limited application because they do not differentiate between active and previous infection or reinfection and they give no indication of intensity of infection. Active infection can be diagnosed by detecting circulating schistosome antigen.

Enzyme immune assays (EIA) to diagnose urinary and intestinal schistosomiasis by detecting circulating schistosome antigens, i.e. CAA (circulating anodic antigen) and CCA (circulating cathodic antigen) in serum and urine have been developed and assessed by van Lieshout *et al.*[13] Antigen tests, however, are not yet available commercially.

TRANSMISSION
1 Metacercariae ingested in raw or undercooked fish.

FRESH WATER
5 Eggs reach water.
Snail host
6 Snail ingests eggs. Miracidia hatch.
7 Miracidia → sporocysts. Multiply → rediae. Rediae → cercariae.
8 Cercariae leave snail.
Fish host
9 Cercariae infect fish. Become metacercariae.

HUMAN HOST*
2 Metacercariae excyst in duodenum. Migrate to bile duct.
3 Become mature flukes in biliary tract.
4 Eggs produced and passed in faeces.

* *O. sinensis* also infects fish-eating animals.

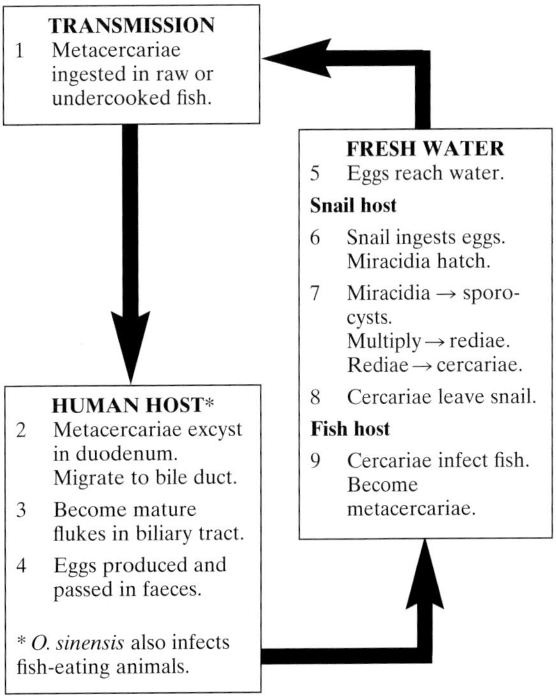

Fig 5.14   Transmission and life cycle of *Opisthorchis sinensis.*

6   *Opisthorchis (Clonorchis) sinensis**

* Although this parasite has been renamed *Opisthorchis sinensis*, the infection is still referred to as clonorchiasis. *O. sinensis* is known as the Chinese or Oriental liver fluke.

O. sinensis is endemic in China, South Korea, Japan, and northern Vietnam and the far east of the Russian Federation. High infection rates are found particularly in areas where human untreated faeces and animal faeces pollute fish culture ponds or other water bodies which contain the snail and fish intermediate hosts.

O. sinensis is transmitted by eating raw, undercooked, smoked, or pickled fish or fish products containing infective metacercariae. Reservoir hosts include fish-eating cats, dogs, pigs, and rodents.

The indirect life cycle of *O. sinensis* is summarized in Fig. 5.14. Following ingestion the metacercariae excyst in the duodenum, migrate to the intrahepatic bile ducts and gall bladder and occasionally to the pancreas where they become egg-producing flukes, about 4 weeks after infection. *O. sinensis* can live for many years in the human host.

Clonorchiasis
Symptoms of infection with *O. sinensis* are rarely serious. In endemic areas, chronic and heavy infections can cause damage to the liver, and bile ducts with jaundice, hepatitis, cirrhosis, and biliary obstruction. The liver frequently becomes enlarged and in some cases cancer of the bile duct (cholangiocarcinoma) can develop. Chronic infection is associated with gall stones (bilirubin stones), recurrent attacks of cholangitis, and pancreatitis.

In heavy infections, symptoms include weakness, weight loss, abdominal fullness, diarrhoea, anaemia, and oedema. In advanced infections, portal hypertension, ascites, and upper gastrointestinal bleeding may occur.

Measures to prevent and control clonorchiasis
- Avoiding eating raw, pickled, smoked, or insufficiently cooked or processed fish or fish products which may contain metacercariae.
- Providing adequate latrines and health education to prevent faecal contamination of fish ponds and other bodies of water that may contain snail hosts.
- Treating those infected.
- Using chemicals or other methods to eradicate snail hosts in areas where this is feasible.

Note: Further information on the distribution, transmission, pathogenic effects, diagnosis, control and prevention of *O. sinensis* infections can be obtained from the WHO publication *Control of foodborne trematode infections,*[14] and in Chapter 81, in *Mansons Tropical Diseases* (see Recommended Reading).

LABORATORY DIAGNOSIS

The laboratory diagnosis of *O. sinensis* infection is by:

- Finding the eggs of *O. sinensis* in faeces.
- Detecting eggs in aspirates of duodenal fluid.

Note: An eosinophilic leukocytosis is common.

Anti-P_1 antibodies: These may be found in the sera of persons infected with *Opisthorchis* flukes who lack antigen P_1 on their red cells, i.e. P_2 positive. The flukes are known to contain P_1 substances that can stimulate the production of anti-P_1 antibodies.

Examination of faeces for *O. sinensis* eggs

The eggs can be few and because they are so small they can be easily missed. A concentration technique should therefore be used if infection is suspected and no eggs are found by direct examination. The method of preparing and examining specimens and the formol ether concentration technique are described in subunit 5.3. Substitution of formol water with a citric acid – Tween solution (Reagent No 18) in the formol ether technique is recommended for the best recovery of *Opisthorchis* eggs.

Note: The 40× objective is required to identify *O. sinensis* eggs and the preparation must not be too thick otherwise the small eggs will be overlooked.

Egg of *O. sinensis*

- It is yellow-brown and *small* measuring 27–32 × 15–18 μm.
- It is shaped like an electric light bulb and contains a ciliated miracidium but this is difficult to see through the surface of the egg.
- Has a clearly seen operculum (lid).
- Often described as having 'shoulders' (rim on which the operculum rests).
- A small projection can sometimes be seen at the other end of the egg.
- When examined with the high power objective, an indistinct outer covering of the shell can often be seen.

Note: The eggs of *O. sinensis* closely resemble those of *O. viverrini* and *O. felineus.*

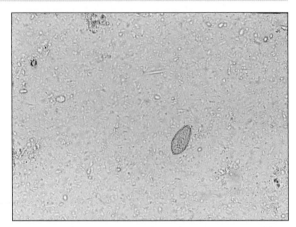

Plate 5.25   Egg of *O.sinensis*. See also Plate 5.1 on p. 194..

Examination of duodenal fluid for *O. sinensis* eggs

A filtration technique can be used to recover the eggs of *O. sinensis* from aspirates of duodenal fluid. A membrane filter of 8 μm pore size is required for filtering the eggs of *O. sinensis*. Staining the membrane with 1% w/v trypan blue in saline helps to show the eggs.

If unable to perform a filtration technique or the specimen is not suitable for filtration, transfer a drop of the aspirate (especially a piece of mucus) to a slide, cover with a cover glass and examine microscopically. Make sure the preparation is sufficiently thin otherwise the eggs will be missed. Use the 40× objective to identify the small eggs. If the aspirate is watery, centrifuge it first and examine a drop of the sediment.

Serological diagnosis of clonorchiasis: Details of antibody tests and tests to detect circulating antigen can be found in Chapter 81, Food-borne trematodes, *Mansons Tropical Diseases* (see Recommended Reading).

## 7	*Opisthorchis viverrini*

O. viverrini is endemic along the Mekong River basin in Thailand, Cambodia, and Lao People's Democratic Republic (also high infection rates occur in Kazakhstan, Ukraine and Russian Federation). It is the commonest trematode infection in Thailand, particularly in the northeast. Prevalence rates up to 90% have been reported.

Transmission, hosts, and life cycle of *O. viverrini* are similar to those of *O. sinensis*. Fish-eating animals especially cats and dogs serve as reservoir hosts. The mature flukes of *O. viverrini*, like those of *O. sinensis*, live in the biliary tract and pancreatic ducts.

Most of the symptoms associated with opisthorchiasis occur in persons with chronic and heavy infections in endemic areas. In Kampuchea and the LAO PDR, co-infection with *S. mekongi* can cause severe liver disease.

Opisthorchiasis

The flukes and deposited eggs cause inflammation and fibrosis around the bile ducts. Symptoms of chronic opisthorchiasis include diarrhoea, flatulence, upper abdominal pain, fatty food intolerance, fever, gall stones, progressive jaundice, enlarged liver, weakness and oedema. Recurrent attacks of cholangitis and pancreatitis can occur. Cancer of the bile duct is associated with chronic infection.

The measures described for *O. sinensis* apply also to the prevention and control of *O. viverrini* infections.

LABORATORY DIAGNOSIS

The laboratory diagnosis of *O. viverrini* infection is the same as that described for *O. sinensis* (see previous text). Eggs can be found in faeces and aspirates of duodenal fluid.

Egg of O. viverrini

It closely resembles that of *O. sinensis* except that it is slightly smaller, measuring 19–29 × 12–17 μm.

Opisthorchis felineus

O. felineus is a common parasite in cats, dogs, and fish-eating wild animals and also infects humans. It is mainly found in the Russian Federation, Kazakhstan, Ukraine, and Poland where it is widely distributed and a major public health problem. The life cycle, clinical features, control, and laboratory diagnosis are similar to those described for *O. sinensis*.

Egg of O. felineus

It closely resembles that of *O. sinensis* except that it is slightly narrower, measuring 26–32 × 11–15 μm. Most of the eggs are asymmetrical, being slightly less convex on one side.

8   *Fasciola hepatica* and *Fasciola gigantica*

F. hepatica and *F. gigantica* are important animal pathogens. They live in the liver and bile ducts of sheep, cattle, and other animals causing the serious disease liver rot. *F. gigantica* infections in cattle lead to considerable economic loss especially in some African countries. Very occasionally *Fasciola* flukes infect humans. Infection with *F. hepatica* is more common than infection with *F. gigantica* which is less adapted to humans.

F. hepatica is found in sheep-raising areas in temperate countries and also in Egypt, parts of the Middle East, and South America, particularly Bolivia.

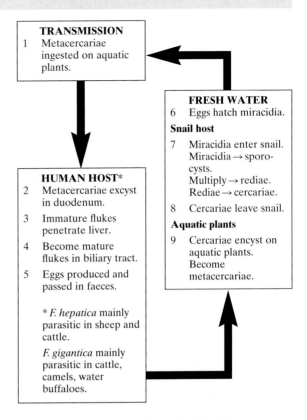

Fig 5.15   Transmission and life cycle of *Fasciola* species.

Sheep, cattle and other herbivores are commonly infected.

F. gigantica is found mainly in tropical Africa, South and South-east Asia, and the Far East. Cattle, camels and water buffaloes are commonly infected. In some areas, e.g. Egypt and the Islamic Republic of Iran, *F. hepatica* and *F. gigantica* occur together.

F. hepatica and *F. gigantica* are transmitted by ingesting metacercariae encysted on wild watercress or other aquatic plants grown in water contaminated with faeces from infected animals.

The indirect life cycle of *F. hepatica* and *F. gigantica* is summarized in Fig. 5.15. Following ingestion the metacercariae excyst in the duodenum and the young flukes migrate through the intestinal wall into the peritoneal cavity. They reach the bile ducts by penetrating through the liver capsule. About 4 months after infection the flukes become mature and produce eggs which are excreted in the faeces. The flukes can live for many years in their host.

Fascioliasis

Light infections are usually asymptomatic. Heavy infections, however, can cause acute disease with serious liver damage during the 4–6 weeks when the immature flukes migrate through the liver. Symptoms during this period include fever, sweating, abdominal pain, dizziness, cough, asthma, urticaria and a *marked* blood eosinophilia. In the bile ducts, the flukes cause inflammation. Occasionally, migrating flukes develop in other organs of the body.

With chronic infection there is thickening of the bile ducts due to a host cellular response. The liver becomes enlarged and blockage of the bile ducts can lead to obstructive jaundice. The gall bladder can also be infected. Anaemia is common in heavy infections.

Measures to prevent and control fascioliasis

- Avoiding eating watercress or other uncooked water plants which may contain infective metacercariae.

- Cultivating watercress in water free from faecal pollution.

- Reducing the infection rate in animals by fencing off grazing land known to be infected with metacercariae. Also treating animals to reduce egg output.

- Identifying and destroying snail habitats where this is feasible.

LABORATORY DIAGNOSIS

The laboratory diagnosis of fascioliasis is by:

- Finding eggs in faeces in chronic infections. *Fasciola* eggs can also be found in duodenal aspirates and in bile.

  Note: Eggs will not be found in faeces in acute fascioliasis when the immature flukes are migrating through the liver and causing serious symptoms but not yet producing eggs. Diagnosis is best made serologically.

- Serological diagnosis by testing serum for antibodies is particularly valuable in the early stages of infection when eggs are not present in the faeces. Cross-reactivity with other trematodes such as schistosomes can occur. In endemic areas where *Fasciola* infections are prevalent, district laboratories should consult with their nearest Public Health Laboratory regarding the availability of a suitable antibody test or faecal antigen test.

Examination of faeces for *Fasciola* eggs

A concentration technique such as the formol ether method described in subunit 5.3 is recommended because the eggs are usually few. Several specimens may also need to be examined to detect the eggs.

Note: If eggs are found in human faeces it must be confirmed that they are present due to a *Fasciola* infection and not from eating animal liver containing *Fasciola* eggs. Repeated finding of the eggs in faeces establishes parasitic infection.

Egg of *F. hepatica* or *F. gigantica*

- It is yellow-brown, *large* and oval.

  F. hepatica eggs measure 130–145 × 70–90 μm.

  F. gigantica eggs are larger, measuring 156–197 × 90–104 μm.

- Has an indistinct operculum (lid).

- Contains an unsegmented ovum surrounded by many yolk cells.

Note: Morphologically *Fasciola* eggs resemble those of *Fasciolopsis buski* and *Echinostoma* species.

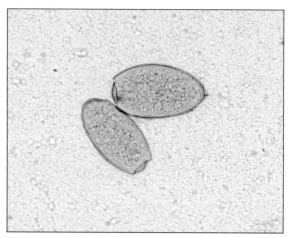

Plate 5.26   Eggs of *F.hepatica*.

---

9   *Fasciolopsis buski*

F. buski is the largest fluke that infects humans. It is known as the giant intestinal fluke. The pig and buffalo are the normal definitive hosts of the parasite.

Human infection with *F. buski* is widespread in Asia including southern and central China, Taiwan, Vietnam and Thailand. It is also found in eastern India, Bangladesh, Malaysia, Borneo, Myanmar and Indonesia. High prevalence rates occur in areas where water plants are cultivated in ponds that are fertilized by untreated infected pig or human faeces. Infection rates are particularly high in children.

Infection with *F. buski* is by ingesting metacercariae from water chestnuts, water caltrop, or other aquatic edible plants grown in water contaminated with faeces. Infections frequently occur when peeling the outer covering off plants with the teeth or eating the fruits of water caltrop on which metacercariae have encysted.

The indirect life cycle of *F. buski* is summarized in Fig. 5.16. Following ingestion, the metacercariae excyst in the duodenum, attach to the wall of the small intestine and within 3 months develop into mature egg-producing flukes. Many eggs are produced and excreted in the faeces. The life span of an adult fluke is only a few months.

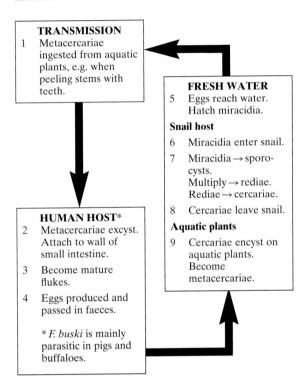

Fig 5.16   Transmission and life cycle of *Fasciolopsis buski*.

Fasciolopsiasis
Most infections with *F. buski* are light and asymptomatic. Heavy infections can cause inflammation and ulceration of the intestinal wall with diarrhoea and abdominal pain. Toxins produced by the flukes can cause oedema of the face and limbs, ascites, and other allergic reactions. Plasma albumin levels may fall due to protein loss. There is usually a blood eosinophilia and slight macrocytic anaemia. Toxic reactions in heavily infected children can be fatal.

Measures to prevent and control *fasciolopsiasis*

- Treating water plants which may be infected using boiling water or cooking them before eating or teeth-peeling.

- Providing latrines and health education to prevent eggs reaching the water (where humans are the main source of infection). Also, treating infected individuals (within a control programme).

- Avoiding the use of untreated human or pig faeces as

fertilizer in cultivation ponds.

- Identifying and destroying snail hosts and their habitats where this is feasible.

LABORATORY DIAGNOSIS

The laboratory diagnosis of *F. buski* infection is by finding the eggs in faeces, examined by direct technique. Concentration techniques are rarely needed. The preparation and direct examination of faecal specimens are described in subunit 5.3.

> ### Egg of *F. buski*
>
> - It is yellow-brown, *large* and oval, measuring 130–154 × 78–98 μm.
>
> - Has a small operculum (lid) which is usually difficult to see.
>
> - Contains an unsegmented ovum surrounded by yolk cells.
>
> *Note:* Morphologically the eggs of *F. buski* resemble those of *F. hepatica*, *F. gigantia* (similar but smaller), and *Echinostoma* species.

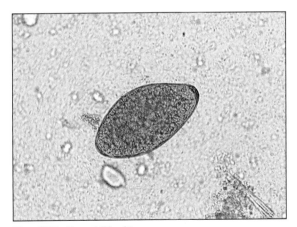

Plate 5.27   Egg of *F.buski*.

Echinostoma species
Echinostoma flukes are mainly intestinal parasites of birds and mammals. About 12 species have been reported as infecting humans in Asia and the Western Pacific often with high prevalences. Human infection is by ingesting metacercariae in raw or undercooked freshwater snails, clams, or fish (e.g. loach). The flukes parasitize the small intestine. Occasionally they cause inflammation and ulceration with diarrhoea, abdominal discomfort, and eosinophilia. The eggs (depending on species) can be smaller or similar in size to those of *Fasciola* species and *F. buski*.

FLUKES OF LESSER MEDICAL IMPORTANCE

Heterophyes heterophyes

H. heterophyes is a small fluke which is normally parasitic in the intestine of rats, cats, dogs, foxes, wolves and jackals. Human infection with *H. heterophyes* occurs mainly in the Far East and Nile delta in Egypt.

Infection is by eating raw or undercooked fish such as the mullet or minnow which contain metacercariae. Following ingestion, the metacercariae excyst and develop into egg-producing flukes in the small intestine. Eggs contain a fully developed miracidium when passed in the faeces. In water, the eggs are ingested by snails (*Pirenella* or *Cerithidia*). In the snail, the miracidia hatch and develop into sporocysts which produce rediae and finally cercariae. The cercariae leave the snail and encyst in a fish host and become infective metacercariae.

Heavy infections can cause intestinal inflammation and necrosis. Rarely the eggs may reach the heart and central nervous system where they can produce serious symptoms. *H. heterophyes* infection is prevented by not eating insufficiently cooked or pickled fish which may contain metacercariae.

LABORATORY DIAGNOSIS

This is by finding the small eggs of *H. heterophyes* in faeces.

Egg of H. heterophyes

Morphologically it resembles the eggs of *Opisthorchis* and *M. yokagawai*.

- It is light brown, *small*, and oval, measuring 23–27 × 14–16 μm.
- Has a less distinct operculum and lacks the 'shoulders' of *Opisthorchis* eggs.
- Small knob can sometimes be seen at the base of the egg.
- It has no outer indistinct coat as seen with *Opisthorchis* eggs.

Metagonimus yokagawai

M. yokogawai is the smallest fluke which parasitizes humans. It lives in the small intestine. Reservoir hosts include dogs, cats, pigs, and pelicans. *M. yokagawai*

is endemic in the Far East (very common) and is also found in the Mediterranean basin.

The transmission and life cycle of *M. yokagawai* are similar to that of *H. heterophyes*. Snail hosts belong to the genera *Semisulcospira* and *Thiara* and second intermediate hosts are cyprinid fish and sweetfish.

LABORATORY DIAGNOSIS

This is by finding the *small* eggs of *M. yokagawai* in faeces. A concentration technique, such as the formol ether method may be necessary to detect and identify the eggs.

Egg of M. yokagawai

Morphologically it resembles the eggs of *Opisthorchis* and *H. heterophyes*.

- It is yellow-brown, *small*, oval, measuring 28–32 × 14–18 μm.
- Has an operculum but lacks the 'shoulders' of *Opisthorchis* eggs.
- Has no outer indistinct coat as seen with *Opisthorchis* eggs.

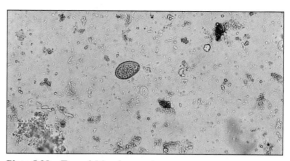

Plate 5.29   Egg of *M. yokagawai*.

Dicrocoelium dendriticum

Dicrocoelium dendriticum is a small fluke which is normally parasitic in the biliary tract of sheep and cattle. It is found in China, North Africa, South America, and Europe.

Human infection is rare. Spurious infection (from ingesting infected beef or sheep liver) is occasionally reported. A person becomes infected with a *Dicrocoelium* fluke by accidentally swallowing ants which contain metacercariae.

Following ingestion, the metacercariae develop into mature egg-producing flukes in the bile ducts and liver. Symptoms of infection are rarely serious.

LABORATORY DIAGNOSIS

This is by finding the eggs of *D. dendriticum* in faeces or duodenal fluid.

> **Egg of D. dendriticum**
> - It is brown, oval, but slightly flattened on one side. It measures 38–48 × 22–30 μm.
> - Operculum is usually clearly seen.
> - Often contains vacuoles.

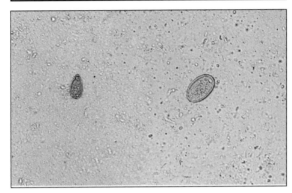

Plate 5.30 *Left*: Egg of *Opisthorchis*. *Right*: Egg of *Dicrocoelium*.

Gastrodiscoides hominis

G. hominis is an amphistome trematode (ventral sucker is situated at the posterior end of the fluke). It is normally parasitic in the intestine of the pig, napu, mouse deer, or rat. Human infections with *G. hominis* are found mainly in India (Ganges river basin) and also in parts of Pakistan, Bangladesh, Vietnam, Malaysia, Guyana, and the Philippines. High infection rates have been reported from Assam (up to 41%).

G. hominis is transmitted by eating water plants or their fruits, frogs, or crayfish on which metacercariae have encysted. The flukes live in the large intestine and eggs containing a miracidium are passed in the faeces. In fresh water, the eggs hatch miracidia which infect snail hosts. In the snail the parasite reproduces and develops (sporocysts, rediae, cercariae). The cercariae leave the snail and mainly encyst on water vegetation and grass, becoming infective metacercariae.

Large numbers of flukes can cause inflammation of the wall of the large intestine with mucus diarrhoea caused by the mechanical and toxic effects of the parasites. Heavy infections can be found in children. Light infections are usually asymptomatic.

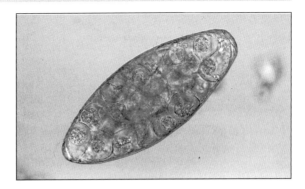

Plate 5.31 Egg of *G.hominis*.

LABORATORY DIAGNOSIS

This is by finding the eggs of *G. hominis* in faeces.

> **Egg of G. hominis**
> - It is spindle shaped and *large*, measuring about 152 × 60 μm.
> - Has a small operculum.
> - Contains an immature ovum and yolk cells.

10 *Taenia saginata and Taenia solium*

T. saginata is often referred to as the beef tapeworm (infection is from eating infected beef) and *T. solium* as the pork tapeworm (infection is by eating infected pork). Humans are the definitive hosts.

Taenia saginata

T. saginata has a worldwide distribution in countries where cattle are raised and beef is eaten. High infection rates are found particularly in the highlands of Ethiopia. In Egypt and Morocco the camel is the main source of human infection.

Mass travel, the migration of workers, and inadequate disposal of sewage have contributed to increases in the prevalence rates of infection with *T. saginata*.

Taenia saginata asiatica: This *Taenia* tapeworm is morphologically similar to but distinct from *T. saginata*. It is found in Indonesia, Korea, Taiwan, the Philippines and Thailand. Pigs not cattle are the main intermediate hosts with cysticerci being found in the liver. *T. saginata asiatica* does not cause human cysticercosis.

T. saginata is transmitted by eating raw or undercooked beef or other animal meat which contains infective cysticercus larvae.*

* Cysticercus (plural: cysticerci): This is the larval form (bladderworm) of *Taenia* tapeworms which is found in the intermediate host (pig or cow) and is infective to humans. It consists of a small fluid-filled bladder containing a single invaginated (inward turning) head, which when ingested and fully developed, evaginates (turns outwards) in the small intestine and grows into a mature tapeworm.

The indirect life cycle of *T. saginata* is summarized in Fig. 5.17. Following ingestion, the scolex (head) in the cysticercus is freed and becomes attached to the wall of the small intestine by its suckers. Segments (proglottides) are formed from the neck region and within 2–3 months the larva has grown into a long tapeworm with the gravid (egg-filled) segments being found at the tail end. Usually only one tapeworm is present but multiple infections can occur.

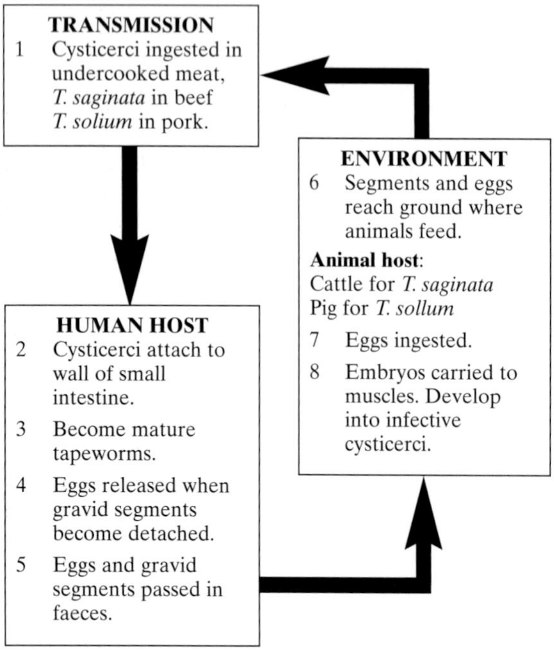

| TRANSMISSION |
| 1   Cysticerci ingested in undercooked meat, *T. saginata* in beef *T. solium* in pork. |

| ENVIRONMENT |
| 6   Segments and eggs reach ground where animals feed. |
| **Animal host:** Cattle for *T. saginata* Pig for *T. sollum* |
| 7   Eggs ingested. |
| 8   Embryos carried to muscles. Develop into infective cysticerci. |

| HUMAN HOST |
| 2   Cysticerci attach to wall of small intestine. |
| 3   Become mature tapeworms. |
| 4   Eggs released when gravid segments become detached. |
| 5   Eggs and gravid segments passed in faeces. |

Cysticercosis: Infection with *T. solium* larvae can occur by ingesting eggs in food or from hands contaminated with faeces. Eggs develop into cysticerci causing cysticercosis and neurocysticercosis.

Fig 5.17 Transmission and life cycle of *Taenia solium* and *Taenia saginata.*

A mature *T. saginata* measures 4–10 metres in length and consists of up to 2 000 segments. When fully developed the gravid segments become detached. Each segment may contain 30 000–50 000

eggs (mature and immature). The eggs are discharged only after the gravid segments have separated from the worm. Gravid segments containing eggs and eggs from ruptured segments are passed in the faeces. *T. saginata* segments also migrate through the anus and release eggs on the perianal skin.

T. saginata taeniasis

Clinically, infection with *T. saginata* rarely produces serious effects. There may be abdominal pain with intestinal disturbances and loss of appetite. Very occasionally migrating segments may cause appendicitis or cholangitis.

Measures to prevent and control *T. saginata* infection

- Avoid eating raw or insufficiently cooked meat which may contain infective cysticerci. The cysticerci can be heat-killed at 56 °C or by deep-freezing meat for a minimum of three weeks.
- Inspecting meat and condemning any found to contain cysticerci.
- Providing health education and adequate latrines to increase the containment of segments and destruction of eggs.
- Not using untreated human faeces to fertilize pastureland.
- Treating infected persons.

LABORATORY DIAGNOSIS

The laboratory diagnosis of *T. saginata* infection is by:

■ Identifying intact gravid segments recovered from clothing or passed in faeces. The segments are usually passed singly.

   Note: Following treatment the head and mature segments may be expelled and collected for identification.

■ Detecting eggs in faeces. Morphologically the eggs of *T. saginata* and *T. solium* are indistinguishable.

Identifying *T. saginata* gravid segments
When freshly passed the segments are white and opaque. Viable (living) segments move by muscular contractions.

Caution: Because viable segments are actively motile, keep them in a closed container until they can be fixed and examined. *Always use forceps to handle the segments* and wear protective gloves.

The method of examining a segment is as follows:

1   If recovered from faeces, wash the segment in clean water. If the segment is dry and shrivelled, soak it first in water before examining it.

2   Press the segment between two slides and hold the slides together with an elastic band or adhesive tape at each end.

3   To kill the eggs, immerse the preparation for 10 minutes in a container of formol saline (Reagent No 29) heated to 70 °C. Remove and wash in water.

Caution: Formaldehyde has an irritating and harmful vapour, therefore when using formol saline make sure the room is well ventilated and cover the container of fixative with a tight fitting lid.

4   Firmly compressing the segment to give a thin preparation, hold it lengthways against the light and count the number of main branches arising from the central stem of the uterus (see Fig. 5.18). The branches are more easily counted with the help of a magnifying lens.

Note: The size of the segment and the number of uterine side branches can usually identify the segment as *T. saginata* or *T. solium*. Differentiation is also possible by examining a mature segment or head of the tapeworm (expelled following treatment).

Gravid segment of *T. saginata*

- Appears white and opaque and measures about 20 mm long by 6 mm wide when freshly passed. It is therefore longer than a *T. solium* gravid segment.

- Uterus has a central stem which has more than 13 main side branches on each side. (*T. solium* has fewer than 13), as shown in Fig. 5.18. The main side branches are subdivided into smaller branches.

Note: If required, the uterine branches can be stained by injecting India ink through the opening (genital pore) on the side of the segment or by staining the segment with haematoxylin (Delafields or Harris'). Staining is not usually necessary to identify fresh segments.

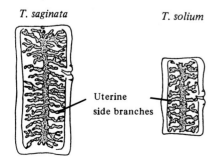

T. saginata   *T. solium*

Uterine side branches

Fig. 5.18   Gravid segments of *T.saginata* and *T.solium*.

Examination of faeces for *Taenia* eggs

A concentration technique and the examination of several specimens may be necessary to detect *Taenia* eggs in faeces. They are usually few because the eggs are not regularly discharged from the tapeworm in the intestine. The eggs can be concentrated by the formol ether technique described in subunit 5.3.

Egg of *T. saginata* or *T. solium*

- It is round to oval, measuring 33–40 μm in diameter.

- Embryo is surrounded by a thick, brown, radially striated wall (embryophore).

- Hooklets are present in the embryo. Careful focusing is necessary to see the three pairs of hooklets.*

    *Embryonic hooklets are present in the eggs of both *T. saginata* and *T. solium*. The term oncosphere is used to describe an embryo with six hooklets.

- Sometimes a clear membrane can be seen surrounding the egg but usually this is lost when the gravid segment disintegrates.

Note: If required the Ziehl-Neelsen staining technique (as used for AFB) can be used to differentiate *Taenia* eggs. The embryophore of *T. saginata* is acid fast (i.e. stains red) whereas that of *T. solium* is not acid fast.

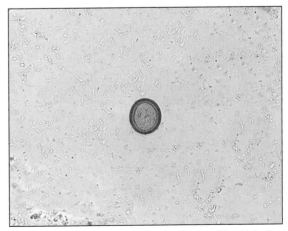

Plate 5.32   Egg of *Taenia* species showing small hooklets. See also Plate 5.1.

Collection of a perianal specimen for Taenia eggs

The clear adhesive tape technique described in subunit 5.5.13 for the recovery of *E. vermicularis* eggs from perianal skin can also be used to collect *Taenia* eggs from skin around the anus.

Identification of the scolex of *T. saginata*

The scolex (head) is very small, measuring only 2 mm across. It may be found among the smallest immature segments with the help of a magnifying lens. The scolex has 4 suckers but no hooks (see Fig. 5.19). The absence of hooks distinguishes the scolex of *T. saginata* from that of *T. solium* which has hooks.

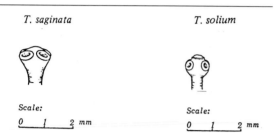

Fig. 5.19   *Left*: Scolex of *T.saginata* showing suckers. *Right*: Scolex of *T.solium* showing suckers and crown of hooks.

Taenia solium

T. solium is not as widely distributed as *T. saginata*. It occurs mainly in southern Africa, China, India, Central America, Chile, Brazil, Papua New Guinea, and non-Islamic South East Asia where human faeces reach pigs and pork is eaten raw or under-cooked. *T. solium* is transmitted by eating raw or insufficiently cooked pork which contains infective cysticercus larvae.

The indirect life cycle of *T. solium* is summarized in Fig. 5.17. Following digestion, the scolex in the cysticercus is freed and becomes attached to the wall of the small intestine by its hooks and suckers and grows into a long tapeworm. Within 2–3 months the tapeworm is mature and gravid segments are formed. Mature worms measure 2–3 metres in length and consist of 800–1 000 segments.

Infection with T. solium larvae (cysticerci)
Human infection with *T. solium* larvae can occur by ingesting viable eggs in infected food or from contaminated fingers. Serious disease can result from infection with *T. solium* cysticerci (see following text).

T. solium taeniasis
Infection with the tapeworm of *T. solium* rarely produces serious effects. There may be abdominal pain with intestinal disturbances and loss of appetite.

T. solium cysticercosis
Infection with the larvae of *T. solium* can cause cystic nodules in subcutaneous tissues and muscles. Usually the cysticerci produce few serious clinical symptoms except when present in the brain where they can cause epilepsy and other central nervous system disorders (neurocysticercosis). Dead and dying cysticerci may cause an inflammatory host response.

Measures to prevent and control *T. solium* infection
● Avoid eating raw or undercooked pork which may contain cysticerci ('measly' pork) and inspecting and condemning any pork found to contain cysticerci. Active surveillance is necessary in areas endemic for *T-solium*.

● Ensuring pigs do not have access to human faeces.

● Treating infected persons, and providing health education and adequate sanitary facilities.

Prevention of cysticercosis: The prevention of cysticercosis caused by internal autoinfection is by diagnosing *T. solium* infection and treating it effectively. Ingestion of eggs can be avoided by personal hygiene and by not eating food which may be contaminated with *T. solium* eggs such as raw vegetables grown on land fertilized with untreated human faeces.

LABORATORY DIAGNOSIS

The laboratory diagnosis of *T. solium* infection is by:

■ Identifying gravid segments passed in faeces.

Note: Following treatment, the head and mature segments may be expelled and collected for identification.

■ Detecting eggs in faeces. Morphologically the eggs of *T. solium* and *T. saginata* are indistinguishable. Examining faecal specimens for *Taenia* eggs is as previously described.

Cysticercosis: This is usually diagnosed serologically. When calcified, the cysts can be detected by X-ray. Cysts in the brain can also be detected by computed tomography (CT scan).[15]

Identifying *T. solium* gravid segments
The segments are often passed in chains. They are less motile than those of *T. saginata*. The segments are examined in the same way as described for *T. saginata* (see previous text).

Gravid segment of *T. solium*

● Appears grey-blue and translucent and measures about 13 mm long by 8 mm wide when freshly passed. It is therefore shorter than a gravid segment of *T. saginata*.

● Uterus has a central stem which has up to 13 main side branches on each side (*T. saginata* has more than 13) as shown in Fig. 5.18. The main side branches are subdivided into smaller branches.

Note: If required the uterine branches can be stained by injecting India ink through the opening (genital pore) on the side of the segment or by staining the segment with haematoxylin (Delafields or Harris'). Staining is not usually necessary to identify fresh segments.

Caution: Use forceps to handle the segments and wear protective gloves to avoid infection of *T. solium* larvae from the eggs. Keep the segments in a closed container until they can be fixed and examined.

Identification of the scolex of *T. solium*

The scolex (head) is very small, measuring only 1 mm in diameter. It may be found among the smallest immature segments with the help of a magnifying lens. The scolex has 4 suckers and a crown of hooks (see Fig. 5.19). The presence of hooks distinguishes the scolex of *T. solium* from that of *T. saginata* which has no hooks.

Caution: Wear protective gloves and use forceps to examine the specimen.

Serological diagnosis of cysticercosis

Tests have been developed to detect parasitic antigen in both serum and cerebrospinal fluid. Garcia *et al* describe a monoclonal antibody-based enzyme-linked immunosorbent assay (ELISA) to assist in the diagnosis, treatment, and follow up of neurocysticercosis patients.[16]

When needing to perform serological tests, district laboratories should consult their regional or central public health laboratory.

11   *Diphyllobothrium latum* *

* Known as the fish tapeworm because its larvae are found in fish. Humans are the important definitive hosts.

D. latum is widely distributed in the lake areas of Europe, North America and the Far East. It is also found in parts of Asia and South America, particularly Chile.

D. pacificum: This tapeworm is found in the coastal countries of South America. It is normally parasitic in seals but occasionally infects humans.

D. latum is transmitted by ingesting plerocercoids (infective larvae) in raw or undercooked fish. The indirect life cycle of *D. latum* is summarized in Fig. 5.20. Definitive hosts include fish-eating carnivores, but humans are the important hosts.

Following ingestion, the plerocercoid becomes attached to the wall of the small intestine and within 2–4 weeks develops into a mature tapeworm up to 10 metres in length with 3 000–4 000 segments. Multiple infections are common. *D. latum* can live for several years in its host. Many eggs are produced which are discharged directly into the lumen of the intestine and passed in the faeces. The eggs are immature when passed.

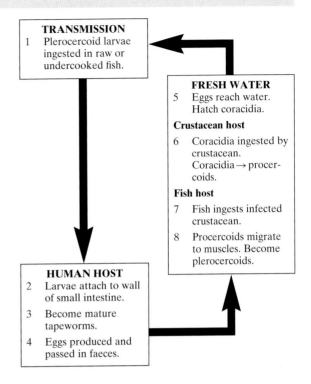

Fig 5.20   Transmission and life cycle of *Diphyllobothrium latum.*

Diphyllobothriasis

Infection with *D. latum* can cause gastrointestinal symptoms, weakness, weight loss, and other clinical features due to toxins released by the tapeworm. Very occasionally a megaloblastic anaemia may develop due to the uptake of vitamin B_{12} by the tapeworm in competition with the host. This is more likely to occur when the tapeworm is situated in the upper part of the jejunum.

Measures to prevent and control *D. latum* infection

- Avoid eating raw or undercooked fish which may contain plerocercoids. Viable plerocercoids may also be found in pickled or smoked fish.

- Killing the plerocercoids in fish by brine saturation or freezing at $-10\,^{\circ}C$ for 24–48 hours.

- Preventing the eggs reaching water by providing adequate latrines combined with health education.

LABORATORY DIAGNOSIS

The laboratory diagnosis of *D. latum* infection is by:

- Finding the eggs of *D. latum* in faeces.
- Occasionally detecting mature segments in faeces.

Examination of faeces for *D. latum* eggs

Many eggs are usually present in the faeces because they are constantly discharged through the uterine pore. They can therefore be easily detected by direct examination of a faecal specimen as described in subunit 5.3.

Egg of *D. latum*

- It is yellow-brown and oval in shape, measuring about 70 × 45 μm.

- Has an operculum (lid) which is usually difficult to see.

- Contains a mass of granulated yolk cells surrounding an undeveloped ovum.

- Sometimes a small projection is visible at the non-operculated end of the egg.

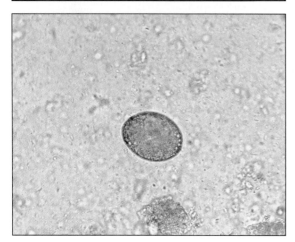

Plate 5.33   Egg of *D.latum* containing yolk cells.

Identification of a *D. latum* segment

Segments are not often found in the faeces because they tend to disintegrate in the intestines. When found, they often appear shrunken and empty. Undamaged mature segments of *D. latum* are wider than they are long, measuring 10–20 mm across by 3–7 mm long. The genital pore is found in the centre of the segment.

---

12   *Vampirolepis nana**

---

*Formerly called *Hymenolepis nana*. It is also known as the dwarf tapeworm, being the smallest (3–4 cm) tapeworm known to infect humans.

V. nana is widely distributed in countries with warm climates including those of South America,

Mediterranean region, Africa, and South East Asia. Children are more commonly infected than adults.

V. nana is transmitted by ingesting eggs in food or water or from hands contaminated with infected faeces. The eggs are infective when passed in the faeces. Internal autoinfection also occurs.

The direct life cycle of *V. nana* is summarized in Fig. 5.21. Unlike other tapeworms, *V. nana* requires no intermediate host. Following the ingestion of eggs, the embryos are freed in the small intestine. They penetrate villi and within a few days develop into infective cysticercoid larvae. When fully mature, the cysticercoids rupture out of the villi into the lumen of the intestine. They become attached to other villi and grow rapidly into mature tapeworms. Eggs are produced after about 4 weeks.

Gravid segments become detached and eggs are released in the intestine. Some of the eggs are passed in the faeces while others remain in the intestine. Those that remain, hatch embryos. These develop into cysticercoids which grow into tapeworms. *V. nana* also infects rodents.

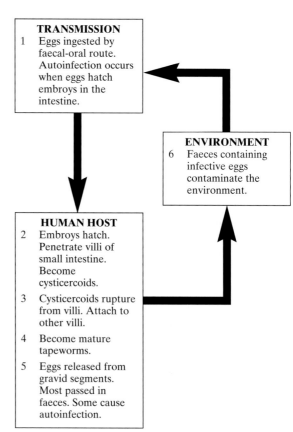

Fig 5.21   Transmission and life cycle of *Vampirolepis nana*.

V. nana infection

Although many *V. nana* tapeworms can be found in the same host due to internal autoinfection, the life-span of the adult worms is only a few months. Symptoms of infection are rarely detected except in children when many tapeworms may cause abdominal pain, diarrhoea, anorexia and lassitude. Toxins released from the worms can cause allergic reactions. Severe and sometimes disseminated infections can occur in malnourished and immunosuppressed persons.

Preventing V. nana infection

- Practising personal hygiene, especially the washing of hands before eating.
- Providing latrines and encouraging their use especially by children to avoid faecal pollution of the ground.
- Avoid eating uncooked food which may be contaminated with infective eggs.

LABORATORY DIAGNOSIS

The laboratory diagnosis of *V. nana* infection is by finding the eggs in faeces. They can usually be found by the direct examination of faeces as described in subunit 5.3. If required the eggs can be concentrated by the formol ether concentration technique or saturated sodium chloride floatation technique.

Caution: Eggs are infective when excreted in the faeces.

> ### Egg of V. nana
> - It is colourless, oval or round, measuring 30–45 μm in diameter.
> - Hooklets are present in the embryo. Careful focusing is necessary to see the three pairs of hooklets.
> - At each end of the egg, thread-like structures called polar filaments are usually visible.

Plate 5.34 Egg of *V. nana* showing hooklets and polar filaments. See also Plate 5.1.

TAPEWORMS OF LESSER MEDICAL IMPORTANCE

Hymenolepis diminuta

H. diminuta is a tapeworm normally parasitic in rodents, with fleas and insects serving as intermediate hosts. Very occasionally humans become accidentally infected by swallowing an intermediate host. Most infections occur in children. Symptoms may include abdominal pain and there is usually an eosinophilia.

The eggs of *H. diminuta* are excreted in the faeces and can be easily distinguished from those of *V. nana*.

> ### Egg of H. diminuta
> - It is yellow-brown, round to oval, and measures 60–80 μm. There are no polar filaments.
> - Contains an embryo which has 3 pairs of hooklets.

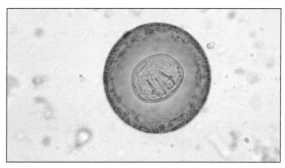

Plate 5.35 Egg of *H.diminuta* showing hooklets.

Dipylidium caninum

D. caninum is a common tapeworm of dogs, foxes, jackals and cats. Very occasionally it infects humans, usually children. Infection is by the accidental ingestion of infected cat or dog fleas which serve as intermediate hosts, and in which the cysticercoid larvae are found. Eggs contained in egg capsules and occasionally gravid segments are excreted in the faeces.

> ### Egg capsule of D. caninum
> - A typical egg capsule measures about 60 × 100 μm and usually contains 8–15 eggs.
> - Each egg contains an embryo which has 3 pairs of hooklets and measures about 35 μm in diameter.

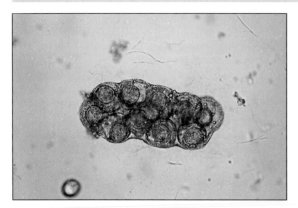

Plate 5.36   Egg capsule of *D.caninum*.

Gravid segment of D. caninum

- Segments resemble melon seeds, measuring about 12 × 27 mm.

- A genital pore is present on each side of the segment (characteristic feature of *Dipylidium* tapeworms).

Caution: Freshly passed segments are motile.

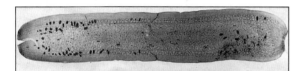

Plate 5.37   Gravid segment of *D.caninum*.

---

13 *Identification of E. vermicularis* eggs in perianal specimens*

---

* Also known as the pinworm or threadworm.

E. vermicularis is a nematode. Eggs can be found in specimens collected from perianal skin. Occasionally eggs can also be found in faeces.

E. vermicularis has a worldwide distribution with children being more commonly infected than adults. Transmission is by ingesting infective eggs. The eggs are deposited on the anal skin usually during night hours and within a few hours of being laid they contain an infective larva. Autoinfection by swallowing infective eggs is common in children because the eggs cause intense irritation and scratching of the infected area leads to the fingers becoming contaminated with eggs. Occasionally larvae hatch from the eggs on the perianal skin and migrate back into the intestine where they grow into mature worms. This type of infection is called retroinfection. Airborne transmission of *E. vermicularis* can also occur.

E. vermicularis has a direct life cycle. Following ingestion of infective eggs, the larvae hatch in the intestine. The larvae develop into fully mature worms in the large intestine. Most worms inhabit the caecum and appendix. The female worms migrate to the rectum, pass out of the anus and lay their eggs on the perianal skin and perineum. The eggs are produced about 6 weeks after infection. They can remain viable on bedding, clothing, household objects, and in dust for several weeks. Warm temperatures and high humidity favour survival.

Enterobiasis

E. vermicularis infection rarely causes serious symptoms. There is usually intense irritation around the anus and in females, infection of the urinary and genital tract can occur. Worms in the appendix can cause appendicitis.

Preventing enterobiasis

Because *E. vermicularis* eggs are infective very soon after being laid, an entire family or community (e.g. in a school or institution) often becomes infected after handling bedding and other articles which have become contaminated. Control and preventive measures therefore include:

- Treating all members of a family in which infection has occurred.

- Washing of the anal skin each morning soon after waking and frequent washing of clothing worn at night.

LABORATORY DIAGNOSIS

The laboratory diagnosis of enterobiasis is by:

- Finding *E. vermicularis* eggs in samples collected from perianal skin or recovered from clothing worn at night.

   Note: Eggs (from perianal skin) may also be found in faeces and occasionally in urine from females.

- Recovering *E. vermicularis* worms from perianal skin or detecting them in faeces or during a clinical examination.

Examination of a perianal specimen for pinworm eggs

The highest number of eggs can usually be recovered in the morning soon after waking and before bathing. The eggs can be collected from skin around the anus or from clothing using clear adhesive tape or a saline swab.

Adhesive tape method

1 Wrap a strip of *clear* adhesive tape (e.g. *Sellotape, Scotch tape*) over the closed end of a tube, sticky side facing out.

2 Wearing protective gloves, apply the tape to skin around the anus. After collecting the eggs, stick the tape lengthways, face down on a microscope slide.

3 Immediately before examining the preparation, lift up the tape and add a drop of xylene to the centre of the preparation. Press down the tape again, smoothing it out with a piece of cotton wool.

   Use of xylene: This is not essential but a drop of xylene will clear any debris and air bubbles, making it easier to detect the eggs. Do not, however, add the xylene until ready to examine the preparation because prolonged contact with xylene may cause the eggs to collapse. Adequate safety precautions should be taken when using xylene (see end of subunit 3.5).

   Note: Adhesive tape-slide preparations of *E. vermicularis* keep well for several days when stored at 2–8 °C should examination of the specimen need to be delayed.

4 Examine the preparation microscopically using the 10× objective to detect the eggs and the 40× objective to identify them. The condenser iris *must* be closed sufficiently to give good contrast otherwise the colourless eggs will not be seen.

   Caution: Most preparations will contain infective eggs by the time they reach the laboratory for examination.

Egg of E. vermicularis

- It is colourless.
- Oval in shape and usually flattened on one side. It measures about 55 × 30 μm.
- Contains a larva.

Swab method

1 Moisten a cotton wool swab in fresh physiological saline. Swab around the perianal area.

2 Agitate the swab in a container of 4–5 ml of saline to wash off the eggs. Cap the container and safely discard the swab.

3 Transfer the saline to a conical tube and cen-

trifuge to sediment the eggs. Discard the supernatant fluid and without delay, transfer the sediment to a slide, cover with a cover glass and examine microscopically as described in step No. 4 of the previous method.

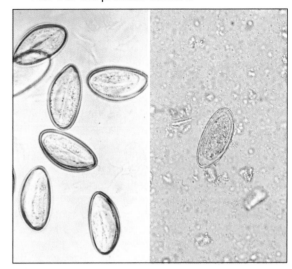

Plate 5.38 *Left*: Adhesive tape preparation showing eggs of *E. vermicularis* recovered from anal skin. *Right*: *E. vermicularis* egg in faeces.

Identification of *E. vermicularis* worms

Worms (females only) may be recovered when collecting eggs from the perianal skin or during a clinical examination. Occasionally the worms can also be found in faecal specimens. They are small, measuring 8–13 mm in length and white resembling a small piece of thread (hence the name threadworm). When examined with a magnifying lens, the long pointed tail will be seen and also the characteristic shaped anterior end (see Fig. 5.23).

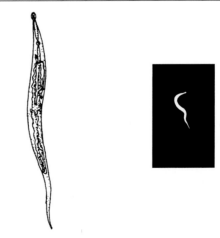

Fig. 5.22 *Left*: Morphology of a female *E. vermicularis* worm. *Right*: actual size of a female *E. vermicularis*.

5.6 Examination of urine for *Schistosoma haematobium* eggs

S. haematobium causes urinary schistosomiasis. The species contains several strains.

Distribution

S. haematobium is endemic in 54 countries, mainly in Africa, and the eastern Mediterranean. It is also found in several Indian Ocean islands and small islands off the coast of East and West Africa. In some areas the distribution of *S. haematobium* overlaps with *S. mansoni* causing double infections.

The development of irrigation schemes and dams for hydroelectric power and flood control have greatly increased the prevalence of *S. haematobium* infections in several countries. The migration of refugees has contributed to an increase in the distribution of the parasite.

Transmission and life cycle

S. haematobium is transmitted by cercariae penetrating the skin when bathing, washing clothes, fishing, or engaged in agricultural work or other activity involving contact with contaminated water. In most endemic areas a large proportion of children and teenagers become infected and reinfected.

S. haematobium has an indirect life cycle similar to that described for other *Schistosoma* species and summarized in Fig. 5.13 in subunit 5.5.6. The snail hosts of *S. haematobium* belong to the genus *Bulinus*.

The flukes pair in the blood vessels of the liver and then migrate to the veins surrounding the bladder (vesical plexus). Mature flukes can also be found in the veins of the liver and rectum. The female lays eggs in the venules (small veins) of the bladder. The estimated egg output of *S. haematobium* is 20–200 eggs per day. Many of the eggs penetrate through the mucosa into the lumen of the bladder and are passed in the urine. Eggs can be found in the urine from about 12 weeks after infection. Each egg contains a fully developed miracidium. About 20% of eggs remain in the wall of the bladder and become calcified. Eggs can also be found in the ureters, rectal mucosa, reproductive organs, and liver.

Urinary schistosomiasis

It is the eggs of *S. haematobium* in the tissues not the adult flukes that stimulate host inflammatory responses that result in the clinical features and damage to the bladder and ureters that characterize urinary schistosomiasis. The degree of illhealth and serious complications that develop later in life are related to the intensity and duration of infection.

S. haematobium infection

Within 24 hours of infection an intense irritation and skin rash, referred to as 'swimmer's itch', may occur at the site of cercarial penetration. Haematuria (blood in urine) caused by eggs penetrating through the wall of the bladder is a feature of urinary schistosomiasis. In endemic areas, up to 50–70% of infected persons (80% of infected children) have symptoms of urinary tract disease with haematuria, dysuria (difficult or painful urination), or frequency.

Eggs trapped in the wall of the bladder and surrounding tissues cause inflammatory reactions with the formation of granulomata. Many of the eggs die and become calcified eventually producing what are known as 'sandy patches' in the bladder. In heavy infections, eggs can be carried to other parts of the body. Following prolonged untreated infection and a marked cellular immune response, the ureters may become obstructed and the bladder wall thickened leading to abnormal bladder function, urinary tract infection, and eventually obstructive renal disease with kidney damage. Complications can arise from genital schistosomiasis.[17]

In some endemic areas, chronic infection of long duration is associated with squamous cell bladder cancer (infection probably promoting rather than directly causing the cancer). *S. haematobium* infection is also linked to an increase in *Salmonella* infections and carriers of *Salmonella typhi* and *Salmonella paratyphi*. Calculi (stones) in the bladder and urinary tract are also found with chronic urinary schistosomiasis.

Anaemia is a common finding in urinary schistosomiasis, particularly in those with a low dietary iron intake, co-existing hookworm infection or malaria. In Africa, urinary schistosomiasis is also reported as impairing the growth and development of children.

Prevention and control

The measures described for *S. mansoni* in subunit 5.5.6 apply to the prevention and control of *S. haematobium* infection.

Further information: Can be found in Chapter 17 *Lecture Notes on Tropical Medicine*, 5th ed,[17] and WHO Report: *Prevention and Control of schistosomiasis and soil-transmitted helminthiasis.*[7]

LABORATORY DIAGNOSIS

Laboratory diagnosis of *S. haematobium* infection is by:

- Finding the eggs or occasionally the miracidia of *S. haematobium* in urine. A quantitative report is required, i.e. number of eggs/10 ml of urine.

- Detecting eggs in a rectal biopsy or bladder mucosal biopsy.

Note: In mixed infections, the eggs of both *S. mansoni* and *S. haematobium* can sometimes be found in urine and occasionally *S. haematobium* eggs can be found in faeces.

Other findings
– Haematuria is a common finding.

> **Haematuria:** In endemic areas, up to 80% of infected children have haematuria, and of those infected with more than 50 eggs/10 ml of urine, 98–100% have haematuria. Questionnaires, asking people about their history of haematuria, have been shown to be accurate, well accepted and cost-effective in screening communities for urinary schistosomiasis.[7]

– Proteinuria is frequently present.
– Eosinophils can often be found in the urine. There is usually also a blood eosinophilia.

> **Identifying eosinophils in urine:** Add a small drop of weak eosin solution (e.g. 1 in 10 dilution of Field's stain B) to a urine sediment. The granules of eosinophils stain bright red whereas those of pus cells remain unstained or stain pale pink.

– Bacteriuria may accompany urinary schistosomiasis.

Detection and counting of *S. haematobium* eggs in urine

The excretion of *S. haematobium* eggs in urine is highest between 10.00 h and 14.00 h, with a peak around midday. Even when persons are heavily infected, eggs may not be present in the urine all the time. It may be necessary to examine several specimens collected on *different* days due to the irregular pattern of egg excretion. The routine examination of urine for schistosome eggs is as follows:

1   Collect 10–15 ml of urine (between 10.00 h and 14.00 h) in a clean dry container.

> *Note:* Neither exercising before passing urine nor collecting terminal urine (last few drops), increase the number of eggs present in the specimen (as once was thought). To avoid the miracidia hatching from the eggs, keep the specimen in the dark if unable to examine it within 30 minutes.

2   Report the appearance of the urine. In moderate to heavy infections, the urine will usually contain blood and appear red or red-brown and cloudy. When visible blood is present, add 2 drops of saponin solution (Reagent No. 54) to lyze the red cells. This will make it easier to detect the eggs.

> If blood is not seen, test the specimen chemically for blood and protein as described in subunit 9.11.

3   Transfer 10 ml of well mixed urine to a conical tube and centrifuge at RCF 500–1 000 g to sediment the schistotome eggs (avoid centrifuging at greater force because this can cause the eggs to hatch).

> *Note:* If a centrifuge is not available, allow the eggs to sediment by gravity for 1 hour.

4   Discard the supernatant fluid. Transfer all the sediment to a slide, cover with a cover glass, and examine the *entire* sediment microscopically using the 10× objective with the condenser iris closed sufficiently to give good contrast.

5   Count the number of eggs in the preparation and report the number/10 ml of urine. If more than 50 eggs are present, there is no need to continue counting. Report the count as 'More than 50 eggs/10 ml'. Such counts indicate a heavy infection.

> In the early stages of urinary schistosomiasis, the egg count is an indicator of the severity of disease.

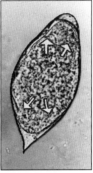 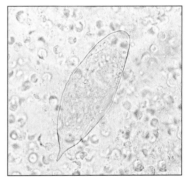

Plate 5.39   Position of flame cells.   Plate 5.40   *S.haematobium* egg and red cells in urine.

Egg of *S. haematobium*

● It is pale yellow-brown, large and oval in shape, measuring about 145 × 55 μm.

● Has a characteristic small spine at one end (terminal spine).

● Contains a fully developed miracidium.

> *Note:* Sometimes the miracidia hatch from the eggs and can be seen 'swimming' in the urine as shown in Plate 5.41.

● A living egg (in fresh unpreserved urine) shows what is called flame cell movement, i.e. flickering of the excretory flame cells (see Plate 5.39).

Miracidia in urine: When the urine is dilute or has been left to stand for several hours in the light, the miracidia will hatch from the eggs. The ciliated miracidia are motile.

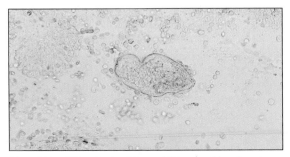

Plate 5.41   Ciliated miracidium of *S.haematobium* in urine.

Other terminally spined Schistosome eggs
Occasionally the eggs of *S. mattheei* or *S. intercalatum* can be found in urine in areas where these species are found and when there is faecal contamination of the urine. They can be differentiated by Ziehl-Neelsen staining. The shell of *S. haematobium* is not acid fast whereas that of other terminally spined *Schistosoma* species is acid fast (red).

Filtration technique for detecting and quantifying *S. haematobium* eggs in urine

Filtration is the most sensitive, rapid, and reproducible technique for detecting and quantifying *S. haematobium* eggs in urine. Polycarbonate membrane filters, however, are expensive although with care they can be reused (see later text). Other types of filters can also be used, e.g. *Nytrel* woven filters.

Required:

– 10 ml Luer syringe.

– Syringe filter holder (Swinnex type), 13 mm diameter. This is suitable for holding filters of 12 mm or 13 mm diameter.

– Polycarbonate membrane filter of 13 mm diameter and 12–14 μm pore size. This is a *clear* filter which can be disinfected in domestic bleach, and reused several times (see end of *Method*).

Availability of filter holders and filters
Millipore Company (see Appendix II) supply reusable plastic 13 mm Swinnex filter holders (10 per pack, catalogue No. SX0001300) and also 13 mm, 12 μm porosity polycarbonate membranes (100 per pack, catalogue No. TKTP 01300).

Method

1   Using blunt-ended (untoothed) forceps, carefully place a polycarbonate filter on the filter support of the filter holder. Re-assemble the filter holder and attach it to the end of a 10 ml Luer syringe (see Plate 5.42).

2   Remove the plunger from the syringe. Fill the syringe to the 10 ml mark with well-mixed urine, and replace the plunger. Holding the syringe over a beaker or other suitable container, slowly pass the urine through the filter.

Note: Filling the syringe is preferred to drawing up the urine into the syringe because it does not require tubing and the air which passes through the membrane after the urine, helps to stick the eggs to the filter.

Clogging of filters
If a membrane filter clogs, remove the filter holder and attach it to another syringe containing 3% v/v acetic acid. Pass the acid through the filter. This may help to clear it. If, however, the blockage does not clear, use another membrane to filter the remaining sample of urine. Both filters must be examined to give the number of eggs in the 10 ml urine sample.

3   Remove the filter holder and unscrew it. Using blunt-ended forceps, carefully remove the filter and transfer it face upwards (eggs on surface) to a slide. Add a drop of physiological saline, and cover with a cover glass.

4   Using the 10× objective with the condenser iris *closed sufficiently* to give good contrast, examine systematically the entire filter for *S. haematobium* eggs. Count the number of eggs and report the number per 10 ml of urine.

Note: If more than 50 eggs are present there is no need to continue counting (50 eggs or more/10 ml of urine is considered a heavy infection). Report the count as 'More than 50 eggs/10 ml'.

Reuse of filters
Immediately after use, carefully remove the filter and soak it for 4–5 hours or overnight in a disinfectant such as domestic bleach diluted 1 in 5 with water (do not use a disinfectant containing phenol). Recover the filter by straining the disinfectant through a small plastic strainer. Wash the filter by agitating the strainer (with filter inside) in warm water containing detergent followed by several rinses in clean water. After the final wash, dry the *underside* of the strainer. Remove the filter from inside the strainer and transfer it to a slide, add a drop of water, and cover with a cover glass. Check microscopically that the filter is clear of eggs and does not appear damaged. If suitable for reuse, dry the filter and return it to its storage box.
Note: the filter holder and syringe should also be soaked in disinfectant before being washed and reused.

Differentiating non-viable from viable schistosome eggs on a filter

In assessing active infection or in judging whether treatment has been successful, it is helpful to know whether the schistosome eggs detected are viable or non-viable.

Although it is often possible to see flame cell

movement in viable eggs (see previous text), a more reliable way of differentiating viable from non-viable schistosome eggs is to examine a preparation stained with 1% w/v trypan blue in physiological saline. A drop of stain is added and the preparation is left for 30 minutes at room temperature (in a damp chamber to prevent drying out).

Non-viable eggs . . . . Stain blue
Viable eggs . . . . Unstained

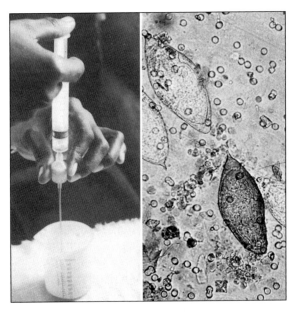

Plate 5.42 *Left*: Filtration concentration technique for detection of *S.haematobium* eggs. *Right*: Trypan blue preparation showing stained non-viable *S.haematobium* egg and unstained living egg.

Examination of total volume of urine collected between 10.00 h and 14.00 h

In light infections to increase the possibility of finding *S. haematobium* eggs, the total volume of urine excreted between 10.00 h and 14.00 h can be examined as follows:

1 Note the appearance of each sample of urine passed over the 4 hours. If blood is not visible test the sample chemically for protein and blood.

2 *After* testing for protein and blood, add about 0.1 ml of 10% v/v formol saline to each sample (50–100 ml) of urine to preserve the eggs. Red cells in the urine will be lyzed.

3 Transfer the urine to a narrow cylinder, cover, and leave for about 2 hours for the eggs to sediment.

4 Discard all but the last approximate 15 ml of urine. Centrifuge to sediment the eggs.

5 Remove the supernatant, and transfer the sediment to a slide, cover with a cover glass and examine microscopically (using 10× objective) for schistosome eggs.

Examination of biopsies for *S. haematobium* eggs

The laboratory examination of rectal and bladder mucosal biopsies is as described for intestinal schistosomiasis in subunit 5.5.6. Non-viable calcified *S. haematobium* eggs appear black. Such eggs are frequently found in rectal biopsies.

5.7 Examination of blood for malaria parasites

Malaria is a major public health problem and cause of much suffering and premature death in the poorer areas of tropical Africa, Asia and Latin America. In many endemic areas it is becoming increasingly difficult to control because of the resistance of the parasite to antimalarial drugs and the failure of vector control measures.

Malaria global situation[18,19]

● Malaria occurs in 100 countries with about 40% of the world's population at risk.

● Each year there are estimated to be 275 million clinical cases of malaria (90% of them in sub-Saharan Africa) resulting in 1.12 million deaths, mostly (75%) in children under 5 years.

● Epidemics are increasing due to man-made conflicts and climate-associated disasters causing the movement of non-immune populations to malaria endemic areas.

● Urban and periurban malaria are now substantial problems in certain areas of Asia and Africa.

● Malaria is becoming more difficult to manage in areas of multidrug resistance where effective drugs are unavailable.

Role of the district laboratory

The diagnosis of malaria based on clinical symptoms alone is not reliable. It can result in unnecessary expenditure and inappropriate use of antimalarial drugs and a delay in establishing the correct diagnosis and treatment of a patient.

Laboratory support is needed to diagnose malaria, especially:

– in children (1–5 y) and pregnant women in areas of stable malaria (intense malaria) transmission.

– in all age groups in areas of unstable transmission where serious epidemics may occur and diagnosis can be difficult during times of low malaria transmission.

The laboratory also has an important role in monitoring response to treatment with antimalarials, and in the investigation and monitoring of anaemia, hypoglycaemia, and other complications of severe malaria.

Terms used to describe the level of endemicity of malaria

The terms used are hypoendemicity (lowest level), mesoendemicity, hyperendemicity and holoendemicity (highest level). These terms define the increasing levels of prevalence of malaria as estimated by surveys of spleen and parasite rates in particular age groups. Holoendemic and hyperendemic malaria are found in areas of stable transmission. Mesoendemic and hypoendemic malaria are found in areas of unstable transmission.

Plasmodium species and their distribution

There are four species of *Plasmodium* that cause human malaria:

Widespread species: *Plasmodium falciparum*
                         Plasmodium vivax

Less widespread species: *Plasmodium malariae*
                         Plasmodium ovale

Subdivision of *Plasmodium*

The genus *Plasmodium* is subdivided into the subgenus *Laverania* and the subgenus of the same name, i.e. *Plasmodium*. *P. falciparum* belongs to the subgenus *Laverania* and *P. vivax*, *P. ovale* and *P. malariae* belong to the subgenus *Plasmodium*.

Plasmodium falciparum

P. falciparum is found mainly in the hotter and more humid regions of the world. It is the main species found in tropical and subtropical Africa and parts of Central America and South America, Bangladesh, Pakistan, Afghanistan, Nepal, Sri Lanka, South East Asia, Indonesia, Philippines, Haiti, Solomon Islands, Papua New Guinea and many islands in Melanesia. It also occurs in parts of India, the Middle East, and eastern Mediterranean.

Varieties of *Plasmodium falciparum*

The species *Plasmodium falciparum* contains several 'varieties' which show differences in geographical distribution, vector susceptibility, human infection pattern, drug susceptibility, morphology and antigenic composition.

Plasmodium vivax

P. vivax is capable of developing in mosquitoes at lower temperatures than *P. falciparum* and therefore has a wider distribution in temperate and sub-tropical areas.

P. vivax is the main *Plasmodium* species in South America (occurring as far south as northern Argentina), Mexico, the Middle East, northern Africa, India, Pakistan, Sri Lanka, Papua New Guinea and the Solomon Islands. It is also found in parts of South East Asia, Indonesia, Philippines, Madagascar, tropical and subtropical Africa, Korea, and China.

Strains of *Plasmodium vivax*

The species *P. vivax* contains many strains which show differences in incubation time, relapsing pattern, morphology, number of parasites in red cells, and response to antimalarials.

Plasmodium malariae

P. malariae has a much lower prevalence than *P. falciparum* and *P. vivax*. It is found in tropical and subtropical regions. In tropical Africa it accounts for up to 25% of *Plasmodium* infections. It is also present in Guyana, India, Sri Lanka and Malaysia. In these countries it accounts for less than 10% of *Plasmodium* infections.

Plasmodium knowlesi: Human infections with *P. knowlesi*, a species that naturally infects monkeys (macaques), have been reported from Malaysia and Thailand. Morphologically *P. knowlesi* resembles *P. malariae* but unlike *P. malariae*, parasite numbers have been reported as high and clinical symptoms more severe.[20]

Plasmodium ovale

P. ovale has a low prevalence. It is found in West Africa where it accounts for up to 10% of malaria infections and has also been reported from other parts of Africa, and from the Philippines, Indonesia, China, and parts of the Far East, South East Asia, and South America.

Transmission and life cycle of malaria parasites

Malaria parasites are transmitted by the bite of an infected female *Anopheles* mosquito. Sporozoites contained in the saliva of the mosquito are inoculated into the blood of a human host when the mosquito takes a blood meal. Infection can also occur by transfusion of infected donor blood, by injection through the use of needles and syringes contaminated with infected blood, and very occasionally congenitally, usually when a mother is non-immune.

The life cycle of malaria parasites is summarized in Fig. 5.24. It involves:

- Asexual reproduction in a human host, i.e. liver cell schizogony* and repeated red cell schizogony* cycles and the formation of gametocytes (gametogony).

  *Schizogony is also referred to as merogony and a schizont as a meront.

- Sexual multiplication (sporogony) in the anopheline mosquito in which male and female gametes fuse to form zygotes which develop into oocysts. Each oocyst produces many sporozoites. The sporozoites are found in the salivary glands of the mosquito and are infective to humans.

Development in humans

Following inoculation, the sporozoites rapidly (within 8 h) leave the blood and enter liver cells. Within 5–15 days (depending on species) they develop into liver schizonts and are referred to as pre-erythrocytic (PE) schizonts. Mature PE schizonts contain many merozoites.

Hypnozoites: Some of the sporozoites of *P. vivax* and *P. ovale* after invading liver cells delay their development into PE schizonts. They become dormant forms called hypnozoites, becoming active and developing into PE schizonts only at a later date, causing relapses.

When mature, a PE schizont ruptures from the liver cell, releasing its merozoites into the blood circulation. The merozoites infect red cells (binding to receptors on the red cell membrane). A proportion are phagocytosed and destroyed. Entry of the parasites into red cells starts a cycle of schizogony in the blood which to complete takes 48 hours for *P. falciparum*, *P. vivax* and *P. ovale* and 72 hours for *P. malariae*. During this time the intracellular merozoites develop into trophozoites ('ring forms') which feed on the contents of the red cells.

Ring forms: Young trophozoites are concave disks which appear ring-shaped in stained preparations because the ring of cytoplasm stains but not the central food vacuole. The ring of cytoplasm contains organelles. The nucleus is clearly visible as a single or sometimes double chromatin dot.

As the trophozoite feeds, malaria pigment (haemozoin) is produced as an end product of haemoglobin breakdown. This accumulates in the trophozoite, appearing as brown-black granules. When the trophozoite is fully developed, the nucleus begins to divide, followed by a division of cytoplasm, resulting in the formation of a schizont containing 8–24 (depending on species) merozoites. The mature schizont ruptures from its red cell releasing merozoites, malaria pigment, and toxins into the plasma (cause of a typical malaria attack).

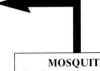

TRANSMISSION
1 Sporozoites inoculated when *Anopheles* mosquito takes a blood meal.
(Malaria parasites can also be transmitted by blood transfusion).

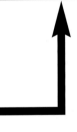

MOSQUITO
6 Gametocytes ingested by mosquito.
7 Male and female gametes fuse. Zygote → oocyst on outside of stomach wall.
8 Sporozoites form in oocyst.
9 Oocyst ruptures. Sporozoites reach salivary glands of mosquito.

HUMAN HOST
2 Sporozoites infect liver cells. Multiply by schizogony.
   Note: Some sporozoites of *P. vivax* and *P. ovale* become dormant hypnozoites in liver. Become active after several months.
3 Liver schizonts rupture. Merozoites enter red cells, become trophozites. Multiply by schizogony.*
   *With *P. falciparum*, schizogony occurs in capillaries deep within the body.
4 Schizonts rupture. Merozoites infect new red cells.
5 Some merozoites develop into male and female gametocytes.

Fig 5.24   Transmission and life cycle of malaria parasites.

Cytoadherence (sequestration) of *P. falciparum*: As *P. falciparum* trophozoites mature, antigens form on the surface of infected red cells which adhere to receptors on endothelial cells lining capillaries in various organs and tissues of the body. Falciparum trophozoites therefore complete their development into schizonts in the capillaries of deep tissues, not in the circulating blood in contrast to *P. vivax*, *P. ovale*, and *P. malariae*.

Merozoites released from schizonts enter the blood circulation and those which are not destroyed by the host's immune system infect new red cells, beginning a further cycle of schizogony with more red cells being destroyed. After several erythrocytic schizogony cycles, some of the merozoites entering red cells develop into male and female gametocytes. For the life cycle to be continued, the gametocytes must be ingested by a female *Anopheles* mosquito in a blood meal (males do not feed on blood). If they are not taken up by a mosquito they die.

Clinical features and pathology of malaria

The characteristic feature of malaria is fever caused by the release of toxins (when erythrocytic schizonts rupture) which stimulate the secretion of cytokines from leucocytes and other cells. In the early stages of infection the fever is irregular or continuous. As schizogony cycles synchronize, fever begins to recur at regular intervals particularly in quartan malaria (every 72 h), vivax and ovale malaria (every 48 h).

Typical malaria fever attack: It starts with a cold stage (rigor) in which the patient shivers and feels cold, even though his or her temperature is rising. A hot stage follows in which the temperature rises to its maximum, headache is severe, and there are back and joint pains, vomiting, and diarrhoea. The final stage is when the patient perspires, the temperature falls, the headache and other pains are relieved, and the patient feels exhausted.

Splenomegaly occurs in all forms of malaria with repeated attacks causing a greatly enlarged spleen. Anaemia and jaundice are also features of malaria, particularly falciparum malaria.

Malaria caused by P. falciparum

Malaria caused by *P. falciparum* is referred to as falciparum malaria, formerly known as subtertian (ST) or malignant tertian (MT) malaria. It is the most widespread, accounting for up to 80% of malaria cases worldwide.

P. falciparum is the most pathogenic of the human malaria species with untreated infections causing severe disease and death, particularly in young children, pregnant women and non-immune adults.

The pathogenicity of *P. falciparum* is mainly due to:

- The cytoadherence of falciparum parasitized red cells (see previous text), causing the cells to adhere to one another and to the walls of capillaries in the brain, muscle, kidneys and elsewhere and in pregnant women, in the placenta. Sequestration of parasitized cells in the microcirculation causes congestion, hypoxia, blockage and rupturing of small blood vessels.

- High levels of parasitaemia resulting in the activation of cytokines and the destruction of many red cells. Falciparum malaria parasitaemia can exceed more than 250 000 parasites/µl of blood. Up to 30–40% of red cells may become parasitized.

Severe falciparum malaria is associated with cerebral malaria, haemoglobinuria, severe anaemia, hypoglycaemia, and complications in pregnancy.

Cerebral malaria

This is the commonest cause of coma and death in falciparum malaria,[22] particularly in children and non-immune adults. Many parasitized cells can be found in the capillaries of the brain and other organs and in the late stages, haemorrhaging from small blood vessels can occur.

Malaria haemoglobinuria

This can occur in severe malaria and in association with glucose-6-phosphate dehydrogenase (G6PD) deficiency. Also as a complication of quinine treatment.[26] In the rare form of malaria haemoglobinuria (formerly known as blackwater fever) there is a rapid and massive intravascular haemolysis of both parasitized and non-parasitized red cells (including transfused cells), resulting in haemoglobinaemia, haemoglobinuria, and fall in haemoglobin. It is accompanied by high fever, vomiting, and jaundice. The parasites are difficult to find in the blood. The urine appears dark red to brown-black due to the presence of free haemoglobin and also contains protein, hyaline and granular casts, and epithelial debris. Haemoglobinuria can occur when persons with glucose-6-phosphate dehydrogenase (G6PD) deficiency are treated with primaquine or other oxidant drug.

Anaemia

This can be severe and occur rapidly, particularly in young children[23]. Anaemia in falciparum malaria is due mainly to the destruction of parasitized red cells. Parasitized cells also lose their deformability and are rapidly phagocytosed and destroyed in the spleen. The production of red cells in the bone marrow is also reduced and there is a slow reticulocyte response. An immune destruction of non-parasitized red cells also occurs. In young children with severe anaemia, tissue anoxia can develop, leading to acidosis.

Hypoglycaemia

This is a common finding particularly in children and pregnant women with severe falciparum malaria, and as a complication of those treated with quinine and quinidine (drugs thought to stimulate the pancreas to produce insulin which lowers blood glucose levels).

Falciparum malaria in pregnancy

Normal immune responses are reduced during pregnancy. In areas of stable malaria transmission, a pregnant woman will have acquired partial immunity to malaria. This will protect her against serious clinical falciparum malaria but not prevent heavy parasitic infection of the placenta and anaemia (often severe) which can result in a low birth weight baby which may not survive. First pregnancies are at greatest risk.

In areas of unstable malaria transmission, pregnant women lack protective immunity and are at serious risk of developing severe life-threatening falciparum malaria, particularly in the last few months of pregnancy and for several weeks after delivery. Untreated infections can result in abortion, still-birth, premature labour or low birth weight. Cerebral malaria, pulmonary oedema, and hypoglycaemia frequently occur. The situation is similar in all pregnancies.

Note: Further information on severe falciparum, malaria-related anaemia and malaria in pregnancy can be found in the references (Nos 22–27) at the end of subunit 5.14.

HIV and falciparum malaria[21]

In those infected with HIV, susceptibility to malaria and parasitaemia increase as immune responses fail. Clinical malaria is more common, particularly in less immune people. Acute falciparum malaria is thought to increase transiently HIV viral concentration. In pregnant women, particularly multigravidae, HIV-associated immunosuppression contributes to more frequent and severe malaria, anaemia, placental malaria, low birth weight, and poor infant survival. Malaria is thought to contribute to increased HIV replication, with possible disease progression and increased risk of mother-to-child transmission of HIV. Antimalarial treatment and responses are often poor.

Malaria caused by P. vivax, P. ovale, P. malariae

Malaria caused by *Plasmodium vivax* is referred to as vivax malaria, formerly known as benign tertian (BT) malaria.

Malaria caused by *Plasmodium ovale* is referred to as ovale malaria, formerly known as ovale tertian malaria.

Malaria caused by *Plasmodium malariae* is referred to as malariae malaria, also referred to as quartan malaria.

Infections caused by *P. vivax*, *P. ovale* or *P. malariae* are rarely life-threatening. Cytoadherence of parasitized cells does not occur and parasitic densities are lower. In vivax and ovale malaria, parasite numbers rarely exceed 50 000/μl or 2% of cells infected, and in quartan malaria (*P. malariae)* parasite numbers are usually less than 10 000/μl with only up to 1% of cells becoming infected.

Relapses are a feature of vivax and ovale malaria due to the delayed development of PE schizonts from hypnozoites in liver cells (see previous text).

Repeated malaria attacks (often over several years) are a feature of *P. malariae* but these are not relapses caused by dormant hypnozoites but recrudescences caused by small numbers of erythrocytic forms of the parasite persisting in the host (recrudescences can also occur in falciparum malaria for up to 1 year following the first attack).

A serious complication of infection with *P. malariae* is nephrotic syndrome which may progress to renal failure. It occurs more frequently in children and is caused by damage to the kidneys following the deposition of antigen-antibody complexes on the glomerular basement membrane of the kidney. It produces oedema, marked proteinuria, and a low serum albumin level.

Hyper-reactive malaria splenomegaly

In this rare condition there is a defective regulation of immune responses associated with recurrent infection by *P. falciparum*, *P. vivax* or *P. malariae*. Those affected are immune adults in malaria endemic areas. The condition is characterized by massive and chronic splenomegaly with high levels of IgM, malaria antibody, and circulating immune complexes, and a moderately enlarged liver with hepatic sinusoidal lymphocytosis. The patient is usually anaemic (normocytic) and has low white cell and platelet counts. Malaria parasites are rarely found in blood films.

Genetic factors that protect against malaria

- *P. vivax* is rarely found in West Africa or other places where the red cells of the population lack the Duffy blood group antigens Fy^a and Fy^b. The glycophorin receptors which *P. vivax* needs to attach to and invade red cells are missing on Duffy negative red cells. The protection is absolute and afforded only to homozygotes.

- Persons with the haemoglobin genotype HbAS (sickle cell trait) are protected against severe falciparum malaria. Parasitaemia is lower because HbAS cells sickle in the circulation and are removed by the spleen before the parasites can develop into schizonts. Sickle cell anaemia (HbSS) is not protective and can cause fatalities in young children with falciparum malaria.

- Persons with ovalocytosis have lower parasite densities of *P. falciparum* and *P. vivax*. Elliptical red cells resist parasitic invasion. In areas of South East Asia and Papua New Guinea where falciparum malaria is endemic there is a high prevalence of ovalocytosis.

- Newborn infants have protection against malaria in their first few months of life when there is a high concentration of HbF in their red cells. Malaria parasites do not grow well in red cells containing HbF.

- β (beta)-thalassaemia trait also appears to protect against severe falciparum infection.

- Possession of certain human leucocyte antigens (HLA) are also thought to protect against severe malaria, such as class I antigen HLA-BW53 and class II antigen HLA-DRB1 1302.

Note: With genes that confer resistance to falciparum malaria but can cause death, such as HbS, there occurs what is called balanced polymorphism in which the death of homozygotes (HbSS) is offset by the survival advantage of heterozygotes (HbAS) in falciparum malaria endemic areas.

Global malaria control

Reducing the suffering and loss of life caused by malaria is possible, providing the financial, political, and technical commitment to achieve this is strengthened.[18,28,29,30] The WHO/UNICEF/UNDP and World Bank *Roll Back Malaria Partnership*, the *Global Fund to fight AIDS, Tuberculosis, and Malaria*, the *Medicines for Malaria Venture*, the *Gates Malaria Partnership* and the *Multilateral Initiative on Malaria* have been established to reduce the burden of malaria by:

- implementing malaria control strategies,
- improving health infrastructures,

- raising awareness of malaria and its effects on poverty and development,
- mobilising communities to combat malaria,
- raising and monitoring funds to effect and sustain malaria control programmes and the development of antimalarial drugs and vaccines.

Strategies to control and prevent malaria[31, 32, 33]
- Providing *accessible* malaria diagnostic facilities and *affordable*, accessible, *effective* drugs to treat promptly active infections and prevent malaria in those at risk such as pregnant women and non-immune persons visiting or going to work in endemic areas. Also, increasing public awareness of the dangers of malaria and how to reduce contact with mosquitoes.
- Avoiding mosquito bites by using long-lasting insecticide-treated bed nets, screening windows and doors with mosquito netting, wearing protective clothing, and using mosquito repellents.
- Preventing the breeding of mosquitoes by removing surface water, filling in ponds, drainage ditches, potholes, etc, altering breeding sites, spraying breeding sites and destroying adult mosquitoes using effective chemicals as part of a control programme.
- Acting more rapidly and effectively to control epidemics in complex emergency situations.[19, 33]

Malaria vaccines: Information on the development of malaria vaccines can be found in *Disease Watch Malaria* 2004,[18] in the papers of Ripley Balbu *et al*,[34] Moree *et al*,[35] and Webster *et al*.[36] Also, *Roll Back Malaria Partnership* website[33] and the *Malaria Vaccine Initiative* website.[37]

Drug resistance of malaria parasites

Effective, affordable, and safe treatment of malaria, particularly falciparum malaria, is becoming increasingly difficult as resistance to quinoline and antifol antimalarial drugs continues to spread throughout the tropics. Multiple drug resistance is common in South East Asia. *P. vivax* resistance to chloroquine is also spreading, with reports of resistance from Thailand, Papua New Guinea, Indonesia, Myanmar, India, Somalia, Brazil and Colombia.

Information on antimalarial drugs used to treat and prevent malaria can be found in the 21st edition of *Mansons Tropical Diseases*, 5th edition *Lecture Notes on Tropical Medicine* (see Recommended reading) and also from the WHO *Roll Back Malaria Partnership*, website www.rbm.who.int

Most resistant strains of *P. falciparum* have developed due to inadequate drug doses mainly as a result of unregulated drug distribution and prescribing, lack of adequate drugs, poor quality of drugs, and incorrect taking of antimalarials by patients. Treatment failure can also occur for reasons other than drug resistance, e.g. vomiting or failure to absorb the drug.

Classifying antimalarial drug resistance[24]

RI   – Following treatment, parasitaemia clears by day 3 but reappears by day 14.

RII   – Following treatment, there is a reduction but not a clearance of parasitaemia. Parasitaemia falls to less than 25% of day-0 density by day 2 or 3, but increases by day 7 or 14.

RIII   – Following treatment there is no reduction of parasitaemia, i.e. parasitaemia never falls below 25% of the day-0 level and may even increase after treatment.

The above method of classifying resistance, based on counting trophozoites in blood films on days 0, 1, 2, 3, 7 and 14, is referred to as *in vivo* testing.

Counting parasite numbers is described under Laboratory Diagnosis.

More recent antimalarial drug resistance classification[24]
Early treatment failure (ETF) – Patient develops severe illness with parasitaemia during the first 4 days after treatment, or patient remains febrile and parasitaemic throughout the 4 days.

Late treatment failure (LTF) – Patient initially improves clinically but both fever and parasitaemia recur by day 14.

Adequate clinical response (ACR) – Patient has neither ETC nor LTF and does not develop febrile parasitaemia by day 14, i.e. patient may have either fever or parasitaemia by day 14, but not both.

In vitro testing
By culturing *P. falciparum*, antimalarial drug susceptibility can be tested by measuring the inhibition of development to the schizont stage. Such a test is useful in epidemiology and control of malaria. Full details can be obtained from WHO Malaria Control Unit, WHO, 1211 Geneva, 27-Switzerland.

    In vitro testing cannot be used to predict a patient's clinical response to treatment.

LABORATORY DIAGNOSIS

The diagnosis of malaria is by:
- Detecting and identifying malaria parasites microscopically in blood films.
- Concentrating parasites in venous blood by centrifugation when they cannot be found in blood films.
- Using a malaria rapid diagnostic test (RDT) to detect malaria antigen.

Other tests
- Measurement of haemoglobin or packed cell volume when there is malaria with heavy parasitaemia particularly in young children and pregnant women, see subunit 8.4 in Part 2.
- Measurement of blood glucose to detect hypoglycaemia, particularly in young children and

pregnant women with severe falciparum malaria. The test is described in subunit 6.5.

- Total white cell count and platelet count (severe falciparum malaria), see subunit 8.6 in Part 2.

- Coagulation tests if abnormal bleeding is suspected in falciparum malaria. Measurement of plasma fibrinogen, FDP's (fibrin/fibrinogen degradation products) and other coagulation tests are described in subunit 8.11 in Part 2.

- Testing urine for free haemoglobin when malaria haemoglobinuria is suspected (see subunit 6.11).

- Blood urea (see subunit 6.4) or serum creatinine (see subunit 6.3) to monitor renal failure.

- Testing urine for protein when nephrotic syndrome is suspected (see subunit 6.11).

- Screening for G_6PD deficiency before treating a patient with an oxidant drug such as primaquine (see subunit 8.9 in Part 2).

Laboratory indices of poor prognosis in falciparum malaria
The following laboratory indices are considered indicative of a poor prognosis in falciparum malaria:

- Heavy parasitaemia with more than 5% of red cells parasitized (250 000 parasites/μl) (lower in non-immune persons).

- Presence of mature trophozoites, malaria pigment in neutrophils, and schizonts in peripheral blood films.

- Peripheral leucocytosis of more than 12 000/μl.

- Low cerebrospinal fluid lactate level (test requires the facilities of a specialist laboratory).

- Low antithrombin 111 levels (test requires the facilities of a specialist laboratory).

- Serum creatinine of more than 265 μmol/l.

- Blood urea nitrogen of more than 21.4 mmol/l.

- Packed cell volume of less than 0.20 or haemoglobin lower than 7.0 g/dl (in previously non-anaemic person).

- Blood glucose of less than 2.2 mmol/l.

- Raised serum aminotransferases (these tests cannot usually be performed in district laboratories).

Blood transfusion in severe falciparum malaria

Blood transfusion may be necessary to correct severe anaemia or to replace deficient clotting factors (fresh blood required). In patients with severe malaria, there may be difficulty in determining the blood group because of autoagglutination of the person's red cells. Testing of the patient's serum as well as red cells is necessary and autocontrols must be used (see Chapter 9 in Part 2).

DETECTING AND IDENTIFYING MALARIA PARASITES IN BLOOD FILMS

It is important for laboratory staff to:

- Process and report malaria blood films with the *minimum of delay.*

- Use standardized and adequately controlled methods for preparing, staining, and reporting blood films.

- Follow a *Safe Code of Practice* when collecting and handling blood specimens and disposing of contaminated lancets, syringes, and needles (see subunits 3.3 and 3.4).

Collection of blood
Malaria blood films are best prepared directly from capillary blood. EDTA (sequestrene) anticoagulated venous blood can also be used providing the blood films are made soon after collecting the blood (within 30 minutes) and thick films are handled with care to prevent the blood being washed from the slide during staining.

Need for thick and thin blood films

Thick film: Compared with a thin film, a thick film is about 30 times more sensitive (detecting about 20 parasites/μl). A thick film is therefore the most suitable for the rapid detection of malaria parasites, particularly when they are few. In areas where *P. malariae* is found, unless a thick film is examined, infection is likely to be missed because parasitaemia is normally low with this species. In a thick film the blood is not fixed. The red cells are lyzed during staining, allowing parasites and white cells to be seen in a much larger volume of blood.

Thin blood film: This is required to confirm the *Plasmodium* species if this is not clear from the thick film. The blood cells are fixed in a thin film, enabling the parasites to be seen in the red cells. Parasitized red cells may become enlarged, oval in shape, or stippled. These features can help to identify *Plasmodium* species. Examination of a thin film greatly assists in the identification of mixed infections.

By counting the percentage of parasitized red cells before and after treatment, thin films are also of value in assessing whether a patient with falciparum malaria is responding to treatment in areas where drug resistance is suspected.

Examination of a thin film also gives the opportunity to investigate anaemia and white cell abnormalities, and in the absence of malaria parasites, suggest an alternative diagnosis, e.g. sickle cell disease.

When to collect blood for malaria parasites

Blood should be collected:

- as soon as malaria is suspected (it may be necessary to collect blood on several occasions to detect the parasites).

- before the patient receives antimalarial drugs.

Note: Always ask an out-patient whether any antimalarial drug has been taken recently.

Making thick and thin blood films

Thick and thin blood films can be made on separate slides or on the same slide which may be more convenient when ward staff are collecting the blood. Whenever possible use slides with frosted ends to facilitate labelling.

Standardizing the amount of blood used and area covered by the thick film

To ensure good staining, reproducibility, and standardization of reporting, the amount of blood used, particularly to make thick films, should be kept as constant as possible and the blood should be spread evenly over a specified area of the slide.

One way of achieving this is to use a plastic bulb pipette to collect the blood and a card which shows a line drawing of a slide, sizes of blood drops, position of the films, and area to be covered by the thick film (see Fig. 5.25). The card can be sealed in a transparent plastic bag to protect it from blood contamination. Such a card can be used by laboratory staff and given to ward staff that collect blood, e.g. paediatric nursing staff.

Capillary blood method (thick and thin films on same slide)

1 Cleanse the lobe of the finger (or heel if an infant) using a swab moistened with 70% v/v alcohol. Allow the area to dry.

2 Using a sterile lancet, prick the finger or heel. Squeeze gently to obtain a large drop of blood. Collect the blood preferably in a small plastic bulb pipette.

3 Using a completely clean *grease-free* microscope slide and preferably a malaria slide card, add a small drop of blood to the centre of the slide and a larger drop about 15 mm to the right (see Fig. 5.25).

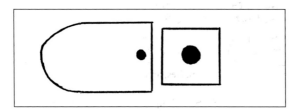

Fig 5.25 Slide card for making thin and thick blood films, showing size of blood drops and area of slide to cover for a thin film and thick film.

4 Immediately spread the thin film using a *smooth* edged slide spreader (see Fig. 5.26). Blood from anaemic patients needs spreading more quickly with the spreader held at a steeper angle.

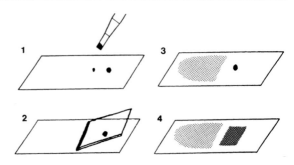

Fig 5.26 Making thin and thick blood films

Spreading a thin blood film: This takes practice. A well made thin blood film should have a smooth tail end (not ragged) and be free of vertical lines and 'holes'. A poorly spread film is extremely difficult to report because the red cells, parasites, and white cells will appear distorted. It is essential to use a spreader which has a smooth ground glass polished edge.

5 Without delay, spread the large drop of blood to make the thick smear. Cover evenly an area about 15 × 15 mm (see Fig. 5.25). It should just be possible to see (but not read) newsprint through the film. When spreading the blood, mix it as little as possible to avoid the red cells forming marked rouleaux which can cause the blood to be easily washed from the slide during staining.

6 Using a black lead pencil, label the slide with the date and the patient's name and number. If a slide having a frosted end is not used, write the information neatly on the top of the *thin* film (after it has dried).

7 Allow the blood to air-dry with the slide in a horizontal position and placed in a safe place.

Drying thick blood films: It is good practice to keep a separate box or deep tray for drying malaria blood films. Cover it with a lid made from netting to protect the films from insects and dust (flies will rapidly 'clean' blood from a slide). If the box or tray is placed in a warm sunny place, the thick film will dry quickly (do not allow the blood to remain in the sun after it has dried). In humid climates, it may be necessary to use a hand dryer or an incubator to dry thick blood films.

Fixing thin blood films

Use absolute methanol (methyl alcohol) or when not available, ethanol (ethyl alcohol) to fix thin blood films. The alcohol must be free from water otherwise it will not fix the cells properly. Always make sure the stock bottle of alcohol is kept tightly stoppered. For routine use, keep a small amount of alcohol in a dispensing bottle, which can be closed in between use.

Method of fixing a thin film when on a slide with a thick film

1 Place the slide horizontally on a *level* bench or on a staining rack.

2 Apply a *small* drop of absolute methanol or ethanol to the thin film, making sure the alcohol *does not touch* the thick film as this will prevent lysis of the red cells and make the thick film unreadable. Alternatively apply the methanol to the thin film using a swab. Allow the thin film to fix for 1–2 minutes.

Staining malaria parasites

Malaria parasites in thick and thin blood films require staining at pH 7.1–7.2 using a Romanowsky stain (contains azure dyes and eosin). The stains most frequently used in district laboratories are:

- Field's stain
- Giemsa stain

Field's stain

This water-based Romanowsky stain is composed of two solutions, Field's stain A and Field's stain B. It is buffered to the correct pH and neither solution requires dilution when staining thick films. When staining thin films, Field's stain B requires dilution. Compared with Giemsa working stain, Field's stains are more stable. They stain fresh blood films well, particularly thick films. The rapid technique is ideally suited for staining blood films from waiting outpatients and when reports are required urgently.

Giemsa stain

This is an alcohol-based Romanowsky stain that requires dilution in pH 7.1–7.2 buffered water before use. It gives the best staining of malaria parasites in thin films. It also stains thick films well providing they are completely dry (overnight drying is recommended), the concentration of stain is low, and the staining time is sufficiently long. Less satisfactory results are obtained when the concentration of Giemsa stain is greatly increased to reduce the staining time. Care must be taken to prevent water from entering the stock stain. Giemsa stain is commonly used in malaria survey work because many films can be stained at one time and differentiation of the different species in thin films is excellent.

Staining thick and thin films on the same slide

When using Field's stain, the thin film should be fixed and stained *first* using Field's thin film staining technique, followed by staining of the thick film using Field's thick film staining technique.

THIN FILM FIELD'S STAINING TECHNIQUE

Required

Field's stain A	Reagent No. 25
Field's stain B, diluted 1 in 5†	
Buffered pH 7.1–7.2 water	Reagent No. 14

† Prepare by mixing 1 ml of Field's stain B (Reagent No 26) with 4 ml of pH 7.2 buffered water. A syringe or graduated plastic bulb pipette can be used to measure the stain and buffered water.

Method

1 Place the slide on a staining rack and cover the methanol-fixed thin film with approximately 0.5 ml of diluted Field's stain B.

2 Add immediately an equal volume of Field's stain A and mix with the diluted Field's stain B. Leave to stain for 1 minute.

Note: The stains can be easily applied and mixed on the slide by using 1 ml graduated plastic bulb pipettes.

3 Wash off the stain with clean water. Wipe the back of the slide clean and place it in a draining rack for the film to air-dry.

Results for malaria thin film

Chromatin of parasite	Dark red
Cytoplasm of parasite	Blue
Schuffner's dots	Red
Maurer's dots (clefts)	Red-mauve
Malaria pigment in white cells	Brown-black
Red cells	Grey to pale mauve-pink
Reticulocytes	Grey-blue
Nuclei of neutrophils	Dark purple
Cytoplasm of mononuclear cells	Blue-grey
Granules of eosinophils	Red

THICK FILM FIELD'S STAINING TECHNIQUE

Required

Container of Field's stain A*	Reagent No. 25
Container of Field's stain B*	Reagent No. 26
Two containers of clean water (need not be buffered)	

* While Field's stains A and B are stable and can be used for staining several thick blood films, it is recommended that the stains are changed frequently to reduce the risk of infection and carry-over of parasites, and also to promote standardized staining.

Caution: Thick blood films are not fixed and the stains do not kill parasites, viruses, or other pathogens which may be present in the blood. See later text for staining *HIGH RISK* blood specimens.

Method

1 Holding the slide with the *dried* thick film facing downwards, dip the slide into Field's stain A for 5 seconds. Drain off the excess stain by touching

a corner of the slide against the side of the container.

2 Wash gently for about 5 seconds in clean water. Drain off the excess water.

3 Dip the slide into Field's stain B for 3 seconds. Drain off the excess stain.

4 Wash gently in clean water. Wipe the back of the slide clean and place it upright in a draining rack for the film to air-dry.

Note: If after staining, the whole of the film appears yellow-brown (usually a sign that too much blood has been used), too blue, or too pink, *do not* attempt to examine it. Restain it by dipping the slide into Field's stain A for 1 second, followed by a gentle wash in clean water, dip into Field's stain B for 1 second and a final gentle wash in clean water.

Results for malaria thick film

Chromatin of parasite . . . . .Dark red
Cytoplasm of parasite . . . . .Blue-mauve
Schuffner's dots around . . . . .Pale red
P. vivax and P. ovale parasites
Malaria pigment . . . . .Yellow-brown
or brown-black
Nuclei of small lymphocytes . . . . .Dark purple
Nuclei of neutrophils . . . . .Dark purple
Granules of eosinophils . . . . .Red
Cytoplasm of mononuclear cells . . . . . . .Blue-grey
Reticulum of reticulocytes . . . . .Blue-grey
stippling in background

Alternative thick film Field's staining technique for HIGH RISK specimens

Thick blood films which may contain highly infectious pathogens, e.g. haemorrhagic fever viruses, hepatitis viruses, or HIV, should not be stained by the dip technique (unless the solutions are discarded after use). A safer alternative staining technique is as follows:

1 Holding the slide, apply a large drop of Field's stain A to cover the thick film.

2 Immediately wash off the stain with water. Apply the water to the back of the slide to prevent loss of the blood. Drain off the excess water.

3 Apply a drop of Field's stain B. Immediately wash off the stain with water.

4 Stand the slide on a piece of absorbent paper to drain, supported against a suitable upright. When the film is dry, wipe the edge of the slide with a piece of absorbent paper soaked in 70% v/v alcohol. Discard this and the drainage piece of paper into hypochlorite disinfectant or bleach solution.

5 Before examining the dried film, mount a cover glass on top of it (immersion oil can be used as the mountant). Even after staining, a thick unfixed blood film containing parasites and pathogenic viruses remains infectious and must be handled with care.

GIEMSA STAINING TECHNIQUE

Required

Giemsa stain	Reagent No. 31
Buffered water, pH 7.1–7.2	Reagent No. 14
or buffered saline, pH 7.1–7.2*	Reagent No. 13

*Buffered physiological saline is recommended because it provides a cleaner background to films and better preservation of parasite morphology.

Method

1 Immediately before use, dilute the Giemsa stain as required:

3% solution for 30 minute staining

Measure 50 ml of buffered water (or saline) pH 7.1–7.2. Add 1.5 ml of Giemsa stain and mix gently. The stain can be measured using a dry graduated plastic bulb pipette or a small volume (2 ml) plastic syringe.

10% solution for 10 minute staining

Measure 45 ml of buffered water, pH 7.1–7.2 in a 50 ml cylinder. Add 5 ml of Giemsa stain (to 50 ml mark) and mix gently.

2 Place the slides *face downwards** in a shallow tray supported on two rods, in a Coplin jar, or in a staining rack for immersion in a staining trough. Thick blood films must be thoroughly dried and thin blood films must be fixed (methanol for 2 minutes).

*This is necessary to prevent fine particles of stain being deposited on the film(s).

3 Pour the diluted stain into the shallow tray, Coplin jar, or staining trough. Stain as follows:

30 minutes if using a 3% stain solution
10 minutes if using a 10% stain solution

4 Wash the stain from the staining container using clean water (need not be distilled or buffered).

Important: Flushing the stain from the slides and staining container is necessary to avoid the films being covered with a fine deposit of stain.

5 Wipe the back of each slide clean and place it in a draining rack for the preparation to air-dry.

Results

Chromatin of parasite . . . . Dark red
Cytoplasm of parasite . . . . Blue
Schuffner's dots . . . . Red
Maurer's dots (clefts) . . . . Red-mauve
Red cells . . . . Grey to pale mauve
Reticulocytes . . . . Grey-blue

Nuclei of neutrophils . . . . Dark purple
Granules of neutrophils . . . . Mauve-purple
Granules of eosinophils . . . . Red
Cytoplasm of mononuclear cells . . . . Blue-grey

Reporting blood films for malaria parasites

Blood films should be examined microscopically using the 40× and 100× objectives. Whenever possible 7× eyepieces should be used in preference to 10× eyepieces (with the 100× oil immersion objective) because these give a brighter and clearer image. WHO and others recommend the use of 7× eyepieces and advize against the use of 10× eyepieces for malaria work.[38,39] Good illumination is *essential* (see subunit 4.3).

REPORTING THICK BLOOD FILMS

1   When the thick film is *completely* dry, apply a drop of immersion oil to an area of the film which appears mauve coloured (usually around the edges).

2   Spread the oil to cover an area about 10 mm in diameter (there is no need to add a cover glass). This is to enable the film to be examined *first* at a lower magnification.

Value of low power magnification examination
Preliminary scanning with the 10× and 40× objectives will:

– indicate quickly the most suitable parts of the film to examine with the 100× objective, i.e. areas of good staining and correct thickness.

– provide information on the white cells, particularly whether they contain pigment and whether there are any marked changes in cell numbers and types, e.g. neutrophilia or eosinophilia.

– avoid missing trypanosomes, microfilariae, and borreliae.

– show whether there is a marked reticulocytosis (heavy blue stippling in the background) which may indicate sickle cell anaemia.

3   Select an area that is well stained and not too thick. Change to the 100× objective (if required add a further small drop of oil).

4   Examine for malaria parasites and malaria pigment. Use the flow chart in Fig. 5.27, boxed texts, and colour plates 5.43–5.46 to help identify the parasites. If necessary, confirm the *Plasmodium* species by examining the thin blood film (see following text).

Examine at least 100 high power (100× objective) microscope fields for parasites. In areas where *P. malariae* exists, examine approximately 200 fields (parasitaemia is usually low).

5   Report the approximate numbers of parasites (trophozoites, schizonts, and gametocytes) and also whether malaria pigment is present in white cells (always mention when the pigment is in neutrophils). The following plus sign scheme can be used to report parasite numbers:

Parasites
1–10   per 100 high power fields . . . .+
11–100   per 100 high power fields . . . .++
1–10   in every high power field . . . . .+++
More than 10 in every high power field . .++++

Note: With falciparum infections, because the gametocytes are easily recognized, it is possible to report separately the asexual and sexual forms e.g. *P. falciparum* trophs +++, gametocytes +, with malaria pigment in white cells.

6   When falciparum malaria parasitaemia is +++ or more (severe infection), perform the following:

–   Count the percentage of *red cells infected* in the thin blood film (see following text). Perform this count on days 1, 2, 3, 7 and 14 following treatment to check for a decrease and clearing of parasites (see previous text, *Classifying antimalarial drug resistance*).

–   Measure the haemoglobin. If the patient is severely anaemic, repeat the test daily particularly if the patient is a child or pregnant woman.

–   Test for hypoglycaemia (see subunit 6.5). This can be a cause of sudden death in severe falciparum malaria.

Important: A low parasitaemia in falciparum malaria does not exclude a serious infection. It can occur when most parasitized red cells are in the capillaries of deep tissues, undergoing schizogony.

7   If no parasites are found after examining 100 fields (or if indicated 200 fields), report the film as:

Malaria thick film: NPF (No parasites found).

Look for other clues in both thick and thin blood films which may help to establish the reason for the patient's fever, e.g. bacterial infection blood picture, other parasitic infection (e.g. trypanosomiasis) or sickle cell disease in a young child (see Colour Plate 5.43).

Patients with malaria but no parasites are found
The commonest causes for not finding parasites (given the reliability of laboratory examination) are that the patient has taken antimalarial drugs or the parasites are too few to be detected in the peripheral blood. Blood films should be collected several hours later when more parasites may be present

(following schizogony). The finding of malaria pigment can help to establish the diagnosis.

Note: Occasionally during routine blood film reporting, parasites may be found when a patient does not have clinical malaria. This is a common finding in adults with protective immunity (areas of stable malaria transmission).

Malaria pigment in white cells

This appears as brown-black granules in monocytes and occasionally in neutrophils. It should always be reported. Pigment in white cells, particularly in neutrophils is associated with severe falciparum malaria. It can give an indication of whole body parasite density, especially when the peripheral blood film shows no parasites or very few (due to cytoadherence). The implications of finding malaria pigment in severe falciparum malaria has been reviewed by Amodu, O.K. *et al.*[40]

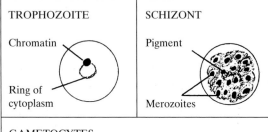

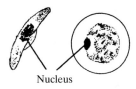

TROPHOZOITE	SCHIZONT
Chromatin	Pigment
Ring of cytoplasm	Merozoites
GAMETOCYTES	
Nucleus	**Note:** Compared with the male gametocyte, the female gametocyte is often larger, stains more deeply, and has a more compact nucleus.

Fig. 5.23   Morphology of trophozoite, schizont, and gametocytes of malaria parasites.

REPORTING THIN BLOOD FILMS

Changes which take place in parasitized red cells can help to identify *Plasmodium* species and to detect mixed infections. Examination of a thin film is also required to count the percentage of parasitized red cells in severe falciparum infections. It also enables a white cell differential count to be performed when required, and the morphology of red cells to be reported in severe anaemia.

The method of examining a thin blood film for malaria parasites is as follows:

1   When the stained thin film is completely dry, apply a drop of immersion oil to the lower third of the film and spread the oil to cover most of this part of the film (serves as a cover glass).

2   Examine the film first with 40× objective to check the staining, morphology, and distribution of the cells and to detect malaria schizonts, gametocytes, and trophozoites (the very small rings of *P. falciparum* may not be seen with this objective). *P. malariae* and *P. ovale* parasites can often be found on the edges of a thin film.

Red cell changes

Look particularly for changes in the appearance of parasitized red cells, such as:

● enlargement and irregular shape, characteristic of *P. vivax.*

● oval cells with ragged ends as seen with *P. ovale.*

● red stippling (Schuffner's dots) as seen with *P. vivax* and *P. ovale* and less distinct irregular stippling (Maurer's clefts) as seen with *P. falciparum.*

● parasites forming a band across red cells, a feature of *P. malariae.*

● several parasites in a single red cell as is common with *P. falciparum* and some strains of *P. vivax.*

3   Change to the 100× objective to examine the parasites. Use the colour plates 5.43–46 to help identify the different *Plasmodium* species.

4   If the thin blood film is well made and well stained, report also:

● any marked increase in white cell numbers and if indicated perform a differential white cell count. Atypical mononuclear cells are often present in falciparum malaria.

● any abnormal red cell morphology and presence of nucleated red cells.

Note: If the film has been made from EDTA anticoagulated *venous* blood, it should also be possible to comment on platelet numbers if the film has been well spread and stained. Do not, however, attempt to report platelet numbers in films made from capillary blood (platelets clump in capillary blood). If thrombocytopenia is suspected, e.g. in severe falciparum malaria, perform a platelet count (see subunit 8.6 in Part 2).

Counting the percentage of parasitized red cells

Count the percentage of parasitized red cells when there is high falciparum malaria parasitaemia (+ + +

or more parasites seen in the thick film). It can help to monitor a patient's response to treatment. A simple method of counting the percentage of parasitized red cells is as follows:

1 Using the 100× objective, select an area of the thin film where the total number of red cells is approximately 250 per field.

2 Count the number of parasitized red cells in 8 fields, i.e. approximately 2 000 cells.

3 Divide by 20 to calculate the percentage (%) of parasitized cells.

Note: WHO considers falciparum parasitaemia to be heavy and to carry a poor prognosis when more than 5% of red cells are parasitized (>250 000 parasites/μl). There is a very high risk of mortality when more than 10% of cells are parasitized (>500 000 parasites/μl).

Counting parasite numbers
The following two methods are commonly used:

Estimating parasite numbers/μl of blood from the thick film

This is carried out by multiplying the average number of parasites per high power field (100× objective and 10× eyepiece) by 500. Between 10–50 fields (depending on parasitaemia) should be examined to determine the average number of trophozoites per high power field (HPF). Ten fields are sufficient when the parasite density is high.

The factor of 500 was proposed by Greenwood and Armstrong.[41] They calculated that 5–8 μl is the volume of blood required to make a satisfactory thick film and that the volume of blood in one HPF (100× objective, 10× eyepieces) of a well-prepared thick film is about 0.002 μl. Therefore the number of parasites per HPF multiplied by 500 gives the estimated number of parasites/μl of blood. This method, Greenwood and Armstrong found to be more accurate and quicker than counting the parasites against white cells as described in the following method.

Estimating parasite numbers/μl of blood by counting parasites against white cells

1 Select a part of the thick film where the white cells are evenly distributed and the parasites are well stained.

2 Using the oil immersion objective, systematically count 100 white blood cells (WBC), estimating at the same time the numbers of parasites (asexual) in each field covered. Counting is best done by using two hand tally counters.

Repeat this in two other areas of the film and take an average of the three counts.

3 Calculate the number of parasites per μl of blood as follows:

$$\frac{\text{WBC count} \times \text{Parasites counted against 100 WBC}}{100}$$

Example
Patient's WBC count = 4000/μl
Parasites counted against 100 WBC = 680

$$\text{Parasite count:} \frac{4000 \times 680}{100} = 27\,200/\mu l$$

Concentrating malaria parasites
Centrifuging EDTA anticoagulated venous blood in a narrow bore tube gives excellent concentration of *P. vivax* parasitized red cells just below the buffy coat layer (white cells and platelets). Other species are less well concentrated but detection of the parasites in stained buffy coat preparations, especially late stage trophozoites and gametocytes, is often possible when no parasites are found in thick and thin blood films.

In buffy coat preparations, the red cells are not destroyed and the parasites stain well and appear more clearly defined than in thick films. Malaria pigment in white cells is more easily detected because the white cells are concentrated.

Method of preparing buffy coat preparations to concentrate malaria parasites

While preparations can be made from centrifuging blood in capillary tubes and then breaking the tubes to obtain the buffy coat layer and red cells below it, this technique can be dangerous and should be avoided.

A safer technique, but one that requires a longer period of centrifugation is as follows:

1 Using a narrow stem plastic bulb pipette or Pasteur pipette, fill two small narrow bore plastic or glass test tubes with EDTA (sequestrene) anticoagulated venous blood. Tubes measuring 6 × 50 mm are suitable (each tube holds about 0.7 ml of blood), or alternatively use *Eppendorf* type microtubes.

Note: A narrow bore tube is best filled by inserting the tip of the pipette containing the blood to the bottom of the tube and withdrawing it as the tube fills.

2 Centrifuge the blood at about RCF 1 000 g for 15 minutes.*

* To judge the best length of time to centrifuge, individual laboratories should try centrifuging at different times, e.g. 10, 15, 20, 25 minutes to evaluate the times which give the best concentration of locally found *Plasmodium* species.

3 Remove and discard (into disinfectant) the supernatant plasma above the buffy coat layer.

Method continued on page 255

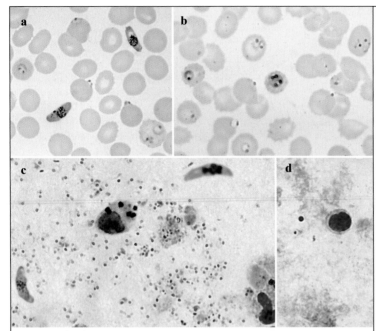

Plate 5.43 *P.falciparum*. **a** Trophozoites and gametocytes in thin film. **b** Young schizont (rare), and trophozoites. **c** Many trophozoites, gametocyte, and white cells containing pigment in Fields stained thick film. **d** Thick film from patient with sickle cell disease and falciparum malaria. Note, blue stippling in background (reticulocytosis) and nucleated red cell nucleus (above trophozoite).

Plasmodium falciparum
- Widespread in tropics.
- Often high parasitaemia.
- Only trophozoites and gametocytes usually seen.

Trophozoites
- Small rings, occasionally larger rings in heavy infections.*
- Often with double chromatin dot.
- May lie on red cell membrane (accolé forms).

* Parasites are difficult to recognize if patient has taken antimalarials. Trophozoites of resistant strains can appear thick and distorted.

Schizonts
- Only seen occasionally in severe infections.
- Usually with 2 or 4 merozoites and pigment.

Gametocytes
- Banana shaped.
- Rounded forms may be seen if film dries slowly.

Host cell
- Often contains several parasites.
- Irregular mauve-red Maurer's dots (clefts) seen in cells with mature rings.

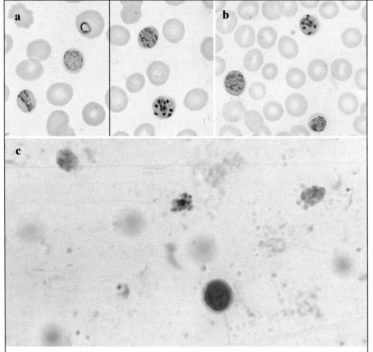

Plate 5.46 *P.malariae*. **a** Trophozoites (Bird's eye and band forms, gametocyte, and schizont in thin film. **b** Schizont, trophozoite, and gametocyte in thin film. **c** Trophozoites, schizonts, and gametocyte in Fields stained thick film.

Plasmodium malariae
- Low prevalence in tropics and subtropics.
- Rarely more than 1% of cells infected (easily missed).
- Trophozoites, schizonts and gametocytes usually seen.

Trophozoites
- Thick, neat, densely stained.
- Yellow-brown pigment in late trophozoites.
- Band forms can be seen in thin films.
- Occasionally 'bird's-eye' ring form may be seen.

Schizonts
- Small with neatly arranged (up to 12) merozoites.
- Yellow-brown pigment.

Gametocytes
- Small, round or oval (can be difficult to differentiate from late trophozoites).
- Yellow-brown pigment.

Host cell
- No changes.
- Older cells parasitized.

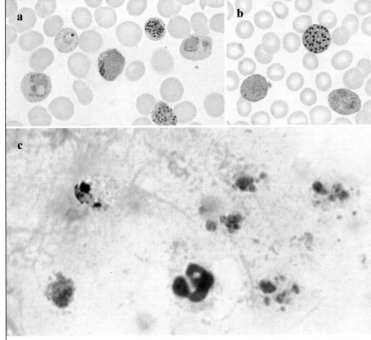

Plate 5.44 *P.vivax*. **a** Trophozoites, gametocytes, and schizonts in thin film. **b** Schizont (mature), gametocyte, and trophozoite in thin film. **c** Trophozoites in Fields stained thick film.

Plasmodium vivax
- Widespread in tropics and temperate areas.
- Rarely more than 2% of cells infected.
- Trophozoites, schizonts and gametocytes, usually seen.

Trophozoites
- Large and amoeboid.
- Cytoplasm fragmented in thick films.
- Fine pigment.

Schizonts
- Large, round or irregular in form.
- Contain up to 24 or more merozoites and fine pigment.

Gametocytes
- Large, round or irregular in form (small forms also).
- Scattered pigment.

Host cell
- Enlarged, irregular in shape, pale staining.
- Schuffner's dots present (pH > 7.1). Seen indistinctly around parasites in thick films.
- Several parasites in a cell with some strains.

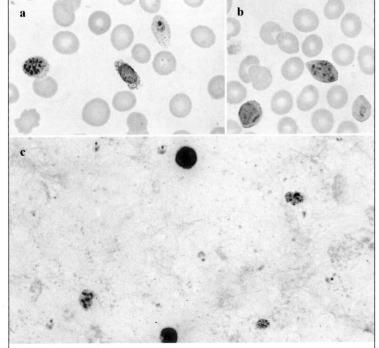

Plate 5.45 *P.ovale*. **a** Trophozoite, schizont, and gametocyte in thin film. **b** Trophozoite, schizont, and gametocyte in thin film. **c** Trophozoite, gametocyte, and schizont in Fields stained thick film.

Plasmodium ovale
- Low prevalence, mainly in West Africa (also elsewhere).
- Rarely more than 2% of cells infected (young cells preferentially parasitized).
- Trophozoites, schizonts and gametocytes usually seen.

Trophozoites
- Small and compact (can resemble *P. malariae* in thick films).
- Small amount of pigment.

Schizonts
- Small and compact.
- Contain up to 12 merozoites.

Gametocytes
- Small and round.
- Difficult to differentiate from late trophozoites.

Host cell
- About 20–30% of cells may become oval with fimbriated (ragged) ends.
- Schuffner's dots are prominent (pH > 7.1). Seen indistinctly around parasites in thick film.

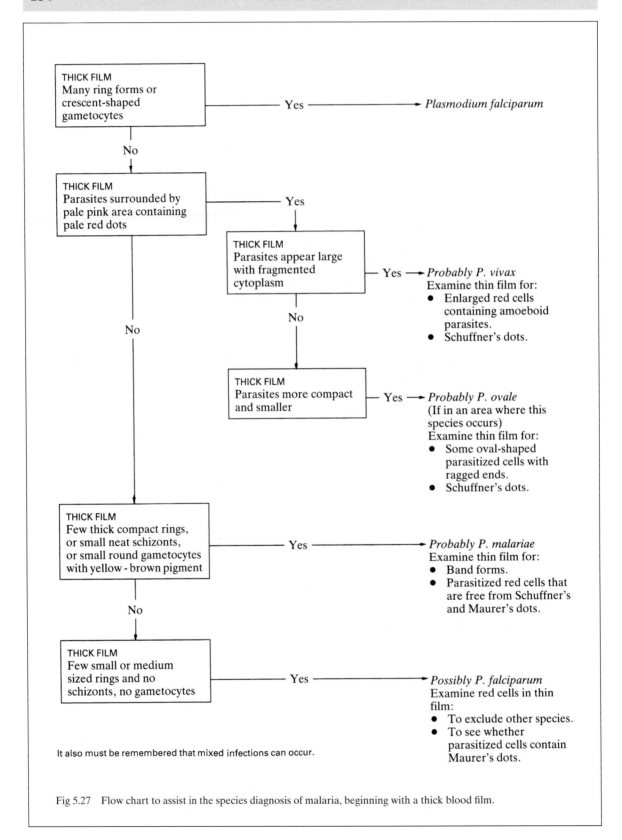

Fig 5.27   Flow chart to assist in the species diagnosis of malaria, beginning with a thick blood film.

4   Transfer the buffy coat layer and red cells immediately below it (to depth of about 1 mm) to one end of a slide and mix with the end of the pipette. Using a smooth edged spreader, make a thin preparation.

5   Allow the preparation to air-dry. When dry, fix with absolute methanol or ethanol for 2 minutes.

6   Stain using Field's thin film staining technique or Giemsa staining method (see previous text). Examine the preparation first with the 40× objective and then with the 100× objective.

Note: Other parasites such as trypanosomes and microfilariae can also be concentrated by this technique. These parasites are concentrated in the plasma immediately above the buffy coat layer. In practice, when withdrawing the buffy coat layer and red cells below it, a small amount of supernatant plasma is always withdrawn and this will contain any trypanosomes or microfilariae which may be in the specimen.

Diagnosing malaria using fluorescence microscopy
In district laboratories fluorescence microscopy is less used than transmitted light microscopy for diagnosing malaria because of the specialist training and expensive equipment required. Interested readers are referred to the paper of Moody[42] and Keiser *et al.*[47] Advice on the equipment needed and AO fluorescent technique to demonstrate malaria parasite, can be obtained from Portable Medical Laboratories Inc. (see Appendix 11). The formerly used Becton Dickinson QBC (quantitative buffy coat) *Paralens* fluorescence system is no longer available (tubes can still be obtained).

DIAGNOSING MALARIA USING A RAPID DIAGNOSTIC TEST (RDT)

In areas and situations where microscopical diagnosis of malaria is not available, the use of malaria rapid diagnostic tests (RDTs) can help to diagnose malaria promptly, improve the accuracy of malaria diagnosis, and avoid the unnecessary use of costly antimalarial drugs (e.g. Artemisinin-based combination therapies).

Users of malaria RDTs, however, need to be aware of the limitations of RDTs, e.g. unlike microscopical diagnosis, most RDTs are less sensitive, are not able to estimate parasite density, cannot indicate when schizonts of *P. falciparum* are present in peripheral blood and cannot provide accurate species identification particularly for non-*P. falciparum* infections.

Principle of malaria RDT
Malaria RDTs are qualitative immunochromatographic lateral flow* tests in dipstick (strip), cassette or card form that detect malaria antigen in peripheral blood.

* Refers to the migration of liquid across the surface of a nitrocellulose membrane.

–   Malaria antigen from a lyzed blood sample is reacted with anti-malaria monoclonal antibody conjugated to colloidal gold (pink-mauve) particles.
–   The antigen–antibody colloidal gold complex migrates along the nitrocellulose membrane where it becomes bound (captured) by a line of specific monoclonal antibody, producing a pink line in the test result area. This line can be seen after a washing buffer has removed the background haemoglobin.

A further pink line, i.e. inbuilt positive control, is produced above the test line indicating that the test reagents have migrated satisfactorily (it is not a malaria antigen control).

Antigens detected by malaria RDTs[42]
RDTs have been developed to detect the following malaria antigens:

● HRP 2 (histidine-rich protein)
● pLDH, (species-specific lactate dehydrogenase) enzyme
● Aldolase enzyme

HRP 2
This is a water-soluble protein produced by asexual stages and young gametocytes of *P. falciparum* only. It is expressed in abundance on the surface membrane of infected red cells.

HRP 2-based RDTs permit a rapid and sensitive ($\geq$100 parasites/μl) diagnosis of *P. falciparum* malaria but they are not suitable for assessing the effectiveness of treatment nor monitoring drug resistance. This is because HRP 2 antigen has been shown to persist for until at least day 7 after successful treatment and has been reported still present on day 28. It remains detectable after the clinical symptoms of malaria have disappeared and the parasites have been cleared from the peripheral blood.

pLDH and aldolase
These metabolic enzymes are found in the glycolytic pathway of malaria parasites. pLDH and aldolase are produced by asexual stages and gametocytes of all four human malaria species. RDTs have been developed with monoclonal antibody specific for *P. falciparum* pLDH and monoclonal antibodies that are pan-specific, i.e. recognizing all four malaria species. This enables non-*P. falciparum* infections to be distinguished from *P. falciparum* or mixed species infections. With the isolation of specific isomers of pLDH, species specific enzyme-based RDTs are becoming available.

Monoclonal antibodies produced against aldolase from *Plasmodium* species are pan-specific and are used with HRP 2 in combination RDTs to detect other *Plasmodium* species as well as *P. falciparum*. Aldolase pan-specific antibodies do not have the same binding sensitivity for *P. falciparum* as HRP 2 and may be negative when an HRP 2 capture line is positive in low parasitaemia.

pLDH and aldolase enzymatic activity correlates with active viable parasites and rapidly disappears with successful treatment. This gives an opportunity to use these enzyme-based RDTs as tests of cure as well as initial detection.

Malaria RDT techniques

Most malaria RDTs are easy to perform and interpret, particularly cassette RDTs. Tests take 10–20 minutes to perform. The following are examples of a dipstick, cassette, and card malaria RDT.

Example of a dipstick (strip) malaria RDT

The malaria RDT shown in Plate 5.47 is the *Paracheck Pf* dipstick which detects *P. falciparum* HRP 2 in whole blood.

Availability: *Paracheck Pf* dipstick is manufactured by and available from Orchid Biomedical Systems (see Appendix 11). Kits contain either 10 or 25 individually packaged dipsticks, clearing buffer, blood collection loops, lancets, and alcohol swabs (test tubes are not provided). Details of other manufacturers and suppliers of *P. falciparum* HRP 2 dipsticks and pan-specific dipsticks can be found on the WHO RDT website www.wpro.who.int/rdt

Method of performing Paracheck Pf dipstick

1. Immediately before use, open the moisture-proof pouch and remove the dipstick and other components.

2. Collect a sample of capillary blood using the sample loop provided. Blot the blood onto the sample pad on the dipstick below the arrows.

3. Dispense 4 drops (200 μl) of the clearing buffer provided into a small 12 × 75 mm test tube.

4. Place the dipstick in the tube, checking that the buffer level is below the blood sample.

5. At the end of 15 minutes read the test result.

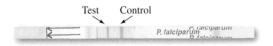

Positive test for *P.falciparum*: Two pink lines appear on the dipstick.

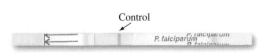

Negative test for *P.falciparum*: Only one pink line (Control) appears on the dipstick.

Plate 5.47   *Paracheck Pf dipstick for P. falciparum.*
Courtesy of Orchid Biomedical systems

Example of a cassette malaria RDT

The RDT shown in Plate 5.48 is the *Paracheck Pf cassette device* which detects *P. falciparum* HRP 2 antigen in whole blood.

Availability: *Paracheck P. falciparum* cassette test is manufactured by and available from Orchid Biomedical Systems (see Appendix 11). Kits are available containing 5, 10, or 25 test cassettes, clearing buffer and other items needed to perform the test including lancets and alcohol swabs. Details of other manufacturers and suppliers of *P. falciparum* HRP 2 cassette RDTs and pan-specific cassette RDTs can be found on the WHO RDT website www.wpro.who.int/rdt

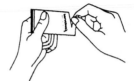 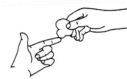

1. Immediately before use open the pouch.

2. Cleanse the finger with the swab provided.

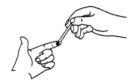 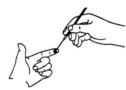

3. Prick the finger with the lancet provided.

4. Collect a blood sample using the loop provided

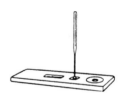 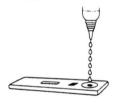

5. Blot the blood onto the sample pad A.

6. Add 2 drops of buffer to the buffer port B.

7. Read the results at the end of 15 minutes.

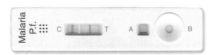

Positive test for *P.falciparum*: Pink line appears in both the C (Control) and T (Test) viewing windows.

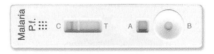

Negative test for *P.falciparum*: Pink line appears in the C (Control) viewing window only.

Plate 5.48   How to perform and interpret *Paracheck Pf* cassette RDT for *P. falciparum*
Courtesy of Orchid Biomedical Systems

Example of a card malaria combination RDT

The RDT shown in Plate 5.49 is the *Binax NOW Malaria* card test which detects *P. falciparum* antigen and an antigen that is common to all four species, *P. falciparum*, *P. vivax*, *P. ovale*, *P. malariae*. The test uses two antibodies, one that is specific for *P. falciparum* HRP 2 antigen (T1 line) and an antibody that is specific for antigen that is common to *P. falciparum*, *P. vivax*, *P. ovale*, *P. malariae*, i.e. aldolase (T2 line). The test distinguishes non-*P. falciparum* infections from *P. falciparum* or mixed species infections.

Availability: The *Binax NOW Malaria* test is manufactured by Binax Inc (see Appendix 11), catalogue number 660–000. It is available as a 25 test kit from Binax distributors. Prices vary depending on country. Being a combination test it is more expensive than most *P. falciparum* RDTs.

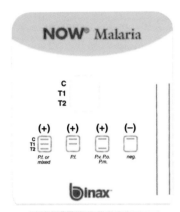

Plate 5.49   *Binax NOW Malaria* RDT.

Misleading malaria RDT results

The WHO publication *The use of malaria rapid diagnostic tests*[43] include the following as possible causes of misleading malaria RDT results:

A negative RDT result does not always exclude malaria with certainty as:

– There may be insufficient parasites to give a positive result.

This may occur when a test that is not sufficiently sensitive is being used, particularly in areas of low malaria transmission.

– The RDT may have been damaged.

This may occur when tests have been exposed to higher than recommended temperatures during transportation or storage, or to humid conditions before use. Enzyme-based RDTs are more susceptible to damage by heat and humidity than HRP 2-based RDTs.

– Illness may be caused by another species of malaria parasite which the RDT is not designed to detect.

This may occur when an HRP 2-based RDT (detecting *P. falciparum*) is used when the malaria is caused by *P. vivax*, *P. ovale*, or *P. malariae* or when an enzyme-based RDT is not sufficiently sensitive to detect other species, particularly *P. ovale* or *P. malariae*.

To the above can also be added:

– The use of an HRP 2 test which is not able to detect the variant of HRP 2 produced by the strain of *P. falciparum* causing the malaria.

– Difficult to read test line (very faint) due to high parasitaemia which may be reported falsely as a negative result.

Important: Guidelines must be in place to advise health workers on the action to take when there are clinical reasons to doubt an RDT result, particularly when an RDT is negative but the patient has symptoms of severe malaria. RDTs must be incorporated into established treatment protocols and health workers made aware of the limitations of malaria RDTs.[44]

A positive RDT result does not always signify malaria illness because:

– Antigen may sometimes be detected after the infecting parasites have died following treatment or there is a persistence of malaria gametocytes which do not cause illness.

The persistence of HRP 2 antigen following treatment (see previous text, HRP 2) is the commonest cause of a false positive *P. falciparum* HRP 2-based RDT.

– The presence of other substances in the blood may occasionally produce a false positive result, for example heterophile antibodies or less commonly, rheumatoid factor affecting both HRP 2 and enzyme-based RDTs.

– The presence of parasites does not always signify clinical malaria in individuals with high immunity. There may be other causes for the fever.

Quality assurance of malaria RDTs

Before purchasing a particular malaria RDT it is important to obtain as much information as possible from the supplier of the test and request copies of any evaluations performed. Purchasers need to be aware that a particular manufacturer's test may be marketed under several names with different suppliers, particularly cassette RDTs. With the increased use of malaria RDTs it has become clear that there exists significant variation between the performance of products in the field, especially with regard to sensitivity and product stability.

WHO malaria RDT website www.wpro.who.int/rdt
This useful website lists some of the malaria RDTs available, the antigens they detect, the contact details for manufacturers/suppliers. The website includes WHO evaluations and the quality assurance of RDTs. Reports of the latest meetings on malaria RDTs are covered. The WHO publications *Malaria rapid diagnosis : making it work (2003)* and *The use of malaria diagnostic tests* (2004) can also be downloaded from this website.

Quality assurance of malaria RDTs includes:

● Purchasing tests from a reliable professional source.

● Ensuring tests kits are transported and stored at the manufacturer's recommended temperature, particularly enzyme-based RDTs.

● Taking precautions to ensure tests are not exposed to conditions of high relative humidity. A test should only be removed from its moisture-proof envelope/pouch when it is ready to be used.

● Checking the performance of newly purchased test kits, e.g. using antigen controls.[45]

● Providing sufficient training and supervision in the performance of tests, including the collection and transfer of blood samples and the interpretation of test results, particularly for combination pan-antigen RDTs.

● Following exactly the manufacturer's written instructions regarding performing tests and when to read the results (these should be translated into the language of the user).

● Instructing health staff never to reuse a malaria RDT, not to mix reagents from different test kit lots, and not to use an RDT beyond its expiry date.

Introducing and selecting a malaria RDT
Factors to consider include the circumstances under which a malaria RDT is to be used, persons who will be performing the test, how test results will be used, how well quality assurance can be implemented, local availability of tests, affordability and cost benefits.

Circumstances of use
Potentially, malaria RDTs have applications in:

– diagnosing malaria in remote areas, particularly severe malaria in young children and pregnant women,

– early investigation and management of malaria epidemics,

– diagnosing malaria in areas of multi-drug resistance (where malaria is being diagnosed clinically).

– diagnosing malaria rapidly in non-immune migrant workers, military personnel, travellers, and displaced communities, e.g. in refugee camps, and in complex emergency situations.

In each of these situations the type of malaria RDT selected will be important, for example:

● Is it appropriate to select an RDT that detects *P. falciparum* only or should a pan-specific test be selected even though it is likely to cost about 40% more and test results more complex to interpret?

● Is there a requirement and are resources available for post-treatment testing which will require the use of an enzyme-based RDT?

● Is the RDT sufficiently sensitive (particularly important in areas of low malaria endemicity)?

● If the test is to be used in the field by community health workers,[46] is an RDT available that has only a few easy to perform procedural steps with easy to interpret test results and are all the items required to perform the test supplied with it or easily obtainable?

● Is it possible to ensure test kits are transported and stored correctly?

● Will the RDT have a sufficiently long shelf-life?

Important: Always obtain as much information as possible from malaria RDT manufacturers/suppliers concerning use, shelf-life, storage requirements, performance characteristics, costs, and kit packaging. Always request a sample kit for evaluation before purchasing.

Cost–benefit
In discussing whether there is a role for malaria RDTs in Africa, Bell comments[44] that cost–benefit ratios depend on the cost of the RDT, cost of treatment, parasite prevalence and the effect of the RDT on treatment practice. In epidemic-prone areas and areas of low malaria endemicity, spending on malaria RDTs would be worthwhile if it avoided giving expensive treatment to many patients with fever who do not have malaria. Where malaria prevalence is high, benefits are less clear with possibly the additional cost of RDT diagnosis not being recouped through treatment cost savings. When costing the use of malaria RDTs it is important to include not just the cost of the tests but also the costs involved in transport, training, and quality assurance.

5.8 Examination of blood, lymph fluid, and c.s.f. for trypanosomes causing African trypanosomiasis

African trypanosomiasis, also known as sleeping sickness (a reference to the comatosed state found in the late stages of the disease), is caused by:

Trypanosoma brucei rhodesiense, causing acute trypanosomiasis.

Trypanosoma brucei gambiense, causing chronic trypanosomiasis.

The parasites are closely related and belong to the *Trypanosoma brucei* group, or complex.

Trypanosoma brucei complex

Trypanosoma brucei brucei, infective to livestock (causing ngana) but not to humans, and the human pathogens *Trypanosoma brucei gambiense* and *Trypanosoma brucei rhodesiense* are morphologically indistinguishable. Each trypanosomiasis endemic area has associated with it several strains of biochemically and antigenically distinct trypanosomes. *T. b. gambiense* appears to be a homogeneous group whereas *T. b. rhodesiense* appears to be made up of many different strains and has a close relationship with *T. b. brucei*.

Distribution

African trypanosomiasis occurs in rural areas in the tsetse fly areas of sub-Saharan Africa between 14 °N and 20 °S. Tsetse flies are found only in Africa.

T. b. gambiense is found in West Africa and western Central Africa, extending from Senegal across to Sudan and down to Angola.

T. b. rhodesiense is found in East Africa, Central Africa, and Southern Africa extending from Ethiopia down to Botswana.

Note: In Uganda both species occur, *T. b. gambiense* in the north-west and *T. b. rhodesiense* in the south-east.

It is estimated that about 60 million people in 36 sub-Saharan countries are at risk of becoming infected with African trypanosomiasis. Interruption in surveillance and vector control measures, combined with population migrations, war, treatment failure, and unavailability of drugs, have lead to a resurgence of African trypanosomiasis in several countries with serious epidemics particularly in Angola, Congo, southern Sudan and Uganda.

Transmission and life cycle

African trypanosomiasis is transmitted by a small number of species of tsetse flies belonging to the genus *Glossina*. Both male and female tsetse flies suck blood and can therefore transmit the disease.

Once infected a tsetse fly remains a vector of trypanosomiasis for the remainder of its life. The lifespan of a tsetse fly is about 3 months.

T. b. rhodesiense

T. b. rhodesiense is transmitted by woodland and savannah tsetse flies, *G. morsitans*, *G. pallidipes* and *G. swynnertoni*. In an epidemic in Uganda, a riverine tsetse fly *G. fuscipes* was found to be the vector.

Rhodesiense trypanosomiasis is a zoonosis with many game animals being naturally infected. Infection can persist for long periods in animals such as the bushbuck, reedbuck, warthog, hartebeest, goat, hyena, giraffe, and lion. Persons at greatest risk are therefore game wardens, honey collectors, fishermen, hunters, wood collectors, tourists, and other persons who enter tsetse fly infested game country in endemic areas. During epidemics, humans are the main sources of infection. In epidemics in East Africa, cattle were found to be reservoir hosts. Cattle movements increase the risk of infection

T. b. gambiense

T. b. gambiense is usually transmitted by lakeside and riverine tsetse flies, including *G. palpalis*, *G. fuscipes*, and *G. tachinoides*. Humans are the main reservoirs of infection. Semidomestic animals may act as reservoir hosts.

Note: Trypanosomiasis can also be transmitted by blood transfusion (fresh blood). In areas where the disease is endemic, blood donors should be checked for infection. Congenital transmission can also occur with *T. b. gambiense* but this is rare.

Life cycle

The life cycle of *T. b. rhodesiense* and *T. b. gambiense* is summarized in Fig. 5.28.

Metacyclic trypomastigotes are inoculated through the skin when an infected tsetse fly takes a blood meal. The parasites develop into long slender trypomastigotes which multiply at the site of inoculation and later in the blood, lymphatic system, and tissue fluid. They are carried to the heart and various organs of the body and in the later stages of infection they invade the central nervous system (CNS).

Trypomastigotes are ingested by a tsetse fly when it sucks blood. In the midgut of the fly, the parasites develop and multiply. After 2–3 weeks, the trypomastigotes migrate to the salivary glands of the tsetse fly where they become epimastigotes, multiply, and develop into infective metacyclic trypomastigotes.

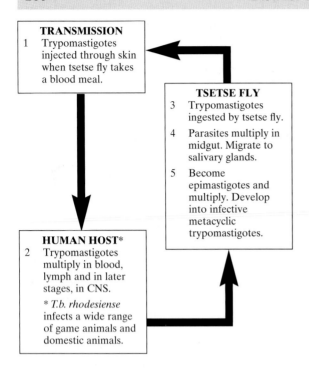

TRANSMISSION
1 Trypomastigotes injected through skin when tsetse fly takes a blood meal.

TSETSE FLY
3 Trypomastigotes ingested by tsetse fly.

4 Parasites multiply in midgut. Migrate to salivary glands.

5 Become epimastigotes and multiply. Develop into infective metacyclic trypomastigotes.

HUMAN HOST*
2 Trypomastigotes multiply in blood, lymph and in later stages, in CNS.

* *T.b. rhodesiense* infects a wide range of game animals and domestic animals.

Fig 5.28   Transmission and life cycle of *T.b. rhodesiense* and *T.b. gambiense.*

African trypanosomiasis

African trypanosomiasis is a wasting disease which is usually fatal unless treated. In rhodesiense trypanosomiasis and less commonly in gambiense infections, a painful swelling called a chancre develops and can be seen at the site of inoculation of the trypomastigotes. It contains multiplying trypomastigotes. It disappears after about 10 days.

Early stage of infection

There is a high irregular fever with shivering, sweating, and an increased pulse rate. There is a persistent headache, and usually pains in the neck, shoulders, and calves, and occasionally a delayed intense pain to knocks and pressure known as Kerandel's sign. The lymph glands become swollen.*

* In gambiense infections the lymph glands at the back of the neck are frequently involved (Winterbottom's sign), while in rhodesiense infections it is usually the glands under the jaw, in the arm-pit, at the base of the elbow, or in the groin which are involved.

As the disease progresses the spleen becomes enlarged, and there is oedema of the eyelids and face, sleeplessness, aimless scratching of the skin, and often a transient rash. In men, impotence may occur and in women, abortion or amenorrhoea. There is a

rapid fall in haemoglobin, reduction in platelet numbers, and a significant rapid rise in the erythrocyte sedimentation rate (ESR). Myocardial symptoms may also develop, especially in rhodesiense infections.

Late stage of the disease

The trypanosomes invade the central nervous system, giving symptoms of meningoencephalitis, including trembling, inability to speak properly, progressive mental dullness, apathy, excessive sleeping, and incontinence. There is usually rapid weight loss, continuing irregular fever, oedema of the limbs and inability to walk without help. If untreated, coma develops and finally death.

Immune responses

The main immune response in African trypanosomiasis is a humoral one with stimulated B lymphocytes producing large amounts of Ig M followed in the later stages of infection by Ig G.

The antibodies are effective in destroying the trypanosomes until the organisms vary their surface antigenic structure, i.e. variant surface glycoproteins (VSG's). The existing antibodies are then ineffective and the parasites multiply once more until the host produces another set of antibodies which are effective against the new VSG antigens. This process can be repeated many times and is thought to explain the temporary disappearance of the trypanosomes from the blood, necessitating repeated blood examinations to detect the parasites.

The level of Ig M rises rapidly and reaches a very high concentration in the blood. As the disease progresses Ig M can also be found in the cerebrospinal fluid. Protection against other diseases, especially bacterial, is reduced due to immune depression and the body's humoral responses being used against the trypanosomes.

Differences between gambiense and rhodesiense trypanosomiasis

T. b. gambiense is more adapted to humans than *T. b. rhodesiense* and therefore gambiense sleeping sickness tends to be a more chronic type of disease showing early lymphatic involvement with swollen glands. Other symptoms develop slowly over several months. The parasites are usually difficult to find in the blood and are more commonly found in aspirates from enlarged lymph glands.

Rhodesiense trypanosomiasis tends to be more acute with a rapid development of encephalitis and symptoms leading to early death from toxaemia or heart failure.

Note: Occasionally infection with *T. b. gambiense* can be acute especially in epidemics and infection with *T. b. rhodesiense* may be chronic. Asymptomatic carriers of both *T. b. gambiense* and *T. b. rhodesiense* have been found in some areas.

Measures to prevent and control African trypanosomiasis
- Detecting and treating human infections at an early stage, and increasing public awareness of the disease. In gambiense trypanosomiasis areas, the card agglutination test (CATT) has been found useful in screening communities for infection (see later text).
- Siting human settlements in tsetse fly infested areas only when there is adequate vector control.
- Reducing tsetse fly numbers by:
  - Using and maintaining insecticide impregnated tsetse fly traps.
  - Identifying and studying the breeding habits of local vectors.
  - Selectively clearing the bush and wooded areas, especially around game reserves, water-holes, bridges, and along river banks.
- Spraying vehicles with insecticide as they enter and leave tsetse fly infested areas.
- Identifying animal reservoir hosts in endemic areas.
- In rhodesiense trypanosomiasis areas, restricting the movement of game animals to within fenced game reserves.

Note: Further information on the prevention and control of African trypanosomiasis can be found in the *WHO Report on African trypanosomiasis*[48] and WHO website www.who.int/tdr

---

LABORATORY DIAGNOSIS

Because of the risks associated with the drug treatment of African trypanosomiasis, particularly if needing to treat for CNS (central nervous system) involvement, it is essential to confirm the diagnosis parasitologically before commencing treatment. The laboratory *must* examine specimens carefully and for a sufficient length of time. Several specimens may need to be examined before detecting the trypanosomes (trypomastigotes).*

* Under *laboratory diagnosis*, the older more familiar term trypanosome is used.

In district laboratories, the diagnosis of African trypanosomiasis and investigation of the stage of infection is by:

- Examining blood for trypanosomes.

- Examining aspirates from enlarged lymph glands for trypanosomes, particularly when gambiense trypanosomiasis is suspected.

- Examining cerebrospinal fluid (c.s.f.) for trypanosomes, cells (including Morula cells), raised protein, and IgM. Testing c.s.f. will provide information on the stage of the disease, i.e. whether the CNS has been involved and further treatment with more toxic drugs is indicated.

Important: To avoid the accidental introduction of trypanosomes into the CNS should the lumbar puncture be traumatic, c.s.f. should not be collected until treatment to kill the parasites in the blood has been started. It is usual to wait 24 h after an injection of suramin before performing a lumbar puncture.

Other tests

- Measurement of haemoglobin. Rapidly developing anaemia with reticulocytosis is a feature of African trypanosomiasis. It develops *early* in the disease and is due mainly to haemolysis and the removal of immune sensitized red cells from the circulation by the spleen.

- Measurement of the erythrocyte sedimentation rate (ESR). A *significant* and *rapid* rise in ESR occurs early in the disease with very high rates being reached as the disease progresses due to changes in plasma proteins.

- Total white blood cell count and differential. A moderate leucocytosis with monocytosis, lymphocytosis and presence of plasma cells are common findings in African trypanosomiasis.

- Checking urine for protein, cells, and casts once treatment has started.

Serological testing using CATT/T.b.gambiense

The card agglutination test for trypanosomiasis (CATT) is described at the end of this subunit.

Blood grouping and crossmatching of blood from patients with trypanosomiasis

The grouping (typing) and crossmatching (compatibility testing) of blood from patients with African trypanosomiasis may cause difficulties due to autoagglutinins and rouleaux formation of red cells. When blood grouping, it is essential to test both the cells and serum of the patient and to check for autoagglutination. When crossmatching, autocontrols must be used and an antihuman globulin crossmatch should be performed.

Screening blood donors for African trypanosomiasis
If donor blood can be stored for a few days at 2–8 °C, the risk of transmitting trypanosomes is removed because when stored at this temperature the parasites rapidly lose their infectivity. If the blood of donors from known trypanosomiasis endemic areas cannot be stored for a few days, such fresh blood should be screened for infection as follows:

- Test for trypanosomes using the microhaematocrit concentration technique (see later text). If unable to perform this test, examine a stained thick blood film (taken at the time of donation).

- Measure the donor's haemoglobin (this test should always

be performed before a person donates blood). Note whether the haemoglobin is lower than would be expected.

- Measure the ESR or alternatively observe the time it takes for the red cells to settle in the unit of donated blood. A rapid sedimentation of the cells should alert laboratory staff as to the possibility of infected blood when taken from a donor living in a trypanosomiasis area, e.g. relative of a patient with the disease.

EXAMINATION OF BLOOD FOR TRYPANOSOMES

Repeated examinations and concentration techniques are often required to detect trypanosomes in the blood because parasite numbers vary at different stages of the infection. At times no parasites will be found (see *Immune responses*).

The following techniques are recommended:

- Examination of a thick stained blood film.

- Microhaematocrit concentration technique (requires a microhaematocrit centrifuge).

- Triple centrifugation tube technique to concentrate trypanosomes when a microhaematocrit centrifuge is not available.

Miniature anion exchange centrifugation (MAEC) technique
This technique is considered by most workers to be the most sensitive for detecting small numbers of *T. b. rhodesiense* or *T. b. gambiense* trypanosomes, but it is an expensive technique and requires careful control. It is mostly used in specialist laboratories.

In the MAEC technique, the patient's heparinized blood is passed through a buffered anion (negatively charged) exchange column of diethyl-aminoethyl (DEAE)-52 cellulose. As the blood is eluted through the column, the strongly charged blood cells are adsorbed onto the cellulose while the less strongly charged trypanosomes are washed through the column with the buffered saline. The eluate is then collected, centrifuged, and the sediment is examined microscopically for motile trypanosomes. The cellulose column requires careful preparation and the pH of the buffer is critical to ensure adsorption of the cells and elution of the trypanosomes.

Note: For further information readers are referred to The Trypanosomiasis Unit, Tropical Diseases Research (TDR) programme, World Health Organization, 1211 Geneva 27–Switzerland. Website www.who.int/tdr

Examination of a thick stained blood film for trypanosomes

Although trypanosomes, when in sufficient numbers, can be detected by their motility in fresh unstained wet blood preparations, examination of a thick stained blood film is recommended because more blood can be examined in a shorter time.

Method

1 Collect a drop of capillary blood on a slide and spread it to cover evenly an area 15–20 mm in diameter.

Avoid making the smear too thick. A thick smear it will not stain well and the trypanosomes will be difficult to detect. The thickness can be taken as correct if this print can be seen but not read when the film is held just above the print.

Rouleaux: Red cells from patients with trypanosomiasis will tend to form rouleaux. To avoid excessive rouleaux, mix the blood as little as possible when spreading it. Marked rouleaux will cause the preparation to be easily washed from the slide during staining. For the same reason it is also best to make thick films from fresh non-anticoagulated blood.

2 Allow the smear to dry completely in a safe place, protected from flies, ants, and dust.

3 Stain the film using Field's rapid technique for thick blood films or Giemsa staining technique (described in subunit 5.7). Allow the preparation to dry.

4 When dry, spread a drop of immersion oil on the film and examine it microscopically for trypanosomes using the 40× objective. Use the 100× objective to confirm that the organisms are trypanosomes (add a further drop of oil if required).

Note: If no trypanosomes are seen, always check the thick film for other possible causes of a patient's fever such as malaria parasites or borreliae (relapsing fever).

T. b. rhodesiense and *T. b. gambiense* trypanosomes

- Trypanosomes measure 13–42 µm in length and may show a variety of forms (pleomorphic).*

  * In the early stages of acute African trypanosomiasis, long slender trypanosomes (often seen dividing) can be found. In the later stages, intermediate and short trypanosomes, some having no free flagellum, may be seen.

- Single flagellum arises from the kinetoplast. It extends forwards along the outer margin of the undulating membrane and usually beyond it as a free anterior flagellum.

- Small dot-like kinetoplast stains darkly.

- Nucleus stains dark-mauve and is usually centrally placed but posterior nuclear forms may also be seen.

- Cytoplasm stains palely and contains granules.

Note: Microscopically, the trypanosomes of *T. b. rhodesiense* and *T. b. gambiense* look the same.

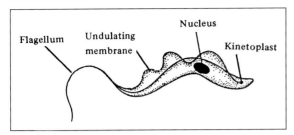

Fig. 5.29 Morphology of a trypanosome of *T.b.gambiense* or *T.b.rhodesiense*.

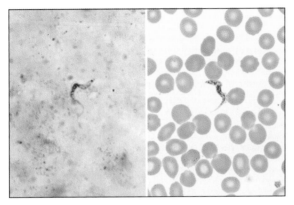

Plate 5.50   *Left*: *T.b.gambiense/T.b.rhodesiense* in thick blood film. *Right*: *T.b.gambiense/T.b.rhodesiense* in thin blood film.

Microhaematocrit technique to concentrate trypanosomes

Although *T. b. rhodesiense* trypanosomes are usually easier to find in the blood than *T. b. gambiense* trypanosomes, they can be very few and difficult to detect in unconcentrated preparations.

The microhaematocrit technique is rapid and recommended for detecting motile trypanosomes in blood when a microhaematocrit centrifuge is available. It also enables the packed cell volume (PCV) to be measured to check whether the patient is anaemic.

Note: The capillary tube technique is not suitable in areas where *Mansonella* or other species of microfilariae are likely to be present with trypanosomes in the blood. In such areas it is best to examine a stained preparation from a test tube concentration technique (see later text).

Method

1 Fill to about 10 mm from the top, two heparinized capillary tubes with capillary blood or two plain capillary tubes with *fresh* anticoagulated (EDTA) blood.

2 Seal the dry top end of each capillary tube by rotating it in a suitable sealant, e.g. *Cristaseal*.

3 Centrifuge the capillaries in a microhaematocrit centrifuge for 3–5 minutes.

   Caution: Handle the blood and capillary tubes with care. Infection can occur if viable organisms penetrate the skin or mucous membranes.

4 Wipe clean the area of each capillary where it will be viewed, i.e. where the red cell column joins the cellular layer (buffy coat) and plasma.

5 Mount the two capillaries on a slide, supported on two strips of plasticine or *Blutak* as shown in Fig. 5.30. Using a cloth or tissue, gently press to embed the capillaries in the plasticine.

6 Fill the space between the two capillaries with clean water and cover with a cover glass.

7 Examine immediately the plasma just above the buffy coat layer for motile trypanosomes. Use a 20× objective or if unavailable use a 10× objective, making sure the condenser iris is *closed sufficiently* to give good contrast, or preferably use dark-field microscopy. Use the 40× objective to confirm that the motility is due to trypanosomes.

The trypanosomes are very small but can be detected with *careful* focusing and providing the light is not too intense and the glass of the capillaries and cover glass is *completely* clean.

Important: The preparation must be examined within a few minutes of the blood being centrifuged

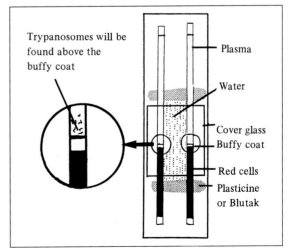

Fig. 5.30   Microhaematocrit centrifugation technique showing capillaries mounted on a microscope slide with close up of the area (circle) in which to look for trypanosomes.

otherwise the trypanosomes will migrate into the supernatant plasma and be missed. Also, the trypanosomes will gradually become less active and therefore more difficult to detect.

Presence of microfilariae
Motile microfilariae will make it impossible to see whether there are also trypanosomes. When this occurs it is best to examine a stained preparation from a test tube preparation as described in the following text. Breaking capillaries to obtain a preparation for staining is *not* recommended for safety reasons.

Triple centrifugation tube technique to concentrate trypanosomes[49]

This technique is appropriate when a microhaematocrit centrifuge technique cannot be performed or when microfilariae are also present in the blood. It requires a bench centrifuge with an adjustable speed control (to give graded RCF).

Method
1 Collect 9 ml of venous blood into a tube containing 1 ml of 6% w/v sodium citrate anticoagulant (Reagent No. 57) and mix gently.

2 With the minimum of delay, centrifuge the fresh blood at *slow* speed, i.e. RCF of about 100 g for 10 minutes. Transfer the plasma and cells above the red cells to a conical centrifuge tube.

3 Centrifuge at a *slightly* higher speed, i.e. RCF of 200–300 g for 10 minutes. Transfer the supernatant fluid to another conical tube.

4 Centrifuge at 700–900 g for 10 minutes. Remove and *discard* the supernatant fluid. Tap the end of the tube to resuspend the sediment and transfer the entire sediment to a glass slide. Cover with a cover glass.

5 Immediately examine microscopically for motile trypanosomes using the 40× objective.

   Microfilariae: If microfilariae are present, remove the cover glass and allow the sediment to dry on the slide. Fix with methanol for 2 minutes and stain the preparation using Field's or Giemsa technique (see subunit 5.7). Examine for trypanosomes as previously described for the examination of a thick stained blood film.

EXAMINATION OF LYMPH GLAND ASPIRATES

In the early stages of African trypanosomiasis, especially in gambiense infections, trypanosomes can often be found in fluid aspirated from a swollen lymph gland.

1 Prepare a small syringe by rinsing it out with sterile isotonic saline. Pull back the plunger half way, ready for use.

   Note: Do not use sterile water to rinse the syringe because trypanosomes are rapidly destroyed in water.

2 Wearing sterile protective gloves, locate the swollen gland and holding it firmly, gently pull it towards the skin surface.

3 Cleanse the swollen area with a spirit swab. Insert a sterile, size 18 gauge needle (without the syringe attached) into the centre of the gland (see Plate 5.51 left).

4 Without moving the needle, gently massage the gland to encourage the fluid to enter the needle. Avoid stirring the needle as this will cause unnecessary pain.

5 Remove the needle, and holding it over a slide, carefully attach the syringe. With care, slowly expel the contents of the needle onto the slide. Immediately cover the specimen with a cover glass to prevent it from drying on the slide.

6 Place a small sterile dressing over the needle wound.

7 With the minimum of delay, examine the entire preparation microscopically for motile trypanosomes using the 40× objective with the condenser iris adjusted to give good contrast.

Note: If only a small amount of fluid is aspirated which is insufficient to examine as a wet preparation, allow the fluid to dry on the slide, fix it with two drops of absolute methanol (methyl alcohol), and stain by Field's rapid technique for thin films or by Giemsa method (see subunit 5.7). Examine the stained preparation as described previously.

Examination of chancre fluid for trypanosomes

When a chancre is present (more commonly seen in early *T. b. rhodesiense* infections than in *T. b. gambiense* infections), trypanosomes can often be detected in fluid aspirated from the swelling. The method of collecting and examining chancre fluid is as follows:

1 Cleanse the chancre with a spirit swab. Wearing sterile protective gloves, puncture the chancre from the side with a small sterile needle. Blot away any blood.

2 Gently squeeze a small amount of serous fluid from the chancre and transfer it to a clean slide. Cover with a cover glass. Examine microscopically for motile trypanosomes as described previously for lymph gland aspirates.

3 Place a sterile dressing over the needle wound.

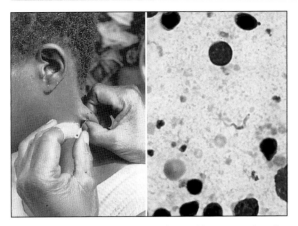

Plate 5.51 *Left*: Collecting lymph fluid to examine for *T.b.gambiense*. *Right*: *T.b.gambiense* in Fields stained smear of lymph fluid

EXAMINATION OF CSF IN AFRICAN TRYPANOSOMIASIS

When there is involvement of the CNS in African trypanosomiasis (see previous text), the following may be found in c.s.f.:

- few trypanosomes
- more than 5 white cells/μl
- morula (Mott) cells (IgM producing plasma cells)
- IgM, usually more than 10% of the total c.s.f. protein
- raised total protein

Caution: As previously mentioned, c.s.f. should only be collected after treatment to kill the trypanosomes in the blood has been started otherwise a traumatic lumbar puncture may introduce trypanosomes into the CNS.

Method of examining c.s.f.

Important: The c.s.f. must be examined *as soon as possible* after it has been collected. This is because the trypanosomes are unable to survive for more than 15–20 minutes in c.s.f. once it has been removed. The organisms rapidly become inactive and are lyzed.

1 Report the appearance of the fluid.

   A normal c.s.f. is clear and colourless. In meningoencephalitis due to trypanosomiasis the c.s.f. usually appears clear to slightly cloudy (large numbers of pus cells are not found as in bacterial meningitis).

2 Gently mix the c.s.f. and perform a white cell count.

   When trypanosomes have invaded the CNS, the c.s.f. will usually contain more than 5 cells/μl and these will be mostly lymphocytes.

3 Centrifuge the c.s.f. at medium to high speed (RCF about 1 000 g) for 10 minutes to sediment the trypanosomes and cells.

4 Using a plastic bulb pipette or other Pasteur pipette, carefully transfer the supernatant fluid to another tube. This can be used for measuring the IgM and total protein concentration.

5 Mix the sediment and if a microhaematocrit centrifuge is available, collect the sediment in a capillary tube. Place 1 drop on a slide (to make a stained smear) and centrifuge the remainder for 2 minutes. Mount the capillary on a slide as described for the blood microhaematocrit technique and examine microscopically near to the sealed end for motile trypanosomes (as soon as possible after centrifuging).

   Alternatively, if unable to concentrate the trypanosomes using a microhaematocrit centrifuge, transfer the sediment to a slide, cover with a cover glass and examine for motile trypanosomes using the 10× and 40× objectives with the condenser iris adjusted to give good contrast. A careful search of the entire preparation is required because only a few trypanosomes will be present. Do *not* use too intense an illumination.

6 If no trypanosomes are found but cells are present, examine a stained smear prepared from the wet preparation (remove the cover glass). Allow the preparation to dry, fix the smear with methanol for 2 minutes, and stain using Field's technique for thin films or Giemsa technique (see subunit 5.7). When dry, spread a drop of immersion oil on the preparation and examine for trypanosomes (may have been missed in the wet preparation) and for morula cells.

Appearance of morula cells

Morula (Mott) cells are larger than small lymphocytes. The nucleus stains dark mauve, and the cytoplasm (may be scanty) stains blue. Characteristic vacuoles can be seen in the cytoplasm as shown in Plate 5.52. When found in

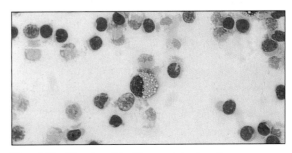

Plate 5.52 Morula cell in Giemsa stained c.s.f.

c.s.f., morula cells usually indicate trypanosome infection of the CNS.

7 If no trypanosomes have been found, using the supernatant fluid, measure the total protein concentration of the c.s.f. as described in subunit 6.12, and if possible test also for IgM (see following text).

When trypanosomes have invaded the CNS, the c.s.f. total protein will be raised. Very occasionally in the early stages of CNS involvement, trypanosomes can be found without a rise in c.s.f. protein but this is rare.

Summary of c.s.f. results in late stage trypanosomiasis with CNS involvement

Pressure . . . . Increased
Appearance . . . . Clear to slightly cloudy
Cell count . . . . More than 5 cells/μl
IgM . . . . Positive (>10% total protein)
Total protein . . . . More than 40 g/l (40 mg%)
Pandy's test* . . . . Positive
Wet preparation . . . . . Trypanosomes may be seen
Stained smear . . . . May contain few
trypanosomes, lymphocytes,
morula cells

*Pandy's test is of value only if unable to measure total protein.

Measurement of IgM in c.s.f.

IgM globulin can be detected in c.s.f. in the late stages of trypanosomiasis when there is CNS involvement. As the disease progresses, amounts of IgM greater than 10% of the c.s.f. total protein may be found. IgM may also be detected in the c.s.f. of patients with viral meningitis, tuberculous meningitis and neurosyphilis but usually in amounts less than 10% of c.s.f. total protein.

Lejon et al have evaluated a simple and rapid to perform latex card agglutination test (LATEX/IgM) for detecting and quantifying IgM in c.s.f. to assist in the detection and treatment of patients with late stage trypanosomiasis.[50] The reagent used in the test consists of anti-human IgM monoclonal antibodies joined to stained latex particles. In the test, c.s.f. (free from blood contamination) is serially diluted, mixed with the reagent, and rotated for 5 minutes. The highest dilution of c.s.f. showing agglutination is the end titre. A chart provided with the test gives the concentration of IgM present in the c.s.f. in mg/l. End titres $\geq$8 indicate central nervous system involvement.

Availability: The LATEX/IgM card agglutination test is manufactured by and available at low cost from Prince Leopold Institute of Tropical Medicine (see Appendix 11). East test kit contains 5 vials of freeze dried reagent, (each sufficient for 50 doses) and 2 vials of phosphate buffered saline. Once reconstituted, the reagent should be used the same day or stored frozen at $-20\,°C$. The buffer requires refrigeration at below

$10\,°C$. An accessory kit is also needed, containing test cards, microplates, mixing sticks and a syringe.

Diagnosis of gambiense trypanosomiasis in field surveys using CATT/T. b. gambiense[51]

The CATT (card agglutination trypanosomiasis test) T.b. gambiense is a simple to perform, rapid, sensitive, latex agglutination antibody test which is used to screen communities for gambiense trypanosomiasis in control programmes in West and Central Africa. It is not suitable for testing in rhodesiense areas.

Antigen used in test: This is variable antigen type LiTat 1.3. Antibodies to this antigen are present in the blood of most T.b. gambiense infected patients. Very occasionally persons with gambiense trypanosomiasis do not produce antibodies to LiTat 1.3 (observed in Ethiope East focus in Nigeria).[51]

In the CATT/T.b. gambiense, one drop of whole blood (screening test) or 25 μl of diluted plasma/serum (confirmatory test to exclude cross-reactions) is mixed with one drop of reconstituted antigen. When antibodies are present, agglutination occurs after 5 minutes rotation at 60 rpm. Antibodies are present in a patient's blood for several months following treatment.

The freeze dried antigen and control sera should be kept at between $2–8\,°C$ during transport and storage. The shelf-life of the antigen, control sera, and buffer is 1 year when refrigerated at below $10\,°C$. The reconstituted reagents can be used for up to 7 days when stored at $2–8\,°C$ or up to 8 hours under field non-refrigerated conditions. The antigen suspension must not be frozen. Each vial of reagent is sufficient for 50 tests.

Availability: CATT/T.b. gambiense is manufactured by and available at low cost from Prince Leopold Institute of Tropical Medicine (see Appendix 11). Kits are available for 250 tests or 500 tests. An accessory kit is also needed. This contains heparinized capillary tubes, test cards, stirring rods, suction bulb, 2.5 ml syringe and droppers (sufficient for 250 tests). For further information, e-mail emagnus@itg.be

Note: The antigen card indirect agglutination test for trypanosomiasis (CIATT) is no longer produced.

5.9 Examination of blood for Trypanosoma cruzi

Trypanosoma cruzi causes Chagas disease, also referred to as American trypanosomiasis.

Trypanosoma cruzi complex
Two principal groups of strains of T. cruzi have been proposed: T. cruzi I and T. cruzi II. Both groups infect humans.

T. cruzi II is associated with more severe disease and higher parasitaemia.

Distribution

T. cruzi is found only in the America's, in tropical and subtropical South and Central American countries from Mexico to Argentina. WHO estimates 13 million people are infected with 3.0–3.3 million symptomatic cases and an annual incidence of 200 000 cases in 15 countries.[53] Large scale initiatives to halt vector-borne and blood transfusion transmission have been successful in many countries of South America.

Transmission and life cycle

T. cruzi is mainly transmitted through contact with the faeces of an infected blood-sucking bug of the family Reduviidae, subfamily Triatominae. The faeces containing infective trypomastigotes are deposited on the skin or mucous membranes as the bug feeds from its host.

Vectors of *T. cruzi*

More than 80 species of triatomine bugs, both adults and nymphs, are capable of transmitting *T. cruzi* but the most important vectors are those that are well adapted to living in human dwellings. These include:

– *Triatoma infestans* in Argentina, Bolivia, Brazil, Chile, Paraguay, Peru and Uruguay.
– *Triatoma brasiliensis* in north-eastern Brazil.
– *Triatoma dimidiata* in Central America and the extreme north of South America.
– *Rhodnius prolixus* in Colombia, El Salvador, Guatemala, Honduras, Mexico, Nicaragua.
– *Panstrongylus megistus* in Argentina, Brazil, Paraguay, and Uruguay.

Adult triatomine bugs are winged and invade houses at night, often attracted by light. All bug stages can also be carried in to houses on roofing or with personal belongings. In houses colonized by bugs, several thousand may be found in the cracks of walls and in roofs, feeding from humans, domestic animals, and rodents. Chickens, although not infected with *T. cruzi*, often provide a source of blood for large numbers of triatomine bugs.

Animal reservoirs of *T. cruzi* include dogs, opossums, cats, small marsupials, rabbits, armadillos, mice, guinea pigs, and bats. *T. cruzi* can also be transmitted by blood transfusion. Less commonly, transplacental transmission occurs with a foetus being infected from an asymptomatic mother. Such infected infants are often stillborn or born prematurely with a low birth weight.

The life cycle of *T. cruzi* is summarized in Fig. 5.31. Following penetration, the metacyclic trypomastigotes invade muscle and other tissue cells near the point of entry and multiply intracellularly as amastigotes. Structurally the amastigotes of *T. cruzi* resemble those of *Leishmania* species. The amasti-

TRANSMISSION

1 Trypomastigotes in bug faeces deposited on skin when a triatomine bug takes a blood meal. They enter through the bite wound or are rubbed in.

(*T. cruzi* can also be transmitted by blood transfusion).

TRIATOMINE BUG

6 Trypomastigotes ingested by bug. Become epimastigotes and round forms. Multiply in gut.

7 Migrate to hindgut. Develop into infective metacyclic trypomastigotes.

HUMAN HOST*

2 Parasites form chagoma in subcutaneous tissue.

3 Parasites enter muscle tissue cells. Become intracellular amastigotes.

4 Multiply, forming pseudocysts.

5 Amastigotes→ epimastigotes. Develop into trypomastigotes. Released into blood. Infect new tissue cells. Some remain in blood.

* Reservoir hosts include opossum, armadillo and some domestic animals.

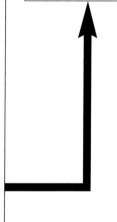

Fig 5.31 Transmission and life cycle of *Trypanosoma cruzi*.

gotes develop into trypomastigotes which are released into the blood. No multiplication of the parasite occurs in its trypomastigote stage in the blood.

The trypomastigotes reach tissue cells, especially those of heart muscle, nerves, skeletal muscle, and smooth muscle of the gastrointestinal tract and elsewhere. The trypomastigotes become amastigotes and multiply, forming pseudocysts.

The amastigotes develop first into epimastigotes and then into trypomastigotes which are released into the blood when the host cell ruptures. Some of these trypomastigotes continue to circulate while the majority infect further tissue cells.

The life cycle is continued when a triatomine bug ingests trypomastigotes in a blood meal. In the vector, the trypomastigotes develop into epimastigotes which multiply by binary fission in the gut of the bug.

Within 10–15 days, metacyclic trypomastigotes are formed and can be found in the hindgut of the bug, ready to be excreted when the vector defaecates as it takes a blood meal.

Chagas disease

Multiplication of *T. cruzi* at the site of infection, together with a host cellular immune response, can produce an inflamed swelling known as a chagoma which usually persists for several weeks. If the site of infection is the eye, usually the conjunctiva becomes inflamed and oedema forms. This is known as Romana's sign.

Geographically, there are differences in the clinical features and pathology associated with *T. cruzi* infection which may be due to variations in the strains of *T. cruzi* found in different areas, and to host factors.

Many people infected with *T. cruzi* remain asymptomatic and free from Chagas disease, or experience only acute infection without progressing to the chronic stage of the disease.

Acute Chagas disease

During the acute phase, trypomastigotes can be found circulating in the blood. They then multiply intracellularly as amastigotes and spread throughout the body.

Symptoms may be minor and pass unnoticed or there may be fever, malaise, an increased pulse rate and enlargement of the lymph glands, liver, and to a lesser extent the spleen. Lymphocytosis is common and peripheral blood films often resemble those seen in glandular fever.

Acute disease is most commonly seen in young children. Occasionally an acute attack can cause serious damage to the heart or result in other complications which may lead to death.

Early detection of *T. cruzi* infection, before there is nerve and muscle fibre damage, reduces the risk of chronic Chagas disease developing. Drugs are available for treating acute Chagas disease.

Chronic Chagas disease

If a person survives an acute attack, chronic Chagas disease may develop with signs of cardiac muscle damage, including a weak and irregular heart beat, enlargement of the heart and oedema. Severe damage to heart muscle leads to heart failure. Approximately 10% of persons infected with *T. cruzi* develop chronic Chagas cardiopathy. In some areas Chagas disease is the leading cause of cardiac death in young adults.

Parasite infection of intestinal muscle may cause damage to nerves in the intestinal wall, causing loss of the muscular action necessary for the movement of food.

The accumulation and slow movement of food leads to enlargement of the oesophagus (megaoesophagus) and colon (megacolon). These features are more commonly seen in central and eastern Brazil.

Co-infection with HIV

This can lead to severe myocarditis, central nervous system involvement with meningoencephalitis, and in the absence of antiretroviral treatment, the reactivation of latent infections.

Measures to prevent and control Chagas disease

- Spraying of bug-infested houses, furniture, sheds, latrines, etc, with insecticides every few months and checking for reinfestation. The insecticides used must be effective against local vectors.

- Using fumigant canisters to control vectors.

- With community support, the improvement of rural housing and household hygiene to eliminate refuges for triatomine bugs, especially the plastering of all creviced wall surfaces with cement or if unavailable with a strong local clay-mud plaster that will not crack. Alternatively, walls can be treated with an insecticide containing paint.

  In areas where *R. prolixus* is found, palm roofing should be replaced by corrugated metal sheets.

- Abandoned bug-infested houses should be burned or sprayed with insecticide. Belongings transferred to new houses should be sprayed with insecticide.

- Removal from houses of animal reservoirs which could harbour *T. cruzi*. Roosting chickens (from which bugs feed) should be removed from houses and encouraged to roost in trees.

- Periodic serological surveys (e.g. among school children) to detect new endemic foci in areas under control, combined with education about the transmission of *T. cruzi*, symptoms of early infection, and importance of treatment at an early stage.

- Screening donor blood for *T. cruzi* infection.

Note: Further information on acute and chronic Chagas disease, prevention and control measures can be found in the WHO Report *Control of Chagas disease*.[52]

LABORATORY DIAGNOSIS

In district laboratories the diagnosis of acute Chagas disease is by finding trypanosomes (trypomastigotes)* in the blood.

*Under *laboratory diagnosis* the older more familiar term trypanosome is used.

Detection of circulating trypanosomes in the early stages of *T. cruzi* infection is of *great importance* because at this stage effective treatment can be given which may prevent damage to heart muscle and the development of chronic Chagas disease in later life. The laboratory must therefore examine specimens carefully and for a sufficient length of time. During the acute stage, large numbers of trypanosomes may be present.

Caution: Laboratory staff should wear protective gloves and a face mask when collecting and handling blood specimens. Infection with *T. cruzi* can occur if parasites (even very few) penetrate the skin, conjunctiva, or mucous membranes.

Other tests
- The ESR is raised in acute infections.
- Blood films in acute Chagas disease often resemble those seen in glandular fever (marked lymphocytosis with atypical mononuclear cells).

Examination of blood for *T. cruzi* in acute disease
The trypanosomes of *T. cruzi* are fragile organisms, easily lyzed in thick blood films (as the blood dries) and easily damaged when spreading blood to make thin films. The following techniques, which are based on detecting motile trypanosomes, are recommended when examining blood for *T. cruzi*:

- Careful microscopical examination of fresh blood for motile trypanosomes.

- Microhaematocrit concentration technique. This is a rapid and sensitive technique.

- Test tube centrifugation concentration technique using clotted whole blood (Strout technique) or lyzed venous blood (Hoff technique).

Miniature anion exchange centrifugation (MAEC) technique: This technique as used for detecting small numbers of *T. b. gambiense* and *T. b. rhodesiense* is not suitable for detecting *T. cruzi* in blood.

Note: In areas where *Trypanosoma rangeli* (non-pathogenic species transmitted by *Rhodnius* bugs) is found with *T. cruzi*, i.e. mainly in Central America,

Venezuela, Brazil, Colombia, all positive preparations should be checked to confirm that the trypanosomes seen are *T. cruzi* and not *T. rangeli* (see later text).

Examination of a wet blood preparation

1   Collect a small drop of capillary blood or fresh venous blood on a slide and cover with a cover glass. Do not make the preparation too thick otherwise the trypanosomes will be missed.

2   Immediately examine the entire preparation microscopically for motile trypanosomes. Use the 40× objective with the condenser iris adjusted to give good contrast or preferably use dark-field or phase contrast microscopy.

Up to 30 minutes may need to be spent examining the preparation to detect *T. cruzi* trypanosomes. The chances of detecting the parasites are increased if several preparations are examined or if a concentration technique is used (see later text).

T. rangeli: If motile trypanosomes are seen, and *T. rangeli* is known to occur in the area, identify the species by examining a stained thin blood film. To minimize damage to the parasites when spreading the blood, hold the spreader at an angle of 60–70° and use as little pressure as possible. Air-dry the film rapidly. Immediately fix the film with absolute methanol for 2 minutes and stain using Field's thin blood film method or Giemsa method (see subunit 5.7). See later text for the features which differentiate *T. cruzi* from *T. rangeli*.

Microhaematocrit concentration technique

This technique is as described for *T. b. gambiense* and *T. b. rhodesiense* in the previous subunit (see 5.8). Examination of four capillary tubes is recommended to increase the chances of detecting the parasites.

If trypanosomes are seen and *T. rangeli* is known to occur in the area, identify the species by examining a stained preparation as described above. For safety reasons, do *not* break the capillary tubes to obtain a specimen for staining. Use either the Strout or Hoff technique to concentrate the trypanosomes and obtain a thin preparation for staining.

Strout concentration technique

1   Collect 5–10 ml of venous blood into a dry glass tube. Incubate for 1 hour at 37 °C.

2   Transfer the serum to a conical centrifuge tube, cap the tube, and centrifuge for 5 minutes at low

speed, i.e. RCF about 400 g.

3　Discard the supernatant fluid and examine the sediment microscopically for motile trypanosomes using the 40× objective. If required to differentiate *T. cruzi* and *T. rangeli*, prepare a thin film, fix with methanol and stain using Field's thin blood film method or Giemsa method as described in subunit 5.7 (see later text for the features which differentiate *T. cruzi* from *T. rangeli*).

Hoff concentration technique

1　Collect 2.5 ml of venous blood into EDTA anticoagulant and mix gently.

2　Dispense 6–7 ml of ammonium chloride lyzing solution (Reagent No. 8) into a conical centrifuge tube. Add the EDTA blood sample and mix.

　　Leave for about 3 minutes to allow time for the red cells to lyze. Cap the tube and centrifuge for 15 minutes at low to medium speed, i.e. RCF of 400–500 g.

　　Continue as described in No. 3 of the previously described Strout technique.

Examination of a stained preparation to differentiate *T. cruzi* from *T. rangeli*

When the stained preparation is completely dry, spread a drop of oil on the film and examine first with the 40× objective to detect the trypanosomes. Use the oil immersion objective to identify the species (adding a further drop of oil if necessary).

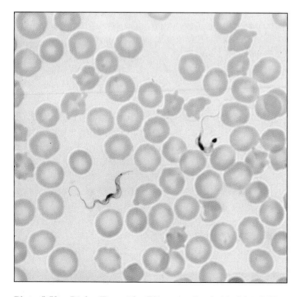

Plate 5.53　*Right*: *T.cruzi* in Giemsa stained thin blood film. *Left*: *T.rangeli*.

The following features can be used to differentiate *T. cruzi* and *T. rangeli* in Romanowsky stained blood films:

T. cruzi trypanosomes
- Usually C-shaped, measuring 12–30 μm in length with a narrow membrane and free flagellum.
- Has a *large*, round to oval, dark-red staining kinetoplast at the posterior end.
- Nucleus is centrally placed and stains red-mauve.

Note: Occasionally slender forms of *T. cruzi* can be seen which have an elongated nucleus, subterminal kinetoplast, and shorter free flagellum.

T. rangeli trypanosomes
Compared with *T. cruzi*, the trypanosomes of *T. rangeli* are longer and thinner, measuring 27–32 μm in length, have a long pointed posterior end and a much smaller kinetoplast which is situated a little way from the posterior end. The nucleus is in the anterior third of the body unlike in *T. cruzi* where it is central.

Note: *T. rangeli* is transmitted by the bite of *R. prolixus* bugs. It is found in Brazil, Venezuela, Colombia, Panama, El Salvador and Guatemala.

Diagnosing chronic Chagas disease

In chronic Chagas disease the number of circulating trypanosomes are too few to be detected using the techniques described for detecting parasites in the acute stage. Specialized techniques are used to demonstrate the parasites in chronic infections, including xenodiagnosis and blood culture.

- **Xenodiagnosis**, in which uninfected, *susceptible*, laboratory-reared triatomine bugs are starved for 2 weeks and then fed on the patient's blood. Ingested trypanosomes multiply and develop into epimastigotes and trypomastigotes which can be found 25–30 days later in the faeces or rectum of the bug. Artificial xenodiagnostic techniques have been developed and are replacing natural xenodiagnosis.

- **Blood culture**, using a blood agar culture medium containing an antibiotic to reduce contamination. After 14–21 days, fluid from the culture is examined for motile epimastigotes.

Most district laboratories will not have facilities for xenodiagnosis or the safe culture of *T. cruzi*. Patients with suspected chronic Chagas disease should be referred to a Chagas Disease Reference Laboratory.

Serological diagnosis of Chagas disease

Once infected with *T. cruzi*, a person remains infected for life and therefore antibodies persist throughout life. Tests to detect anti-*T. cruzi* antibodies in serum include an indirect fluorescent antibody test (IFAT), an indirect haemagglutination (IHAT), and an enzyme-linked immunosorbent assay (ELISA). These tests become positive about 1 month after infection and usually remain positive after treatment.

ELISA techniques can be performed on finger-prick blood collected onto filter paper. Filter paper blood samples should be stored frozen in a sealed bag containing a desiccant (e.g. silica gel) until they can be tested. Most antigens cross-react with *Leishmania* species and with *T. rangeli*. In most South American countries, there are Chagas disease immunodiagnostic centres to which district laboratories can send blood samples for testing.

When diagnosing congenital Chagas disease, the tests used must distinguish between IgM antibodies produced by an infected infant and maternal IgG antibodies which have crossed the placenta and are present in the serum of the infant.

Further information on the immunodiagnosis of Chagas disease: Readers are referred to the WHO Report *Control of Chagas disease.*[52]

Screening donor blood for *T. cruzi* infection

T. cruzi can be transmitted in infected donor blood (whole blood, red cell concentrates, and plasma), and therefore in endemic areas, it is essential to screen all units of donated blood for infection with *T. cruzi*. In many countries this is now a legal requirement.

Simple to perform rapid latex and red cell agglutination tests have been developed for the screening of blood. District laboratories should consult their nearest Chagas Disease Reference Laboratory or Regional Transfusion Centre regarding which test is appropriate to use in their area.

In some areas, gentian violet is added to donor blood (125 mg/500 ml blood) followed by storage at 2–8 °C for 24 h to kill *T. cruzi*. The main disadvantages are that the dye stains (reversibly) the tissues of the recipient of the blood and it can also be toxic to blood components. New more acceptable agents to add to blood to kill *T. cruzi* are being researched by the World Health Organization.

5.10 Examination of specimens for *Leishmania* parasites

The following are the principal *Leishmania* species that cause the different clinical forms of leishmaniasis:

Visceral leishmaniasis (VL)	*L. donovani*[1] *L. infantum*[1] (*L. chagasi*)* **L. infantum* and *L. chagasi* are now recognised as the same organism. Some workers, however, prefer to use the name *L. chagasi* for South American parasites.
Cutaneous leishmaniasis (CL)	*L. tropica*[2] *L. major*[3] *L. aethiopica*[4] *L. mexicana*[5] *L. peruviana*[6] *L. guyanensis*[7] *L. panamensis*[7]
Diffuse cutaneous leishmaniasis (DCL)	*L. aethiopica*[4] *L. amazonensis*[5] *L. mexicana*[5]
Mucocutaneous leishmaniasis (MCL)	*L. braziliensis*[6] *L. panamensis*[7]

[1] Belong to the *L. donovani* complex. [2,3,4] Each species belongs to a separate complex of the same name. [5] Belong to the *L. mexicana* complex. [6] Belong to the *L. braziliensis* complex. [7] Belong to the *L. guyanensis* complex (classification based on isoenzyme studies).

Distribution

Leishmaniases are endemic in 88 countries with an estimated 350 million people at risk of infection. The overall prevalence of the leishmaniases is estimated at 12 million cases with 0.5 million new visceral leishmaniasis cases per year and 1.0–1.5 million new cutaneous leishmaniasis cases per year (these figures are thought to under-estimate true case-load).[54] More than 90% of visceral leishmaniasis occurs in Sudan, Bangladesh, Nepal, Brazil and India, and more than 90% of cutaneous leishmaniasis in Brazil, Peru, Afghanistan, Syria, Iran and Saudi Arabia. In recent years there have been major epidemics of visceral leishmaniasis in southern Sudan, eastern India, Bangladesh, and north-east Brazil. Increased infections and the spread of leishmaniases are related to environmental and behavioural changes and development, conflict and war, bringing non-immune people into closer contact with vectors and reservoir hosts.[54] An increase in the incidence of *Leishmania* infections is also being reported from HIV prevalent areas.

Leishmania species are widespread in the Old World and New World:

OLD WORLD (Africa, Asia, Europe)

L. donovani: Bangladesh, northeast India, Burma, Sudan, Kenya and Horn of Africa. Infections are anthroponotic, i.e. from one human to another (rodents and dogs may serve as reservoirs in some areas of Africa).

L. infantum: Endemic in central Asia, northeast China, Middle East and the Mediterranean basin. Infections are zoonotic, i.e. from animal to human, with dogs, foxes, and jackals serving as reservoir hosts.

L. major: Widespread distribution, being found in sub-Saharan Africa from Senegal across to central Sudan, north India, Pakistan, central Asia, Middle East and north Africa. Infections are zoonotic with rats and gerbils serving as reservoir hosts.

L. tropica: Middle East, eastern Mediterranean countries, north Africa, northwest India and Afghanistan. Infections are anthroponotic.

L. aethiopica: Found only in the highlands of Ethiopia and Kenya. Infections are zoonotic with rock and tree hydraxes serving as reservoir hosts.

NEW WORLD (South America and Central America)

L. infantum (L. chagasi): Central America and parts of South America, especially Brazil and Venezuela. Infections are zoonotic with dogs, foxes and marsupials serving as reservoir hosts.

L. mexicana: Tropical forests in Mexico (Yucatan), Guatemala and Belize. Forest rodents are the reservoir hosts.

L. amazonensis: Tropical forests of Brazil and Venezuela and also in Trinidad. Forest rodents are the reservoir hosts.

L. braziliensis: Tropical forests of South America, especially Amazon forest and also in Central America. Reservoir hosts are possibly rodents and some domestic animals.

L. guyanensis: Guyanas, Brazil, Surinam. Sloths and anteaters are reservoir hosts.

L. panamensis: Panama, Costa Rica, Colombia. Sloths are reservoir hosts.

L. peruviana: Andes in Peru, Argentinian highlands. Dogs are naturally infected but there is also probably a wild animal host.

Transmission and life cycle

Leishmania species are transmitted by the bite of an infected female sandfly, belonging to the genus *Phlebotomus* in Africa, Asia and Europe, and the genus *Lutzomyia* in the Americas. About 30 species of sandflies act as vectors, infecting humans and animal reservoir hosts.

Sandfly vectors

The feeding, breeding and flight habits of sandflies are species specific. Most sandflies feed mainly on plant juices, but female

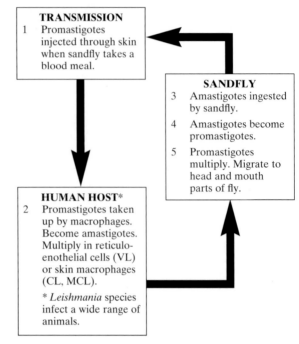

Fig 5.32 Transmission and life cycle of *Leishmania* parasites. VL: Visceral leishmaniasis, CL: Cutaneous leishmaniasis, MCL: Mucocutaneous leishmaniasis.

flies also require blood meals for egg development. Most species feed at night, dusk or dawn. Sandfly habitats include rotting leaves under trees, excreta, termite hills, and rodent burrows. They are weak fliers and tend to fly in short hops. The sandfly species that transmit *Leishmania* parasites in the Old World and New World are described in the 21st edition *Mansons Tropical Diseases* (see Recommended Reading).

The life cycle of *Leishmania* species is summarized in Fig. 5.32. A person becomes infected when promastigotes are inoculated at the time a female sandfly takes a blood meal. The promastigotes are taken up by macrophages and develop into intracellular forms called amastigotes. They multiply, rupture from the macrophages, and infect new cells.

In visceral leishmaniasis the amastigotes multiply in the macrophages of the spleen, liver, bone marrow, lymph glands, mucosa of the small intestine, and other tissues of the reticuloendothelial system. Blood monocytes are also infected. In cutaneous leishmaniasis the parasites multiply in skin macrophages (histiocytes).

The life cycle is continued when intracellular and free amastigotes are ingested by a female sandfly. After about 72 hours, the amastigotes become flagellated promastigotes in the midgut of the sandfly. They multiply and fill the lumen of the gut. After 14–18 days (depending on species), the promastigotes move forward to the head and mouth-parts of the sandfly. The salivary glands are not parasitized.

Note: Parasites of the *L. braziliensis* complex develop in both the midgut and hindgut of the vector.

Visceral leishmaniasis (VL)

This is the most severe form of leishmaniasis. It is caused by *L. donovani* and *L. infantum (L. chagasi)*. In endemic areas, the disease is more chronic with young adults and children being more commonly infected. About twice as many males are affected than females. In epidemics, all age groups are susceptible (except those with acquired immunity), and the disease is often acute. Without treatment, VL is usually fatal. Significant advances have been made in the treatment of visceral leishmaniasis.[56]

Symptoms in chronic VL include irregular fever, splenomegaly, hepatomegaly, and, or, lymphadenopathy, loss of weight with wasting, diarrhoea, low white cell and platelet counts, and anaemia. Skin changes are common. The local Indian name for VL, *kala-azar* (meaning black sickness) is a reference to the greyish colour which the patient's skin becomes. In acute VL there is splenomegaly, high undulating fever, chills, profuse sweating, rapid weight loss, fatigue, anaemia, and leucopenia. Often there is epistaxis (nose bleed) and bleeding from the gums.

In the New World, VL is endemic or sporadic. Asymptomatic infections and subclinical forms of the disease are more common. Malnutrition and other infections increase the risk of developing symptomatic VL.

In active visceral leishmaniasis there is a poor cell-mediated immune response and therefore the parasites multiply rapidly. There is, however, a humoral response with large amounts of polyclonal non-specific immunoglobulin especially IgG being produced and also specific anti-leishmanial antibody. Patients who have recovered from visceral leishmaniasis are immune from reinfection but relapses can occur, particularly in those coinfected with HIV.

Post kala-azar dermal leishmaniasis (PKDL)

In India and occasionally in East Africa, a cutaneous form of leishmaniasis can occur about 2 years after treatment and recovery from visceral leishmaniasis. This is referred to as post kala-azar dermal leishmaniasis and affects about 20% of patients in India. Hypopigmented and raised erythematous patches can be found on the face, trunk of the body, and limbs. These may develop into nodules and resemble those of lepromatous leprosy, fungal infections or other skin disorders. Occasionally there is ulceration of the lips and tongue. Amastigotes are present in the papules and nodules.

HIV coinfection

In areas where both leishmaniasis and HIV infection occur, visceral leishmaniasis (VL) is being increas-ingly reported in those with immunosuppression caused by HIV. Frequently parasites infect not just the reticuloendothelial system but also the lungs, central nervous system, normal skin, and blood. Parasites have been found in phagocytic cells in the peripheral blood in up to 75% of patients (98% in bone marrow aspirates).

Patients with VL/HIV coinfection do not respond well to treatment. In most patients, VL is rapidly progressive and VL accelerates the onset of AIDS in the absence of antiretroviral treatment. Relapses are common.

There are also reports of severe VL being caused by *Leishmania* strains normally of low or no virulence. The results of different serological tests need to be interpreted with care as up to 42% of coinfected patients have been found to have a negative antibody response.

In southern Europe between 25–70% of adult VL cases are estimated to be HIV-related. Intravenous drug users are particularly at risk. In other parts of the world, e.g. India, East Africa and Brazil, the risk of *Leishmania*/HIV coinfection is increasing as VL is becoming more urbanized, and HIV infection is becoming more common in rural areas.[55]

Cutaneous leishmaniasis (CL)

The clinical forms of CL vary according to the species of parasite, region, and response of the patient.

OLD WORLD CL

L. tropica: Infection is often referred to as dry urban oriental sore. Dry painless ulcers 25–70 mm in diameter are produced which are self-healing usually after 1–2 years but often leave disfiguring scars. The patient is immune to reinfection. Rarely there may develop multiple unhealing lesions, often on the face. This condition is known as leishmaniasis recidivans (LR) and is thought to be an allergic state. It can last many years and is difficult to treat. Untreated LR is destructive and disfiguring.

L. major: Infection is often referred to as wet oriental sore. The early papule is often inflamed and resembles a boil of 5–10 mm in diameter which rapidly develops into a large uneven ulcer which is self-healing in as little as 3–6 months. Multiple lesions may occur in non-immune persons. *L. major* infections protect against reinfection and also against infection with *L. tropica*.

L. aethiopica: A cutaneous lesion is produced that is similar to typical oriental sore with healing in 1–3 years. *L. aethiopica* however, can cause diffuse cutaneous leishmaniasis (DCL) in patients with little or no cell-mediated immunity against the parasite. This is an incurable condition characterized by the formation of disfiguring nodules over the surface of the body. The nodules contain large numbers of amastigotes. *L. aethiopica* can also cause mucocutaneous leishmaniasis.

NEW WORLD CL

L. mexicana: Causes chiclero's ulcer or 'bay sore'. Lesions of the body tend to be self-healing but those on the ear may last up to 30 years and entirely destroy the pinna of the ear.

L. peruviana: Mainly infects children. The single or few lesions are painless and usually heal spontaneously after about 4 months. The infection is known locally as 'uta'. It occurs at high altitudes in dry valleys.

L. guyanensis: May give rise to painless dry single ulcers or multiple lesions scattered all over the body. The disease is often referred to as 'forest yaws' ('pian bois'). Spontaneous healing is rare and relapses are frequent.

L. panamensis: Causes single or few skin ulcers which are not self-healing. Lymphatic involvement is common, resulting in secondary nodules.

Diffuse cutaneous leishmaniasis (DCL)

DLC is usually caused by *L. aethiopica* (Old World) and *L. amazonensis* (New World). Skin lesions develop over a large area of the body. The lesions on the eyebrows, nose and ears resemble those of lepromatous leprosy. At first the lesions are smooth, and firm. Later they become scaly and rough. They do not heal spontaneously. DCL caused by *L. amazonensis* is resistant to treatment. With *L. aethiopica*, relapses tend to occur after treatment.

Mucocutaneous leishmaniasis (MCL)

Also known as 'espundia', MCL is caused by New World *Leishmania* species, *L. braziliensis*, *L. panamensis* and occasionally by *L. guyanensis*. In immunosuppressed persons, mucosal lesions can be caused by *L. donovani*, *L. major*, or *L. infantum*.

MCL is the most severe and destructive form of cutaneous leishmaniasis in South America. Lesions are similar in development to those of oriental sore and the resulting ulcers may become very large and long-lasting. Early in the infection, parasites may migrate to tissues of the nasopharynx of the palate and sometimes after many years when the first lesion has healed there begins a slow continuous erosion of these tissues. Disfiguration is often extreme with complete destruction of the nasal septum, perforation of the palate, and damage to the tissues of the lips and larynx.

Patients with a history of inadequate treatment and prolonged scarring, tend to develop MCL. Mucosal lesions do not heal spontaneously and secondary and often severe bacterial infections can occur. A Sudanese form of MCL is referred to as oronasal leishmaniasis.

Measures to prevent and control leishmaniasis

- Early detection and treatment of infected persons, especially in areas where humans are the only or important reservoirs of infection.
- Personal protection from sandfly bites by:
  - Using insect repellants, although in hot and humid conditions they are of limited use due to profuse sweating.
  - Avoiding endemic areas especially at times when sandflies are most active.
  - Use of insecticide impregnated bednets and curtains.
- Vector control by the use of light traps, sticky paper traps, or residual insecticide spraying of houses and farm buildings where this is practical, or alternatively using insecticide paints in a slow-release emulsifiable solution.
- Destruction of stray dogs and infected domestic dogs in areas where dogs are the main reservoir hosts.
- Elimination and control of rodents in areas where these are sources of human infections.
- Whenever possible, siting human dwellings away from the habitats of animal reservoir hosts where sandflies are known to breed, e.g. rodent burrows or rocks where hydraxes live.

Further information: Readers are referred to the 21st edition *Mansons Tropical Diseases* (see Recommended Reading) and the WHO/TDR website www.who.int/tdr

LABORATORY DIAGNOSIS

DIAGNOSIS OF VISCERAL LEISHMANIASIS

The laboratory diagnosis of visceral leishmaniasis (VL) in district laboratories is by:

- Finding amastigotes in:
  - material aspirated from the spleen, bone marrow or an enlarged lymph node,
  - nasal secretions,
  - peripheral blood monocytes and less commonly in neutrophils (buffy coat preparations).

The positivity rates for aspirates and peripheral blood (buffy coat) preparations are as follows:

% Positive

Spleen aspirate	95–98%
Bone marrow aspirate	64–86%
Enlarged lymph node aspirate	55–64%

Buffy coat (India) 67–99%
Buffy coat (Africa) . . . . About 50%

Note: In VL patients coinfected with HIV, amastigotes are frequently found in blood monocytes and neutrophils in buffy coat preparations and also in aspirates from *enlarged* lymph nodes.

■ Testing for leishmanial antibodies using antigen known to detect local parasite strains.

■ Testing for leishmanial antigen in urine.

Culturing aspirates and peripheral blood and examining cultures for promastigotes.

District laboratories wishing to culture *Leishmania* parasites should contact their Regional Laboratory or specialist Leishmaniasis Reference Laboratory for advice.

Other tests

■ Formol gel (aldehyde) test. This is a non-specific screening test which detects marked increases in IgG. Large amounts of polyclonal non-specific immunoglobulin are produced by patients with active VL.

■ Haematological investigations including:
  – measurement of haemoglobin,
  – total and differential white cell (leukocyte) count,
  – platelet (thrombocyte) count.

In VL, the reticuloendothelial system becomes parasitized and the spleen greatly enlarged. Patients become anaemic, leukopenic, and thrombocytopenic. During treatment, a rising haemoglobin and white cell count indicate a good response.

Other haematological findings usually include a raised ESR, positive direct antiglobulin test and often auto-agglutination of red cells. Well washed red cells must be used when slide and tube blood grouping and an indirect antihuman globulin technique when crossmatching.

■ Plasma albumin levels are greatly reduced (often below 2 g/l) and total protein raised in patients with VL.

Examination of buffy coat preparations for amastigotes

In up to 50% or more of patients with VL, parasites can be detected in stained buffy coat smears prepared from EDTA (sequestrene) anticoagulated venous blood. The same EDTA blood sample can be used to measure the haemoglobin, and perform white cell and platelet counts.

Method

1 Collect 2.5 ml of venous blood, dispense into an EDTA container (see Reagent No. 22) and mix gently.

2 After performing a haemoglobin, white cell count, and platelet count, and making a thin blood film, centrifuge the EDTA blood in narrow bore tubes, e.g. *Eppendorf* plastic tubes or glass tubes 6 × 50 mm. Centrifuge for 15 minutes at medium to high speed, i.e. RCF about 1 000 g to obtain the buffy coat (cream coloured layer of white cells and platelets above the red cells).

Filling narrow bore tubes: Using a long stemmed plastic bulb pipette or Pasteur pipette, aspirate the blood from the EDTA container. Insert the tip of the pipette to the *bottom* of the tube and fill the tube(s) with blood, withdrawing the pipette as the tube fills.

3 Using a plastic bulb pipette or Pasteur pipette, carefully remove and discard the plasma above the buffy coat. Transfer the buffy coat to a slide and mix. Place a drop of this on another slide and spread to make a thin smear. Air-dry the smear and fix it with methanol for 2 minutes.

4 Stain the smear by Giemsa technique or Field's rapid technique for thin films as described in subunit 5.7.

5 When dry, spread a drop of immersion oil on the film and examine microscopically. Use the 40× objective to scan the smear for monocytes containing groups of amastigotes. Occasionally amastigotes can be detected in neutrophils. Use the 100× objective to identify the intracellular amastigotes (add a further drop of oil if necessary). The small amastigotes may also be seen lying between cells.

Examination of aspirates for amastigotes

Splenic aspiration

The technique is described by Zijlstra.[57] A splenic aspiration must *not* be performed without training and experience because it may lead to fatal haemorrhage if done incorrectly. Whenever possible, laboratory staff should assist the medical officer performing the aspiration, to ensure films of the correct thickness are made, air dried rapidly, and methanol fixed immediately. Before performing a splenic aspiration, the following tests must be performed:

● Platelet count and prothrombin time to check for abnormal bleeding. The aspiration should *not* be performed if the patient's platelet count is below 40 × 10⁹/l (40 000/mm³) or the prothrombin time is 5 seconds or more longer than that of the control.

Amastigotes of Leishmania species

Structurally, the amastigotes of *Leishmania* species that cause VL, CL and MCL are similar. There are variations in size between species.

- *Small*, round to oval bodies measuring 2–4 μm.
- Can be seen in groups inside blood monocytes (less commonly in neutrophils), in macrophages in aspirates or skin smears, or lying free between cells.
- The nucleus and rod-shaped kinetoplast in each amastigote stain dark reddish-mauve.
- The cytoplasm stains palely and is often difficult to see when the amastigotes are in groups.

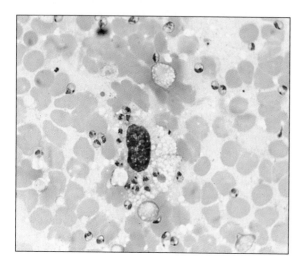

Plate 5.54   *Leishmania* amastigotes in monocyte in a Giemsa stained blood film.

- Haemoglobin to check that the patient is not severely anaemic.

Note: After collecting a splenic aspirate, the patient's pulse and blood pressure should be monitored for up to 8 hours.

Method of examining splenic, bone marrow, lymph node aspirates

1 Immediately after aspiration, make at least 2 thinly spread smears of the aspirate on *clean* slides. Only a small quantity of aspirate is required. Dilution with blood should be avoided.

   Note: If culturing facilities are available, aseptically dispense any remaining aspirate into sterile culture medium.

2 Air-dry the smears as rapidly as possible. Fix by covering each smear with a few drops of absolute methanol (methyl alcohol) or if more convenient, immerse the slides in a container of methanol. Fix for 2-3 minutes.

3 Stain the smears by the rapid Field's technique for thin films or by the Giemsa staining technique as described in subunit 5.7.

4 When dry, spread a drop of immersion oil on the smear and examine microscopically. Use the 40× objective to scan the smear for large mononuclear phagocytic cells containing groups of amastigotes. Use the 100× objective to identify the amastigotes (add a further drop of oil if necessary).

Other findings in aspirates

Other parasites which may be found and should be reported in aspirates include malaria parasites and trypanosomes. If a smear contains pigment and eosinophils this may indicate *Schistosoma* infection. Eosinophils are absent or scanty in visceral leishmaniasis.

Note: Smears that contain abnormal cells which could be malignant cells should be sent to a Cytology Laboratory for reporting. Any remaining aspirate and unstained fixed smears should also be sent.

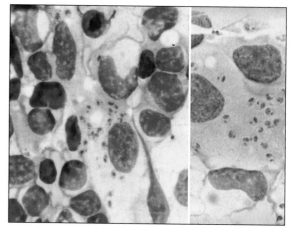

Plate 5.55   Giemsa stained amastigotes of *L.donovani*. *Right*: As seen in bone marrow. *Left*: As seen in splenic aspirate.

Detection of anti-leishmanial antibody

In visceral leishmaniasis, specific antibody as well as non-specific polyclonal Ig G and Ig M are produced. Several techniques have been developed to detect and measure specific anti-leishmanial antibodies in patients' sera. Those being used in district laboratories and field surveys include:

– Direct agglutination test (DAT)
– rK39 dipstick to detect anti-rK39 antibody.

Direct agglutination test

The DAT is widely used in field surveys in endemic areas to screen large numbers of people for VL. The antigen used in the test is available in a heat-stable freeze-dried form. It consists of a suspension of trypsin-treated fixed promastigotes, stained with Coomasie brilliant blue. The test is performed in V shaped wells in microtitration plates with the patient's serum, or eluate from whole blood collected on filter paper, being serially diluted. The test requires incubation at room temperature for about 18 hours. It is read visually against a white background. The endpoint of the test (titre) is taken as the last well where agglutination is seen, i.e. the well before a clear sharp-edged blue spot 'button in the bottom of the well' (like that seen in the control well). The titre which is taken as indicating a positive test must be decided locally. As with other leishmanial antibody tests, the DAT is unable to distinguish active VL from subclinical or past infection. The sensitivity and negative predictive value of the DAT is reported as >90% and specificity 72–95%.[58] Sera from patients coinfected with HIV may be (but not always), nonreactive.

Availability of DAT: A complete DAT kit at cost price is available from the Prince Leopold Institute of Tropical Medicine (see Appendix 11). Freeze dried DAT antigen only is available from Kit Biomedical Research (see Appendix 11). An experimental fast agglutination screening test (FAST) antigen is also available from Kit Biomedical Research.

rK39 dipstick to detect anti-rK39 antibody

Several rapid immunochromatographic dipstick (strip) and cassette format tests have been developed to detect anti-rK39 antibody in patients with VL. Circulating antibody to rK39 antigen has high sensitivity and specificity for active VL. The antigen used in the test is a recombinant (r) antigen rK39 derived from *L. chagasi*. The patient's serum is applied to the strip and reacts with the colloidal gold dye conjugate. A buffer solution is added. As the antibody-colloidal gold complex migrates up the strip it is captured by a line of rK39 antigen in the test area, producing a pink line. A positive pink control line above the test area indicates satisfactory migration of the reagents. Most rK39 tests take 10 minutes to perform.

Several studies in India in VL endemic areas have reported the test to be 100% sensitive and 88–98% specific.[58] Lower sensitivities have been reported

from the Sudan, Brazil and southern Europe. Evaluations in Nepal have reported sensitivities of 87–100% and specificities of greater than 93%.[59] Positive results may be found after successful treatment but to a lesser extent than with the DAT. In HIV coinfected patients, antibody response to rK39 antigen is variable. Evaluations on recently developed commercially available dipstick and cassette tests in VL endemic and low prevalence areas are underway.

Availability: Dipstick and cassette rK39 tests called *Kala-azar Detect* are available from InBios (see Appendix 11), individually pouched and in packs of 25 dipsticks/vial or 25 cassettes/box. They require storage below 30 °C and must be protected from exposure to humid conditions. The buffer solution requires storage at 2–8 °C.

rK39 dipsticks called *Leishmania RapiDip InstTest* are available from Cortex Diagnostics (see Appendix 11). Each kit contains 25 dipsticks individually pouched or contained in a vial. They must be stored below 30 °C and protected from humidity. The buffer solution requires storage at 2–8 °C.

Katex test to detect leishmanial antigen in urine

The *Katex* test is a recently developed latex agglutination test which detects leishmanial antigen in the urine of patients with VL. The test uses latex particles sensitised with antibodies raised against *L. donovani* antigen. A urine sample is first boiled for 5 minutes to inactivate substances capable of causing false positive reactions with the latex reagent. After allowing the urine to cool to ambient temperature, 50µl of sample is mixed with 1 drop of the latex reagent. Results are read after mixing for 2 minutes. Agglutination indicates a positive test for VL. A negative control is run with the test samples to distinguish between a weak positive and negative test result.

The *Katex* test has been shown to perform better than any serological test when compared to microscopy.[60] It has been reported as a sensitive test and specific for active VL infections and is also a useful test in indicating treatment failure and detecting VL in HIV coinfected patients.[61] Field trials are ongoing to determine the performance of the test in different VL endemic areas.

Availability: The *Katex* test is manufactured by and available from Kalon Biological (see Appendix 11). The latex reagent, positive and negative controls and other items required to perform the test are included in the test kit. Reagents require refrigeration at 2–8 °C.

Formol gel (aldehyde) test

Although not a reliable test for diagnosing VL,[59] because of its simplicity and low cost, the formol gel test remains in use in some remote areas. The test is non-specific. It detects large amounts of non-specific polyclonal globulin in the patient's serum. It becomes positive about 3 months after infection and negative about 6 months after successful treatment.

Method

1 Collect about 5 ml of venous blood in a dry glass tube and leave to clot. When the clot begins to retract (30–60 minutes after collection), centrifuge the blood to obtain clear serum. If a centrifuge is not available, leave the specimen to separate overnight.

2 Transfer about 1 ml of red cell free serum to a small tube. Add 2 drops of concentrated formalin solution and mix. Allow to stand for 30 minutes. Most positive tests, however, can be read after a few minutes.

Positive test: Serum whitens and gels within 30 minutes (often within 5 minutes).

Negative test: Serum remains unchanged or gelling *only* occurs. A negative test cannot exclude VL (test only becomes positive about 3 months after infection).

Note: Patients with multiple myeloma may also give a positive formol gel test. Other conditions such as chronic liver disease, malaria, trypanosomiasis, and leprosy are also associated with raised globulin levels. In typhoid, haemolytic anaemia, chronic myeloid leukaemia, and infective endocarditis, the formol gel test is negative. Variable results are found in VL patients infected with HIV.

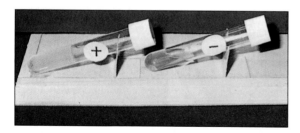

Plate 5.56   Formol gel test showing positive (+) and negative (−) reactions.

DIAGNOSIS OF CUTANEOUS AND MUCOCUTANEOUS LEISHMANIASIS

The *Leishmania* species that cause cutaneous leishmaniasis (CL) and mucocutaneous leishmaniasis (MCL) are listed at the beginning of this subunit. The laboratory diagnosis of CL and MCL is by:

- Detecting amastigotes in smears taken from infected ulcers or nodules. In MCL, the parasites are scanty and difficult to find in smears.

- Culturing ulcer material and examining cultures for promastigotes.

Serological diagnosis of CL and MCL

Because of the poor antibody response in CL, serological tests are of little value in diagnosis. There is, however, a cellular response which is the basis of the leishmanin skin test (see later text). In MCL, antibodies can be found in the serum. District laboratories should contact their nearest Leishmaniasis Reference Laboratory for information on the most appropriate test to use.

Collection and examination of slit skin smears for amastigotes

Material for examination should be taken from the inflamed *raised swollen edge* of an ulcer or nodule. Care should be taken to avoid contaminating the specimen with blood.

Smears taken from the centre of a lesion

Ramirez *et al* in a study carried out in Colombia found that the diagnosis of CL by microscopy improved significantly when a smear was taken from the centre of a lesion. They recommend that smears be taken from *both* the edge and centre of lesions.[62]

Note: Secondary bacterial contamination makes it difficult to find parasites and therefore if bacterial infection is present, examination for *Leishmania* amastigotes is best delayed until antimicrobial treatment has been completed and the bacterial infection has cleared.

Method

1 Cleanse the area with a swab soaked in 70% v/v alcohol. Allow to dry completely.

2 Firmly squeeze the edge of the lesion between the finger and thumb to drain the area of blood (protective rubber gloves should be worn).

3 Using a sterile scalpel blade, make a small cut into the dermis and blot away any blood. Scrape the cut surface in an outward direction to obtain tissue juice and cells.

4 Spread the material on a clean slide using a circular motion and working outwards to avoid damaging parasites in those parts of the smear that have started to dry.

 The smear must be thinly spread and not left as a thick 'dab' smear. Parasites will be difficult to find in thick smears.

5 When dry, fix the smear by covering it with a few drops of absolute methanol (methyl alcohol). Fix for 2–3 minutes.

6 Stain the smear using the Giemsa technique or rapid Field's technique for thin films as described in subunit 5.7.

7 When the smear is dry, spread a drop of immersion oil on it and examine first with the 10× and 40× objectives to detect macrophages which may contain amastigotes (the parasites can also be found outside macrophage cells). Use the 100× oil immersion objective to identify the amastigotes, adding a further drop of oil if required.

Note: The features which identify *Leishmania* amastigotes are described in the previous text. *L. mexicana* amastigotes are larger than those of *L. braziliensis* and have a more centrally placed kinetoplast.

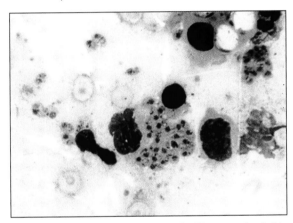

Plate 5.57 *Leishmania* amastigotes in Giemsa stained skin slit smear.

Culture of ulcer material

Culture is of value when cutaneous leishmaniasis is suspected and parasites cannot be found in smears. In leishmaniasis recidivans, culture is usually required to detect parasites.

Material for culture is best obtained by injecting and then aspirating a small quantity of sterile physiological saline in and out of the hardened margin of the ulcer. A few drops of the final aspirate is used to inoculate the culture medium. *L. tropica* grows rapidly in culture. *L. brazilliensis* grows more slowly in culture than *L. mexicana* and the promastigotes are smaller.

Note: District laboratories wishing to culture *Leishmania* parasites should contact their nearest Leishmaniasis Reference Laboratory for advice on the type of culture media to use, details of technique, and how to minimize contamination of cultures.

Leishmanin skin test

The antigen used in the leishmanin test, or Montenegro reaction, is prepared from killed culture forms (promastigotes) of *L. braziliensis, L. mexicana,* or *L. tropica,* with a concentration of 10×10^6 parasites per ml.

The antigen is available from centres of leishmaniasis studies or from commercial manufacturers. In the test, 0.1 ml of well-shaken antigen is injected intradermally into the inner surface of the forearm. It is preferable to perform tests with an accompanying control solution. The diameter of induration is measured at 48 and 72 hours.

Positive reaction

The reaction is considered positive when the area of induration is 5 mm in diameter or more.

A positive reaction may be found in many persons from endemic areas who show no visible skin lesions but have been exposed to infection (test remains positive for life). A positive leishmanin test in children under 10 years of age from endemic areas, is highly suggestive of the disease.

In persons entering an endemic area for the first time, the development of skin lesions and positive leishmanin test indicate cutaneous leishmaniasis.

In South American MCL, the leishmanin test is positive and the reaction may be sufficiently violent to cause necrosis in the centre of the area of induration.

Negative reaction

A negative reaction may be found in some 15% of patients with uncomplicated cutaneous leishmaniasis, especially in patients infected with *L. aethiopica.* The test is usually negative in *active* visceral leishmaniasis and diffuse cutaneous leishmaniasis.

There are no significant cross-reactions with other diseases.

Differentiation of *L. braziliensis* and *L. mexicana*

There are differences in the prognosis and treatment of diseases caused by parasites of the *L. braziliensis* and *L. mexicana* complexes. It is therefore important to know which organism is causing infection. Whenever possible, positive cultures or serum for serological testing should be sent to a Leishmaniasis Reference Laboratory for identification of the species.

5.11 Examination of blood for microfilariae in lymphatic filariasis and loiasis

Lymphatic filariasis is caused by the filarial worms *Wuchereria bancrofti*, *Brugia malayi*, and *Brugia timori* which live in the lymphatic vessels and lymph nodes. Loiasis, also known as Calabar swelling, is caused by the filarial worm *Loa loa* which lives in subcutaneous tissues. *L. loa* is often referred to as the 'eye worm' because the adult worms sometimes migrate across the conjunctiva or eyelid.

The microfilariae (1st stage larvae) of filarial worms that cause lymphatic filariasis and loiasis can be found in the blood and often show what is called periodicity, i.e. they are present in the peripheral blood in greater numbers during certain hours which correspond to the peak biting times of their insect vectors.

Nocturnal periodicity: Microfilariae are present in greatest numbers in the peripheral blood during night hours, e.g. periodic *Wuchereria bancrofti*, *Brugia malayi* and *Brugia timori*.

Diurnal periodicity: Microfilariae are present in greatest numbers in the peripheral blood during day hours, e.g. *Loa loa*.

Nocturnal subperiodicity or diurnal subperiodicity: Microfilariae can be found in the peripheral blood throughout the 24 hours with only a slight increase in numbers during day or night hours, e.g. subperiodic *W. bancrofti* and subperiodic *B. malayi*.

Note: The blood collection times for *W. bancrofti* (periodic and subperiodic nocturnal and subperiodic diurnal), *B. malayi* (periodic and subperiodic nocturnal), *B. timori* (nocturnal), and *L. loa* (diurnal) are summarized under *Laboratory diagnosis*.

Distribution
LYMPHATIC FILARIASIS
Lymphatic filariasis is one of the most prevalent tropical diseases with 120 million people infected in 83 countries. Most infections (90–95%) are caused by *W. bancrofti*.[63] An estimated 40 million people have severe chronic disease.

W. bancrofti
Nocturnal periodic *W. bancrofti* is endemic in tropical America, Caribbean, tropical Africa, Egypt, the Middle East, India and South East Asia, southern and eastern China, the Far East and New Guinea.

The diurnal subperiodic variant of *W. bancrofti* is found mainly in the eastern Pacific (Polynesia). The nocturnal subperiodic variant is found especially in Thailand and Vietnam.

W. bancrofti is found with *B. malayi* in parts of South East Asia and South India.

B. malayi and *B. timori*
B. malayi is endemic in parts of South East Asia including many of the islands of the Malay Archipelago. It also occurs in south west India, the Philippines, Vietnam, China, and South Korea.

Periodic *B. malayi* is commonly found in open swamps and the rice-growing areas of coastal regions. The subperiodic variant is found mostly in fresh water swamps in forests along major rivers.

B. timori shows a nocturnal periodicity. It is found only in the Lesser Sunda Islands of Indonesia. The species takes its name from the island of Timor which forms part of the group. It is found in low lying riverine and coastal areas.

LOIASIS
L. loa is restricted to the equatorial rain forest areas of West and Central Africa particularly Congo, Gabon, Cameroon, southern Nigeria, and equatorial Sudan. It is endemic in many areas where *W. bancrofti* also occurs.

Transmission and life cycle
LYMPHATIC FILARIASIS
W. bancrofti, *B. malayi*, *B. timori* are transmitted by female mosquitoes belonging to the genera *Culex*, *Anopheles*, *Aedes*, and *Mansonia*. Infection occurs when infective larvae are deposited on human skin when a mosquito vector takes a blood meal. The larvae penetrate the skin through the bite wound.

Vectors
Periodic *W. bancrofti* is transmitted by *Culex*, *Anopheles*, and *Aedes* mosquitoes. Subperiodic *W. bancrofti* is transmitted by *Aedes* mosquitoes.

Nocturnal periodic *B. malayi* is transmitted mainly by mosquitoes belonging to the genera *Anopheles* and *Mansonia*.

Subperiodic *B. malayi* is transmitted by *Mansonia* and *Coquillettidia* mosquitoes. Monkeys are important reservoirs of subperiodic *B. malayi* in parts of Malaysia, Sumatra, and Kalimantan. Domestic cats, dogs and possibly other animals are also thought to be reservoir hosts of subperiodic *B. malayi*.

B. timori (nocturnal periodic) is transmitted by *Anopheles* mosquitoes.

Note: Further information on the mosquitoes that transmit *W. bancrofti* and *Brugia* species can be found in the 21st edition *Mansons Tropical Diseases* (see Recommended Reading).

The life cycle of *W. bancrofti*, *B. malayi* and *B. timori* is summarized in Fig. 5.33.

Development of the larvae takes place in the lymphatics. Within 3–15 months, the larvae become mature male and female worms. The females produce many sheathed microfilariae which can be found in the blood about 9 months after infection for *W. bancrofti* and after about 3 months for *Brugia* species.

The mature worms can live for many years in their host depending in part on the extent of the host's immune response. Their mean lifespan is 4–6 years but they can survive up to 15 years or more.

The microfilariae are taken up by a mosquito vector when it sucks blood (microfilariae which are not ingested die within 6–24 months). In the stomach of the mosquito the microfilariae lose their sheath and migrate from the midgut to the thorax of the vector where they develop into infective larvae. Development in the mosquito takes 1–2 weeks. Mature infective larvae migrate to the mouth-parts of the mosquito ready to be transmitted when the insect next takes a blood meal.

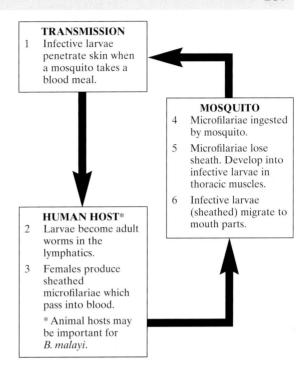

Fig 5.33   Transmission and life cycle of *W. bancrofti* and *Brugia* species.

LOIASIS

L. loa is transmitted by blood-sucking daytime biting tabanid flies of the genus *Chrysops*. They are often referred to as horseflies.

Infective larvae (often in large numbers) enter human skin through the deep wound made by an infected *Chrysops* fly when it sucks blood. The larvae penetrate subcutaneous connective tissues and within 6–12 months they develop into mature male and female worms. The viviparous females produce sheathed microfilariae which can be found in the blood during day hours.

The mature worms may live for 4–12 years in their host. They wander in subcutaneous tissue and occasionally under the conjunctiva of the eye.

The microfilariae are taken up by a female *Chrysops* when sucking blood. In the stomach of the *Chrysops* the microfilariae lose their sheath. They pass through the stomach wall, penetrate thoracic muscles, and develop into infective larvae. Development in the insect vector takes about 10 days. Mature infective larvae migrate to the mouth-parts of the insect ready to be transmitted when the *Chrysops* takes a blood meal.

Lymphatic filariasis
Clinical features and pathology depend on the sites occupied by developing and mature worms, the number of worms present, length of infection, and the immune responses of the host especially to damaged and dead worms. Symptoms of infection differ from one endemic area to another. Infections can be asymptomatic, acute, or chronic.

Asymptomatic lymphatic filariasis

In endemic areas a proportion of infected persons develop no clinical symptoms although microfilariae can be found in their blood (microfilaraemia). Such persons can remain asymptomatic for several years or progress to acute and chronic filariasis.

Acute lymphatic filariasis

In the acute form there are recurrent attacks of fever (filarial fever) with painful inflammation of the lymph nodes (lymphadenitis) and lymph ducts (lymphangitis). The lymphatics involved are those of the limbs, genital organs (especially spermatic cord) and breasts.

In bancroftian filariasis, the lymph glands in the groin and lymphatics of the male genitalia are frequently affected. Inflammation of the spermatic cord and repeated attacks can lead to blockage of the spermatic lymph vessels, leading to accumulation of fluid in the scrotal sac which becomes distended (hydrocele). In brugian filariasis, the affected lymph nodes are mostly situated in the inguinal and axillary regions with inflammation of distal lymphatics.

Acute attacks can last for several days and are usually accompanied by a rash and eosinophilia. Damage to the lymphatics leads to thickening and eventual blockage of lymphatic vessels with lymphoedema (lymph fluid in surrounding tissues). Infections with subperiodic *W. bancrofti* and *B. timori* are associated with ulcers which form along the inflamed lymph vessels.

Chronic lymphatic filariasis

This is characterized by hydrocele, lymphoedema and elephantiasis. Hydrocele is common in bancroftian filariasis. Microfilariae are rarely found in the blood of patients with hydrocele or elephantiasis but can be found occasionally in hydrocele fluid.

Elephantiasis is a complication of advanced lymphatic filariasis. It is seen as a coarse thickening, hardening, and cracking of the skin overlying enlarged fibrosed tissues. The legs are more commonly affected than the arms and in *W. bancrofti* endemic areas, the thigh also is often involved. Grossly enlarged limbs make walking difficult. Secondary bacterial and fungal infections of the skin can occur. Elephantiasis is more commonly seen in filariasis endemic areas of Africa, China, India, and the Pacific region.

In brugian filariasis, symptoms of infection develop more rapidly and children are often infected. Elephantiasis occurs less frequently and tends to involve only the lower limbs. In male adults, the scrotum and spermatic cord are not usually affected and hydrocele is rare.

Non-filarial elephantiasis

In tropical countries, causes of elephantiasis other than filarial worms include tuberculosis and siliceous deposits. Endemic elephantiasis of the lower legs associated with siliceous deposits has been reported from the highlands of Kenya, Tanzania, Ethiopia, Ruanda, Burundi, western Sudan, Cape Verde Islands, Cameroon and Rajastan in India. Damage to local lymphatics with obstruction occurs when silica from the soil is absorbed through bare feet, usually resulting in bilateral elephantiasis.

Chyluria

An uncommon complication of chronic bancroftian filariasis is chyluria. It occurs when the urogenital lymphatic vessels which are linked to those that transport chyle from the intestine become blocked and rupture. Chyle and occasionally blood and microfilariae can be found in the urine especially in early morning specimens. Microfilariae are usually present in the fibrin clots which form.

Occult filariasis and tropical pulmonary eosinophilia

The term occult filariasis refers to a rare condition which is caused by a hypersensitivity reaction to filarial antigens. The features of lymphatic filariasis are not present and microfilariae are not detected in the blood but may be found in tissues.

Tropical pulmonary eosinophilia is a form of occult filariasis in which there is a hypersensitive reaction to the destruction of microfilariae in pulmonary capillaries. It is found particularly in filariasis endemic areas of India and South-East Asia. Males are more commonly affected than females. It interferes with breathing and can lead to chronic pulmonary fibrosis. Symptoms are worse at night. There is a marked eosinophilia, raised erythrocyte sedimentation rate, and high levels of filarial antibody including high titres of IgE. Eosinophils often appear vacuolated.

Measures to prevent and control lymphatic filariasis

- Controlling mosquito vectors by:

  - Studying the ecology and behaviour of local vectors to reduce mosquito numbers and eradicate breeding sites, e.g. reducing the breeding of *C. quinquefasciatus* (important vector of *W. bancrofti*) in stagnant and polluted water by improving the maintenance of pit latrines and septic tanks and covering the surface water with polystyrene beads. The use of selective weed killers has proved an effective measure against *Mansonia* mosquitoes that transmit *B. malayi*.

  - Using insecticides known to be effective against local vectors (*C. quinquefasciatus* is resistant to most insecticides).

- Avoiding mosquito bites by wearing suitable clothing, using mosquito nets, and as far as possible making houses mosquito-proof. The use of insecticide impregnated bed-netting is proving successful in many areas where the mosquito vector is a night feeder.

- Treating infected individuals as part of a mass control programme in *W. bancrofti* endemic areas (to prevent mosquitoes becoming infected). DEC cannot be used in areas where *O. volvulus* and *L. loa* occur because of life-threatening adverse reactions to the drug (further details from WHO/TDR unit www.who.int/tdr).

- Informing those living in endemic areas about the cause, early symptoms, detection and control of lymphatic filariasis.

- Clearing trees around houses in brugian filariasis areas where monkeys are important reservoir hosts.

Global programme to eliminate lymphatic filariasis (GPELF)

The WHO GPELF provides technical assistance to countries who are implementing mapping activities and mass drug administration campaigns. It also coordinates efforts to promote appropriate prevention and control of clinical symptoms of lymphatic filariasis.

Further information: Readers are referred to the *Report on Lymphatic Filariasis*. WHO/CDS/CPE/CEE/2002.28, Geneva. Can be downloaded from the *Global alliance to eliminate lymphatic filariasis* website www.filariasis.org

Also recommended is the *Liverpool lymphatic filariasis support centre* website www.filariasis.net

Loiasis

Many people infected with *L. loa* do not develop clinical symptoms. The disease is characterized by the formation of swellings known as Calabar swellings which may last from a few days up to 3 weeks and measure from 3–10 cm in diameter. The arms are most frequently affected. The inflamed areas are an allergic response to adult *L. loa* worms migrating in the subcutaneous tissue. Worms are not usually present in the swellings but they can occasionally be seen migrating below the skin surface. In non-immune persons, infection with *L. loa* can cause severe allergic reactions.

Adult worms also migrate in subconjunctival tissues. They can be seen under the eyelids and occasionally slowly crossing the white of the eye. They can cause inflammation and irritation but not blindness. The microfilariae do not seem to cause any serious symptoms although it has been reported that encephalitis can occur following treatment of heavy infections.

An eosinophilic leucocytosis and high titres of specific anti-filarial antibodies are found in patients with loiasis. Occasionally an immune complex related glomerulonephritis can occur with blood and protein being found in urine.

Measures to prevent and control loiasis
- Avoiding the bites of *Chrysops* flies (daytime feeders) by:

  - Wearing protective clothing, e.g. long trousers. Light-coloured clothing also gives some protection.

  - Siting settlements, including adequate water supplies, away from forest areas.

- Destroying *Chrysops* flies by:

  - Changing the character of breeding places wherever possible, e.g. clearing vegetation to allow in sunlight to dry out muddy areas which were previously heavily shaded.

  - Using insecticides as part of a control programme where this is feasible.

- Detecting and treating individuals, including using a rapid assessment procedure based on clinical signs (history of eyeworm or Calabar swelling) to assess the endemicity of loiasis to help identify those at risk of severe adverse reactions to invermectin treatment.[64, 65]

LABORATORY DIAGNOSIS

Lymphatic filariasis is diagnosed by:
- Finding and identifying the microfilariae of *W. bancrofti* or *Brugia* species in blood collected at the correct time.
- Occasionally detecting the microfilariae of *W. bancrofti* in hydrocele fluid or in the urine of patients with chyluria.
- Detection of *W. bancrofti* specific antigen in whole blood, serum or plasma to diagnose bancroftian filariasis (cannot diagnose brugian filariasis).

Loiasis is diagnosed by:
- Finding and identifying *L. loa* microfilariae in blood collected at the correct time. In 60–70% of patients with occult loiasis it is not possible to find microfilariae in the blood.
- Occasionally by finding *L. loa* microfilariae in joint fluid.

Note: Calabar swelling is accompanied by a marked eosinophilia.

Mansonella microfilariae that can be found in blood
In areas where *W. bancrofti* and *L. loa* occur, patients may also be infected with microfilariae of *Mansonella* filarial worms. These parasites are mostly non-pathogenic or of low pathogenicity causing allergic reactions, fever, and sometimes arthralgia and cutaneous swellings. Their microfilariae show no periodicity, i.e. they can be found in the peripheral blood both during day and night hours.

M. perstans is found in tropical Africa, Central America and South America. It therefore requires differentiation from *W. bancrofti* and *L. loa* (see later text).

M. ozzardi is found in the West Indies, Central America, and South America. It therefore requires differentiation from *W. bancrofti* (see later text).

EXAMINATION OF BLOOD FOR MICROFILARIAE

Even when specimens are collected at the correct time, the numbers of microfilariae in the blood are often few and therefore concentration techniques are frequently needed. Microfilariae are rarely found in the blood of patients with hydrocele or elephantiasis once the lymphatics become blocked. Occasionally in endemic areas microfilariae can be present in the blood of asymptomatic persons. In *L. loa* endemic areas, microfilariae can be found in the blood of only 30–40% of infected persons.

In *W. bancrofti* and *Brugia* infections, microfilariae numbers are higher in capillary blood than in venous blood.

Summary of distribution of microfilariae that can be found in blood

AFRICA	INDIA
W. bancrofti	*W. bancrofti*
L. loa	*B. malayi*
M. perstans	
	SOUTH EAST ASIA PHILIPPINE ISLANDS
CENTRAL AMERICA	*W. bancrofti*
SOUTH AMERICA	*B. malayi*
W. bancrofti	*B. timori* (Lesser Sunda Is.)
M. perstans	
M. ozzardi	CHINA
	W. bancrofti
PACIFIC REGION	*B. malayi*
W. bancrofti	

Note: Onchocerca volvulus, normally found in skin (see subunit 5.12), can also be found in blood and other body fluids in heavy infections and after treatment with diethylcarbamazine (DEC). *O. volvulus* is found in Africa, South America and Central America (described in subunit 5.12).

Correct time to collect blood to detect pathogenic blood microfilariae

Blood specimens must be collected during the hours when the numbers of microfilariae circulating in the peripheral blood are at their highest, i.e. to coincide with their periodicity (see beginning of subunit).

SPECIES	COLLECTION TIME
Wuchereria bancrofti	
Periodic, nocturnal Asia, Africa, Caribbean South America, west Pacific	22.00–04.00 h Peak 24.00 h
Subperiodic, nocturnal Thailand, Vietnam	20.00–22.00 h Peak 21.00 h
Subperiodic, diurnal South east Pacific	14.00–18.00 h Peak 16.00 h
Brugia malayi	
Periodic, nocturnal South and east Asia	22.00–04.00 h Peak 24.00 h
Subperiodic, nocturnal South East Asia	20.00–22.00 h Peak 21.00 h
Brugia timori	
Nocturnal	22.00–04.00 h Peak 24.00 h
Loa loa	
Diurnal	10.00–15.00 h Peak 13.00 h

Note: Mansonella microfilariae are nonperiodic, i.e. can be found in day and night blood.

Selection of technique

The following techniques are recommended to detect, quantify, and identify microfilariae in blood in district laboratories:

- *Lyzed capillary blood technique*

  100 μl (0.1 ml) of capillary blood (preferably taken from the ear lobe) is haemolyzed in saponin-saline. The microfilariae are concentrated by centrifugation. The addition of a blue nuclear stain helps to identify the species. The number of microfilariae counted multiplied by 10 gives the approximate number per ml of blood (mf/ml). If no microfilariae are detected by this technique, a concentration should be carried out.

  Ear lobe blood: More microfilariae can often be found in capillary blood collected from the ear lobe than from the finger.

CONCENTRATION TECHNIQUES

- *Tube centrifugation lyzed venous blood technique*

  10 ml of venous blood is lyzed in saponin-saline. The microfilariae are concentrated by centrifugation. The addition of a blue nuclear stain helps to identify the species. The number of microfilariae (mf) counted divided by 10 gives the number of mf/ml.

- *Microhaematocrit tube technique*

  Capillary blood (preferably ear lobe blood) is collected in two heparanized capillary tubes or about 100 μl is first collected into EDTA anticoagulant and transferred to plain capillary tubes. The blood is centrifuged in a microhaematocrit centrifuge and the buffy coat examined microscopically for motile microfilariae (see subunit 5.8). In areas where the species is known and *Mansonella* microfilariae are not found, this is a rapid technique for detecting microfilariae.

- *Membrane filtration technique*

  10 ml of venous blood is collected into sodium citrate anticoagulant and the blood passed through a polycarbonate (clear) membrane filter of 3 μm or 5 μm porosity. The microfilariae are retained and the membrane is examined microscopically. The number of microfilariae counted divided by 10 gives the number of mf/ml. This is the most sensitive method of detecting small numbers of microfilariae but it is expensive for routine use.

Other diagnostic and field techniques used to detect microfilariae in blood

- *Thick stained smear technique*

  20 μl (0.02 ml) of capillary blood is collected from the ear lobe, allowed to dry and stained by Giemsa stain. It is less sensitive than the lyzed capillary blood technique in which 100 μl of blood is examined. The same smear can be used to detect both malaria parasites and microfilariae. Smears should be stained within 48 hours of collecting the blood to prevent shrinkage and distortion of the microfilariae. Providing 20 μl of blood is used to make the smear,

the number of microfilariae counted in the entire smear multiplied by 50 will give an approximate number of mf/ml.

■ *Wet slide preparation*
$20 \mu l$ (0.02 ml) of capillary blood is mixed with 2 drops of water (to lyze the red cells) on a slide. The preparation is covered with a cover glass and examined for motile microfilariae using the $10\times$ objective, preferably by dark-field microscopy. This technique is sometimes used as a screening test but it is not as sensitive as techniques in which $100 \mu l$ of blood is examined.

■ *Counting chamber technique*
This is similar to the lyzed capillary blood technique except that the $100 \mu l$ of blood is lyzed with water in a simple ruled chamber (prepared from strips of glass slides). The technique is not as convenient as the saponin-saline lyzed blood technique. In the counting chamber, microfilariae are more difficult to focus in such a large depth of red fluid. The preparation also takes longer to examine because the microfilariae are not concentrated and methylene blue cannot be added to assist in identifying the microfilariae.

Lyzed capillary blood technique

Required

Saponin-saline solution to lyze the red cells.	Reagent No. 54
Methylene blue-saline Azur B, or Field's stain A*	Reagent No. 42

* This will stain the nuclei and show whether the microfilariae are sheathed. The sheaths do not stain but can be seen as unstained extensions at the head and tail end (see Plate 5.58).

Method

1 At the correct time (see previous text), collect $100 \mu l$ (0.1 ml) of capillary blood (preferably from the ear lobe) and dispense it into a centrifuge (conical) tube containing 1 ml of saponin-saline lyzing solution.

Note: If saponin-saline is not available, dispense the blood into 1 ml of water. When water is used, the microfilariae remain motile as in saponin-saline but the haemolysate is not as clear (contains red cell stroma).

Field surveys
Collect 0.1 ml of capillary blood into 3% v/v acetic acid. This will fix and preserve the microfilariae, enabling the specimen to be examined several days later if necessary.

2 Mix the blood gently in the lyzing solution and leave for about 2 minutes to allow time for all the red cells to lyze (leave for 10 minutes if using water).

3 Centrifuge for 5 minutes at slow to medium speed, i.e. RCF 300–500 g. Do not centrifuge at high speed because this may cause the loss of sheaths from pathogenic microfilariae.

If a centrifuge is not available, add a small drop of concentrated formaldehyde solution to kill and preserve the microfilariae. Leave the haemolysate undisturbed for at least 4 h or preferably overnight to allow the microfilariae time to sediment by gravity.

4 Using a plastic bulb pipette or Pasteur pipette, remove and discard the supernatant fluid. Transfer all the sediment to a slide, add a *small* drop of methylene blue-saline, Azur B, or Field's stain A, and cover with a cover glass.

5 Examine the *entire* preparation microscopically for motile microfilariae (non-motile if formaldehyde has been used), using the $10\times$ objective with the condenser iris *closed sufficiently* to give good contrast, or preferably examine by dark-field microscopy.*

* When using dark-field microscopy, the sheaths of the pathogenic microfilariae can be clearly seen when viewed with the $40\times$ objective. The preparation must be sufficiently thin and the cover glass and slide, completely clean.

6 Count the number of microfilariae in the entire preparation. Multiply the number counted by 10 to give an approximate number of microfilariae per ml of blood (mf/ml).

Value of microfilaria count in routine diagnosis
In heavy infections, especially in loiasis, severe reactions can occur during treatment and therefore it is helpful for the medical officer to know whether the microfilaria concentration is high before starting treatment.

7 If unable to identify the species, examine a fixed stained preparation with the $100\times$ objective as follows:

– Remove the cover glass and add a *small* drop of plasma, serum, or albumin solution.* Mix and spread thinly. Allow the preparation to dry completely.

* The addition of albumin, plasma, or serum (known to be microfilaria-free) will help to prevent the preparation from being washed from the slide during staining.

– Fix with absolute methanol or ethanol for 2–3 minutes.

– Stain using Field's technique for thin films or Giemsa technique as described in subunit 5.7. If looking for *L. loa*, use Delafield's haematoxylin technique as this will stain the sheath of *L. loa*.

Note: See Plate 5.58 for the identifying features of *W. bancrofti*, *B. malayi*, *B. timori*, *L. loa* and *Mansonella* microfilariae.

DIFFERENTIATION OF MICROFILARIAE THAT CAN BE FOUND IN BLOOD

Species	Sheath	Main Features	Other Points
W. bancrofti Lymphatic filariasis	+	• Large, measuring 275–300 × 8–10 μm. • Body curves are few, nuclei are distinct. • Sheath stains pink with Giemsa and palely with haematoxylin. *Tail:* There are no nuclei in the tip.	Test night blood (14–18 h: Pacific strain) Differentiated from *Brugia* species and *L. loa* by its tail features. Differentiated from *Mansonella* species by its larger size and sheath.
B. malayi Lymphatic filariasis	+	• Large, measuring 200–275 × 5–6 μm • Body has many angular curves, nuclei are dense and stain darkly. • Sheath stains dark pink with Giemsa and palely with haematoxylin (may be absent). *Tail:* There are 2 nuclei in the end of the tail which tapers irregularly.	Test night blood. Differentiated from *W. bancrofti* by its darker stained sheath and nuclei, kinked body, and tail features. Differentiated from *B. timori* by its shorter length and darker stained sheath.
B. timori Lymphatic filariasis	+	The following features distinguish *B. timori* from *B. malayi*: • It is longer, measuring 290–325 × 5–6 μm. • Sheath stains palely or not at all with Giemsa (often absent). • Body nuclei are less dense and the space at the head end (cephalic space) is longer. *Tail:* Similar to *B. malayi*, i.e. has 2 nuclei in end.	Test night blood. Only found in Lesser Sunda Is.
L. loa Loiasis (Calabar swelling)	+	• Large, measuring 250–300 × 8–10 μm • Body has several curves and kinks. Nuclei are not distinct. • Sheath stains best with haematoxylin. *Tail:* Nuclei extend to end of tail.	Test day blood. Differentiated from *W. bancrofti* by its tail features. Differentiated from *M. perstans* by its larger size and sheath.
M. perstans Non-pathogenic or of low pathogenicity	−	• Small and thin, measuring 190–240 × 4.5 μm • Body nuclei are irregular. *Tail:* Nuclei extend to end of tail which is rounded. Large nucleus in tip.	In day and night blood. Differentiated from *L. loa* and *W. bancrofti* by its smaller size, absence of sheath, tail features, and non-periodicity.
M. ozzardi Non-pathogenic or of low pathogenicity	−	• Small and thin measuring 150–200 × 4.5 μm. • Body nuclei are not distinct. Anterior nuclei are positioned side by side. *Tail:* No nuclei in the end of the tail which is long and pointed.	In day and night blood. Differentiated from *W. bancrofti* by its smaller size, absence of sheath, and non-periodicity.

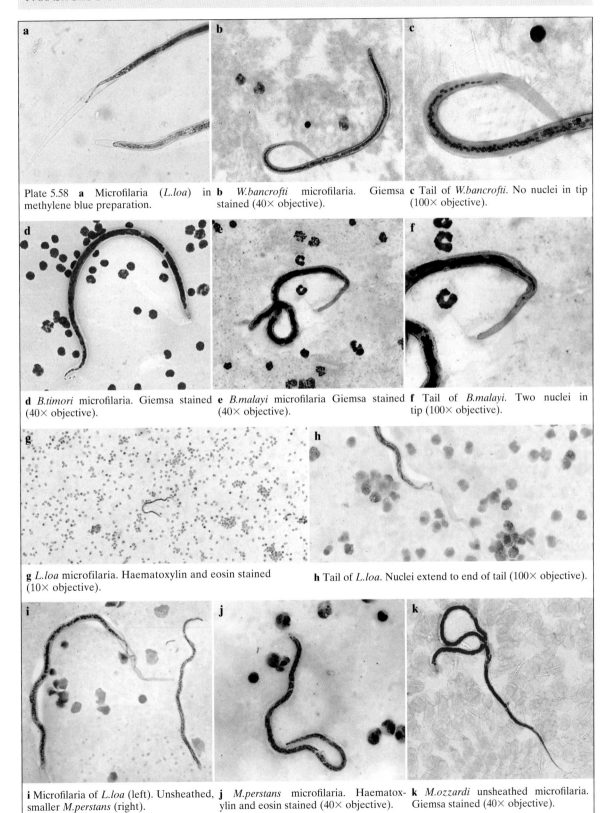

Plate 5.58 **a** Microfilaria (*L.loa*) in methylene blue preparation.

b *W.bancrofti* microfilaria. Giemsa stained (40× objective).

c Tail of *W.bancrofti*. No nuclei in tip (100× objective).

d *B.timori* microfilaria. Giemsa stained (40× objective).

e *B.malayi* microfilaria Giemsa stained (40× objective).

f Tail of *B.malayi*. Two nuclei in tip (100× objective).

g *L.loa* microfilaria. Haematoxylin and eosin stained (10× objective).

h Tail of *L.loa*. Nuclei extend to end of tail (100× objective).

i Microfilaria of *L.loa* (left). Unsheathed, smaller *M.perstans* (right).

j *M.perstans* microfilaria. Haematoxylin and eosin stained (40× objective).

k *M.ozzardi* unsheathed microfilaria. Giemsa stained (40× objective).

Delafield's rapid haematoxylin staining technique

This stains the nuclei and sheath of *L. loa* and other pathogenic species.

Required

Field's stain A	Reagent No. 25
Field's stain B, diluted 1 in 5†	
Buffered water, pH 7.1–7.2	Reagent No. 14
Delafield's haematoxylin, diluted 1 in 10‡	

† Prepare by mixing 1 ml of Field's stain B with 4 ml of pH 7.2 buffered water. If preferred, 0.5% w/v eosin can be used.

‡ Prepare by mixing 1 ml of Delafield's haematoxylin (Reagent No. 20) with 9 ml of distilled water or clean filtered water.

Method

1 Place the methanol-fixed preparation on a staining rack and cover with approximately 1 ml of diluted Field's stain B. Add immediately an equal volume of Field's stain A and mix with the diluted Field's stain B. Stain for 1 minute.

Note: The stains can be easily applied and mixed on the slide by using plastic bulb pipettes.

2 Wash off the stains with clean water. Cover the preparation with diluted Delafield's haematoxylin and stain for 5 minutes. Wash off with pH 7.1–7.2 buffered water. Wipe the back of the slide clean and place it in a draining rack for the smear to dry.

3 When dry, spread a drop of immersion oil on the smear and examine microscopically. Use the 10× objective (with the condenser iris closed sufficiently to give good contrast) to scan the preparation for microfilariae and the 40× and 100× objectives to identify the species.

Results

Nuclei of microfilariae	Blue
Sheath of *W. bancrofti*	Blue-grey
Sheath of *B. malayi*	Blue-grey
Sheath of *B. timori*	Blue-grey
Sheath of *L. loa*	Pale blue-grey
Granules of eosinophils	Orange-red

CONCENTRATION TECHNIQUES

Tube centrifugation lyzed blood technique
Required

Saponin-saline solution	Reagent No. 54
Methylene blue-saline, Azur B, or Field's stain A	Reagent No. 42

Method

1 Collect 10 ml of venous blood and dispense it into 10 ml of saponin-saline lyzing solution.

Note: If saponin-saline is not available, dispense the blood into 10 ml of water.

2 Mix the blood gently in the lyzing solution and leave for 5 minutes to give time for all the red cells to lyze (10 minutes if using water).

3 Centrifuge the haemolysate for 10 minutes at slow to medium speed, i.e. RCF 300–500 g.

4 Using a plastic bulb pipette or Pasteur pipette, immediately remove and discard the supernatant fluid. Transfer the sediment to a slide, add a *small* drop of methylene blue, Azur B, or Field's stain A, and cover with a cover glass. The stain will be taken up by the nuclei and show whether the microfilariae are sheathed.

5 Examine the entire preparation microscopically for motile microfilariae using the 10× objective with the condenser iris *closed sufficiently* to give good contrast.

6 Count the number of microfilariae in the entire preparation. Divide the number counted by 10 to give the approximate number of microfilariae per ml of blood (mf/ml).

7 If unable to identify the species with certainty, examine a fixed stained preparation with the 100× oil immersion objective as described under the *Lyzed capillary blood technique.*

Membrane filtration technique
Required

Nuclepore or other polycarbonate (e.g. *Isopore*) membrane filter, 25 mm diameter 5 μm pore size, available from Millipore (see Appendix 11), catalogue TMTP 02500 (pack of 100).

Note: To prevent the filters from sticking to each other, they are usually packaged between white paper discs. The filters are the thin *transparent* discs. Handle with *blunt-ended* forceps to avoid damaging them.

Reuse of polycarbonate filters
With care, polycarbonate filters can be disinfected, washed, and reused several times when no microfilariae are detected. Before reuse, the filters should be checked for damage. Positive filters should not be reused because microfilariae become trapped in the small pores of the filter.

Syringe filter holder, 25 mm diameter available from Millipore (see Appendix 11), catalogue SX00 02500 (pack of 12).

Syringe, Luer, 10 ml capacity.

Sodium citrate anticoagulant	Reagent No. 57
Methylene blue saline, or Azur B	Reagent No. 42

Method

1 Collect 10 ml of venous blood and dispense it into 1 ml of sodium citrate anticoagulant. Mix well but do not shake.

   Caution: Blood may contain highly infectious viruses and other pathogens, therefore handle the blood, needle, and syringe with great care.

2 Withdraw the plunger of a clean 10 ml Luer syringe.

3 Unscrew the filter holder, and using blunt-ended forceps, *carefully* position the membrane filter (25 mm diameter, 5 μm pore size) on the filter support of the filter holder. Re-assemble the filter holder and attach it to the end of the syringe barrel.

4 Fill the syringe barrel with the anticoagulated blood, holding it over a beaker or other suitable container. Carefully replace the plunger of the syringe and slowly pass the citrated blood through the filter.

5 Remove the filter holder and attach a needle or small length of tubing to the syringe. Draw up about 10 ml of the methylene blue or Azur B saline solution, re-attach the filter holder, and pass the solution through the filter.

6 Remove the filter holder and draw air into the syringe. Re-attach the filter holder and pass the air through the filter. This will help to stick the microfilariae to the filter.

7 Detach the filter holder, unscrew it, and using blunt-ended forceps, carefully remove the filter and place it *face upwards* on a slide. Add a small drop of physiological saline, and cover with a cover glass.

8 Examine the entire filter microscopically for motile microfilariae using the 10× objective with the condenser iris *closed sufficiently* to give good contrast.

   Use the 40× objective to see whether the microfilariae are sheathed (seen as unstained extensions at the head and tail end of the microfilariae) and whether the blue stained nuclei extend into the tip of the tail.

   Count the number of microfilariae in the entire preparation. Divide the number counted by 10 to give the approximate number of microfilariae per ml of blood (mf/ml).

9 If unable to identify the species of microfilariae, prepare a stained preparation and examine with the 100× objective as follows:

   – Wash the filter off the slide into a bottle containing about 2 ml of physiological saline. Stopper and shake to dislodge the microfilariae from the filter.

   – Transfer the washings to a conical tube and centrifuge for 5 minutes at slow to medium speed (300–500 g).

   – Using a plastic bulb pipette or Pasteur pipette, immediately remove and discard the supernatant fluid. Transfer the entire sediment to a slide, mix with a small drop of albumin, plasma or serum (known to be microfilariae-free) and spread thinly. Allow the preparation to dry completely.

   – Fix with absolute methanol or ethanol for 2–3 minutes.

   – Stain using Field's technique for thin films or Giemsa technique as described in subunit 5.7. If looking for *L. loa*, use Delafield's haematoxylin technique as this will stain the sheath (see previous text).

Examination of urine for *W. bancrofti* microfilariae

In chronic bancroftian filariasis a condition called chyluria can occur, i.e. passing of chyle in urine. Chyle consists of lymph and particles of digested fat (soluble in ether). Urine containing chyle appears creamy white. When blood is also present, the urine appears pinkish-white. Microfilariae can often be found in the fibrin clots which form.

Specimen: Collect 10–20 ml of early morning urine, i.e. first urine passed by the person after waking.

Method

1 Report the appearance of the urine. Add about 2 ml of ether and shake to dissolve the chyle.

   Caution: Ether is highly flammable, therefore use well away from an open flame and make sure the room is well-ventilated.

2 Centrifuge the specimen at slow to medium speed, i.e. RCF 300–500 g (high speed centrifugation may cause the microfilariae to lose their sheath).

3 Remove and discard the supernatant fluid. If the sediment contains blood, lyze the red cells by adding an equal volume of saponin-saline solution (Reagent No. 54) or if unavailable add an equal volume of water. Mix and centrifuge again. Discard the supernatant fluid.

4 Transfer the sediment to a slide, add a *small* drop of methylene blue-saline, Azur B, or Field's stain

A, and cover with a cover glass. Examine microscopically for motile microfilariae using the 10× objective with the condenser aperture closed sufficiently to give good contrast.

Note: O. volvulus microfilariae may also be found in urine in heavy infections and after treatment with diethylcarbamazine. Unlike *W. bancrofti*, the microfilariae of *O. volvulus* are unsheathed.

Examination of aspirates for W. bancrofti microfilariae

The method described above for examining urine (omitting the addition of ether) can also be used to examine aspirates of hydrocele fluid or lymph gland fluid for *W. bancrofti* microfilariae.

DETECTION OF *W. BANCROFTI* ANTIGEN

A rapid easy to perform, sensitive and specific immunochromatographic filarial antigen test is available for the diagnosis of active bancroftian filariasis. The test is called *NOW ICT Filariasis* and has a card format. The test detects circulating *W. bancrofti* antigen in whole blood, serum or plasma. The specimen can be collected at any time during the day unlike blood specimens for the detection of microfilariae which, for nocturnal periodic *W. bancrofti*, require collection during night hours.

Principle and method

The *NOW ICT Filariasis* test uses a polyclonal antibody (PAb) in the sample pad. The PAb is attached to colloidal gold (pink colour). A monoclonal antibody (MAb) specific for *W. bancrofti* is impregnated in a line across the strip above the test pad.

The specimen (100 μl) is added to the pink sample pad. Any *W. bancrofti* antigen present binds to the colloidal gold-labelled antibody. When the card is closed, antigen joined to the colloidal gold-labelled antibody, travels along the strip. When the MAb line is reached the antigen-antibody complex binds to (is captured by) the monoclonal antibody, forming a pink line T in the viewing window. A positive control is included which is seen as a pink line above the test, indicating that the reagents have migrated satisfactorily.

Test results are read at 10 minutes (not beyond this time). A positive test indicates infection with *W. bancrofti*.

Specimens from persons infected with other filarial worms, e.g. *Brugia* species, *L. loa*, *O. volvulus*, and *Mansonella* species give a negative test result.

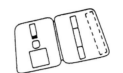

1. Open card and lay it flat on work surface.

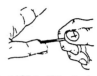

2. Collect 100μl of blood using heparinized capillary.

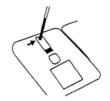

3. Apply blood slowly to top of pad.

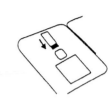

4. Wait until the blood has flowed into pink area.

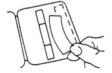

5. Remove and discard the adhesive strip liner.

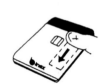

6. Close the card and press firmly to seal it.

7. Read the test result through the viewing window at 10 minutes (see below).

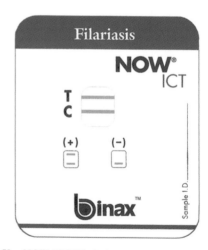

Plate 5.59   *NOW ICT Filariasis* test.
Positive test: Two pink lines T (Test) and C (Control) in viewing window.
Negative test: Single pink line C (Control) in viewing window.
Courtesy of Binax Inc.

Compared to microfilaria detection tests, the *NOW ICT filariasis* antigen test is more sensitive. Furthermore, antigen can be detected when microfilariae are not circulating but living adult worms are present in the lymphatics. Following treatment, antigen can be detected for up to 18 months or more. The test can be performed easily in field situations. The manufacturer's instructions *must be followed exactly*.

Availability of NOW ICT Filariasis Test: The test is available from Binax Inc (see Appendix II). A similar test was formerly available from ICT Diagnostics and Amrad. It is available as a 25 or 50 test kit with a shelf-life, from date of manufacture, of about 12 months. It is recommended that kits be stored refrigerated (4-8 °C) but the kits are also stable at ambient room temperature for a limited period of time (further information from Binax Inc). The kit includes heparinized capillaries. Prices depend on the country of use and application.

5.12 Examination of skin for *Onchocerca volvulus* microfilariae

Onchocerca volvulus is a filarial worm that causes onchocerciasis. The disease is also known as river blindness because invasion of the eye can lead to loss of vision. There are several strains of *O. volvulus* which differ in virulence and the type and severity of disease they cause.

Distribution
It is estimated that there are more than 17.7 million people with onchocerciasis with most infections (99%) occurring in tropical Africa.[66] *O. volvulus* occurs most widely along the courses of fast running rivers and streams in rain forests and savannah areas.

It is found in 28 countries in Africa from Senegal in the west to Uganda and Ethiopia in the east and as far south as Zambia. Following the success of the *Onchocerciasis Control Programme* (1974–2002), onchocerciasis has been eliminated as a public health problem in 11 countries in West Africa (see later text).

Smaller onchocerciasis endemic areas occur in the Yemen Arab Republic, in central America (Mexico and Guatemala), and in South America (Brazil, Ecuador, Venezuela, Columbia). In central America, the vectors of *O. volvulus* breed in slow running streams.

Transmission and life cycle
O. volvulus is transmitted by *Simulium* blackflies. The commonest vectors belong to the *Simulium damno-* *sum* complex. The infective larvae enter through the bite wound after an infected blackfly takes a blood meal. The larvae take several months to develop into mature worms.

The life cycle of *O. volvulus* is summarized in Fig. 5.35. The adult worms live in subcutaneous tissue and in lymph spaces, occurring singly or in tangled masses. In the later stages of infection a proportion of the worms become encapsulated in fibrous nodules. The worms can live up to 10 years or more in their host. The females produce many unsheathed microfilariae which can be found just below the surface of the skin in the lymph spaces and in connective tissue. They can also be found in the fluid of nodules. Microfilariae are thought to be present in the skin from about 7 months onwards after infection. The microfilariae also migrate to the eye and other organs of the body.

The microfilariae are ingested by a blackfly as it feeds. After passing through the stomach wall of the fly, the microfilariae migrate to the thoracic muscles where they develop into infective larvae. Development in the blackfly vector takes about 10 days. The mature infective larvae pass to the mouth-parts of the blackfly ready to be transmitted when the fly next takes a blood meal.

Onchocerciasis
Onchocerciasis is a major health and socioeconomic problem, especially in endemic areas in Africa. The

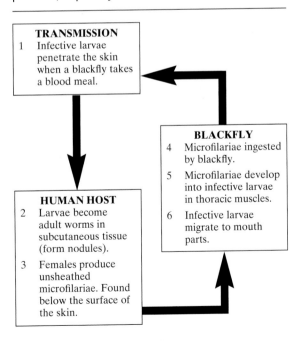

Fig 5.35 Transmission and life cycle of *Onchocerca volvulus.*

clinical features and pathology of onchocerciasis are caused mainly by the inflammatory reactions around damaged and dead microfilariae. The disease varies from one area of infection to another and within a particular population. Variations are due to differences in parasitic strains, degree and frequency of infection, and host differences which include nutritional state and immune responses to parasite antigens. The main clinical features are the formation of nodules, dermatitis, and inflammatory reactions in the eye leading to blindness. Onchocerciasis is also thought to be a risk factor for epilepsy.

Nodule formation

Nodules form under the skin when the adult worms become encapsulated in subcutaneous tissue. The nodules are called onchocercomas. They are firm, smooth and rubbery, round or elongated and measure from 5 mm across up to 50 mm when found in clusters. They may contain large numbers of microfilariae.

In many endemic areas of Africa, nodules are commonly found on the lower part of the body around the pelvis. In Central America and the savannah areas of Africa, nodules are often found on the upper part of the body. In young children (below 9 y), the nodules are found mainly on the head. In Yemen the lower limbs are mainly affected.

Skin disease

There is an inflammatory dermatitis which is usually accompanied by intense irritation, raised papules on the skin, and subsequently alteration in the pigmentation of the skin. The term 'sowda' (black disease) is used to describe a severe allergic response usually affecting only one limb with darkening of the skin. The lymph nodes draining the limb become swollen and painful.

In chronic onchocerciasis, the skin loses its elasticity and becomes wrinkled which makes people look more aged than they are (known as 'elephant skin'). When the skin around the groin becomes affected 'hanging groin' develops. The term 'leopard skin' refers to a spotted depigmentation of the skin which is associated with chronic onchocerciasis.

Blindness

The most serious complication of onchocerciasis is when microfilariae in the skin of the face migrate into the eye. In early eye infections the microfilariae can be found in the cornea and in the anterior chamber. There is redness and irritation of the eye. Progressive changes caused by inflammatory reactions around damaged and dead microfilariae can cause sclerosing keratitis which can lead to blindness. Often the iris is also affected. Inflammation of the choroid and retina can also lead to blindness.

Possible role of *Wolbachia* bacteria in the pathogenesis of onchocerciasis

Wolbachia are intracellular bacteria found in filarial nematodes. Endosymbiotic *Wolbachia* may play a role in *Onchocerca* ocular and skin disease.[66] Deoxycycline antibiotic directed at *Wolbachia* in *O. volvulus* leads to the sterility of adult worms and elimination of skin microfilaria.

Measures to prevent and control onchocerciasis
- Identification of infected communities followed by treatment with ivermectin. Careful monitoring is required in areas where *L. loa* also occurs.
- Interruption of transmission by the destruction of *Simulium* including: the selective use of insecticides, e.g. aerial spraying to destroy blackfly larvae in rivers and streams.
- Avoiding *Simulium* bites by covering as far as possible those parts of the body most at risk and siting human dwellings away from areas where blackflies breed. This often leads to the abandonment of fertile river valleys.

Global initiatives to control onchocerciasis
The *Onchocerciasis Control Programme* (OCP), from 1974–2002, encompassed 35 million people in 11 countries in West Africa. It succeeded in eliminating onchocerciasis as a public health problem by aerial insecticide spraying to destroy blackfly larvae. Fertile land free from onchocerciasis became available for resettlement and agriculture. Individual countries have assumed responsibility for surveillance and managing any recrudescence of infection.

The ongoing *African Programme for Onchocerciasis Control* (APOC), began in 1995 with the objective by 2007 of creating sustainable community-directed ivermectin distribution systems in the remaining 17 run-OCP countries where onchocerciasis remains a serious public health problem. The Programme also includes selective insecticide spraying in a few isolated foci to eradicate local vectors.

The *Onchocerciasis Elimination Programme in the Americas* (OEPA) began in 1992 and is being coordinated by the Pan American Health Organization (PAHO). It is also using community-based invermectin treatment.

Further information: Readers are referred to the WHO TDR website www.who.int/tdr and to the article of Lazdins – Helds *et al*[66] and paper of Pion *et al*.[67]

LABORATORY DIAGNOSIS

Diagnosis of onchocerciasis in district laboratories is by detecting and identifying the microfilariae of *O. volvulus* in skin snips.

Note: In heavy infections and following treatment, *O. volvulus* microfilariae can also be found in urine, blood, and most body fluids.

Method of collecting and examining skin snips for *O. volvulus* microfilariae

Skin snips should be taken from those sites most likely to be heavily infected. In Africa and South America, the highest number of microfilariae can usually be found in skin snips taken from the buttocks, iliac crests or calves of the legs, in Mexico and Guatemala from behind the shoulders or trunk, and in Yemen from the lower limbs.

Important: A bloodless skin snip is required. It can be collected using a sterile needle and razor blade (or scalpel).

Method

A tube centrifugation-technique is recommended if a centrifuge is available. Alternatively, a slide technique can be used (skin snip immersed in saline on a slide and covered with a cover glass).

1   Cleanse the skin using a spirit swab. Allow the area to dry.

2   Insert a sterile fine needle almost horizontally into the skin. Raise the point of the needle, lifting with it a small piece of skin measuring about 2 mm in diameter.

3   Cut off the piece of skin with a sterile razor blade (or scalpel). Immerse the skin snip in a conical centrifuge tube containing about 1 ml of fresh physiological saline and leave it at room temperature for up to 4 hours. Do not tease (pull apart) the skin because this is not necessary and can damage the microfilariae.

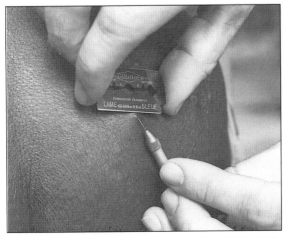

Plate 5.60   Taking a skin snip for the detection of *O.volvulus* microfilariae.

Incubation time and the emergence of microfilariae
In some areas it has been shown that after 1 hour, up to 90% of microfilariae contained in a skin snip (saline preparation) will have emerged, whereas in other areas an incubation time of more than 4 hours is needed for most of the microfilariae to emerge.

4   Using forceps, remove the skin snip, place it on a slide, and cover with a cover glass. Centrifuge the contents of the tube at medium to high speed, i.e. RCF 500–1000, for 5 minutes. Remove and discard the supernatant fluid. Transfer the entire sediment to a slide.

5   Examine both the skin snip and sediment microscopically for microfilariae using the 10× objective with the condenser iris *closed sufficiently* to give good contrast. Report the number of microfilariae as scanty, few, moderate numbers, or many.

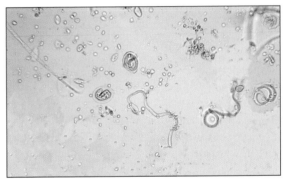

Plate 5.61   Saline preparation showing *O.volvulus* microfilariae from a skin snip.

Note: If no microfilariae are seen, immerse the skin snip in a further 1 ml of saline and reincubate. If after overnight incubation no microfilariae are seen, report the preparation as 'Negative'.

If microfilariae are present identify them as *O. volvulus* as follows:

–   Remove the cover glass and allow the preparation to dry *completely*.

–   Fix the dried preparation with absolute methanol or ethanol for 2–3 minutes.

–   Stain with Giemsa as described in subunit 5.7. Cover the preparation with a drop of immersion oil and examine it microscopically using the 40× and 100× objectives to identify the microfilariae (see Plate 5.62).

Differentiation of *O. volvulus* from *Mansonella* species
■   In West Africa and Central Africa, *O. volvulus* requires differentiation from *M. streptocerca*.

■   In the West Indies, Central America, and South America, *O. volvulus* requires differentiation from *M. ozzardi*.

DIFFERENTIATION OF MICROFILARIAE THAT CAN BE FOUND IN SKIN

Species	Sheath	Main Features in Stained Preparations	Other Points
O. volvulus Onchocerciasis	−	• Large, measuring 240–360 × 5–9 μm. • Head is slightly enlarged. • Anterior nuclei are positioned side by side. *Tail:* No nuclei in the end of the tail which is long and pointed.	Differentiation from *M. streptocerca* is easy. Differentiation from *M. ozzardi* is mainly on its larger size and enlarged head.
M. streptocerca Non-pathogenic or of low pathogenicity	−	• Small and thin, measuring 180–240 × 4.5 μm. • Anterior nuclei are positioned in single file. *Tail:* Nuclei extend to the end of the tail which is usually hooked. Tip is rounded or forked (West Africa).	Differentiation from *O. volvulus* is by its smaller size, single file anterior nuclei, and tail features. Less motile than *O. volvulus* in wet preparations.
M. ozzardi Non-pathogenic or of low pathogenicity	−	• Small and thin, measuring 150–200 × 4.5 μm. • Anterior nuclei are positioned side by side. *Tail:* No nuclei in the end of the tail which is long and pointed.	Differentiation from *O. volvulus* is mainly by its smaller size and different shaped head. Less motile than *O. volvulus* in wet preparations.

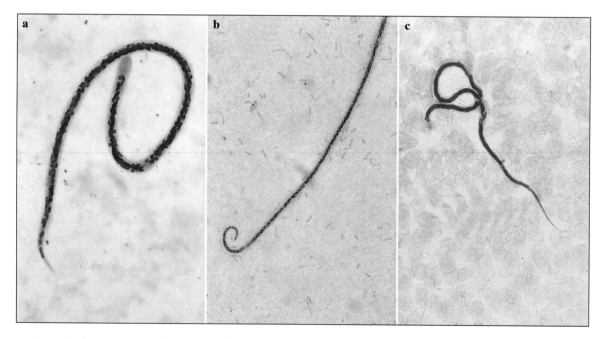

Plate 5.62   **a** *O.volvulus* microfilaria. **b** *M.streptocerca* microfilari. Smaller than *O.volvulus* usually with hooked tail. **c** *M.ozzardi* microfilaria. Smaller than *O.volvulus* with long pointed tail. Giemsa stained as seen with 40× objective.

Mansonella species

M. streptocerca is a filarial worm that produces small unsheathed microfilariae that can be found in the skin. Most infections are asymptomatic or sometimes cause an itching dermatitis, hypopigmented macules, and thickening of the skin. *M. streptocerca* is transmitted by *Culicoides* midges and is found only in the rain forests of Africa, especially in Ghana, Nigeria, Zaire, and Cameroon.

M. ozzardi is a filarial worm that produces small unsheathed microfilariae that can be found both in the skin and blood (non-periodic). Most infections are asymptomatic or cause chronic arthritis, skin rashes, and other symptoms. *M. ozzardi* is transmitted by *Culicoides* midges and *Simulium* blackflies. It is found in the West Indies, Surinam, Guyana, Colombia, Brazil, northern Argentina, Mexico and Panama.

Note: Other species of microfilariae may be found if the skin snip becomes contaminated with blood at the time it is collected.

Counting microfilariae in surveys

In onchocerciasis epidemiological surveys, the microfilariae from skin snips may need to be counted. To do this, a Walser corneoscleral punch can be used to collect skin snips weighing about 1.0 mg. Each skin snip is immersed in 200 μl (0.2 ml) of physiological saline in the well of a microtitration plate or in a small tube, and the plate or tube covered with *Parafilm* or cling film. After overnight incubation, the contents of the well or tube are transferred to a slide, the microfilariae counted, and the number reported per mg of skin. If it is not possible to count the microfilariae the following day, the microfilariae can be preserved by adding 1 small drop of 20% v/v formalin to the preparation.

5.13 Examination of sputum for *Paragonimus* eggs

Paragonimus flukes cause paragonimiasis, also known as lung fluke disease.

Distribution

About 21 million people are infected with *Paragonimus* species in areas where crabs and crayfish are eaten raw or undercooked. Species which cause paragonimiasis in tropical and subtropical countries include:

ASIA
- *P. westermani* (Oriental lung fluke) in the Far East and South East Asia (Korea, China, Philippines, Japan, Malaysia, Thailand, Indonesia, Vietnam), and also parts of India, and some Pacific Islands.

- *P. heterotremus*, also in Thailand, Lao Peoples Democratic Republic, and South China.

- *P. philippinensis*, in the Philippines.

AFRICA
- *P. uterobilateralis*, in the west and south of Africa. It is the main species in Nigeria. Also occurs in Burkina Faso, Central African Republic, Congo, Côte d'Ivoire, Equatorial Guinea, Gabon, Liberia, Sierra Leone, Zaire, Zambia.

- *P. africanus*, in Cameroon and also in Nigeria, and parts of central Africa.

CENTRAL AND SOUTH AMERICA
- *P. mexicanus*, in Central and South America, especially Ecuador and Peru. Also found in limited foci in Colombia, Costa Rica, Cuba, El Salvador, Guatemala, Honduras, and Mexico.

Transmission and life cycle

Infection with *Paragonimus* flukes is by ingesting the flesh or juice of raw, undercooked, or pickled crab or crayfish which contains metacercariae. In China, shrimps have also been found to be infected.

Infection can also occur by ingesting metacercariae from fingers contaminated during food preparation.

The life cycle of *Paragonimus* species is summarized in Fig. 5.36. Following ingestion, the metacercariae excyst in the duodenum and the young flukes penetrate the intestinal wall. They migrate across the abdominal cavity, penetrate through the diaphragm into the pleural cavity and into the lungs, where they become mature flukes. In the early stages of infection the flukes migrate in the lungs. Eventually they become encapsulated. Occasionally the young flukes migrate to the liver, spleen, brain, and other organs of the body.

About 3 months after infection, eggs are produced. These pass into the sputum or are excreted in the faeces after being swallowed in sputum. For the life cycle to be continued the eggs must reach water. In water the miracidia develop, hatch from the eggs and swim in the water in search of suitable snail hosts.*

* Snails of the genera *Semisulcospira* and *Thiara* serve as first intermediate hosts of *P. westermani*. Snail hosts of other *Paragonimus* flukes include species of the genera *Brotia*, *Assiminea*, *Oncomelania*, *Tricula*, and *Potadoma*.

In the snail, the miracidia develop into sporocysts which produce rediae and finally cercariae. Development and reproduction in the snail takes about 8 weeks. The cercariae are shed from the snail and encyst in crabs or crayfish, becoming metacercariae. The metacercariae of *Paragonimus* species

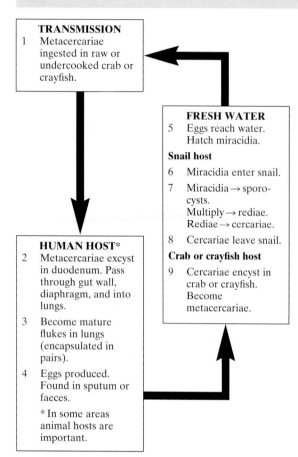

Fig 5.36 Transmission and life cycle of *Paragonimus* species.

that infect humans are also infective to crustacean-eating animals. In some areas animal reservoir hosts are important in transmission.

The life-span of a *Paragonimus* fluke is usually 6–7 years but human infections of up to 20 years have been reported.

Paragonimiasis

Light to moderate *Paragonimus* infections are usually asymptomatic. Heavy infections, however, can cause pulmonary disease with inflammatory responses to the flukes and eggs. The flukes become encapsulated.

Symptoms of severe pulmonary paragonimiasis often resemble those of pulmonary tuberculosis with chest pain, cough, night sweats, pleural effusion, and haemoptysis (coughing up blood).

Paragonimus flukes in the intestine and liver cause liver disease, pain, diarrhoea, and vomiting. The most serious complications occur when *Paragonimus* flukes parasitize the central nervous system causing severe headache, cerebral haemorrhage, oedema, mental confusion, and meningitis.

Measures to prevent and control paragonimiasis

- Not eating raw, undercooked, or pickled crabs or crayfish which may contain infective metacercariae.

- Not contaminating water with sputum or faeces.

- Detecting and treating infected persons in endemic areas.

- Identifying and destroying the snail hosts of local *Paragonimus* species where this is feasible.

Further information: Readers are referred to the 21st edition *Mansons Tropical Diseases* (see Recommended Reading).

LABORATORY DIAGNOSIS

The diagnosis of paragonimiasis in district laboratories is by:

■ Finding *Paragonimus* eggs in sputum or occasionally in aspirates of pleural fluid.

■ Examining faeces for *Paragonimus* eggs that have been swallowed in sputum.

Other findings

With heavy infections there is a raised ESR and moderate blood eosinophilia. In *Paragonimus* pericarditis many eosinophils can be found in aspirates of pleural fluid. Charcot Leyden crystals may also be seen in specimens.

Examination of sputum for *Paragonimus* eggs

Sputum from patients with pulmonary paragonimiasis, often contains blood, mucus, and stringy particles of rusty-brown gelatinous material in which masses of eggs can be found. Sputum from less heavily infected patients may contain very few eggs and a concentration technique may be necessary to detect the eggs.

Method

1 Report the appearance of the sputum, i.e. whether watery, mucoid, mucopurulent, or red and jelly-like, and whether it contains blood and rusty-brown particles.

2 If rusty-brown gelatinous particles are present, transfer a sample of this material to a slide and cover with a cover glass. Using a cloth or tissue, gently press on the cover glass to make a thin evenly spread preparation.

If no rusty-brown particles are present or if no eggs are found when the particles are examined, carry out a concentration technique (preferably using sputum collected over 24 h).

Concentration technique
- Add an equal volume of 30 g/l (3% w/v) sodium hydroxide solution to the sputum, shake, and leave for 15–30 minutes to allow time for the sodium hydroxide to dissolve the mucus.
- Shake well and centrifuge in a conical tube at slow to medium speed, i.e. not over RCF 500 g (approx. 2 000 rpm) for 5 minutes. Using a plastic bulb pipette or Pasteur pipette, remove and discard the supernatant fluid and transfer a drop of the sediment to a slide. Cover with a cover glass.

3 Examine microscopically for eggs using the 10× objective with the condenser iris *closed sufficiently* to give good contrast. Use the 40× objective to identify the eggs.

Note: The eggs of *Paragonimus* species are identified from a knowledge of locally occurring species and by differences in egg size, shape and shell thickness.

FAR EAST
Egg of P. westermani
- Yellow-brown and usually asymmetrical in shape, being slightly flattened on one side. It measures 70–100 × 50–65 μm.
- Has a flat operculum (lid).
- Thickness of the shell varies. It is thicker at the end opposite the operculum.
- Contains an unsegmented ovum and mass of yolk cells.

Note: Details of the eggs of other *Paragonimus* species that occur in the Far East can be found in SEAMIC *Color Atlas of Human Helminth Eggs.*

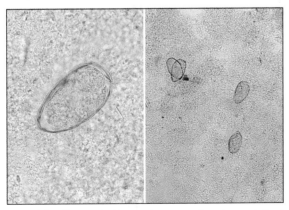

Plate 5.63 Eggs of *Paragonimus* species in unstained sputum. *Right:* As seen with the 10× objective. *Left:* As seen with the 40× objective.

AFRICA
Egg of P. uterobilateralis
Similar to the egg of *P. westermani* but smaller, measuring 50–98 × 35–52 μm.

Egg of P. africanus
This egg is larger than that of *P. uterobilateralis*, measuring 72–124 × 42–59 μm. It is similar to *P. westermani* but slightly thinner.

SOUTH AND CENTRAL AMERICA
Egg of P. mexicanus
Similar to that of *P. westermani* except that it has a thin irregularly undulating shell. It measures 73–92 × 47–53 μm.

Examination of pleural fluid for *Paragonimus* eggs
Aspirates of pleural fluid can be examined in the same way as described for sputum, except that there is no need to treat the fluid with sodium hydroxide before centrifuging. The fluid may contain many eosinophils.

Examination of faeces for *Paragonimus* eggs
A concentration technique should be used because only a few *Paragonimus* eggs are likely to be present in faeces. The formol ether concentration technique is recommended. Floatation techniques are not suitable. A *Paragonimus* egg in sputum is shown in Plate 5.1 (p. 194).

5.14 Less frequently needed parasitology tests

This subunit contains the following tests that occasionally may need to be performed in district laboratories:

1 Investigation of amoebic liver abscess.

2 Investigation of primary amoebic meningoencephalitis.

3 Diagnosis of toxoplasmosis.

4 Diagnosis of hydatid disease.

5 Examination of muscle tissue for *Trichinella* larvae.

6 Detection of *Dracunculus medinensis* (Guinea worm) larvae.

1   Investigation of amoebic liver abscess

Amoebic liver abscess is a rare complication of infection with *Entamoeba histolytica*. It occurs when amoebae are carried to the liver by way of the portal circulation. Usually the right liver lobe is affected (clinical features are described in subunit 5.4.1).

Serological tests used to assist in the diagnosis of amoebic liver abscess in district laboratories include:

■   Latex slide test to detect antibodies to *E. histolytica.*

Fumouze Bichro-Latex Amibe test
The above 5-minute latex test is manufactured and supplied by Fumouze Diagnostics (see Appendix II). It is available as a 25 test kit. Its approximate shelf-life is 12 months. All the reagents are supplied in the kit, including positive and neagtive controls. It is positive in invasive amoebiasis.

■   Cellulose acetate precipitin (CAP) test to detect significantly raised levels of anti-*E.histolytica* antibodies in serum. The test is highly specific for invasive amoebiasis.

Other tests

Haematology tests, including total and differential white cell count and ESR. A leucocytosis with neutrophilia is found in about 80% of patients with amoebic liver abscess. The ESR is always raised, usually over 50 mm/h and often over 100 mm/h.

Examination of pus from liver abscess

The centre of an amoebic liver abscess contains a viscous pink-brown or grey-yellow fluid consisting of digested liver tissue. It is referred to as 'pus' but contains very few pus cells. As *part of treatment* (not diagnosis) the fluid is often aspirated and is usually sent to the laboratory. Occasionally it is possible to detect motile *E. histolytica* trophozoites in the 'pus'. This, however, is rare because the trophozoites are found around the periphery of an abscess, not in its centre.

Cellulose acetate precipitin (CAP) test to investigate invasive amoebiasis

This is a simple inexpensive technique which is of value in confirming a diagnosis of amoebic liver abscess. It has a high specificity with positive results being obtained only if invasive amoebiasis is present. The test becomes positive early and negative 3–14 days after successful treatment.

The CAP test relies on the surface diffusion of specific globulins and soluble antigen to produce a line of precipitation where they meet which can be visualized by staining.

Required

–   Plastic box containing foam sponge (reusable).

   Preparation of the box
   1 Take a shallow medium size plastic box with an airtight lid.
   2 Take a piece of foam sponge (about 10–15 mm depth) and cut it to the size of the box. Cut a 5 cm square from the centre of it.
   3 Place the sponge in the box.
   4 Cut a piece of thick filter paper to cover the sponge with a 5 cm square cut out in the same position as the cut out area in the sponge. Moisten the filter paper with buffer (PBS).

–   Piece of cellulose acetate paper cut to 60 mm square, obtainable from Sartorius AG (see Appendix 11), code SM 12200–78–150–K.

–   Template to make wells in the CAP to contain the antigen.

   Making a template
   1 Take a piece of perspex or other thin rigid plastic.
   2 Drill 5 bevelled holes, a central hole measuring 3 mm across the bevel, and four holes measuring 6 mm across the bevel and situated 1 cm apart and 1 cm from the central hole (see Fig. 5.37).

–   Soluble amoebic antigen.

   Sources of amoebic antigen
   Information can be obtained from Chief Biomedical Scientist, Protozoology Dept, London School Hygiene and Tropical Medicine, Keppel Street, London WC1E 7HT, UK.

–   Phosphate buffered saline   Reagent No. 48
    (PBS), pH 7.0

–   Nigrosin stain   Reagent No. 43

Method

1   Float the square of cellulose acetate paper onto PBS, pH 7.0 (contained in a shallow dish), and allow it to adsorb the buffer evenly. Immerse the paper in the buffer, remove, and blot to take up the excess buffer.

2   Using the template and a rod (e.g. wire loop holder), make 5 wells in the paper (avoid puncturing the paper). Label one of the outer wells + (positive control) and another outer well − (negative control), and the other two wells with the patient's initials, e.g. 'AG' as shown in Fig. 5.37.

3   Moisten the filter paper on the sponge with PBS, pH 7.0 and place the paper in the box over the hole.

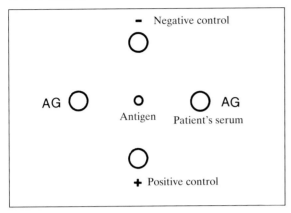

Fig. 5.37 Position of wells in the CAP test (AG = Patient's initials).

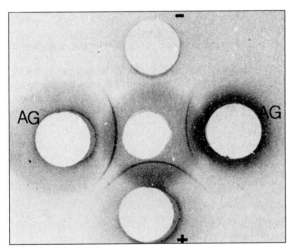

Plate 5.64 Result of a positive CAP test from a patient with amoebic liver abscess. Precipitin arcs (black curved lines) can be seen between the antigen well and patient's serum wells (left and right). There is no precipitin arc between the negative control serum well and the antigen well. A precipitin arc is shown with the positive control serum.

4 Using a fine capillary, place one drop (approx. 5 μl) of the patient's serum in each of the initialled wells, a positive serum in the positive well, and a negative serum in the negative well. Place one drop (approx. 3 μl) of amoebic antigen in the centre well.

5 Close the lid of the box and leave it at room temperature for 4 hours.

6 Remove the paper and wash it in physiological saline for 5 minutes.

7 Immerse the paper in nigrosin stain for 2 minutes. Rinse in water or 2% v/v acetic acid to clear the paper.

8 Holding the paper against a strong light, look for precipitin arcs. Check the positive and negative controls.

Results

A positive test is indicated by seeing a precipitin arc between the serum and the antigen as shown in Plate 5.64.

Report the test as 'CAP test Positive' or 'CAP test Negative'.

2 Investigation of primary amoebic meningoencephalitis

Primary amoebic meningoencephalitis is a very rare condition caused by *Naegleria fowleri*. Most infections have been traced to bathing in stagnant freshwater lakes, pools contaminated with sewage or other decaying matter, and under-chlorinated swimming pools. The organism feeds on bacteria.

N. fowleri attacks healthy persons, causing an acute meningoencephalitis. It is the trophozoites of *Naegleria* which infect the brain. The organisms enter through the nose and are thought to invade the brain via the olfactory nerve.

The cysts of *Naegleria* (round in form) are free-living and not found in humans. *Naegleria* (which is an amoeboflagellate) develops a flagellated form for dispersal in the environment.

Unless diagnosed and treated at an early stage, irreversible brain damage occurs and the infection is fatal. Death almost always occurs within a few days of the onset of symptoms.

Examination of c.s.f. for amoebae

The cerebrospinal fluid (c.s.f.) is purulent with a cell count similar to that found in pyogenic bacterial meningitis. When the c.s.f. is examined microscopically, the motile amoebae can usually be seen.

Look especially for *Naegleria* amoebae if the c.s.f. contains polymorphonuclear neutrophils but no bacteria can be detected in a Gram stained smear. The c.s.f. may also contain eosinophils and red cells. As in bacterial meningitis, the c.s.f. glucose will be reduced and protein raised.

Method

1 Transfer a drop of uncentrifuged purulent c.s.f., or a drop of sediment from a centrifuged specimen, to a slide and cover with a cover glass.

2 Examine the specimen, using the 10× objective

with the condenser iris *reduced sufficiently* to give good contrast.

Look for small, clear, motile elongated forms among the pus cells.

Use the 40× objective to identify the rapidly moving amoebae (even if the amoebae are not detected first with the 10× objective, *always* examine the preparation with the 40× objective).

Important: If amoebae are seen in the c.s.f., immediately notify the medical officer attending the patient. Amoebic meningoencephalitis is a rapidly fatal condition.

Naegleria amoeba

- Elongate in form, measuring 10–22 × 7 μm.
- Rapidly motile (more than 2 body lengths per minute). Pseudopodia are lobulate and show characteristic explosive protrusion.
- When viewed with the 40× objective, vacuoles can often be seen in the cytoplasm (the small nucleus with its nucleolus is not usually visible in an unstained preparation).
- Does not contain ingested red cells.

Note: Naegleria amoebae will remain motile for several hours at room temperature and up to 24 hours at 35–37 °C.

The amoebae can be stained with Giemsa stain, but they do not stain well by the Gram technique. They can also be seen in acridine orange stained preparations examined by fluorescence microscopy (cytoplasm appears red and foamy).

In distilled water, the amoebae develop flagella after 2–4 hours.

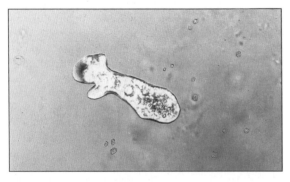

Plate 5.65   Trophozoite of *Naegleria*.

Acanthamoeba species
Other free-living amoebae belonging to the genus *Acanthamoeba* have been reported as causing chronic granulomatous amoebic encephalitis and skin abscesses, in immunocompromised persons. The brain is probably infected via the blood-stream, possibly from infected skin, eye, or lung. *Acanthamoeba* species can also cause chronic amoebic keratitis in healthy people.

Acanthamoeba cysts as well as the amoebae are thought to be infective. Dry cysts can survive for several years in dust. They are angular in shape with a double wall. The amoebae are slow moving with spiky projections. Cerebrospinal fluid from patients with amoebic encephalitis usually contains only a few cells (polymorphs).

Balamuthia mandrillaris
This free-living amoeba has been reported as causing necrotising granulomatous encephalitis and skin abscesses in patients with AIDS. The living trophozoites can be distinguished from *Naegleria* and *A. canthamoeba* by their extremely irregular form.[68]

---

3   Diagnosis of toxoplasmosis

Toxoplasma gondii is an animal coccidian parasite which causes toxoplasmosis, with congenital toxoplasmosis being the most serious form of human infection. *T. gondii* has a worldwide distribution.

The definitive hosts in which oocysts are formed are the cat and the lynx. *T. gondii* is transmitted by the ingestion of oocysts in food, water, or from hands contaminated with faeces from an infected cat. Transmission can also occur by transplacental transmission, by blood transfusion, or by ingesting the parasites in undercooked meat of an infected animal intermediate host.

Humans, with rodents, chickens, lambs and other animals, act as intermediate hosts of *T. gondii*. Following ingestion of infective oocysts, the parasites become intracellular and multiply in the lymph glands, liver, muscle, central nervous system, and other internal organs.

Toxoplasmosis
In the early acute stages of infection, the parasites (referred to as tachyzoites) invade phagocytic cells and mononuclear leucocytes. In the chronic stages of infection, the parasites (referred to as bradyzoites) multiply intracellularly in the tissues, forming cysts (bradycysts).

Although adult acquired infections are often asymptomatic, they can cause fever, a rash, enlargement of lymph glands with lymphocytosis, and occasionally inflammation of the eye (ocular toxoplasmosis), myocarditis, meningoencephalitis, and atypical pneumonia. In some infected persons the only clinical symptom is fever.

HIV associated toxoplasmosis

Serious and often fatal opportunistic *Toxoplasma* infections can occur in those with abnormal immune responses, especially in patients with acquired immunodeficiency syndrome (AIDS). Most infections are due to the reactivation of cysts and cause encephalitis with fever, headache, mental deterioration and seizures.

Congenital toxoplasmosis

Intra-uterine infection with *T. gondii* due to active parasitaemia during pregnancy, can cause severe and often fatal cerebral damage to a foetus. Infants who recover often show evidence of mental defects. The risk of foetal infection from an infected mother increases as pregnancy progresses. About 10–15% of infections acquired in the first trimester of pregnancy result in foetal infection. This increases to 30% for those acquired in the second trimester and 60% for those acquired in the third trimester.

Infection occurring in early pregnancy may result in abortion or the still-birth of a foetus, while infection late in pregnancy may cause symptoms of infection to develop in the infant 2–3 months after birth, including blindness and mental retardation. Immunocompromised mothers can transmit *Toxoplasma* to the foetus from infections acquired prior to pregnancy and reactivated during pregnancy.

LABORATORY DIAGNOSIS

Most infections with *T. gondii* are diagnosed serologically. Serological testing, however, has only a limited value in diagnosing *Toxoplasma* encephalitis in AIDS patients. The diagnosis is usually made clinically, supported by computerized tomography or magnetic imaging scans where these facilities are available.

Trophozoites may occasionally be found, e.g. in c.s.f. of AIDS patients with *Toxoplasma encephalitis*. A blood lymphocytosis with many atypical lymphocytes is usually found in acute *Toxoplasma* infections. The blood picture often resembles that seen in infectious mononucleosis (glandular fever). A low platelet count may also be found.

Serological diagnosis of toxoplasmosis

The most reliable test for the diagnosis of acute toxoplasmosis in pregnancy, and to test neonates, is the Sabin-Feldman dye test. This highly sensitive and specific test is a complement-mediated neutralizing antigen-antibody reaction which uses live trophozoites to measure *Toxoplasma* specific antibody. It is performed in Reference Laboratories.

The Eiken *Toxoreagent latex agglutination test* is a simpler test. It shows 94.4% agreement with the dye test and is performed as a quantitative test in microtitration plates. The latex particles are coated with inactivated *T. gondii* soluble antigen. The test detects all immunoglobulin classes. The test does not require heat inactivation of serum samples. A positive control is included in each test kit.

Availability of the *Toxoreagent* latex agglutination test
The test is available as a 50 test kit. It has a shelf life of about 12 months when stored at 2–8 °C. It is manufactured by Eiken Chemical Co Ltd (see Appendix II) and available from a network of distributors including Mast Diagnostics (see Appendix 11).

Interpretation of test results

The interpretation of *Toxoplasma* serological test results is often difficult because of the high prevalence of antibodies in most populations due to past and subclinical infections. A rising antibody titre helps to establish a diagnosis, but this is often 'missed' due to a rapid immune response (in persons with normal immune responses) and often a delay in investigating patients. Detection of *Toxoplasma* specific IgM is indicative of recent infection, but IgM antibody testing is expensive and normally only available in Reference Laboratories.

In diagnosing congenital toxoplasmosis, the presence of IgM (which does not cross the placenta) in the infant's circulation is diagnostic but often this is not found. Specific IgG in the infant's circulation may be of maternal origin or due to infection. Testing of the infant's blood at 2 monthly intervals will show whether the IgG antibody level is decreasing. At 6–10 months, the infant's circulation should not contain maternal IgG and therefore persistence of IgG beyond this time is indicative of infection in the infant. In seriously affected infants, the diagnosis of congenital toxoplasmosis can usually be made clinically with the help of X-rays.

In AIDS patients, *Toxoplasma* encephalitis can be excluded if IgG antibody is not detected while the presence of IgG in serum does not establish active infection. By testing both serum and cerebrospinal fluid, comparison of the ratio of specific and non-specific levels in both samples may indicate the production of *Toxoplasma* specific antibody in the central nervous system. IgG and IgM specific *Toxoplasma* antibody tests are available from Cortez Diagnostics (see Appendix 11).

Further information on diagnosing toxoplasmosis encephalitis in AIDS: A recent study carried out in India of HIV-associated toxoplasmosis encephalitis, antibody response, and the value of *Toxoplasma* antigen detection in the diagnosis of encephalitis can be found in the paper of Malla N *et al*: Antigenaemia and antibody response to *T. gondii* in HIV-infected patients. *British Journal of Biomedical Science*, 2005, 62 (1), pp. 19–23.

Detection of *T. gondii* parasites in c.s.f.

Occasionally *T. gondii* tachyzoites can be found in specimens such as c.s.f. in AIDS patients with cerebral involvement. The c.s.f. usually contains neutrophils and mononuclear cells.

Method

1 Centrifuge the c.s.f. in a conical tube at medium to high speed, i.e. RCF about 1 000 g for 5 minutes. Transfer the supernatant fluid to another tube. This can be used for protein testing (raised in *Toxoplasma* encephalitis).

2 Tap the bottom of the tube to mix the sediment. Spread a drop on a slide and allow the smear to air-dry. Fix with methanol for 1–2 minutes.

3 Stain the smear using Giemsa technique or Field's technique for thin films (described in sub-unit 5.7).

4 When dry examine the preparation microscopically using the 40× objective to detect the parasites and the 100× objective to identify the tachyzoites.

Toxoplasma in tissue sections

Toxoplasma may occasionally be found in a tissue section in which the organisms may appear round and resemble *Leishmania* amastigotes, but the infected tissue will have a characteristic histological appearance. The parasites can be identified using a direct fluorescent antibody test.

Tachyzoites of *T. gondii* in c.s.f.

- Parasites are frequently seen in neutrophils and mononuclear cells.

- They are crescent shaped and small, measuring about 3 × 7 μm. One end is rounded and the other end more pointed.

- Nucleus is situated towards the rounded end and stains dark red.

- Cytoplasm stains blue.

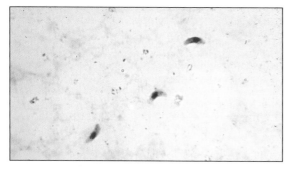

Plate 5.66 Giemsa stained trophozoites (tachyzoites) of *T.gondii*.

---

4   Diagnosis of hydatid disease

Hydatid disease is caused by the accidental ingestion of eggs of the tapeworm *Echinococcus granulosus* in food or water or from hands contaminated with dog faeces. The dog is the definitive host of *E. granulosus* (harbours adult tapeworm). Following ingestion, the embryos are freed in the small intestine. They migrate through the intestinal wall into a blood vessel and are carried in the circulation to the liver, peritoneal cavity, lungs, kidneys, bone, and other sites in the body where they develop into hydatid cysts (larval form of *E. granulosus*).

Humans are not the natural intermediate hosts of *E. granulosus*. When a human becomes infected there is no transfer of the parasite except in places where definitive hosts are able to feed on human remains. The normal intermediate hosts are sheep, cattle, camels, pigs and goats with dogs becoming infected by eating tissue containing hydatid cysts from these animals.

Distribution

Hydatid disease is known to occur in many parts of the world where sheep are in close association with dogs and humans or where dogs and wild carnivores are associated with livestock and wild herbivores. High infection rates occur in China, East Africa (especially the Turkana region in Kenya), North Africa, South Africa, India, Nepal, eastern Mediterranean, Middle East, and parts of South America, and Australasia.

Hydatid disease

Infections can produce serious symptoms depending on the site and size of the hydatid cyst and host response. The cyst grows slowly but continuously. Obstruction and pressure on vital organs or rupture of the cyst with subsequent anaphylactic shock can be fatal. Some cysts may grow for only a short time and then die and calcify.

Different strains of the parasite are thought to cause disease in different organs. Up to 60% of hydatid cysts are found in the right lobe of the liver where they cause pain, fever and hepatomegaly. In the lungs, hydatid cysts can cause pulmonary symptoms. Sputum may contain blood and cyst fluid. When hydatid cysts develop in bone there is no fibrous wall formed and therefore the cyst spreads causing pain and bone fractures. Other sites include the brain, kidneys, or spleen but these organs are only rarely infected.

Hydatid disease (especially when cysts are in the liver and abdomen) is usually diagnosed clinically with the assistance of ultrasound scanning and other imaging techniques in places where these facilities are available.

LABORATORY DIAGNOSIS

Laboratory investigations include:

- Testing serum for antibodies produced in response to infection and where available, testing for cystic fluid antigens.

- Examining cyst fluid for brood capsules, protoscoleces and hooks following the surgical removal of a cyst or fine needle aspiration under ultrasound guidance.

Note: During surgery, care must be taken not to puncture a hydatid cyst because leakage of the fluid can cause anaphylaxis and massive reinfection from released protoscoleces. A solution that kills the scoleces is used during the surgery.

Histology of the cyst wall: Tests should include PAS staining to show the laminated membrane and Ziehl-Neelsen staining to show the acid fast hooks of the protoscoleces.

PROTOSCOLEX   HYDATID CYST

Invaginated

Fibrous wall
from host

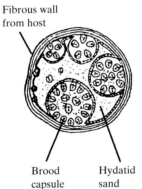

Evaginated

Brood   Hydatid
capsule   sand

Fig. 5.38   *Right*: Morphology of hydatid cyst of *E.granulosus*. *Left*: An invaginated protoscolex (upper) and evaginated protoscolex (lower) of *E.granulosus*.

Protoscoleces can occasionally be found in sputum when pulmonary hydatid cysts rupture.

Useful tests to differentiate liver hydatid disease from hepatoma

Serum glycoproteins, serum aminotransferases, and other liver function tests are usually normal with hydatid disease of the liver but abnormal with cancer of the liver. The erythrocyte sedimentation rate (ESR) is usually moderately raised with hydatid disease whereas with cancer of the liver it is markedly raised.

Examination of cyst fluid for protoscoleces

Hydatid cyst: Structurally the cyst consists of an outer thick laminated cyst wall and an inner, thin, nucleated germinal layer. From the germinal layer, brood capsules are produced inside which small protoscoleces form (see Fig. 5.38).

The brood capsules may break off and sink down through the fluid which fills the cyst. Free brood capsules and individual protoscoleces released from the capsules, form what is called hydatid sand.

There is a marked cellular response by the host to the presence of the hydatid cyst which leads eventually to it being surrounded by a fibrous wall. Older cysts may become calcified.

Method

After centrifuging the cyst fluid (hydatid sand), transfer a drop of the sediment to a slide and cover with a cover glass. Examine the preparation microscopically for evaginated and invaginated protoscoleces using the 10× objective to identify the hooks of the scolex (double row).

Note: If the hydatid cyst is sterile, no protoscoleces will be found.

Viability of protoscoleces

To test whether the protoscoleces are viable (living), prepare an eosin preparation (Reagent No. 23) of the fluid. Viable protoscoleces remain unstained whereas dead (non-viable) protoscoleces have a damaged membrane and take up the eosin.

Protoscolex of *E. granulosus*

- It is colourless, round to oval in shape, measuring about 140 × 80 μm. May be invaginated or evaginated (see Fig. 5.38).

- With focusing the hooks of the scolex can be easily seen.

- Viable protoscoleces do not stain with eosin.

- Non-viable protoscoleces stain red with eosin.

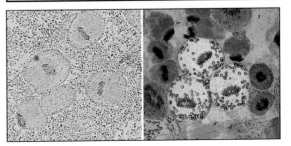

Plate 5.67   *Left*: Invaginated and evaginated protoscoleces of *E.granulosus* in hydatid cyst fluid. *Right*: Eosin preparation showing viable (unstained) protoscoleces and non-viable (red stained) protoscoleces.

Serological diagnosis of hydatid disease

In general the sensitivity of serological tests is affected by the site and condition of a hydatid cyst. Sensitivity is higher with liver cysts than with lung cysts. Dead or calcified cysts may give negative results. False negative results may be obtained from patients with circulating immune complexes. For most of the tests that have been developed, reagents are not generally available. In high prevalence areas district laboratories should contact their nearest Reference Laboratory for availability of reagents and advice on the most appropriate test to perform.

A review of antibody and antigen tests used in the serological diagnosis of hydatid disease can be found in the 21st edition of *Mansons Tropical Diseases* (see Recommended Reading).

Echinococcus multilocularis

Human infection with the hydatid cyst of this species causes multilocular or alveolar hydatid disease. Infections have been reported mainly from Canada, Alaska, USSR and Europe. The hydatid cyst of *E. multilocularis* is invasive and spreads like a malignant tumour causing cavities and necrosis. It is not encapsulated like the hydatid cyst of *E. granulosus*. The liver is commonly infected. Surgical removal is rarely possible and the disease is usually fatal.

Multiceps species

The larval stage of these tapeworm species is a coenurus cyst and human infection with the larva is referred to as coenuriasis. Infection occurs following the ingestion of eggs in food or from hands contaminated with dog faeces.

Multiceps multiceps is found in North and South Africa and the coenurus infects the brain. There is no treatment and infection is usually fatal. *Multiceps brauni* is found in tropical Africa and causes a less serious disease because the coenurus does not infect the brain. The eyes and other parts of the body are infected.

The definitive hosts of *Multiceps* species are dogs and jackals. The intermediate hosts of *M. multiceps* are sheep and the intermediate hosts of *M. brauni* are rodents.

---

5   Examination of muscle tissue for *Trichinella spiralis* larvae

---

Trichinella spiralis is a tissue nematode normally parasitic in domestic and wild pigs, rats, and many wild carnivores. Human infection is called trichinosis (trichinellosis) and is a zoonosis.

Distribution

T. spiralis contains three subspecies: *T. s. spiralis* which is found in temperate regions, *T. s. nativa* which is found in the Arctic, and *T. s. nelsoni* which is found in Africa and southern Europe.

Transmission

Human infection occurs when encysted *Trichinella* larvae are eaten in raw or undercooked meat, usually from an infected wild pig (Africa). The larvae become mature worms in the small intestine. The females produce larvae which are carried in the blood circulation to skeletal muscle where they encyst and often become calcified. Humans are not the natural hosts of *T. spiralis*. When a human becomes infected there is no transfer of the parasite. In the natural cycle (in Africa) the flesh of a wild pig containing infective cysts is eaten by a wild carnivore such as a jackal, lion, hyena, or leopard.

Trichinosis

Within 48 hours of ingesting *Trichinella* larvae, intestinal disturbances may occur. These can include abdominal pain, nausea and vomiting. During migration of the larvae, allergic symptoms develop including fever, oedema of the face, headache, and eosinophilia. Encystment of the larvae often causes muscle pain.

Heavy infections with widespread migration of larvae may cause neurological disorders and occasionally a fatal myocarditis.

LABORATORY DIAGNOSIS

The laboratory diagnosis of trichinosis is by:

- Detecting *Trichinella* larvae in striated muscle.
- Testing serum for *Trichinella* antibodies (in Reference laboratories).

Note: An eosinophilic leucocytosis is found in the acute stage of the disease and serum aminotransferases are often raised.

Examination of muscle for *Trichinella* larvae

The larvae can be found in muscle tissue from the second or third week after infection.

Specimen: A striated muscle biopsy (collected under local anaesthesia) is required. Suitable sites to biopsy include the muscles of the shoulder, outer thigh, or calf of the leg. A biopsy measuring about 20×10 mm is adequate.

Techniques used to detect *Trichinella* larvae in muscle include:

- Direct slide technique
- Digestion technique

Direct slide technique

1   Place the fresh biopsy on a glass slide and cut the tissue into thin pieces. Cover with another slide. Press the slides together and keep them together by binding each end with adhesive tape or an

elastic band.

Caution: Wear protective rubber gloves and handle the biopsy with forceps.

2 Examine the entire preparation microscopically for coiled larvae using the 10× objective with the condenser iris *closed sufficiently* to give good contrast.

Note: If larvae are not seen, run a drop of glycerine (glycerol) between the slides and leave the preparation until the tissue begins to clear. This will make it easier to see any larvae which may be present.

Trichinella larva in unstained tissue

- It is usually seen coiled inside a lemon-shaped cyst.
- Most cysts lie longitudinally along the muscle fibres.
- Calcified larvae appear black.

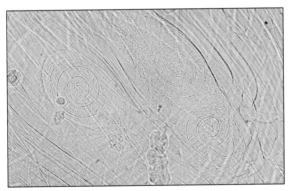

Plate 5.68   Encysted *Trichinella* larvae in unstained muscle biopsy.

Digestion technique

In this technique, pepsin is used to digest the muscle and the larvae are concentrated by centrifugation.

1 Cut the tissue into pieces about 2–3 mm in size and transfer to a bottle containing about 20 ml of acid pepsin solution (Reagent No. 4). Incubate overnight at 35–37 °C.

Caution: Wear protective rubber gloves and use forceps to handle the tissue.

2 Mix well and transfer the contents of the bottle to two conical tubes. Centrifuge at medium to high speed, i.e. RCF about 1 000 g for 2–5 minutes to sediment the larvae.

3 Using a plastic bulb pipette or Pasteur pipette, remove and discard the supernatant fluid from each tube. Wash and fix the sediments as follows:

- Resuspend the sediment and fill each tube with formol saline solution (Reagent No. 29). Mix well.
- Centrifuge to sediment the larvae. Remove and discard the supernatant fluid.

4 Transfer the two sediments to a slide and cover each preparation with a cover glass. Examine microscopically for *Trichinella* larvae using the 10× objective with the condenser iris *closed sufficiently* to give good contrast.

Intradermal tests

Skin tests are of little value in the diagnosis of acute trichinosis because they show positive reactions for many years following an infection. Cross-reactions with other nematodes may also occur.

---

6 Detection of *Dracunculus medinensis* (Guinea Worm) larvae

Dracunculus medinensis is a tissue nematode that causes dracunculiasis (Guinea worm ulcer disease). Infection occurs by drinking water which contains crustaceans that are infected with the larvae of *D. medinensis.*

Distribution

In recent years dracunculiasis eradication has been achieved in several countries in Asia and the Middle East. The disease is still found among rural communities in areas without safe water supplies in sub-Saharan Africa. The three most endemic countries are Sudan (73% of infections), Nigeria and Ghana.[69] In 2000 WHO reported 75 223 cases of dracunculiasis from sub-Saharan Africa (compared to 3.6 million in 1986).

Dracunculiasis

Following infection, the larvae are freed and penetrate through the duodenal wall. The larvae become adult worms in the connective tissues. The female worm migrates to the subcutaneous tissues (usually of the lower limbs) and buries its anterior end in the dermis causing inflammation. A blister forms which eventually breaks to form an ulcer. When the affected area is bathed in water the female protrudes through the ulcer and large numbers of larvae are released into the water. The larvae are taken up by a *Cyclops* or related crustacean.

Heavy infections can cause serious disease. The female worms (1 metre or more in length) cause severe pain and allergic reactions including urticaria, fever, nausea and vomiting. Damage to the worms in the skin can produce severe inflammation. Secondary infection may also occur leading to cellulitis and occasionally septicaemia. If a joint is involved, arthritis may develop. The disease can have crippling effects with serious consequences to the economical viability of a community.

D. medinensis larva

- It is large, measuring 500–700 μm in length.
- Anterior end is rounded.
- Tail is long and pointed. In wet preparations the tail can be seen coiling and uncoiling.

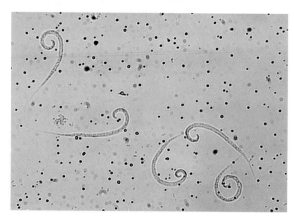

Plate 5.69 Larvae of *D.medinensis* as seen with 10× objective.

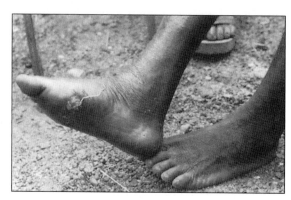

Plate 5.70 Female *D.medinensis* worm protruding from ulcer.

LABORATORY DIAGNOSIS

Laboratory tests to investigate dracunculiasis are limited because the larvae of *D. medinensis* are normally washed into water. A diagnosis is usually made when the blister has ruptured and the anterior end of the female worm can be seen.

If required, laboratory confirmation of the diagnosis can be made as follows:

1 Place a few drops of water on the ulcer to encourage discharge of the larvae.

2 After a few minutes collect the water in a plastic bulb pipette or Pasteur pipette.

3 Transfer the water to a slide and examine microscopically for motile larvae using the 10× objective with the iris diaphragm *closed sufficiently* to give good contrast.

REFERENCES

1 WHO TDR website www.who.int/tdr and TDR 2004 CD-ROM, obtainable free of charge from TDR (see Appendix 11).

2 **Casemore DP et al.** Laborataory diagnosis of cryptosporidiosis. *J. Clinical Pathology*, 1985, 38, pp. 1337–1341.

3 **Jackson TFHG, Ravdin JI.** Differentiation of *Entamoeba histolytica* and *Entamoeba dispar* infections. *Parasitology Today*, 1996, Vol. 12, No. 10, pp. 406–411.

4 **Sargeaunt PG.** *Entamoeba histolytica* is a complex of two species. *Transactions Royal Society Tropical Medicine and Hygiene*, 1992, 86, p. 348.

5 **Sharma A K et al.** Evaluation of newer diagnostic methods for the detection and differentiation of *Entamoeba histolytica* in an endemic area. *Transactions Royal Society Tropical Medicine and Hygiene*, 2003, 97, pp 396–397.

6 Method kindly supplied by Smith H. V. and Suresh K. Further information can be obtained from Professor H. V. Smith, Scottish Parasite Diagnostic Laboratory, Stobhill Hospital, Glasgow, G21 3UW, Scotland.

7 *Prevention and control of schistosomiasis and soil-transmitted helminthiasis.* Report of WHO Expert Committee, Geneva World Health Organization, 2002 (WHO Technical Report Series No 912).

8 **Ashford RW et al.** *Strongyloides füelleborni kellyi*: Infection and disease in Papua New Guinea. *Parasitology Today*, 1992, Vol. 8. No. 9, pp. 314–318.

9 Disease Watch No 4: Schistosomiasis, 2004. *TDR Nature Reviews Microbiology*.

10 WHO website www.who.int/health-topics/schisto.htm

11 **Crompton et al.** Preparing to control schistosomiasis and soil-transmitted helminthiasis in the twenty-first century. *Acta Tropica*, 2003, 86, pp 121–347.

12 **Marshall I et al.** Comparison of potassium hydroxide digestion and a modified Kato technique for the semi-quantitative estimation of *Schistosoma mansoni* eggs in faeces. *Annals Tropical Medicine and Parasitology*, 1989, Vol. 83, No. 1, pp. 31–35.

13 **Van Lieshout *et al*.** Immunodiagnosis of schistosomiasis by determination of the circulating antigens CAA and CCA, in particular in individuals with recent or light infections. *Acta Tropica: special issue, Schistosomiasis in the post-transmission phase*, 2000, 77, No 1, pp 69–80. Available from WHO/TDR, Geneva.

14 *Control of food-borne trematode infections.* Report of a WHO Study Group, Geneva, World Health Organization, 1995 (WHO Technical Report Series, No. 849).

15 **Garcia H H *et al*.** *Taenia solium* cysticercosis. *Lancet*, 2003, 361, pp 547–556.

16 **Garcia H H et al.** Serum antigen detection in the diagnosis, treatment, and follow-up of neurocysticercosis patients. *Transactions Royal Society Tropical Medicine and Hygiene*, 2000, 94, pp 673–676.

17 Chapter 17 in *Lecture Notes on Tropical Medicine*, 5th edition, 2004, pp 129–140, Blackwell Science.

18 Disease Watch No. 7, Malaria, 2004. *TDR Nature Reviews Microbiology*.

19 **Delacollette C.** Malaria epidemic response: what the clinician needs to know. *Mera*, 2004, July, iii.

20 **Singh B *et al*.** A large focus of naturally acquired *Plasmodium knowlesi* infections in human beings. *Lancet*, 2004, 363, pp 1017–24.

21 *Technical consultation meeting on malaria, HIV/AIDS interactions and policy implications*, June, 2004, WHO, Geneva.

22 **WHO.** Severe falciparum malaria. *Transactions Royal Society Tropical Medicine and Hygiene*, 2000, 94, Supplement.

23 **Crawley J.** Reducing the burden of anaemia in infants and young children in malaria-endemic countries of Africa: From evidence to action. *American Journal Tropical Medicine and Hygiene*, 2004, pp 25–34, Supplement 2.

24 Malaria, Chapter 9 in *Lecture Notes on Tropical Medicine*, 5th edition, 2004, pp 55–72. Blackwell Science.

25 **Marchesini P *et al*.** Reducing the burden of malaria in pregnancy. *Mera*, 2004, January, iii–iv.

26 **Rogier C. *et al*.** Epidemiological and clinical aspects of blackwater fever among African children suffering frequent malaria attacks. *Transactions Royal Society Tropical Medicine and Hygiene*, 2003, 97, pp 193–197.

27 **White N. J.** Malaria, Chapter 71 in *Mansons Tropical Diseases*, 21st edition, 2003, pp 1205–1295, Saunders, Elsevier Science.

28 **Alnwick D.** Meeting the malaria challenge. *Africa Health*, supplement, Sept 2001, pp 18–19.

29 The intolerable burden of malaria: What's new, what's needed? *American Journal Tropical Medicine and Hygiene*, 2004, 71, 2 Supplement.

30 **Klausner R, Alonso P.** An attack on all fronts. *Nature*, August 2004, 430, pp 930–931.

31 **Beales P F, Gilles H M.** Rationale and technique of malaria control. Ch. 6 in 4th ed. *Essential Malariology*, 2002, pp 107–190.

32 **Williams, J E.** Integrated vector management of malaria. *Mera*, November 2004, pp iii–iv.

33 **Roll Back Malaria Partnership** website www.rbm.who.int

34 **Ripley Ballou W et al.** Update on the clinical development of candidate malaria vaccines. *American Journal Tropical Medicine and Hygiene*, 2004, 71, pp 239–247.

35 **Moree M et al.** Strength in unity. *Nature*, August 2004, 430, pp 938–939.

36 **Webster D et al.** Progress with new malaria vaccines. *Bulletin World Health Organization*, 2003, 81(12), pp 902–909.

37 **Malaria Vaccine Initiative** website www.malariavaccine.org

38 *Basic malaria microscopy. Part 1 Learners Guide*. WHO, Geneva 1991.

39 **Payne D.** A lens too far? *Transactions Royal Society Tropical Medicine and Hygiene*, 1993, 87, p. 496.

40 **Amodu O K et al.** Intraleucocytic malaria pigment and clinical severity of malaria in children. *Transactions Royal Society Tropical Medicine and Hygiene*, 1998, 92, pp 54–56.

41 **Greenwood B M and Armstrong J R M.** Comparison of two simple methods for determining malaria parasite density. *Transactions Royal Society Tropical Medicine and Hygiene*, 1991, 85, pp 186–188.

42 **Moody A.** Rapid diagnostic tests for malaria parasites. *Clinical Microbiology Reviews*, January 2002, Vol 15, No 1, pp 66–78.

43 *The use of malaria rapid diagnostic tests*. World Health Organization, Geneva, 2004. Can be downloaded from the WHO website www.wpro.who.int/rdt

44 **Bell D.** Is there a role for malaria rapid diagnostic tests in Africa. *Mera*, September 2004, pp iii–iv.

45 *Malaria rapid diagnosis, making it work. Informal consultation on field trials and quality assurance on malaria rapid diagnostic tests*. World Health Organization, 2003. Can be downloaded from WHO website www.wpro.who.int/rdt

46 **Guthmann J P et al.** Validity, reliability and ease of use in the field of five rapid tests for the diagnosis of *P. falciparum* malaria in Uganda. *Transactions Royal Society Tropical Medicine and Hygiene*, 2002, 96, pp 254–257.

47 **Keiser J et al.** Acridine orange for malaria diagnosis: its diagnostic performance, its promotion and implementation in Tanzania, and the implications for malaria control. *Annals of Tropical Medicine and Parasitology*, 2002, 96, No 7, pp 613–654.

48 *Report of the Scientific Working Group on African trypanosomiasis, 2001*. World Health Organization, Geneva, 2003, TDR/SWG/01.

49 **Ash L R and Orihel T C.** Parasites: A guide to laboratory procedures and identification, 1987, p. 109. ASCP Press, American Society Clinical Pathologists, Chicago.

50 **Lejon V et al.** IgM quantification in the cerebrospinal fluid of sleeping sickness patients by latex card agglutination test. *Tropical Medicine International Health*, 2002, 7 pp 685–692.

51 *CATT/T.b. gambiense*. Explanatory note and instructions for use. Prince Leopold Institute of Tropical Medicine, Applied Technology and Production Unit (see Appendix 11 for contact details).

52 *Control of Chagas disease.* Second report of the WHO Expert Committee, WHO Technical Report Series, 905, 2002. World Health Organization, Geneva.

53 *Chagas disease.* TDR Nature Reviews Microbiology. Disease Watch No 1, 2003.

54 **Des jeux P.** Focus leishmaniasis. Disease Watch. *Nature Reviews Microbiology* 2004, 2, pp 692–693.

55 *The leishmaniases and Leishmania/HIV co-infections.* World Health Organization 2000, Fact sheet No 116. Website www.who.int/mediacentre/factsheets

56 **Croft S L, Coombs G H.** Leishmaniasis, current chemotherapy and treatment and recent advances in search for novel drugs. *Trends in Parasitology*, 2003, Vol 19, pp 502–508.

57 **Zijlstra E.** Leishmaniasis, Chapter 32, p. 468 in *Principles of Medicine in Africa*, 3rd edition, 2004. Cambridge University Press.

58 **Sundar S Rai M.** Laboratory diagnosis of visceral leishmaniasis. *Clinical and diagnostic laboratory immunology*, Sept 2002, pp 951–958.

59 **Boelaert M et al.** A comparasitive study of the effectiveness of diagnostic tests for visceral leishmaniasis. *American Journal Tropical Medicine and Hygiene*, 2004, 70(1), pp 72–77.

60 **Sayda el-Safi.** Field evaluation of the latex agglutination test for the detection of urinary antigens of visceral leishmaniasis in Sudan. Project SGS00/32. Can be downloaded from WHO website www.emro.who.int/tdr (Evaluation of rapid diagnostic tests, SGS00/32).

61 **Attar Z J et al.** Latex agglutination test for the detection of urinary antigens in visceral leishmaniasis. *Acta Tropica*, 2001, Vol 78, Issue 1, pp 11–16.

62 **Ramirez J R et al.** The method used to sample ulcers influences the diagnosis of cutanerus leishmaniasis. *Transactions Royal Society Tropical Medicine and Hygiene*, 2002, 96 Supplement 1, pp 169–171.

63 *Lymphatic filariasis. Disease burden and epidemiological trends*, 2002, World Health Organization TDR website www.who.int/tdr

64 *Guidelines for rapid assessment of Loa loa*, 2002. WHO TDR/IDE/RAPLOA/02.1, Geneva. Website www.who.int/tdr

65 *Rapid assessment procedures for Ioiasis*, 2001. WHO/TDR/IDE/RP/RAPL/01.1, Geneva: Website www.who.int/tdr

66 **Lazdins-Helds, J K et al.** Onchocerciasis Disease Watch. *TDR/Nature Reviews Microbiology*, No 3, December 2003. Can be downloaded from WHO/TDR website www.who.int/tdr

67 **Pion S D S et al.** Impact of four years of large scale invermectin treatment with low therapeutic coverage on the transmission of *Onchocerca volvulus* in Mbam Valley focus, central Cameroon. *Transactions Royal Society Tropical Medicine and Hygiene*, 2004, 98, pp 520–528.

68 Infection with free-living amoebae. *Tropical Medicine and Parasitology*, 5th edition 2002, pp 254–255. Mosby, Elsevier Science.

69 *Dracunculiasis eradication.* WHO website www.who/int/ctd (follow links to Dracunculiasis Eradication, Disease status).

RECOMMENDED READING

Parry E, Godfrey R, Mabey D, and Gill G. *Principles of Medicine in Africa*, 3rd edition, 2004. Cambridge University Press. Low price edition available.

Cook G and Zumla A. *Manson's Tropical Diseases*, 21st edition, 2003. W B Saunders and Elsevier Science. Low price edition available.

Peters W and Pasvol G. *Tropical Medicine and Parasitology*, 5th edition, 2002. Mosby and Elsevier Science.

Eddleston M, Davidson R, Wilkinson R, and Pierini S. *Oxford Handbook of Tropical Medicine*, 2nd edition, 2004. Oxford University Press.

Gill G V and Beeching N J. *Lecture Notes on Tropical Medicine*, 5th edition, 2004. Blackwell Science.

Lucas A O and Gilles H M. *Short Textbook of Public Health Medicine for the Tropics*, 4th edition, 2003. Arnold, Hodder Headline Group. Low price edition available.

Warrell D A and Gilles H M. *Essential Malariology*, 4th edition, 2002. Arnold, Hodder Headline Group. Low price edition available.

Service M. *Medical Entomology*, 3rd edition, 2004. Cambridge University Press.

Lankester T. *Setting up Community Health Programmes*, 2nd edition, revised 2002. TALC, Macmillan, TearFund.

Chiodini P L, Moody A H and Manser D. W. *Atlas of Medical Helminthology and Protozoology*, 4th edition, 2001.

Garcia L S. *Diagnostic medical parasitology*, 4th edition, 2001. American Society for Microbiology.

Walley J, Wright J and Hubley J. *Public Health: An Action Guide to Improving Health in Developing Countries*, 2001. Oxford University Press.

McCusker J. *Epidemiology in Community Health: Rural Health Series 9*, revised edition 2001. AMREF, Nairobi.

Dreyer G, Addiss D, Dreyer P and Noroes J. *Basic Lymphodema: Management, treatment and prevention of problems associated with lymphatic filariasis*, 2002. Hollis Publishing (USA).

MSF. *Refugee Health – An approach to emergency situations*, 1997. MSF and Macmillan Publishers.

Cheesbrough M. *Microscopical Diagnosis of Tropical Diseases, No 1–9 Colour learning brochures*, revised 2002. No. 1 Malaria. 2 African and South American trypanosomiasis, leishmaniasis. 3 Filariasis, Ioiasis, onchocerciasis. 4 Amoebiasis, giardiasis, *Cryptosporidium, Isospora*. 5 Meningitis, tuberculosis, relapsing fever, staphylococci, *Campylobacter*, ringworm, gonorrhoea, donovanosis, leprosy, plague, cholera, syphilis. 6 Urinalysis. 7 Blood. 8 Intestinal helminth infections. 9 Infections associated with HIV disease and AIDS. Available from Tropical Health Technology (see Appendix 11).

Compton D W T et al. Preparing to control schistosomiasis and soil-transmitted helminthiasis in the 21st century, 2003. *Acta Tropica*, 86, (2–3), pp 121–347.

WHO PUBLICATIONS AND REPORTS

TDR publications and reports are available free of charge (see TDR, Appendix 11). For the price of other WHO publications, apply to WHO Publications, Geneva.

Crompton D W T, Montresor A, Nesheim M C, Savioli L. *Controlling Disease due to Helmith Infections*, 2004. WHO Geneva.

Wisner B, Adams J. *Environmental health in emergencies and disasters*, 2002. WHO, Geneva.

Malaria: Scientific Working Group Report, 2003. TDR/SWG/03. Available on website www.who.int/tdr

The Use of Malaria Rapid Diagnostic Tests, 2004. WHO Regional Office for the Western Pacific. Available on website www.rbm.who.int

Insect Vectors and Human Health, 2002. TDR/SWG/VEC/03.1. Available from TDR World Health Organization (see Appendix 11).

Global Programme to Eliminate Lymphatic Filariasis: Annual Report, 2001. WHO/CDS/CPE/CEE 2002.28. Available on website www.filariasis.org

Rapid Assessment Procedures for Loiasis, 2001. TDR/IDE/RP/RAPL/01.1. Available from TDR World Health Organization (see Appendix 11).

Control of Chagas Disease: Second Report of WHO Expert Committee, 2002. WHO, Geneva.

Report of the Scientific Working Group on Leishmaniasis, 2004. TDR/SWG/04.

WHO TDR CD-ROM, May 2004. Available from TDR World Health Organization (see Appendix 11).

WHO Bench Aids:

– Diagnosis of malaria, 2nd edition 2000.

– Diagnosis of intestinal parasites, 1994.

– Diagnosis of filarial infections, 1997.

TDR News: WHO TDR Newsletter, published three times a year. Available from TDR World Health Organization (see Appendix 11).

Useful WHO websites

Tropical Diseases Research Programme (TDR) www.who.int/tdr

Roll back malaria www.rbm.who.int

Malaria vaccine initiative www.malariavaccine.org

Malaria rapid diagnostic tests (RDT) www.wpro.who.int/rdt

Global alliance to eliminate lymphatic filariasis www.filariasis.org

Also Liverpool School of Tropical Medicine *Lymphatic filariasis support* website www.filariasis.net

CDC DPDx CD-ROM Laboratory identification of parasitic diseases, 2nd edition 2004

This free of charge CD-ROM includes summaries of parasitic diseases (including life cycles, geographical distribution, treatment and prevention), an interactive quiz, diagnostic procedures, image library, and case studies.

It is available from DPDx (Dept Parasitic Diseases), Centers for Disease Control and Prevention, MS-F36, 4770 Buford Highway NE, Atlanta, Georgia 30341–3724, USA. E-mail dpd.cdc.gov

6

Clinical chemistry tests

6.1 Clinical chemistry in district laboratories

The clinical chemistry tests performed in district laboratories will depend on:

■ The health needs of the community and the requirement for clinical chemistry tests to assist in disease diagnosis and prognosis, monitoring of treatment, and screening to prevent illhealth.

■ The training and experience of laboratory staff and the support that can be provided by the district laboratory coordinator to ensure clinical chemistry tests are performed correctly with adequate control and safety.

■ Whether the appropriate equipment is available and affordable (purchasing and running costs) and can be maintained by the user.

■ Whether the required chemicals and products to make reagents, standards, and controls are available and affordable, and whether the more complex reagents can be provided to district laboratories in ready-made form or in easy to prepare packs that have sufficient stability.

■ Whether the laboratory has access to or can make its own supply of chemically pure water (see subunit 4.4).

■ Whether the numbers of tests performed are sufficient to avoid reagents, standards, and controls from being wasted due to their expiry. In some situations it may be possible and more appropriate to send patients' samples to a larger laboratory for clinical chemistry tests.

Tests
The following tests are described in this chapter:

Whole blood, serum, or plasma tests
– albumin, to investigate disorders of water balance, liver diseases, protein energy malnutrition.

– urea or preferably creatinine, to investigate disorders of renal function and monitor uraemia.
– glucose, to diagnose and monitor diabetes.
– bilirubin, to diagnose and monitor jaundice, e.g. in newborn.
– amylase, to assist in the diagnosis of acute pancreatitis.
– alanine aminotransferase, to investigate liver disease.
– potassium and sodium, to investigate and monitor disorders causing electrolyte disturbances.

Note: In district hospitals with a specialized clinical chemistry laboratory, blood, serum, or plasma tests may also include the measurement of alkaline phosphatase, aspartate aminotransferase (AST), calcium, cholesterol, cholinesterase, iron, and triglycerides.

The recommended manual methods of performing the above extended range of blood/serum/plasma tests together with details of how to prepare the required reagents, standards, and controls can be found in the 1995 WHO publication, *Production of basic diagnostic laboratory reagents.*[1]

Urine clinical chemistry tests
– protein, to diagnose and monitor proteinuria, e.g. in pregnancy or nephrotic syndrome.
– glucose, to screen for and monitor diabetes.
– bilirubin, to assist in the diagnosis of hepatocellular and obstructive jaundice.
– urobilinogen, to investigate haemolytic jaundice.
– ketones, to detect and monitor ketonuria, e.g. in diabetes.
– haemoglobin, to investigate intravascular haemolysis, microbial infection and glomerulonephritis.
– nitrite and leukocyte esterase, to assist in the diagnosis of urinary tract infection.
– relative mass density (specific gravity), occasionally needed to investigate the concentrating and diluting power of the kidneys.

Faecal clinical chemistry tests
– Occult blood, to investigate bleeding lesions of the gastrointestinal tract.
– Lactose, to investigate lactase deficiency.
– Examining faeces for excess fat to investigate disorders of fat absorption.

Cerebrospinal fluid (c.s.f.) clinical chemistry tests

- Protein to investigate meningitis and African trypanosomiasis.
- Glucose, occasionally needed to assist in diagnosing meningitis.

CLINICAL CHEMISTRY METHODS USED IN DISTRICT LABORATORIES

The following clinical chemistry methods are used in district laboratories:

- Manual techniques.

- Test kits using ready-made reagents.

- Rapid solid phase (dry reagent) technologies, e.g. reagent strip tests.

- Direct read-out analyzers for use with ready-made liquid reagents..

Manual techniques

Manual colorimetric techniques are possible and recommended in district laboratories when:

- the chemicals needed can be obtained and the reagents and standards correctly and economically made or preferably supplied to district laboratories from the regional or central laboratory.

- the required control material can be obtained and the quality of test methods monitored.

- the manual technique for a particular test is an approved test method.

For some tests where the reagents are stable and not complex and the manual technique is easy to perform, it will be more economical for district laboratories to prepare their own reagents and standards. When, however, reagents are complex to make or contain several chemicals which are not easily obtainable or available only in large quantities (often the situation), it will be difficult and expensive for district laboratories to use manual techniques.

Whenever possible the regional or central laboratory should procure the chemicals, prepare the reagents and standards, and distribute them with the necessary controls and approved testing procedure to district laboratories.

Use of test kits

Commercially produced clinical chemistry test kits are used by district laboratories, particularly when there is no local reliable production and distribution of reagents. In these situations test kits are used because all the reagents are ready-made or easily reconstituted, standards are often also provided, and the test method is usually rapid and simple to perform.

Compared with manual techniques, some test kits are expensive, particularly when the standards or working reagents have poor stability and have to be discarded before they are finished. When manual tests require complex reagents each containing several chemicals, the use of test kits for measuring analytes can be less expensive and preferable.

Many clinical chemistry test kits are designed either for use with automatic analyzers, which are not suitable for manual techniques, or as manual kits that require the use of a spectrophotometer or colorimeter fitted with interference filters to provide a specific wavelength. The use of a calculation factor in such a test kit is dependent on reading the test at the wavelength stated in the method.

Selecting test kits appropriately

Before purchasing a test kit, check the following:

- The type of instrument that is required, e.g. is the kit a colorimetric end-point method that can be used with a colour filter colorimeter measuring within the visible wavelength range 400–700 nm, e.g. Biochrom CO 7000 colorimeter described in subunit 4.10. If not, what type of instrument is required?

- Whether the test method is clearly presented and easy to follow.

- Whether the total volume of the sample and reagents is sufficient to read in the instrument being used, e.g. for some test kits the total volume is only 1.1 ml. Volumes can be doubled but this will increase the cost of each test.

- Prices and local availability. Try to find out whether there is more than one local agent and whether prices of kits vary between suppliers.

- Size, format, and stability of kits, e.g. how many tests can be performed, are all the reagents provided, how are they packaged, and what are the expiry dates of reagents (stock and *working*) and standards, both from their date of manufacture and from when they are opened. Also check the storage requirements for the different reagents and standards.

- Whether a control is available.

- References for the kit method and if available, field evaluations.

Important: Before purchasing a test kit, obtain from the supplier a copy of the insert leaflet that accompanies the kit. This will provide much of the information that is needed regarding the stability and storage of reagents, and also details of the specimen required, test method, calculation, and safety recommendations. It should also suggest a quality control serum to use and advize on the linearity of the method and reference ranges.

Dry reagent systems and liquid reagent analyzers

Direct readout clinical chemistry analyzers that use ready-made dry or liquid reagent technologies are available for the rapid measurement of a wide range of analytes in whole blood or serum. In response to the requirements of 'point of care' ('near patient testing'), many of the analyzers are small battery operated instruments designed for rapid single specimen testing and easy to use, calibrate, and maintain.

Dry reagent analyzers

Most of the analyzers that use a dry reagent system measure analyte concentration by:

- Reflectance photometry in which the specimen reacts with the reagents multilayered on a strip or film or contained in a cartridge type device. Light is directed on the surface of the testing device and that light which is not absorbed by the reaction is reflected, measured, and converted to the required units of concentration to give a direct read-out of the result.

   Simple low cost reflectance meters are available for the measurement of blood glucose, cholesterol and triglycerides (see subunit 6.5). Reflectance analyzers that measure a wide range of analytes are also available but expensive, e.g. *Reflotron Plus* manufactured by Roche Diagnostics.

   Reflotron Plus: This is a reflectance meter that uses reagent strips. All the information needed to measure the different analytes is coded on each strip. No separate test modules or calibrators are required. Within 2–3 minutes, test results are displayed digitally and printed from the integral printer. It is possible to use capillary or venous whole blood as well as serum and plasma. The *Reflotron Plus* operates from mains electricity 115–230 V AC and also from a car battery (10–30 V direct current).

   The reagent strips have a shelf-life of $1\frac{1}{2}$–2 years and are available (15 or 30 tests/pack, depending on test) for the measurement of alkaline phosphatase, amylase, bilirubin, cholesterol, CK, creatinine, glucose, GOT, GPT, HDL cholesterol, haemoglobin, triglycerides, urea, and uric acid. A potassium reagent strip is also available. Controls are available in pack sizes 4 × 2 ml. Full details of prices and distributors can be obtained from Roche Diagnostics (see Appendix 11).

- Transmittance photometry in which the specimen reacts with the dry reagents contained in a special disposable microcuvette. Absorbance is measured and converted into concentration units for the analyte being measured.

   Examples of meters that measure by transmittance photometry using dry reagents include the *HemoCue* meters manufactured by HemoCue AB for the direct measurement of haemoglobin and glucose. Both these meters and test microcuvettes, however, are expensive when compared with other technologies for measuring haemoglobin and glucose.

- Biosensor technology in which electrodes are used to measure electrochemically analytes such as sodium, potassium, chloride, urea, and glucose. While low cost glucose measuring biosensor analyzers are available, most multitest biosensor analyzers that measure electrolytes are very expensive, e.g. the *i-Stat* analyzer. Most cartridges used to measure blood gases and electrolytes have a shelf-life of only a few months.

Wet reagent analyzers

Most wet reagent system analyzers measure analytes by transmittance photometry and can be used only with the manufacturer's reagents. To use such analyzers in developing countries, the test reagents need to be available locally at affordable prices, have good stability, and the test method must be reliable and easy to perform.

Clin-Check Plus analyzer

One of the few manufacturers that produces clinical chemistry analyzers that can be used both with the manufacturer's ready-made reagents, other test kits and locally produced reagents, is Biochemical Systems International (see Appendix II). The *Clin-Check Plus* analyzer as shown in Plate 6.1 has a built-in two-place 37 °C heat-block and 6 interference filters (wavelengths: 340, 405, 505, 546, 578, 630 nm). It operates from mains electricity or from rechargable batteries. The light source is a long-life tungsten lamp. The analyzer is able to read in the UV range. Calculations are performed automatically with results displayed digitally in the required concentration units.

Clin-Check Plus measures analytes by colorimetric end-point, kinetic, or fixed time methods. All the enzyme tests are kinetic (absorbance varying linearly with time). The *Clin-Check Plus* analyzer can be programmed for up to 40 tests.

Biochemical Systems International make available cuvettes with prefilled reagents for the following tests: albumin, alkaline phosphatase, *alpha*-amylase, calcium, creatine kinase, chloride, cholesterol, HDL cholesterol, creatinine, haemoglobin, iron, glucose, AST (GOT), APT (GPT), LDH, proteins, inorganic phosphorous, magnesium, potassium, sodium, urea, total bilirubin, triglycerides, and uric acid. Control serum, normal and pathological, are also available.

When using the manufacturer's reagents, the operator uses the factor programmed in the analyzer for each test. When using other reagents, the operator needs to use a standard to calculate the factor to enter in the analyzer for each test. Most of the manufacturers' reagents have a shelf-life of 12–24 months.

The *Clin-Check Plus* analyzer is designed for use in district, regional, or central clinical chemistry laboratories where staff have been trained in basic clinical chemistry techniques.

Availability: Details of the *Clin-Check Plus* analyzer and its availability through local distributors can be obtained from the manufacturer Biochemical Systems International (see Appendix 11). It measures 275 × 210 × 90 mm and weighs 3.8 kgs.

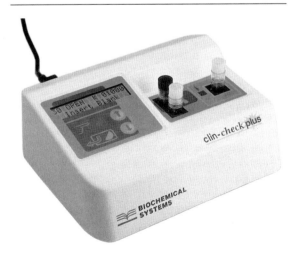

Plate 6.1 *Clin-Check Plus* clinical chemistry analyzer for use with ready-made or laboratory made reagents. *Courtesy of Biochemical Systems International.*

6.2 Quality assurance of clinical chemistry tests

As discussed in subunits 2.2 and 2.4 the purpose of quality assurance (QA) is to provide tests that are relevant and affordable, and test results that are reliable, timely, and used correctly in patient and community health care. QA includes therefore all those activities both outside and inside the laboratory that are required to achieve and sustain the objectives of QA and ensure resources are used as efficiently and effectively as possible. Staff must be adequately trained and the competence of staff must be monitored.

Well written and implemented Standard Operating Procedures (SOPs) covering the pre-analytical, analytical and post-analytical stages of testing are key to ensuring that:

– tests are selected appropriately and performed using standardized methods with adequate quality control.
– results are verified and reported within the target turn around time, using a standardized format.

Note: The information that needs to be contained in SOPs can be found in subunit 2.4.

QUALITY ASSURANCE: PRE-ANALYTICAL STAGE OF CLINICAL CHEMISTRY TESTS

The pre-analytical stage covers the reasons for performing a particular test, preparation of the patient, collection and transport of the specimen, the request form, and checks which need to be made when the specimen reaches the laboratory.

The reasons for performing a particular clinical chemistry test can be found at the beginning of each test as described in the subsequent subunits of this chapter (see also subunit 2.2).

The correct collection of specimens is essential for reliable test results. A summary of the collection of specimens for clinical chemistry tests can be found in Chart 6.1 and also at the beginning of individual test methods for those tests included in this chapter. The Chart also includes details of how to collect and stabilize specimens for transport to a specialist clinical chemistry laboratory.

Note: The safe transportation of specimens is described at the end of subunit 3.3.

Collection of blood specimens

Factors regarding the collection of blood specimens that can affect the correctness of clinical chemistry test results include:

- incorrect venepuncture technique,
- haemolysis of red cells,
- collection into the wrong container,
- instability of some chemical substances in whole blood, serum, and plasma.

Venepuncture technique

The following precautions need to be followed when collecting venous blood:

- Do not apply the tourniquet too tightly or for too long a period because this will cause venous stasis leading to a concentration of substances in the blood such as haemoglobin, plasma proteins, potassium, and calcium.

- Do not collect the blood from an arm into which an intravenous (IV) infusion is being given.

- If an anticoagulated specimen is required, add the correct amount of blood to the tube or bottle and mix the blood with the anticoagulant by gently inverting the container several times.

- Follow a safe technique and wear protective gloves (see subunit 8.3 in Part 2).

Note: A vein which can be felt is usually easier to enter than one which can only be seen.

Avoiding haemolysis

The haemolysis (rupture) of red cells can be a serious source of unreliable test results. If red cells are haemolyzed, substances from the cells are released into the serum or plasma leading to a false increase in the concentration of analytes, e.g. potassium. Haemolysis also interferes with many chemical reactions.

Haemolysis can be avoided by:

- Checking that the syringe and needle are dry and that the barrel and plunger of the syringe fit well.

- Not using a needle with too fine a bore.

- Not withdrawing the blood too rapidly or moving the needle once it is in the vein. Frothing of the blood must be avoided.

- Removing the needle from the syringe before dispensing the blood into the specimen container. Allow the blood to run gently down the inside wall of the container.

- Adding the correct amount of blood to anticoagulant. Do not shake the blood but gently mix it with the anticoagulant.

- Using clean dry tubes or bottles for the collection of blood from which serum is required and by allowing sufficient time for the blood to clot *and* clot retraction to take place. Red cells are very easily haemolyzed by the rough use of an applicator stick to dislodge a clot.

- Centrifuging blood samples for a minimum period of time. Centrifuging for 5 minutes at about 1000 g is adequate to obtain serum or plasma.

- Not storing whole blood samples in, or next to, the freezing compartment of a refrigerator.

Specimen containers and anticoagulants

Specimen containers for clinical chemistry tests must be leakproof and chemically clean. They should be well washed with detergent, rinsed in several changes of clean water, and finally rinsed in distilled or deionized water before being allowed to dry.

To avoid the confusion which often arises from the use of several different types of container, the following system is recommended:

Non-urgent blood tests (excluding glucose): Dispense about 5 ml of blood (see Chart 6.1) into a dry tube or bottle and allow to clot.† When the clot has retracted, centrifuge the specimen and transfer the serum to a labelled container. Tightly cap the container to avoid water evaporating from the specimen in dry warm conditions or moisture entering in humid environments.

† Avoid collecting blood into a plastic container if serum is required. Blood takes much longer to clot and clot retraction is poorer in a plastic tube or bottle than in a glass one.

Urgent blood tests (excluding glucose) and paediatric blood tests: Dispense the correct amount of blood into a tube containing lithium heparin anticoagulant.‡ *Gently* mix the blood with the anticoagulant. Centrifuge the specimen and transfer the plasma to a labelled container.

‡ Lithium heparin does not interfere with most chemical reactions and helps to minimize haemolysis. It does not contain sodium or potassium. Anticoagulants such as EDTA and fluoride-oxalate contain sodium or potassium salts and therefore these cannot be used when electrolytes are to be measured. Prior to analysis, stored plasma samples from heparinised blood often require re-centrifuging to remove clots.

Blood glucose (non-urgent or urgent): Dispense the correct amount of blood into a tube containing fluoride-oxalate.* *Gently* mix the blood with the anti-coagulant. Centrifuge the specimen to obtain plasma.

*Fluoride is an enzyme inhibitor. It prevents the break down of glucose to lactic acid by enzyme action (glycolysis). Blood collected into fluoride-oxalate (Reagent No. 27) can also be used for measuring protein, urea and bilirubin but not for electrolytes or enzymes. Fluoride-oxalate must not be used if measuring glucose using a reagent strip test.

Important: The regional or central clinical chemistry laboratory should advize on the collection of specimens for the tests referred to it for analysis.

Stability of analytes in blood specimens

Biochemical substances in blood are found in both plasma and cells but not necessarily in equal concentrations:

More concentrated in cells	Potassium Phosphate Aspartate amino-transferase (AST) Lactate dehydrogenase
More concentrated in plasma	Sodium Chloride Carbon dioxide
Concentration about equal in cells and plasma	Creatinine Glucose Urea Urate

Some of the chemical changes which may occur in blood specimens within a few hours of being collected include:

- Diffusion of potassium and some enzymes through the red cell membrane into the serum or plasma.

- Diffusion of carbon dioxide off the surface of the blood, leading to a lowering in the concentration of bicarbonate with a compensatory increase in plasma chloride (the 'chloride shift').

- Decrease in the concentration of glucose by glycolysis (when fluoride-oxalate is not used).

- Reduction or loss in the activity of certain enzymes, for example acid phosphatase.

- Decomposition of bilirubin in daylight or fluorescent light.

Some of these changes can be prevented by separating the plasma or serum from the red cells as soon as possible (within 1 hour) after the blood has been collected. The blood should not be refrigerated before the serum or plasma is separated because this can lead to falsely raised potassium values. Glycolysis can be prevented by using fluoride-oxalate anticoagulant (see previous text). The decomposition of bilirubin can be avoided by protecting specimens from light.

To minimize any alteration in the concentration of substances due to the ingestion of food or day-time variation, most blood specimens are best collected at the beginning of the day before a patient takes food.

Collection of urine specimens
Depending on the type of investigation, a single specimen may be adequate or it may be necessary to collect urine over a 24 hour period.

Collection of single urine specimen

A fresh, cleanly collected midstream 10–20 ml urine sample is required to test for protein, glucose, ketones, urobilinogen, bilirubin, specific gravity, leukocyte esterase, and nitrite. The container should be clean, dry, leak-proof, and sufficiently wide-necked for the patient to use. It must be free from all traces of disinfectants. The container must be sterile if the urine is also to be cultured.

Whenever possible, the sample should be the first urine passed by the patient at the beginning of the day because this will generally contain the highest concentrations of substances to be tested.

Collection of a 24 hour urine

A 24 hour urine specimen is required for the quantitative analysis of substances such as hormones, steroids, phosphate, calcium, and protein. The successful collection of a 24 hour urine depends on explaining the procedure fully to the patient. The procedure is as follows:

1 At a specified time, usually 08.00 hours, instruct the patient to empty his or her bladder. *Discard* this urine. This should not form part of the collection.

2 Give the patient a large (2 litre capacity) bottle containing a preservative or stabilizer as required (see later text).

3 Instruct the patient to collect into the bottle all the urine he or she passes in the next 24 hours, up to and *including* the urine passed at 08.00 hours the following morning.

A 24 hour urine should reach the laboratory as soon after collection as possible. If a delay is unavoidable, the specimen must be refrigerated at 2–8 °C until it can be delivered to the laboratory. The bottle must be labelled with the patient's name, hospital number, and the date and time when the collection was started and completed.

Stability of analytes in urine

The chemical changes which may occur in urine specimens stored at room temperature include:

- Breakdown of urea to ammonia by bacteria, leading to an increase in the pH of the urine. This may cause the precipitation of calcium and phosphates.
- Oxidation of urobilinogen to urobilin.
- Destruction of glucose by bacteria.
- Precipitation of urate crystals in acidic urine.

These chemical changes can be slowed down by refrigerating the urine at 2–8 °C. Chemicals can also be added to urine to preserve it, especially to 24 hour specimens. Urine preservatives and stabilizers include:

- *Hydrochloric acid:* This can be used to preserve urine for determinations such as amino acids, inorganic phosphate, calcium, and catecholamines. It must not be used to preserve urine for the measurement of protein or urate.
  15–20 ml of 6 mol/l hydrochloric acid is required to preserve a 24 hour urine specimen for measurements such as total protein and creatinine.
- *Thymol (few crystals):* This can be used to preserve a 24 hour urine specimen for measurements such as total protein and creatinine.

Important: Urine which contains the above preservatives cannot be cultured.

Collection of cerebrospinal fluid

The biochemical analysis of cerebrospinal fluid (c.s.f.) includes the measurement of total protein and occasionally, glucose.

c.s.f. for measuring glucose

To prevent the breakdown of glucose in the c.s.f. (leading to a falsely low value), collect 0.5–1.0 ml of the fluid into fluoride-oxalate preservative (Reagent No. 27).

c.s.f. for measuring protein

For total protein, collect about 1 ml of fluid into a dry tube or bottle. Total protein can also be measured using the supernatant fluid which remains after the bacteriological tests have been completed. Great care must be taken when handling c.s.f. because the specimen is obtained by lumbar puncture. Only a limited amount of fluid can be withdrawn from a patient at any one time.

Collection of faeces for occult blood testing

Instruct the patient to collect a small amount of faeces into a clean, dry, wide-necked container such as a waxed carton. It is usual to collect three specimens on different days. The patient should be on a diet free from meat and vegetables containing peroxidases for at least 2 days before collecting the specimen (see subunit 6.13).

The specimen should be tested as soon after collection as possible. If a delay is unavoidable, the specimen should be refrigerated at 2–8 °C. No preservative should be added to the faeces.

Note: If using a kit test, follow the instructions supplied with the kit.

Request form for clinical chemistry tests

The request form should be as simple and clear as possible in a standardized format. It should provide essential information concerning the patient and a clinical note regarding diagnosis and treatment (see also subunit 2.2).

It is particularly important that details of drug therapy are supplied. Several drugs are known to interfere with the chemical reactions of certain test methods and a change of method may have to be considered if the interfering drug cannot be withheld.

The form must specify the actual tests required and avoid general requests e.g. 'liver function tests'.

The form must also state the date and time of specimen collection.

Checking of clinical chemistry specimens

Before specimens reach the laboratory, those responsible for collecting samples must check that every specimen is labelled clearly with the patient's name and hospital number and that the name and number agree with what are written on the request form. Clerical mistakes can lead to serious errors and cause delays in the testing of specimens and subsequent treatment of patients.

A specimen should be rejected by the laboratory if:

- It is unlabelled or the identity on the form does not match that on the specimen.
- It is not correct for the test being requested or it has been collected in the wrong container, e.g. containing the incorrect anticoagulant.
- The specimen container is leaking.
- There is evidence of contamination.
- A blood sample appears haemolyzed or an anticoagulated specimen contains clots.
- There is too long a delay in the specimen reaching the laboratory or it has not been transported correctly.

Abnormal appearances of specimens

Any abnormal appearance of a specimen should be reported and investigated if indicated. Such action on the part of a technician may lead to a condition being diagnosed more rapidly and a patient receiving appropriate treatment at an earlier stage. The following are examples of abnormal specimen appearances and their possible significance:

- A dark coloured urine may be positive for bilirubin or haemoglobin.
- A urine that contains whole blood may contain *S. haematobium* eggs.
- A black faecal specimen may contain occult blood due to gastrointestinal bleeding.
- A dark brown serum may indicate intravascular haemolysis due to sickle cell disease, severe malaria, or an incompatible blood transfusion.
- A lipaemic (fatty) serum is associated with raised triglycerides (above 3.4 mmol/l).
- A deep yellow (icteric) serum indicates that a patient is jaundiced.
- A serum sample that is abnormally viscous (thick) or turbid may contain paraproteins.
- A serum that becomes markedly turbid after being refrigerated may contain cryoglobulins or cold agglutinins.
- A blood sample that contains a high concentration of red cells from which little serum or plasma can be obtained indicates severe dehydration or a blood disorder.

Chart 6.1 COLLECTION AND DISPATCH OF SPECIMENS FOR CLINICAL CHEMISTRY TESTS

The following chart gives information regarding the collection of specimens and minimum stability of substances for biochemical analysis[2]. Although guidelines are also provided regarding the referral and dispatch of specimens, each laboratory must obtain detailed instructions from its own referral centre. If special specimen containers are required, these should be obtained from the referral laboratory. Where an automated analyzer is used, follow the manufacturer's instructions regarding the collection of individual specimens.

Notes
- 'Room temperature' refers to 20–28 °C.
- The term 'kept cool' refers to the transportation of specimens in an insulated flask or box that contains a freezer pack or ice cubes.

Sterile container: When a blood specimen is likely to take longer than 24 h to reach its destination, to reduce the risk of bacterial contamination, collect the specimen into a sterile container. Aseptically transfer the plasma or serum to a sterile tube or bottle for transport.

Further information: Readers are referred to the WHO document *Use of anticoagulants in diagnostic laboratory investigations, and stability of blood, plasma and serum samples*[2].

BLOOD SPECIMENS

Test	Specimen	Container	Stability
Alanine aminotransferase (ALT) Previously SGPT	3–5 ml clotted blood. Haemolysis interferes with test. *Referral:* Send 1 ml serum, kept cool, to reach destination within 24 h.	Dry container.	Stable in whole blood at room temperature up to 3 h or at 2–8 °C up to 12 h. *Sterile serum:* Stable up to 7 days at 2–8 °C.
Albumin	2 ml clotted blood. Haemolysis interferes with test. *Referral:* Send 0.5 ml serum to reach destination within 72 h	Dry container.	Stable in whole blood at room temperature or at 2–8 °C up to 8 h. *Sterile serum:* Stable up to 5 months at 2–8 °C.

BLOOD SPECIMENS

Test	Specimen	Container	Stability
Alcohol (Ethanol)	2.5 ml anticoagulated blood. *Referral:* Send whole blood kept cool, to reach destination within 3 h.	Fluoride-oxalate container.	Stable in whole blood at room temperature or at 2–8 °C up to 3 h. *Sterile plasma:* Stable up to 6 months at 2–8 °C.
Alkaline phosphatase	see Phosphatase, alkaline		
alpha Amylase	3–5 ml clotted blood. *Referral:* Send 1–2 ml serum kept cool, to reach destination within 24 h.	Dry container.	Good stability in whole blood. *Sterile serum:* Stable up to 7 days at 2–8 °C.
Aspartate aminotransferase (AST) Previously SGOT	3–5 ml anticoagulated blood. Haemolysis interferes with test.	Preferably lithium heparin container	As for alanine aminotransferase. *Sterile plasma:* Stable up to 7 days at 2–8 °C.
Bicarbonate	see Carbon dioxide		
Bilirubin, total	3–5 ml clotted blood. *Infants:* 1–2 ml anticoagulated Haemolysis interferes with test. *Referral:* Send 0.5–1.0 ml serum or plasma, kept cool and protected from light, to reach destination within 6 h.	Dry container. *Infants:* Lithium heparin or EDTA container.	Protect from light. Stable in whole blood at room temperature or at 2–8 °C up to 2 h. *Sterile serum/plasma:* Stable up to 7 days in the dark at 2–8 °C.
Calcium, total	1–2 ml clotted blood. Collect fasting blood and avoid venous stasis. Patient must not be receiving EDTA therapy. *Referral:* Send 0.5 ml serum kept cool, to reach destination within 48 h.	Dry container which must be chemically clean.	Stable in whole blood at room temperature or at 2–8 °C for up to 3 h. *Sterile serum:* Stable up to 3 weeks at 2–8 °C.
Carbon dioxide (biocarbonate) Blood pH PCO_2	5 ml anticoagulated blood. Perform venepuncture with great care. Avoid introducing air bubbles into sample (make sure barrel and plunger of syringe fit well).	Lithium heparin container.	Very poor stability. Plasma must be separated from cells and analyzed as soon as possible (within 2 hours). *Sterile plasma:* Stable up to 7 days at 2–8 °C.
Cholesterol	3–5 ml clotted blood. *Also:* 2.5 ml of blood into EDTA. *Referral:* Send 0.5–1.0 ml serum and 2.5 ml EDTA blood to reach destination within 72 h.	Dry container.	Stable in whole blood at room temperature or at 2–8 °C up to 12 h. Stable in serum at 2–8 °C up to 72h. *Sterile serum:* Stable up to 7 days at 2–8 °C.

BLOOD SPECIMENS

Test	Specimen	Container	Stability
Cholesterol, HDL	3–5ml clotted blood	Dry container	As above
Cholinesterase	1–2 ml clotted blood. *Referral:* Send 0.2–0.5 ml serum to reach destination within 24 h.	Dry container.	Stable in whole blood at room temperature or at 2–8 °C up to 3 h. Stable in serum at 2–8 °C up to 3 h. *Sterile serum:* Stable for up to 1 year at 2–8 °C.
Creatinine	2–3 ml clotted blood. Haemolysis interferes with test. *Referral:* Send 0.5–1.0 ml serum kept cool, to reach destination within 18 h.	Dry container.	Stable in whole blood at room temperature or at 2–8 °C up to 12 h. Stable in serum at 2–8 °C up to 24 h. *Sterile serum:* Stable for up to 7 days at 2–8 °C.
Electrolytes: Sodium Potassium	5–7 ml clotted blood or 5 ml anticoagulated blood. Haemolyzed blood cannot be used. Do not collect blood from an arm receiving an I.V. infusion. *Referral:* Send about 1 ml serum or plasma, kept cool, to reach destination within 12 h.	Dry container or lithium heparin container.	Stable in whole blood at room temperature up to 1 h. Do not refrigerate sample before removing serum or plasma. Stable in serum or plasma at 2–8 °C up to 24 h. *Sterile plasma:* Potassium stable up to 6 weeks, sodium up to 2 weeks, at 2–8 °C.
Glucose	1 ml anticoagulated blood (fasting, post-prandial, or random specimen). Do not collect blood from an arm receiving an I.V. infusion. *Referral:* Send 0.5 ml plasma from fluoride/oxalated blood, kept cool, to reach destination within 36 h.	Fluoride-oxalate container.	Stable in fluoride/oxalated blood at room temperature up to 3 h. Stable in plasma at 2–8 °C up to 48 h. *Sterile plasma:* Stable for up to 7 days at 2–8 °C.
Iron Total iron-binding capacity (TIBC)	10–12 ml clotted blood. Collect at the beginning of the day. Haemolyzed samples cannot be used. *Referral:* Send at least 4 ml serum, kept cool, to reach destination within 18 h.	Dry preferably plastic container. Must be chemically clean.	Stable in whole blood at room temperature up to 2 h or in serum at 2–8 °C up to 24 h. *Sterile serum:* Stable for up to 3 weeks at 2–8 °C.
Lactate dehydrogenase (LDH)	3–5 ml anticoagulated blood. Blood which is haemolyzed (even slightly) cannot be used. *Referral:* Send 1–2 ml plasma to reach destination within 48 h.	Lithium heparin container.	Unstable in whole blood. Stable in plasma at 2–8 °C for up to 48 h. *Sterile plasma:* Stable for up to 4 days at 2–8 °C.

BLOOD SPECIMENS

Test	Specimen	Container	Stability
Phosphatase, alkaline	3–5 ml anticoagulated blood. Haemolysis interferes with test. *Referral:* Send 1 ml plasma to reach destination within 24 h.	Lithium heparin container.	Stable in whole blood at room temperature up to 12 h. Stable in plasma at 2–8 °C up to 24 h. *Sterile plasma:* Stable for up to 7 days at 2–8 °C.
Phosphate, inorganic (Phosphorus)	3–5 ml anticoagulated blood. Haemolyzed blood cannot be used. *Referral:* Send 1 ml plasma to reach destination within 24 h.	Lithium heparin container.	Unstable in whole blood. Stable in plasma at room temperature up to 24 h. *Sterile plasma:* Stable up to 4 days at 2–8 °C.
Potassium	see Electrolytes		
Protein, total	3 ml anticoagulated blood. Avoid venous stasis. Haemolysis interferes with test. *Referral:* Send 0.5 ml plasma to reach destination within 24 h.	Preferably lithium heparin container.	Stable in whole blood at room temperature or at 2–8 °C up to 8 h. *Sterile plasma:* Stable up to 4 weeks at 2–8 °C.
Protein, electrophoresis: *alpha* Fetoprotein Paraproteins	3–5 ml clotted blood. *Referral:* Send 1 ml serum, kept cool, to reach destination within 8 h.	Dry container.	Separate serum from cells. *Sterile serum:* Stable up to 7 days at 2–8 °C.
Sodium	see Electrolytes		
Thyroxine (T_4) and TSH	5 ml clotted blood.	Dry container.	As for ALT. *Sterile serum:* Stable up to 3 days at 2–8 °C.
Triglycerides	3–5 ml clotted blood (fasting specimen). *Also:* 2.5 ml of blood into EDTA. *Referral:* Send 1 ml serum and 2.5 ml EDTA blood, kept cool, to reach destination within 48 h.	Dry container.	Stable in whole blood at room temperature or at 2–8 °C up to 3 h. Stable in serum at 2–8 °C up to 72 h. *Sterile serum:* Stable up to 7 days at 2–8 °C.
Urate (Uric acid)	5 ml clotted blood. *Referral:* Send 1–2 ml serum to reach destination within 72 h.	Dry container.	Protect from daylight. Stable in whole blood at room temperature or at 2–8 °C up to 12 h. Stable in serum at 2–8 °C for up to 72 h. *Sterile serum:* Stable up to 7 days at 2–8 °C.

| Urea | 1–2 ml clotted blood. Plasma from EDTA or fluoride/oxalate blood can also be used. *Referral:* Send 0.2–0.5 ml serum to reach destination within 48 h. | Dry container. | Stable in whole blood at room temperature or at 2–8 °C up to 12 h. Stable in serum at 2–8 °C for up to 48 h. *Sterile serum:* Stable up to 7 days at 2–8 °C. |

URINE SPECIMENS

Test	Specimen	Container	Stability
Amino acids	*Adults:* 24 hour urine. *Infants:* First morning urine. *Referral:* Measure volume of urine, mix, and send 20 ml aliquot kept cool to reach destination within 24 h.	Large bottle containing 5 ml HCl, 6 mol/l. Dry container.	Stable for several hours at 2–8 °C.
delta Aminolaevulinic acid (ALA)	24 hour urine.	Large bottle containing 10 ml glacial acetic acid.	Stable for up to 4 days at 2–8 °C.
Bence Jones protein	10–20 ml midstream first morning urine. *Referral:* For protein electrophoresis, send urine (and serum sample) kept cool, to reach destination within 6 h.	Dry container.	Stable for up to 1 month at 2–8 °C.
Bilirubin	5–10 midstream urine.	Dry container.	Stable for a few hours at room temperature if protected from light.
Calcium	24 hour urine. *Referral:* Measure volume of urine, mix, and send 5 ml aliquot, kept cool, to reach destination within 6 h.	Large bottle containing 20 ml HCl, 6 mol/l.	Stable for up to 4 days at 2–8 °C.
Glucose	5–10 ml midstream urine.	Dry container.	Test as soon as possible after collection. Bacteria decrease stability.
Haemoglobin	5–10 ml midstream urine. *Referral:* Send urine, kept cool, to reach destination within 6 h.	Dry container.	Stable at room temperature for a few hours.
Ketones	5–10 ml midstream urine.	Dry container.	Test as soon as possible after collection.
3-Methoxy-4-hydroxy mandelic acid (HMMA), (VMA)	24 hour urine.	Large brown bottle containing 10 ml glacial acetic acid.	Stable up to 7 days at 2–8 °C.

URINE SPECIMENS

Test	Specimen	Container	Stability
Morphine and other opium-containing compounds	20–30 ml urine. *Referral:* Send urine, kept cool to reach destination within 6 h.	Dry container.	Contact Referral laboratory for stability information
pH	3–5 ml midstream urine.	Dry container.	Test as soon as possible after collection.
Phosphate, inorganic	24 hour urine.	Large bottle containing 20 ml HCl, 6 mol/l.	As for amino acids.
Protein, semi-quantitative:	10–20 ml midstream urine.	Dry container.	Stable for up to 7 days at 2–8 °C.
quantitative:	24 hour urine. *Referral:* Send 50 ml well-mixed aliquot, kept cool to reach destination within 6 h.	Large dry container.	Measure volume of urine.
Relative mass density (specific gravity)	50–60 ml if using a urinometer or 1 ml if using a refractometer. Midstream, first morning urine.	Dry container.	Test as soon as possible after collection.
Urobilinogen	5–10 ml midstream urine.	Dry container.	Test as soon as possible after collection.
Xylose absorption test	Contact the Referral Laboratory for details.		

FAECAL SPECIMENS

Test	Specimen	Container	Stability
Lactose	5–10 ml *fluid* faecal specimen.	Dry container.	Test as soon as possible after collection.
Occult blood	Collect a small sample each day for 3 days. Patient should not eat meat or vegetables containing peroxidases for 2 days before the test.	Dry wide-necked container, e.g. a waxed carton.	Test as soon as possible after collection. If a delay is inevitable the sample can be preserved by storing at 2–8 °C.

CEREBROSPINAL FLUID SPECIMENS

Test	Specimen	Container	Stability
Glucose	0.5 ml c.s.f. *Referral:* Send c.s.f. kept cool, to reach destination within 18 h.	Fluoride-oxalate container.	Stable at room temperature up to 3 h, or at 2–8 °C up to 24 h.
Protein, total	1 ml c.s.f. *Referral:* Send c.s.f. to reach destination within 24 h.	Dry container (sterile, if c.s.f. for culture also).	Stable at room temperature up to 3 h, or for 6 days at 2–8 °C.

QUALITY ASSURANCE: ANALYTICAL STAGE OF CLINICAL CHEMISTRY TESTS

The analytical stage covers the principle of the test method, the reagents, standards, control materials and equipment used, details of the test method, and quality control procedures (described in the subsequent subunits of this chapter).

Quality control of quantitative chemical tests

Quality control procedures are needed to detect and minimize errors in the performance of tests. As explained in subunit 2.4 (*Sources of error in district laboratory practice*), reliable test results depend on laboratory staff detecting and correcting errors at an early stage and keeping errors of imprecision and inaccuracy to a minimum by good laboratory practice and quality control.

Errors of imprecision, or scatter: Precision refers to the reproducibility of a result. A test, however can be precise without being accurate as described in the following text. Errors of imprecision are often referred to as errors of scatter because they are irregular or random. Results differ from the correct result by varying amounts.

Errors of inaccuracy, or bias: Accuracy is defined as closeness of agreement between a test result and the accepted true value. Errors of inaccuracy are often referred to as errors of bias because they are consistent or regular. All the test results differ from their correct result by approximately the same amount.

Story to help understand the differences between imprecision and inaccuracy
The story is about the owners of three village stores (the storekeepers have English names but you may like to substitute your own local names):

- *Mr Smith:* He was a jolly man but unfortunately very careless.
- *Mr Jones:* He was a helpful man but always so inefficient and disorganized.
- *Mr Brown:* He was a friendly man who was both careful and efficient.

All three shopkeepers stocked salt and sold it in 1 kg bags but whereas the service given by *Mr Brown* was of a high quality, that given by *Mr Smith* and *Mr Jones* was not all it should have been:

- The bags of salt sold by *Mr Brown* always contained the same amount of salt and as near to the correct weight as *Mr Brown* could make them. *Mr Brown* checked regularly the equipment he was using and kept a careful eye on his assistant to make sure he was not getting careless in the amount of salt he was putting into each bag.

- The bags of salt from *Mr Smith*'s store contained different amounts of salt due to the careless way *Mr Smith* and his assistant worked.

- The bags of salt from *Mr Jones*'s shop all contained the same amount of salt (his assistant weighed the salt carefully) but they were underweight. *Mr Jones* never checked his scales.

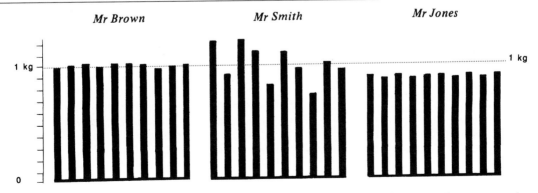

Fig. 6.1   Weights of individual bags of salt sold by Messrs. *Brown*, *Smith*, and *Jones*. The dotted line represents the correct weights of 1 kg. It can be seen that *Mr Brown*'s customers received a high standard of service whereas *Mr Smith*'s and *Mr Jones*'s customers received a poor service. *Courtesy of BJ Seaton.*

Fig. 6.1 shows the weights of salt in 10 of the bags sold from the three different stores and Table 6.1 lists the weights.

One day *Mr Smith* and *Mr Jones* had occasion to visit *Mr Brown* (they had run out of a few essential supplies) and after seeing the way he worked they resolved to improve the quality of service they gave to their customers.

Mr Smith after visiting *Mr Brown* wanted to improve the reliability of his 1 kg bags of salt and decided to find out just how good he could be if he really tried. So he chose a time when he was not usually busy with customers, closed his shop, cleaned and adjusted his scales and weighed out 20 bags of salt. *Mr Smith* knows that he will not always be able to weigh the salt so well when the shop is busy with customers but the exercise has shown him what he is capable of under optimal (ideal) conditions and gives him a standard to strive for.

Mr Jones after visiting *Mr Brown* realized that if he were to obtain an exact 1 kg weight then he too would be able to make sure that his customers received the correct amount of salt. His assistant was pleased when the new 1 kg weight was obtained because although he had always weighed the salt carefully he had never had a way of checking that he was in fact weighing exactly 1 kg.

After improving their way of working and introducing various checks, the service given by *Mr Smith* and *Mr Jones* to their customers became very much better. They noticed however, that even with careful weighing and using equipment now known to be reliable, it was much more difficult to provide customers with exactly 1 kg of potatoes than 1 kg of salt. Even *Mr Brown* experienced the same difficulty. The customers, however, understood that it was not easy to weigh such large items and were not surprised to find quite large variations in weights at different times (see Fig. 6.2 and Table 6.2).

Applying the story of the storekeepers

- Medical laboratory workers (storekeepers in the story) want to provide the best possible service to their patients (customers in the story).

Table 6.1. Actual weights of '1 kg' bags of salt sold by *Messrs Smith, Jones and Brown.*

BAGS	WEIGHTS (kg)		
	Mr Smith	*Mr Jones*	*Mr Brown*
1	1.069	0.952	0.991
2	0.955	0.947	1.000
3	1.076	0.954	1.002
4	1.031	0.947	0.995
5	0.920	0.951	1.004
6	1.031	0.952	1.006
7	0.978	0.949	1.002
8	0.883	0.954	0.990
9	0.997	0.948	0.999
10	0.971	0.959	1.002
Total weight	9.911 kg	9.513 kg	9.991 kg
Average weight:*	0.991 kg	0.951 kg	0.999 kg
Bias:†	−0.009	−0.049	−0.001
Scatter:‡	0.062	0.003	0.005

* Calculated by dividing the total weight of all the bags by their number, i.e. by 10.
† Bias is the difference between the average weights of the bags of salt and their correct weight, i.e. 1 kg.
‡ Scatter is calculated as the standard deviation (SD) of the weights (see Fig. 6.3).

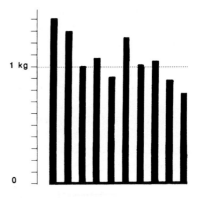

Fig. 6.2   Weights of individual 1 kg bags of potatoes achieved by *Mr Brown. Courtesy of BJ Seaton.*

Table 6.2. Actual weights of '1 kg' bags of potatoes sold by *Mr Brown.*

BAGS	WEIGHTS (kg)
1	1.169
2	1.126
3	1.007
4	1.032
5	0.962
6	1.102
7	1.007
8	1.029
9	0.961
10	0.918
Total weight	10.310 kg
Average weight:*	1.031 kg
Bias:†	+0.031
Scatter:‡	0.079

* Calculated by dividing the total weight of all the bags by their number, i.e. by 10.
† Bias is the difference between the average weights of the bags of potatoes and their correct weight, i.e. 1 kg.
‡ Scatter is calculated as the standard deviation (SD) of the weights (see Fig. 6.3).

- 'Customers' will expect any errors in results to be kept down to reasonable levels depending on the type of test. As with weighing salt and potatoes, not all tests can be performed equally well.
- Errors of imprecision, or scatter, are irregular with results differing from the correct test result by varying amounts like *Mr Smith's* bags of salt. His bags were unacceptable because of large scatter even though his bias was low. (See Fig. 6.1 and Table 6.1.)
- Errors of inaccuracy, or bias, are regular with all test results differing from the correct result by approximately the same amount like *Mr Jones's* bags of salt. His bags were unacceptable because of high bias even though his amount of scatter was low (see Fig. 6.1 and Table 6.1).

- *Mr Brown*'s bags of salt were acceptable (consistently near to 1 kg) because his precise and accurate way of working produced both small scatter and a low bias (see Fig. 6.1 and Table 6.1). He worked both precisely and accurately.
- Laboratory test results will only be acceptable if both scatter and bias are kept to a minimum. If results are charted regularly (quality control chart) it will be easy to see whether errors are being kept to reasonable levels and when a test method is drifting out of control.
- Some tests will be easier than others to perform reliably, like weighing 1 kg of salt compared with weighing 1 kg of potatoes (see Fig. 6.2 and Table 6.2).

Common causes of errors in clinical chemistry work

Errors of imprecision (scatter)

The causes of these can be summarized as follows:

- Incorrect and variable pipetting and dispensing.
- Inadequate mixing of sample with reagents.
- Samples are not incubated consistently at the correct temperature (when incubation of tests is required).
- Individual items of glassware or plastic-ware are not clean or dry before reuse.
- Equipment malfunctioning (erratic performance).
- Incomplete removal of interfering substances, e.g. red cells when measuring analytes in serum or plasma.

See also subunit 2.4.

Errors of inaccuracy (bias)

The causes of these can be summarized as follows:

- Incorrect calibration of a test method.
- Tests being read at the incorrect wavelength or the wrong filter being used.
- An automatic pipettor is used that has been set to measure an incorrect amount.
- Consistent calculation error (e.g. incorrect factor is used).
- Use of unsatisfactory reagents, standards, or controls.

See also subunit 2.4.

Important: In the performance of clinical chemistry analytical tests it is essential to check regularly for imprecision and inaccuracy and to detect at an early stage when errors are being introduced that are going to lead to incorrect test results. When such errors are found their cause must be identified and the necessary corrective action(s) taken.

Establishing performance standards

Before any test method is used for patients, the laboratory must *first* ensure that the method is working reliably and that it can be performed within acceptable limits of variability. After a test has been introduced it must be adequately controlled.

Some tests will be easier than others to perform reliably, e.g. serum albumin can be measured (bromocresol green method) with less variability than serum aspartate aminotransferase (Reitman Frankel method) using a manual colorimetric technique.

The following procedure is used to assess precision by confirming that the analytical coefficient of variation (CV) under optimal and routine conditions (within and between batches) is acceptable.

Establishing the coefficient of variation

1 Obtain sufficient quantity of a control serum that contains a known amount of the substance being measured.
2 Under optimal conditions, perform 20 measurements on the same control serum. Follow the method as carefully as possible using the same reagents and equipment for each of the 20 measurements.
   Note: The analyst should be a well-trained experienced clinical chemistry analyst. He or she should not be assigned any other task at the time.
3 Read off the values from the calibration graph (details of calibration are given at the beginning of each test method).
4 List the values for each of the 20 estimations as shown in the example in Table 6.3.
5 Calculate the mean (average value) by adding up all the results and dividing the total by 20.
6 For each result, work out the difference in value from the mean, entering the differences in the second column of the chart.
7 Multiply each difference value by itself to give the squared difference values, entering these figures in the third column of the chart.
8 Add up the figures in column three, to give the sum of the squared differences (see Table 6.3).
9 Calculate what is called the standard deviation (SD) using the formula:

$$SD = \sqrt{\frac{\text{Sum of the squared difference}}{n-1}}$$

Where n is the number of results, i.e. 20.

Example: Follow the SD calculation in Table 6.3.

10 Calculate the optimal CV using the formula:

$$CV = \frac{SD}{\text{Mean}} \times 100$$

Example: Follow the CV calculation in Table 6.3.

Table 6.3   Example of how to calculate the SD and CV for a glucose assay

27 MARCH 2003   GLUCOSE   ANALYST: SB

Test No.	Test Results in mmol/l	Differences from mean	Squared differences	Calculations
1	6.5	−0.2	0.04	
2	6.7	0.0	0.00	$SD = \dfrac{0.44}{20\text{-}1}$
3	6.5	−0.2	0.04	
4	6.6	−0.1	0.01	
5	6.8	+0.1	0.01	$= \sqrt{0.023}$
6	6.9	+0.2	0.04	
7	6.5	−0.2	0.04	$= 0.15$ mmol/l
8	6.5	−0.2	0.04	
9	6.7	0.0	0.00	
10	6.8	+0.1	0.01	
11	6.7	0.0	0.00	$CV = \dfrac{0.15}{6.7} \times 100$
12	6.8	+0.1	0.01	
13	6.4	−0.3	0.09	
14	6.8	+0.1	0.01	$= 2.2\%$
15	6.5	−0.2	0.04	
16	6.7	0.0	0.00	
17	6.9	+0.2	0.04	
18	6.6	−0.1	0.01	
19	6.8	+0.1	0.01	
20	6.7	0.0	0.00	

Total = 133.4   Total = 0.44

Mean = 133.4 ÷ 20
         = 6.7 mmol/l

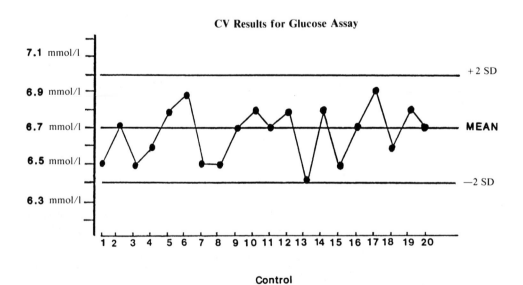

Fig. 6.3   Plotting CV glucose values from the results shown in Table 6.3.

Note: In correct statistical terms, the formula

$$\frac{SD}{Mean} \times 100$$

gives the coefficient of variation (CV). It is simply expressing the SD (which is given in substance units) as a percentage of the mean.

11 Check whether the optimal CV is below the maximum allowed for the particular test, e.g.

Test	Suggested optimal CV maximum %
Albumin	3%
Alkaline phosphatase	10%
Amylase	6%
Aspartate aminotransferase	8%
Bilirubin (total)	6%
Calcium	1.5%
Cholesterol	7%
Creatinine	4%
Glucose	2%
Total protein	2%
Urate	5%
Urea	3%

Note: The above figures are those for manually performed colorimetric tests.[3]

12 Chart the results as follows:
– Take a sheet of graph paper and draw on it three horizontal lines corresponding to the mean, +2 SD and −2 SD as shown in Fig. 6.3.
– Work out the values for +2 SD and −2 SD as follows:

    +2 SD = Mean +2 SD
    −2 SD = Mean −2 SD

    Example
    Using the mean of 6.7 mmol/l and SD of 0.15 mmol/l as shown in Table 6.3:

    +2 SD = 6.7 + 0.3
          = 7.0 mmol/l
    −2 SD = 6.7 − 0.3
          = 6.4 mmol/l

– Enter the mean, +2 SD, −2 SD, and other values on the left hand side of the chart.
– Mark the horizontal axis 'Control' and number it 1 to 20.
– Chart the result of each test as shown in the example chart.

13 Examine the chart for the distribution of values around the mean. The chart should show a fairly even distribution of values on each side of the mean within +2 SD and −2 SD (see Fig. 6.3).

Establishing the routine CV

When a test is performed under routine conditions of work the degree of variability, i.e. routine CV, will inevitably be higher than the optimal CV and therefore the range of acceptable values will be wider.

Although the CV can be determined in a single experiment it takes some time to accumulate enough information from routine tests to calculate the routine CV, i.e. repeatability (variation from day to day). When, therefore, a new test is first introduced, it is usual to set up the first control chart using twice the optimal SD and CV.

How to use a quality control chart

Having established that a test method is reliable and has an acceptable CV, it can be put into routine use providing it can be controlled adequately. A control serum must be used with *every* batch of tests.

The use of a control chart will enable most faults to be identified and corrected at an early stage before patients' results are affected and reporting has to be delayed.

Setting up a daily quality control chart

The daily control chart is similar to the CV control chart illustrated in Fig. 6.3 except that the horizontal axis is numbered for the days of the month as shown in Fig. 6.4, and the ±2 SD are calculated from the routine conditions standard deviation.

1 Calculate the +2 SD and −2 SD values for the assay and prepare a control chart as shown in Fig. 6.4.

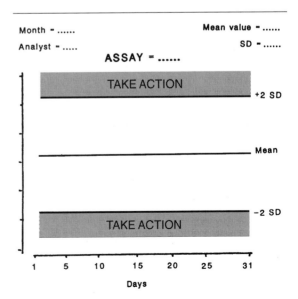

Fig. 6.4 Example of a layout for a quality control chart.

First control chart

When setting up the first control chart, the performance of the test under routine conditions will not be known. To obtain a realistic routine conditions SD value from which to establish acceptable limits, it is usual to double the optimal conditions SD value obtained as previously described.

Example: If the optimal SD value is 0.15 mmol/l, the routine SD should be taken as 0.30 mmol/l.

Once the test method has been performed 20 times a revised routine CV can be calculated and this value can then be used instead of the 2 × optimal CV value.

2   Using the same control serum for each batch of tests, plot the values on the daily control chart as shown for the CV chart in Fig. 6.3.

3   Each day after charting the control value, check that it is within the acceptable limits of ±2 SD and that there is no marked change in the distribution of results above or below the mean or a movement (drift) towards the TAKE ACTION zones.

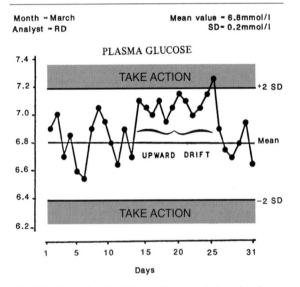

Month = March   Mean value = 6.8mmol/l
Analyst = RD   SD = 0.2mmol/l

Fig. 6.5   Example of a daily quality control chart showing an upward drift due to the deterioration of a reagent.

Interpretation of results

Control value within ±2 SD limits: This is a good sign. It can be assumed that the patients' results are reliable and therefore they can be reported with confidence.

Control value outside ±2 SD limits: This is unacceptable and the patients' results must *not* be reported. A fresh control serum should be measured together with a few of the patients' samples. If the result of the fresh control serum is within ±2 SD limits and the results of the repeated tests agree with those of the first testing, all the patients' results can be reported.

If, however, the control result is still not acceptable, the patients' results must *not* be reported. The error(s) must be found and put right and the batch of tests repeated. Check particularly for:

– Reagent deterioration or the incorrect preparation of a working reagent.

– Faulty equipment, e.g. heat-block or water-bath not at the correct temperature.

– Wrong filter being used or the colorimeter giving fluctuating readings or readings different from those given previously for the control or standard solutions.

Control value moving towards TAKE ACTION zone: The patient's results can be reported but a drift of values upwards or downwards is a warning that the test is becoming unreliable and the cause(s) must be investigated before the next batch of tests is performed (see Fig. 6.5).

Preparation of a new quality control chart

When the first quality control chart is almost completed, prepare a new one using the most recent 20 control results to re-calculate the CV. If, as is to be hoped, the test is being performed better, i.e. with less imprecision, then the new CV will be lower than the previous one.

Re-calculate the +2 SD and −2 SD values using the new SD value.

Quality control sera

Commercially produced liquid or lyophilized assayed quality control (QC) sera are expensive and not always available for use in district laboratories. An alternative to the routine use of commercially produced QC sera is for district laboratories to be provided with an ethylene glycol stabilized QC serum that has been prepared, and calibrated in the district's clinical chemistry reference laboratory. Full details can be found in the WHO document *Preparation of stabilized liquid quality control serum to be used in clinical chemistry laboratories.*[4]

When it is not possible for a district laboratory to be supplied from a reference laboratory with an assayed stabilized QC serum, an ethylene glycol stabilized QC serum can be prepared in the laboratory from pooled sera of human origin, providing a member of staff is sufficiently well trained.

A method that can be used is as follows:

1   Collect venous blood aseptically from several volunteers that have tested negative for hepatitis antigen(s) and HIV antibody. Collect the blood into screw cap glass bottles without anticoagulant. Obtain sufficient blood that will provide a serum pool of about 100 ml.

2   Allow the blood to clot at room temperature. Refrigerate overnight at 2–8 °C. Protect the bottles from light by surrounding them with tin foil or thick paper.

3   Collect the separated serum from each bottle and centrifuge it for 15 minutes at 1 000–2 000 g.

4   Transfer 100 ml of the clear centrifuged serum into a screw cap plastic container (premark the 100 ml level). Exclude from the pool, serum that appears cloudy (lipaemic), icteric, haemolyzed or abnormally coloured due to dyes.

5   Immediately freeze the pooled serum at −20 °C.

6   The following day (or at a later stage), thaw completely the pooled serum at room temperature, keeping the container upright and not mixing the serum. Protect the container from light by surrounding it with tin foil or thick paper.

7   Using a 10 ml syringe and wide bore needle, remove and discard the top 15 ml of fluid from the 100 ml of pooled serum. This will contain mainly water and a weak concentration of analytes.

8   Replace the fluid with 15 ml of ethylene glycol (ethanediol).

Ethylene glycol: This is an effective bacteriostatic and stabilizing agent when added to serum at a 15% concentration. No other preservative need be added. Commonly assayed blood substances are stable in ethylene glycol preserved serum for at least 4 months at 2–6 °C and some analytes for up to 12 months. Most analytes remain unchanged for 6 days at ambient temperatures, allowing an ethylene glycol control serum to be used in external quality assessment programmes.

Note: Serum containing ethylene glycol must not however be used as a control serum in ISE analyzers because the chemical can damage the electrodes.

9   Mix well for 15–30 minutes, preferably using a magnetic stirring mixer or other electric mixer (not a vortex mixer).

10 Immediately dispense the pooled stabilized serum in 2 ml or other convenient amounts into brown screw cap bottles. When dispensing, keep the serum well mixed. Label, date, and store the bottles at 2–8 °C.

11 Assign values to the pooled stabilized serum for each analyte measured in the laboratory. Measure carefully in duplicate each analyte in the new pooled serum in the same way as test samples.

For each analyte include an assayed QC serum. If the results obtained are correct for the assayed QC serum it can be assumed that the values for the new stabilized pooled QC serum will be correct. List the analytes and their values and date the list. Give the QC serum a batch number.

Note: The assayed QC serum used to calibrate the new QC control can be a previously calibrated ethylene glycol stabilized QC serum or if this is not available, it will be necessary to use a commercially produced QC serum, preferably a liquid product. If needing to use a lyophilized QC serum, ensure it is correctly reconstituted.

Reconstitution of a lyophilized (dried) QC serum

–   Read carefully the manufacturer's instructions.

–   Open the bottle slowly to avoid any loss of material (the serum is often vacuum packed).

–   Reconstitute with good quality glass-distilled water or with the special diluent supplied by the manufacturer. Pipette accurately using a chemically clean pipette.

–   After adding the water or diluent, stopper the container and gently *swirl* the contents. Allow to stand for 10 minutes and then swirl again. Repeat the process until the main solid 'plug' of serum has dissolved. Invert gently three or four times to ensure that any remaining powder on the stopper will be washed into the solution. Stand for 2–3 minutes and then invert again three or four times.

–   Allow reconstituted serum to stand at room temperature (20–28 °C) for the time specified by the manufacturer (usually 30–60 minutes). After the waiting period, *gently* remix the serum.

–   Dispense the serum in 0.5–1 ml amounts, or as required, into small sterile brown/amber containers. To reduce the risk of contamination, it is advisable to transfer the serum by pouring, not by pipetting.

–   Label each container with the date and Lot No. (Batch No.) of the serum. Freeze immediately and store at −20 °C or below until required.

    For use, allow the serum to warm to room temperature. When completely thawed, mix gently but well.

Quality control of enzyme tests

In addition to the quality control procedures described previously for the quantitative measurement of blood analytes, the measurement of enzymes requires careful attention to technique. Small errors of technique can lead to grossly unreliable and misleading test results.

Enzymes are usually present in very small

amounts in plasma or serum, therefore they cannot be measured directly like other substances. They are assayed indirectly by measuring either the reduction in concentration of the substrate upon which the enzyme acts or the amount of product formed from the substrate. It is therefore enzyme activity that is being measured.

International unit of enzyme activity:
This is the amount of enzyme which under defined assay conditions will catalyze the conversion of 1 μmol of substrate per minute. Results are expressed in International Units per litre (U/l). In accordance with this definition the assay conditions for enzyme analysis must be specified. These include:

- Substrate used, including its concentration.
- pH and buffer system.
- Time of incubation.
- Temperature of the reaction.
- Presence of activators or inhibitors.
- Direction in which the reaction proceeds.

The reporting of enzyme activity in katals is preferred by some clinical chemists because the katal refers to the conversion of 1 mol of substrate per *second* whereas the International Unit refers to the conversion of 1 μmol of substrate per *minute*. The second (s) is the SI unit of time (the minute is a non-SI unit).

The relationship between katals and International Units is 1 nkatal = 16.7 U.

The following are the most important factors that can affect the measurement of enzyme activity:

Temperature

Reaction rate increases with temperature. Most enzymes show their optimal activity between 30 °C and 50 °C. Above 60 °C, enzyme denaturation occurs. The incubation temperatures in test methods must be strictly followed.

Time

The substrate concentration falls with time as the product concentration increases. Timing is therefore important because substrate and product concentrations are changing all the time and it is one of these that is being measured. An accurate timer must be used to measure the incubation time of an enzyme and its substrate.

pH

Any increase or decrease in pH away from the optimum will cause a decrease in enzyme activity. A marked change in pH can lead to the denaturation of an enzyme. The pH of buffers and substrates used in enzyme tests must therefore be correct.

Light rays

Ultraviolet light tends to inhibit enzyme activity while blue or red light tends to increase it. Samples for enzyme analysis must therefore be protected from direct light.

Enzyme stability

Many enzymes do not have good stability. Specimens for enzyme analysis should not be left at room temperature for long periods.

Serum should be separated from cells as soon as possible after the blood has clotted and the clot retracted. With the loss of carbon dioxide the pH of fresh blood rises rapidly. This leads to enzyme inactivation. Haemolyzed specimens are generally unsuitable for enzyme analysis.

Glassware

Glassware contaminated with traces of heavy metals or detergents can inhibit enzyme activity. The use of chemically clean glassware is essential. Cuvettes must be clean and their optical surfaces dry and free from scratches and finger marks.

Reagents

Test results can be seriously affected when reagents, particularly substrates and buffers, are not prepared correctly. Precautions should be taken to avoid bacterial contamination of reagents.

Quality control of qualitative chemical tests
The reagents used in qualitative and semi-quantitative chemical tests must also be controlled, e.g. those used to detect or measure semi-quantitatively substances in urine, c.s.f. and faeces. A known positive and negative control must be used to check that a particular reagent is giving the correct results and has not deteriorated or been prepared incorrectly.

Note: The quality control of urine reagent strip tests is described at the end of subunit 6.11.

QUALITY ASSURANCE: POST-ANALYTICAL STAGE OF CLINICAL CHEMISTRY TESTS

The post-analytical stage includes the reporting, checking (verifying), timeliness, and interpretation of test results and procedure to follow should a result be seriously abnormal or unexpected. Clinical chemistry test reports must include the following:

- Type of specimen analyzed, e.g. whole blood, serum, plasma, urine, c.s.f., faeces.
- Analyte (substance) measured.
- Test results clearly and informatively presented using SI units (with conversion factors to former units if needed).
- Reference range for quantitative tests.

Reports should have a standardized format and include as much information as possible to help those requesting tests to interpret the results correctly.

Laboratory staff must know the expected reference ranges for the tests they perform and the biological and laboratory factors that need to be considered when deciding the reference range for each test.

Note: Subunit 2.2 describes in detail the reporting, recording, and interpretation of test results, meaning and assessment of reference ranges, and what action needs to be taken when test results are seriously abnormal.

Chart 6.2 lists the reference ranges commonly given for clinical chemistry tests.

Chart 6.2 APPROXIMATE REFERENCE RANGES FOR CLINICAL CHEMISTRY TESTS

The reference ranges given in this publication have been compiled from accepted Western values and those received by the author from a small number of tropical countries. They should be used *only* as a guideline.

Test	SI units	Old units	Factor*	Notes
*To convert from SI units to old units, *multiply* by the factor. To convert from old units to SI units, *divide* by the factor.				
BLOOD TESTS				
Acid phosphatase	0–0.3 U/l	Expressed in King Armstrong units/100 ml		
Albumin	30–45 g/l	3.0–4.5 g/100 ml	0.1	Lower when lying down. Lower in infants.
Alkaline phosphatase	*Adults* 20–90 U/l	Expressed in King Armstrong units/100 ml		
	Children Up to 350 U/l			Rapidly growing children have highest values.
alpha Fetoprotein	<1.0 μg/l	<1.0 ng/ml	1	
alpha Amylase	70–340 U/l	Expressed in Caraway units per 100 ml	See 6.9	
Aspartate amino-transferase (AST)	Up to 42 U/l at 37 °C	Expressed in Reitman-Frankel units/ml		
Bicarbonate	23–31 mmol/l	23–31 mEq/l	1	
Bilirubin, total	*Adults* 3–21 μmol/l	0.2–1.3 mg/100 ml	0.06	
	Newborns 8–67 μmol/l	0.5–4.0 mg/100 ml	0.06	Highest values in first 3–5 days of life.
Calcium	*Adults* 2.25–2.60 mmol/l	9.0–10.4 mg/100 ml	4	Lower when lying down.
	Newborns 1.85–3.45 mmol/l	7.4–13.8 mg/100 ml	4	Values influenced by diet.
PCO_2	4.6–6.1 kPa	35–46 mmHg	7.5	SI units not often used.
Chloride	96–107 mmol/l	96–107 mEq/l	1	
Cholesterol	3.0–7.8 mmol/l	116–300 mg/100 ml	38.7	Influenced by age and diet. Female values slightly higher than those of males.
Cholinesterase	*Males* 2.60–5.53 U/l			Acylcholine acyl-hydrolase method.
	Females 1.93–4.60 U/l			

Test	SI units	Old units	Factor*	Notes

*To convert from SI units to old units, *multiply* by the factor.
 To convert from old units to SI units, *divide* by the factor.

Test	SI units	Old units	Factor*	Notes
Creatinine	*Males* 60–130 µmol/l	0.7–1.4 mg/100 ml	0.011	Lower in children depending on muscle mass.
	Females 40–110 µmol/l	0.4–1.2 mg/100 ml		
Glucose	*Adults* – fasting (plasma) 3.6–6.4 mmol/l	65–115 mg%	18	Whole blood values are about 15% lower than those of plasma.
	– random (plasma) 3.3–7.4 mmol/l	59–133 mg%	18	Capillary blood values are slightly higher than those of venous blood (post-prandial).
	Newborns 1.1–4.4 mmol/l	20–80 mg%	18	
	Children – fasting (plasma) 2.4–5.3 mmol/l	43–95 mg%	18	
Iron (serum)	11–27 µmol/l	61–150 µg/100 ml	5.58	Take sample at 09.00 h.
Iron binding capacity (TIBC)	41–74 µmol/l	229–413 µg/100 ml	5.58	Take sample at 09.00 h.
Lactate dehydrogenase(LDH)	120–365 U/l	Expressed in Karmen units/ml		
pH	7.36–7.42	7.36–7.42	1	
Phosphate, inorganic	*Adults* 0.8–1.5 mmol/l	2.5–4.7 mg/100 ml	3.1	
	Children 1.3–2.2 mmol/l	4.1–7.0 mg/100 ml	3.1	Highest value when fed on cows milk.
Potassium	*Adults* 3.6–5.0 mmol/l	3.6–5.0 mEq/l	1	
	Newborns 4.0–5.9 mmol/l	4.0–5.9 mEq/l	1	Highest levels immediately after birth.
Protein, total	60–81 g/l	6.0–8.1 g/100 ml	0.1	Lower when lying down.
Sodium	134–146 mmol/l	134–146 mEq/l	1	
Thyroxine (T$_4$)	60–145 nmol/l	4.7–11.2 µg/100 ml	0.077	
Triglycerides	*Fasting* 0.4–2.0 mmol/l	35–175 mg/100 ml	87.5	Take sample after 12–16 h fast.
Urate (Uric acid)	*Males* 206–460 µmol/l	3.5–7.8 mg/100 ml	0.017	
	Females 135–382 µmol/l	2.3–6.5 mg/100 ml	0.017	
	Children 60–290 µmol/l	1.0–4.9 mg/100 ml	0.017	
Urea	*Adults* 3.3–7.7 mmol/l	20–46 mg/100 ml	6.01	Values are higher in the elderly and slightly lower in females.
	Infants 1.3–5.8 mmol/l	8–35 mg/100 ml	6.01	

URINE TESTS

Amino acids	*Adults* 12–38.0 μmol/24 h	0.9–2.8 μg/24 h	0.075	As glycine
	Infants 2.0–36.5 μmol/24 h	0.1–2.7 μg/24 h		
delta Aminolaevulinic acid (ALA)	9.1–42.0 μmol/24 h	1.2–5.5 mg/24 h	0.13	
Calcium, total	1.6–7.0 mmol/24 h	65–280 mg/24 h	40	
Creatinine	7–16 mmol/24 h	0.8–1.8 g/24 h	0.113	Lower in children. Values depend on muscle mass.
3-Methoxy-4-hydroxy mandelic acid (HMMA) (VMA)	<50 μmol/24 h	<10 mg/24 h	0.198	
Protein	<0.15 g/24 h			

Note: There is great variation in the accepted range of reference values for urine tests.

CEREBROSPINAL FLUID TESTS

Glucose	2.5–4.0 mmol/l	45–72 mg/100 ml	18	c.s.f. (lumbar) glucose is usually 60–80% of blood glucose.
Protein	0.1–0.4 g/l	10–40 mg/100 ml	100	

6.3 Measurement of serum or plasma creatinine

Analyte: Creatinine is a nitrogenous waste product formed from the metabolism of creatine in skeletal muscle. Creatinine diffuses freely throughout the body water. It is filtered from the extracellular fluid by the kidney and excreted in the urine. The excretion of creatinine is mainly renal and in the absence of disease, relatively constant.

Value of test

Measurement of serum or plasma creatinine is an important test of kidney function. It is recommended in preference to the measurement of serum or plasma urea because it is a better indicator of overall renal function and progress in renal failure. Serum creatinine levels are less affected than urea levels by age, dehydration, and catabolic states, e.g. fever, sepsis, and internal bleeding. Creatinine levels are also less influenced by changes in diet such as low intake of protein (providing this is not prolonged).

Increasingly the measurement of serum creatinine is being used to investigate HIV associated renal disease and to monitor patients being treated with nephrotoxic antiretroviral drugs, e.g. tenofovir.

TEST SELECTION AND CALIBRATION

In district laboratories, the Jaffe-Slot modified alkaline picrate colorimetric method of measuring serum or plasma creatinine is recommended.[5] This reduces interference from non-creatinine substances, making the test more specific. A further modification made by Seaton and Ali eliminates the need for a precipitation stage.

Creatinine test kits

An end-point colorimetric creatinine test kit based on the Jaffe-Slot alkaline picrate method is available from Span Diagnostics, code 25921 (see Appendix 11). Using a test kit avoids the need for district laboratories to stock picric acid which can be a hazardous chemical (explosive if allowed to dry).

Principle of the Jaffe-Slot alkaline picrate creatinine method

Creatinine reacts with picric acid in an alkaline medium. The absorbance of the yellow-red colour produced is measured in a colorimeter using a blue-green filter 490nm (Ilford No. 603) or in a spectrophotometer at 490 nm wavelength.

A number of other compounds similarly react with picric acid giving artificially high results for creatinine if one simply measures the total yellow-red colour produced. A second reading is therefore made after making the solution acid. The colour produced by creatinine is quickly destroyed by acid whereas that given by non-creatinine chromogens is destroyed more slowly. By subtracting the second reading which is due to non-creatinine substances from the first reading (due to creatinine and non-creatinine substances), the colour produced by the true creatinine can be obtained.

Calibration
The creatinine method is calibrated from a solution of creatinine. This is prepared and diluted to make a series of standards as follows:

Stock creatinine standard, 10 mmol/l

1 Weigh accurately 0.113 g of anhydrous creatinine or 0.362 g of creatinine zinc hydrochloride. Transfer the chemical to a 100 ml volumetric flask.

2 Half fill the flask with 100 mmol/l hydrochloric acid (Reagent No. 34) and mix to dissolve the creatinine. Make up to the 100 ml mark with the hydrochloric acid reagent and mix well.

The creatinine concentration in the flask is 10 mmol/l (10 000 μmol/l).

3 Transfer the stock creatinine standard solution to a storage bottle. Label and store at 2–8 °C. The solution is stable for about 2 months.

Working creatinine standards, 100, 200, 300, 400, 500 μmol/l

1 Take five 100 ml volumetric flasks and number them 1 to 5. Pipette accurately into each flask as follows:

Flask	Stock creatinine, 10 mmol/l
1	1 ml
2	2 ml
3	3 ml
4	4 ml
5	5 ml

2 Make the contents of each flask up to the 100 ml mark with 1 g/l benzoic acid (Reagent No. 12) and mix well.

The concentration of creatinine in each standard is as follows:

Flask 1 = 100 μmol/l
2 = 200 μmol/l
3 = 300 μmol/l
4 = 400 μmol/l
5 = 500 μmol/l

3 Transfer each solution to a storage bottle, label, and store at 2–8 °C. The working standards are stable for about 2 months.

Preparation of creatinine calibration graph
1 Take *two sets* of six tubes and label each set 'B' (reagent blank) and 1 to 5.

Pipette 2 ml of freshly prepared creatinine working reagent (see *Reagents*) into each tube.
2 Add to each tube as follows:

Tube
B .... 0.2 ml (200 μl) acetic acid, 60% v/v
1 .... 0.2 ml standard, 100 μmol/l
2 .... 0.2 ml standard, 200 μmol/l
3 .... 0.2 ml standard, 300 μmol/l
4 .... 0.2 ml standard, 400 μmol/l
5 .... 0.2 ml standard, 500 μmol/l

3 Mix well the contents of each pair of tubes and continue as described in steps 4 to 8 of the creatinine test method.

4 Take a sheet of graph paper and plot the absorbance of each standard (vertical axis) against its concentration in μmol/l (horizontal axis), as described in subunit 4.10. A linear calibration should be obtained.

The useful working limit (linearity) of the Slot creatinine method is about 500 μmol/l.

Important: Check the calibration graph by measuring a control serum using the creatinine method. A new calibration graph should be prepared and checked against controls whenever stock reagents are renewed.

TEST METHOD

Reagents
– Sodium dodecyl sulphate,   Reagent No. 58
40 g/l (sodium lauryl sulphate)
– Phosphate borate buffer,   Reagent No. 46
pH 12.8
– Picric acid reagent   Reagent No. 51
– Acetic acid, 60% v/v   Reagent No. 2

The above reagents can be stored at room temperature (20–28 °C). Details of their shelf-life can be found under the preparation of each reagent.

Creatinine working reagent
Mix equal volumes of the sodium dodecyl sulphate

reagent, phosphate borate buffer, and picric acid reagent. Allow 2 ml of working reagent for each tube.

Note: The creatinine working reagent is not stable. Once prepared it can be used for one day only.

Specimen:

The method requires 0.4 ml (400 μl) of patient's fresh serum or plasma which must be free from haemolysis (see also chart 6.1 in subunit 6.2).

Method

1 Take *two sets* of four or more test tubes (depending on the number of tests) and label each set as follows:

    B .... – Reagent blank
    S .... – Standard, 200 μmol/l
    C .... – Control serum (see 6.2)
    1,2, etc ..... – Patients' tests

Two sets of tubes are required in this assay because one set is read after the addition of acid.

2 Pipette 2 ml of *freshly* prepared creatinine working reagent into each tube.

3 Add to each tube as follows:
    Tube
    B .... 0.2 ml (200 μl) distilled water
    S .... 0.2 ml standard, 200 μmol/l
    C .... 0.2 ml control serum
    1,2, etc ..... 0.2 ml patient's serum or plasma

4 Mix well the contents of each pair of tubes and leave at room temperature for 90 minutes.

5 Read the absorbances of one set of solutions in a colorimeter using a blue-green filter 490mm (e.g. Ilford No. 603) or in a spectrophotometer set at wavelength 490 nm. Zero the instrument with the blank solution in tube B.

    Note: For some colorimeters it may be necessary to use a modified cuvette holder to measure small volumes. No modification is required if using the Biochron CO 7000 colorimeter (see subunit 4.10).

6 Add 50 μl (0.05 ml) of 60% v/v acetic acid reagent to each of the second set of tubes and leave for 6 minutes.

7 Read the absorbances of the second set of solutions. Zero the colorimeter with the acidified blank solution in tube B (second set). Subtract the readings of the second set of tubes from the readings of the first set of tubes. This will give the absorbance of creatinine in the standard, control, and test solutions.

8 Calculate the concentration of creatinine in the control and patients' samples by:
  – Reading the values from the calibration graph providing the reading of the 200 μmol/l standard agrees with the calibration, or if not by:
  – Using the following formula:

$$\text{Creatinine } \mu\text{mol/l} = \frac{AT}{AS} \times 200$$

where AT = Absorbance of test(s) or control
       AS = Absorbance of 200 μmol/l standard

Creatinine results over 500 μmol/l

Repeat the assay using a 1 in 3 dilution of the patient's serum or plasma in distilled water. Multiply the result by 3.

9 Report the patients' results if the value of the control serum is acceptable.

Quality control
The principles of quality control in clinical chemistry are described in subunit 6.2.

TEST RESULTS

Approximate creatinine reference (normal) range

Males: 60–130 μmol/l (0.7–1.4 mg%)
Females: 40–110 μmol/l (0.4–1.2 mg%)

To convert μmol/l to mg%, multiply by 0.011.
To convert mg% to μmol/l, divide by 0.011.

Note: Reference values for serum or plasma creatinine are slightly lower in children. Values depend on muscle mass.

Interpretation of serum or plasma creatinine results

Increases

Any disease or condition that causes a fall in the glomerular filtration rate (GFR) will increase plasma creatinine levels. Because creatinine is so readily excreted, blood levels rise more slowly than do urea levels in renal disease with slight increases occurring when there is moderate renal damage.

Urinary creatinine clearance: Formerly GFR was assessed by measuring urinary creatinine clearance. This has now been largely replaced by measuring serum/plasma creatinine levels.

Summary of Creatinine Method

For detailed instructions, see text

Two sets of tubes are required.
- Pipette into each set of tubes as follows:

	BLANK B	STANDARD S	CONTROL C	TEST 1, 2, etc
Creatinine working reagent (fresh)	2 ml	2 ml	2 ml	2 ml
Distilled water	0.2 ml	–	–	–
Standard, 200 μmol/l	–	0.2 ml	–	–
Control serum	–	–	0.2 ml	–
Patient's serum or plasma	–	–	–	0.2 ml

- Mix well.

- Leave at room temperature for 90 minutes.

- READ ABSORBANCES OF FIRST SET OF TUBES, i.e. *Reading 1*

  Colorimeter: Blue-green filter 490mm, e.g. Ilford No. 603
  Spectrophotometer: 490 mm

- Zero instrument with blank solution in tube B (first set of tubes).

- Pipette into *second set of tubes:*

Acetic acid, 60% v/v	50 μl	50 μl	50 μl	50 μl

- Leave *second set of tubes* for 6 minutes.

- READ ABSORBANCES OF SECOND SET OF TUBES, i.e. *Reading 2*

  Colorimeter: Blue-green filter 490 nm, e.g. Ilford No. 603
  Spectrophotometer: 490 nm

- Zero instrument with blank solution in tube B (second set of tubes).

- Subtract *Reading 2* from *Reading 1.*

- Obtain values from calibration graph if the reading of the 200 μmol/l standard agrees with the calibration. If not, calculate the result as follows:

$$\text{Creatinine } \mu\text{mol/l} = \frac{\text{Absorbance of test or control}}{\text{Absorbance of 200 } \mu\text{mol/l standard}} \times 200$$

- Report patients' results if control value is acceptable.

$$200 \ \mu\text{l} = 0.2 \text{ ml}$$
$$50 \ \mu\text{l} = 0.05 \text{ ml}$$

Diseases that can cause renal failure with a reduced GFR include glomerulonephritis (inflammation of the kidney glomeruli), pyelonephritis (inflammation of the pelvis of the kidney), and renal tuberculosis.

Diseases causing obstruction of urine outflow may also lead to kidney failure, e.g. urethral structures, prostatic enlargement, cancer of the bladder, and urinary schistosomiasis.

Acute renal failure is often due to sudden reduced blood flow to the kidney occurring in haemorrhage, obstetrical and surgical emergencies, malaria, and septicaemia.

Non-renal causes of increased plasma creatinine levels include strenuous exercise and the effect of drugs such as salicylates. Falsely high serum/plasma creatinine levels can be due to large amounts of acetoacetate in specimens from patients with diabetic ketoacidosis. Other substances that can cause analytical interference resulting in raised creatinine levels include ascorbic acid and cephalosporin antibiotics.

Uraemia: Term used to describe the presence of excessive amounts of creatinine, urea, and other nitrogenous waste products in the blood, as occurs in renal failure. It causes nausea, vomiting, lethargy, and if untreated, coma and death. Burr cells can be seen in the peripheral blood film.

Decreases

Diseases associated with muscle wasting reduce the level of creatinine in the blood. In general, however, decreases in concentration are of little significance because serum or plasma creatinine levels are proportional to the muscle mass of an individual.

6.4 Measurement of serum or plasma urea

Analyte: Urea is the main waste product of protein breakdown. It is formed in the liver by the reactions of the Krebs urea cycle. Amino acids are deaminated (nitrogenous amine group is removed), releasing ammonia. The ammonia, which is toxic to the body, is detoxified by combining with carbon dioxide to form urea which passes into the circulation and is excreted by the kidneys. Not all the urea that is filtered by the glomeruli is excreted in the urine. Depending on a person's state of hydration, 40–70% of the urea is passively reabsorbed with water and returned to the blood. The rate of reabsorption is inversely related to the rate of urine flow. When the rate of urine flow is low, more urea is absorbed.

Value of test
As a test of renal function, the measurement of plasma urea is less useful than the measurement of plasma creatinine. Urea levels are affected by several factors including state of hydration and dietary intake. These factors have little affect on plasma creatinine levels. Whenever possible therefore, creatinine should be measured in preference to urea in the investigation and monitoring of renal function (see subunit 6.3).

TEST SELECTION AND CALIBRATION
The direct measurement of urea by the diacetyl monoxime method is recommended as a manual colorimetric technique in district laboratories.[6] The stock reagents have good stability at room temperature, but care must be taken when preparing and using the acid working colour reagent because it is *highly corrosive.*

Urea test kits
Very few test kits are available using the diacetyl monoxime method. An endpoint colorimetric test kit based on the diacetyl monoxime method is available from Span Diagnostics, code 25927 (see Appendix 11).

Other colorimetric (non-UV) manual test kits use the urease-Berthelot reaction. This uses the enzyme urease to hydrolyze urea at 37 °C. The ammonia produced reacts with alkaline hypochlorite and phenol in the presence of a catalyst to form indophenol which is measured at 570 nm. The reagents in most of these kits do not have sufficient stability to allow them to be used economically in most district laboratories.

Principle of the diacetyl monoxime urea method
Urea reacts with diacetyl monoxime at high temperature in an acid medium in the presence of cadmium ions and thiosemicarbazide. The absorbance of the red colour produced is measured in a colorimeter using a green filter 520 nm (Ilford No. 604) or in a spectrophotometer at 530 nm wavelength.

Calibration
The diacetyl monoxime urea method is calibrated from a solution of urea. This is prepared and diluted to make a series of standards as follows:

Stock urea standard, 125 mmol/l

1 Weigh accurately 0.75 g (750 mg) of pure urea. Transfer the chemical to a 100 ml volumetric flask.

2 Half fill the flask with 1 g/l benzoic acid (Reagent No. 12) and mix to dissolve the urea. Make up to the 100 ml mark with the benzoic acid reagent and mix well.

The urea concentration in the flask is 125 mmol/l.

3 Transfer the stock urea standard to a storage bottle, label, and store at 2–8 °C. The solution is stable for several months.

Working urea standards 2.5, 5, 10, 15, 20 mmol/l

1 Take five 50 ml volumetric flasks and number them 1 to 5. Pipette accurately into each flask as follows:

Flask	Stock urea, 125 mmol/l
1	1 ml
2	2 ml
3	4 ml
4	6 ml
5	8 ml

2 Make the contents of each flask up to the 50 ml mark with 1 g/l benzoic acid (Reagent No. 12) and mix well. The concentration of urea in each standard is as follows:

Flask	1 = 2.5 mmol/l
	2 = 5 mmol/l
	3 = 10 mmol/l
	4 = 15 mmol/l
	5 = 20 mmol/l

3 Transfer each standard solution to a storage bottle, label, and store at 2–8 °C. The working standards are stable for several months.

Preparation of urea calibration graph

1 Take six tubes and label them 'B' (reagent blank) and 1 to 5.

Pipette 4 ml of freshly prepared urea colour reagent (see *Reagents*) into each tube.

2 Add to each tube as follows:

Tube	
B	20 μl (0.02 ml) distilled water
1	20 μl standard, 2.5 mmol/l
2	20 μl standard, 5.0 mmol/l
3	20 μl standard, 10 mmol/l
4	20 μl standard, 15 mmol/l
5	20 μl standard, 20 mmol/l

3 Mix well and continue as described in steps 4 to 6 of the urea assay method.

4 Take a sheet of graph paper and plot the absorbance of each standard (vertical axis) against its concentration in mmol/l (horizontal axis), as described in subunit 4.10. A linear calibration should be obtained. The useful working limit (linearity) of the diacetyl monoxime urea method is about 20 mmol/l (120 mg%).

Important: Check the calibrated graph by measuring a control serum. A new calibration graph should be prepared and checked against controls whenever stock reagents are renewed.

TEST METHOD

Reagents

– Urea acid reagent   Reagent No. 68
– Diacetyl monoxime, 4 g/l   Reagent No. 21

The above reagents can be stored at room temperature (20–28 °C).

Urea colour reagent

Mix equal volumes of the urea acid reagent and diacetyl monoxime reagent. Allow 4 ml of colour reagent for each tube.

Note: The colour reagent is not stable. Once prepared it can be used for one day only. Handle it with care because it is *highly corrosive.*

Specimen

The method requires 20 μl (0.02 ml) of patient's serum or plasma. For details of urea stability in serum and plasma, see chart 6.1 in subunit 6.2.

Method

1 Take four or more tubes (depending on the number of tests) and label as follows:

B	– Reagent blank
S	– Standard, 10 mmol/l
C	– Control serum (see 6.2)
1, 2, etc.	– Patients' tests

2 Pipette 4 ml of freshly made urea colour reagent into each tube.

Caution: The colour reagent is highly corrosive, therefore *do not* mouth-pipette.

3 Add to each tube as follows:

Tube	
B	20 μl (0.02 ml) distilled water
S	20 μl standard, 10 mmol/l
C	20 μl control serum
1, 2, etc	20 μl patient's serum or plasma

4 Mix well the contents of each tube and incubate at 100 °C for 15 minutes, preferably in a heat-block set at 100 °C or if unavailable in a container of boiling water. Stopper each tube using a *loose* fitting cap or plastic stopper having a small hole through which the steam can escape.

Summary of Urea Method

For detailed instructions, see text

Pipette into tubes as follows:	BLANK B	STANDARD S	CONTROL C	TEST 1, 2, etc
Urea colour reagent (fresh)	4 ml	4 ml	4 ml	4 ml
Distilled water	20 μl	–	–	–
Standard, 10 mmol/l	–	20 μl	–	–
Control serum	–	–	20 μl	–
Patient's serum or plasma	–	–	–	20 μl

- Mix well.

- Incubate at 100 °C for *exactly* 15 minutes.

  Do not let water enter the tubes.

- Cool.

  Protect tubes from light.

- READ ABSORBANCES

  Colorimeter: Green filter 520 nm, e.g. Ilford No. 604
  Spectrophotometer: 530 nm

- Zero instrument with blank solution in tube B.

- Obtain values from the calibration graph if the reading of the 10 mmol/l standard agrees with the calibration. If not, calculate the results as follows:

$$\text{Urea mmol/l} = \frac{\text{Absorbance of test or control}}{\text{Absorbance of 10 mmol/l standard}} \times 10$$

- Report patients' results if control value is acceptable.

20 μl = 0.02 ml

5 Remove the tubes and cool the contents by placing the tubes in a container of cold water for about 5 minutes, making sure no water enters the tubes.

Important: Protect the tubes from direct light because the red compound is sensitive to light. When protected from light, the colour of the solution is stable for up to 1 hour.

6 Read the absorbances of the solutions in a colorimeter using a green filter 520 nm (e.g. Ilford No. 604) or in a spectrophotometer set at wavelength 530 nm. Zero the instrument with the blank solution in tube B.

7 Calculate the concentration of urea in the control and patients' samples by:

– Reading the values from the calibration graph providing the reading of the 10 mmol/l standard agrees with the calibration, or if not by

– Using the following formula:

$$\text{Urea mmol/l} = \frac{AT}{AS} \times 10$$

where: AT = Absorbance of test(s) or control
       AS = Absorbance of 10 mmol/l standard

Urea results over 20 mmol/l
Repeat the assay using a 1 in 2 dilution (or more if necessary) of the patient's serum or plasma in distilled water. Multiply the result by the dilution factor.

8 Report the patients' results if the value of the control serum is acceptable.

Quality control
The principles of quality control in clinical chemistry are described in subunit 6.2.

TEST RESULTS

Approximate urea reference (normal) range
Adults: 3.3–7.7 mmol/l (20–46 mg%)
Infants: 1.3–5.8 mmol/l (8–35 mg%)

To convert from mmol/l to mg%, multiply by 6.
To convert from mg% to mmol/l, divide by 6.

Note: Reference values for serum or plasma urea increase with age. Values are slightly lower in females and also in children.

Interpretation of serum or plasma urea results
Increases
A marked and prolonged increase in serum or plasma urea is indicative of damaged renal function. The causes of renal failure leading to increases in urea levels are the same as those described in subunit 6.3 under increases in serum or plasma creatinine.

Non-renal causes: Slight increases in urea (not more than three times the upper limit of the reference range) may occur when there is:
– Dehydration
– Diuretic therapy
– Gastrointestinal blood loss
– Any condition associated with increased protein breakdown such as pneumonia, malaria, meningitis, typhoid, major trauma, and surgical operations.

Decreases
Low urea levels may be found in:
– Pregnancy
– Malnutrition and AIDS
– Severe liver disease
– Water overload

6.5 Measurement of blood or plasma glucose

Analyte: Glucose provides the energy for life processes. It is the main end product of carbohydrate digestion. Oxidation of glucose by the glycolytic and tricarboxylic acid pathways provides the chemical energy needed for cellular activity. When not required for the body's immediate energy needs, glucose is converted to glycogen and stored in the liver and muscles (glycogenesis). When required to maintain the blood glucose level, liver glycogen is converted back to glucose (glycogenolysis). Muscle glycogen provides the glucose for muscular activity. Excess glucose is oxidized to fatty acids and stored as fat in the tissues. If needed, glucose can also be formed from fats and protein (gluconeogenesis). An increase in the breakdown of fats to provide energy, results in an increase in the production of ketones.

Insulin is the most important hormone that regulates the amount of glucose in the blood, the rate at which glucose is taken up by the tissues, and the conversion of glucose to glycogen. It is made and secreted by the beta-islet cells of the pancreas. Only insulin is capable of reducing the concentration of glucose in the blood.

Value of test
Plasma or blood glucose is measured mainly in the diagnosis and management of diabetes mellitus. Good control of blood glucose levels in diabetic

patients helps to prevent or delay the development of complications which may lead to premature disability or death from blindness, kidney failure, coronary thrombosis, stroke, bacterial infections (particularly mycobacterial and anaerobic infections), and fungal infections.

Diabetes mellitus

In diabetes mellitus there is an absolute or relative deficiency of insulin action and or insulin secretion. This causes a rise in blood glucose, depression of glucose metabolism in the tissues, an increase in glycogenolysis, and the stimulation of gluconeogenesis. Symptoms include excessive thirst, polyuria, pruritus, and often unexplained loss of weight. The disease, however, may be discovered accidentally (by a "routine" blood glucose test) or may be detected from the complications associated with untreated diabetes.

There are major geographical and ethnic differences in the prevalence of the different forms of diabetes mellitus in tropical countries. Distribution, prevalence and incidence are linked to genetic susceptibility and environmental factors. In many areas and populations, changes in lifestyles and diet associated with modernization and westernization are contributing to major increases in the prevalence and incidence of diabetes and linked disorders.

Different forms of diabetes mellitus based on the WHO clinical classification[7]

Diabetes mellitus is defined by the World Health Organization as a group of aetiologically different metabolic defects. It can be classified as follows:

- *Type 1 diabetes : formerly known as insulin-dependent diabetes (IDDM):*
  Insulin treatment is required to sustain life. There is an absolute insulin deficiency due to the immune destruction of pancreatic beta-cells possibly triggered in genetically susceptible persons by a viral infection (e.g. congenital rubella), consumption of cows milk early in life, or possibly by chemical toxins. The onset of type 1 diabetes is abrupt with severe symptoms, often including ketosis. Type 1 diabetes is the commonest form of diabetes among children and young adults in European countries but has a low prevalence in tropical countries.

- *Type 2 diabetes : formerly known as non-insulin dependent diabetes (NIDDM):*
  Individual or ethnic genetic factors lead to susceptibility. There is some secretion of insulin but a decrease in insulin action (insulin resistance). Several factors are associated with the development of type 2 diabetes in susceptible individuals. These include dietary changes, overnutrition with increased intake of saturated fats and decreased intake of dietary fibre, obesity, physical inactivity, and ageing. There is often arterial hypertension and dyslipidaemia. Some drugs and hormones can also cause glucose intolerance and diabetes.
  Type 2 diabetes has high prevalence rates in some

populations in developing countries, e.g. migrant Asian Indians, Polynesians, Melanesians, Mauritians and Creoles. It is the commonest form of diabetes also in developed countries. In general, prevalence rates are lower, but rapidly increasing, in much of tropical Africa, Latin America, and Asia, where traditional lifestyles are followed.

- *Malnutrition-related diabetes mellitus (MRDM):*
  MRDM is a controversial entity, and current WHO classifications of diabetes[7] does not include MRDM. It is also known as 'tropical pancreatic diabetes', and is seen in localized areas throughout tropical countries. It is related to pancreatic damage and is characterized by young age of onset and past or present malnutrition. Steatorrhoea may occur due to exocrine pancreatic deficiency. Pancreatic calcification can occur in some cases. The cause is unknown; toxicity from the cyanide content of the root crop cassava has been suggested but not definitely substantiated.

- *Gestational diabetes mellitus (GDM):*
  This is defined as diabetes first recognized in pregnancy. Glucose values often return to normal postpartum but glucose intolerance and type 2 diabetes may occur later in life.

- *Other forms of diabetes:*
  These rarer forms can be found with pancreatic disease, some hormonal diseases and genetic syndromes, abnormalities of insulin or its receptors, and as a result of treatment with certain drugs or exposure to certain chemical toxins.

Measuring plasma or blood glucose in district laboratories

Methods include:

- Measuring glucose in capillary blood using a reagent test strip and glucose meter. This method provides a rapid result and is appropriate for health centres and small district laboratories where the numbers of glucose tests required are low. Inexpensive, simple to use reliable blood glucose meters are widely available.

- Measuring glucose in plasma using a glucose-oxidase colorimetric test method. This method is appropriate when the number of glucose tests makes it more cost-effective to use a colorimetric method, staff are trained in clinical chemistry techniques, and the standards, controls, and reagents needed for the colorimetric assay are available locally or provided by the district's clinical chemistry reference laboratory.

Important: Blood glucose measurements must be carried out on the day and at the time requested. Collection times are usually related to food intake, insulin treatment, or both. Provision must be made for urgent glucose tests which may be necessary outside the normal working hours of the laboratory.

Terms used to describe the collection of blood glucose specimens

Fasting specimen: This refers to blood collected after a period of no food intake. For adults the fasting time is usually 10 to 16 hours. For children the fasting time is 6 hours unless a longer time is indicated, e.g. when investigating hypoglycaemia. The drinking of plain water is permitted.

Post-prandial specimen: This describes blood collected after a meal has been taken. The sample is usually taken as a 2 h postprandial specimen.

Random specimen: This refers to a blood sample collected at any time, regardless of food intake.

BLOOD GLUCOSE METERS

A wide range of portable electronic blood glucose meters is available. Most are designed for home use by diabetic patients and to obtain test results quickly in clinics and point-of-care testing situations. The meters are therefore small and battery-operated, require only a small volume of blood, are easy to operate, and provide blood glucose values usually within 30 seconds. Some meters have automatic downloading and a memory facility. Blood glucose is measured electrochemically using electrode biosensor technology or photometrically by reflectance. Electrochemical meters use sensor test strips and reflectance metes use glucose-oxidase peroxide or glucose-dehydrogenase reacting test strips. *Strips are not interchangeable between meters.* Capillary blood, EDTA or heparinised venous blood can be used. Fluoride preserved blood is not suitable.

Most modern blood glucose meters have good accuracy and precision providing the manufacture's instructions are followed exactly as regards use and operational limits. Test results can be affected when the amount of blood used is either insufficient or too much. Measurement of blood glucose using a glucose meter may be affected when a blood specimen is lipaemic. Haematocrit values may also affect the accuracy of results.

Screening neonates for hypoglycaemia
When intending to use a glucose meter to screen newborns for hypoglycaemia, staff must ensure that the meter is capable of reading low glucose values accurately. Overestimation of a blood glucose concentration may lead to a newborn with significant hypoglycaemia not being treated.

Selecting and using a blood glucose meter
The following are important considerations when selecting a blood glucose meter:

- Are the test strips available locally and at an affordable price? How sensitive are they to high temperatures?

- How easy is it to obtain the batteries needed to operate the meter? Some meters are powered by AAA batteries while others use a button J type battery, e.g. 3V CR2032.

- Can the system be controlled adequately, e.g. are glucose control solutions available?

*Accu-Chek Advantage meter**
* Known in some countries as *Accu-Chek Sensor*

Accu-Chek Advantage is an example of an amperometric biosensor meter which measures glucose electrochemically using *Accu-Chek Advantage 11* test strips.

Test strip reaction
Glucose in the blood sample is oxidized in the reactive zone of the strip to gluconolactone. During this reaction, oxidized hexacyanoferrate 111 is reduced to hexacyanoferrate 11. A voltage is applied between the two palladium electrodes contained in the strip. This leads to the hexacyanoferrate 11 being reoxidized to hexacyanoferrate 111 with release of electrons. The small electric current that is generated is measured by the meter and converted into a glucose concentration reading.

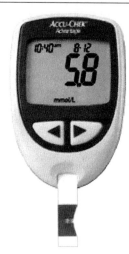

Plate 6.2 *Accu-Chek Advantage* meter for use with *Accu-Chek Advantage 11* test strips.
Courtesy of Roche Diagnostics.

Inserting a strip in the meter, turns on the meter. Blood is applied to the side of the strip which is curved to fit the shape of the finger. This not only makes it easy for the small drop of blood (about 4µl) to be drawn into the strip but also avoids any blood contaminating the meter. Capillary blood, venous blood (using EDTA, heparin, but not fluoride oxalate), cord blood, neonate and arterial blood can be used. Results are digitally displayed after 26 seconds. The meter measures within the glucose range 0.56–33.3 mmol/1 (10–600 mg/dl). A memory facility enables 480 test readings to be stored. The meter operates reliably between a temperature range of 14–40 °C and relative humidity below 85%.

The *Accu-Chek Advantage* is powered from one CR2032 or DL2032 3 volt lithium button battery. To conserve the life of the battery the meter automatically turns off after 90 seconds of non-use or 5 seconds after taking a strip out of the meter following a test. The display incorporates a low battery symbol indicator.

Calibration and quality control of Accu-Chek Advantage

The *Accu-Chek Advantage* meter requires calibration each time a new batch of strips is used. This is performed automatically by using the lot-specific code key included with each vial of test strips. The key is inserted in the back of the meter and the code number is displayed which is the same as that shown on each test strip of the batch.

To ensure that the meter is performing reliably it is necessary to perform a quality control check using *Accu-Chek Advantage 11 Glucose Control Solution* (Level 1 and Level 2). Once opened the glucose solutions are stable for up to 3 months. When the control test results are within the correct range, the meter reads "OK". Test strips must be kept tightly stoppered and protected from moisture and high temperatures. They should be stored at room temperature and not refrigerated. A desiccant is enclosed with the strips to maintain a dry environment. Test strips must not be used beyond their expiry date. Only *Accu-Chek Advantage 11* strips must be used with the meter.

Limitations of Accu-Chek Advantage

Falsely elevated glucose results may be obtained when a person's blood contains bilirubin (unconjugated) >340 μmol/l (>20 mg/dl), triglycerides >57 mmol/l, galactose >0.56 mmol/l or maltose >0.47 mmol/l. Abnormal uric acid levels may also interfere with test results. Caution is needed in the interpretation of neonate blood glucose values <2.8 mmol/l (<50 mg/dl).

Abnormal haematocrit values may affect test results. *Accu-Chek Advantage* operates reliably within haematocrit ranges 0.20–0.65 (20–65%) for glucose values, <11.1 mmol/l (<200 mg/dl) and 0.20–0.55 (20–55%) for glucose values >11.1 mmo/1 (>200 mg/dl). Haematocrit levels below 0.20 may cause falsely low glucose values when the glucose concentration is less than or equal to 11.1 mmol/l. Values above 0.55 may cause falsely low glucose values when the glucose is above 11.1 mmol/l.

Availability: *Accu-Chek Advantage* meter, *Accu-Chek Advantage 11* test strips, *Accu-Chek Advantage 11 Glucose Control Solutions* are manufactured by Roche Diagnostics (see Appendix 11). Test strips are available in vials containing 10 or 50 test strips. Each meter is supplied with a well written and illustrated User Manual. The meter measures $84 \times 56 \times 20$ mm and weighs 57 g.

Glucose meters that also measure cholesterol

Roche Diagnostics also manufactures meters that measure both glucose and cholesterol. The *Accutrend GC* measures glucose (1.1–33.3 mmol/l) using *Accutrend Glucose* strips, and cholesterol (3.88–7.76 mmol/l) using *Accutrend Cholesterol* strips. The *Accutrend GCT* meter measures both glucose and cholesterol (using the same strips as for *Accutrend GC*) and also triglycerides (0.8–6.86 mmol/l) using *Accutrend Triglycerides* strips. Both meters measure by reflectance photometry, operate from 3×1.5 V batteries, type micro LR 03 (AAA), measure $115 \times 62 \times 185$ mm and weigh 90g (without batteries). Further details can be obtained from Roche Diagnostics (see Appendix 11).

Interpretation of test results

The approximate reference range for blood glucose and the reasons for increased and decreased values can be found at the end of this subunit.

Betachek **visually read glucose strips**

Betachek Visual test strips enable glucose to be measured semi-quantitatively over the range 0.55 mmol/l (9 mg/dl) to 55 mmol/l (991 mg/dl). A drop of blood is placed on the strip and allowed to react for 30 seconds. The blood is then wiped from the strip and the colour matched after a further 30 seconds with the pink and blue colour chart provided. Colour matching is facilitated by the twin pad technology and the small increments used in the colour chart. *Betachek Visual* is manufactured by and available from National Diagnostic Products Pty Ltd (see Appendix 11).

COLORIMETRIC GLUCOSE METHOD

The glucose-oxidase enzymatic method is recommended because it is specific for glucose.[8] A protein precipitation stage is included because this removes substances such as urate which may be present in blood samples in sufficient concentration to interfere in the final stage of the reaction.

Other methods: The *o*-toluidine colorimetric method should be avoided because the reagent is highly corrosive and toxic, and the chemical *o*-toluidine is carcinogenic. Copper and ferricyanide blood glucose reduction methods are not recommended because they are not sufficiently selective for glucose.

Principle of glucose oxidase-peroxidase method

Glucose oxidase (GOD) catalyzes the oxidation of glucose to give hydrogen peroxide (H_2O_2) and gluconic acid. In the presence of the enzyme peroxidase (POD), the hydrogen peroxide is broken down and the oxygen released reacts with 4-aminophenazone (4-aminoantipyrine) and phenol to give a pink colour.

The absorbance of the colour produced is measured in a colorimeter using a green filter 520 nm (Ilford No. 604) or in a spectrophotometer at 515 nm.

Calibration

The glucose oxidase method is calibrated from a solution of glucose. This is prepared and diluted to make a series of standards as follows:

Stock glucose standard, 100 mmol/l

1   Weigh accurately 1.8 g of dry anhydrous glucose (analytical reagent grade).

    Note: To ensure the glucose is dry, heat it in an open container in an oven at 60–80 °C for about 4 hours. Remove and close the container immediately. When cool, weigh the glucose.

2   Transfer the glucose to a 100 ml volumetric flask. Half fill the flask with 1 g/l benzoic acid (Reagent No. 12) and mix until the glucose is fully dissolved. Make up to the 100 ml mark with the benzoic acid reagent and mix well.

    The glucose concentration in the flask is 100 mmol/l.

3   Transfer to a storage bottle and label. When stored at 2–8 °C the stock standard is stable for about 6 months. If stored frozen in tightly stoppered containers the stock standard is stable for at least 1 year.

Working glucose standards 2.5, 5, 10, 20, 25 mmol/l

1   Take five 100 ml volumetric flasks and number them 1 to 5. Pipette accurately into each flask as follows:

Flask	*Stock glucose, 100 mmol/l*
1	2.5 ml
2	5.0 ml
3	10.0 ml
4	20.0 ml
5	25.0 ml

2   Make the contents of each flask up to the 100 ml mark with 1 g/l benzoic acid (Reagent No. 12) and mix well.

The concentration of glucose in each standard is as follows:

Flask		
1	=	2.5 mmol/l
2	=	5.0 mmol/l
3	=	10.0 mmol/l
4	=	20.0 mmol/l
5	=	25.0 mmol/l

3   Transfer each solution to a storage bottle and label. Store at room temperature (20–28 °C). The working standards are stable for about 2 months.

Preparation of glucose calibration graph

1   Take six tubes and label them 'B' (reagent blank) and 1 to 5. Pipette 1.5 ml of protein precipitant reagent into each tube.

    Note: The use of the protein precipitant reagent is required because it forms part of the buffer system and contains phenol which is needed for the colour reaction.

2   Add to each tube as follows:

    Tube
    B .... 50 µl (0.05 ml) distilled water
    1 .... 50 µl standard, 2.5 mmol/l
    2 .... 50 µl standard, 5 mmol/l
    3 .... 50 µl standard, 10 mmol/l
    4 .... 50 µl standard, 20 mmol/l
    5 .... 50 µl standard, 25 mmol/l

3   Continue as described in steps 5 to 7 of the glucose method.

4   Take a sheet of graph paper and plot the absorbance of each standard (vertical axis) against its concentration in mmol/l (horizontal axis) as described in 4.10. A linear calibration should be obtained.

    The useful working limit (linearity) of the glucose oxidase method is about 25 mmol/l.

Important: Check the calibration graph by measuring a control serum. A new calibration graph should be prepared and checked against controls whenever stock reagents are renewed.

TEST METHOD

Reagents

– Protein precipitant reagent   Reagent No. 53
– Colour reagent   Reagent No. 19

The protein precipitant reagent can be stored at room temperature (20–28 °C). It is stable indefinitely. The colour reagent requires storage at 2–8 °C. When refrigerated it has a shelf-life of about 3 months.

Specimen

The method requires 50 μl (0.05 ml) of patient's plasma from a fluoride-oxalate specimen. Serum can also be used providing the assay is carried out within 30 minutes of collecting the blood (without fluoride preservative the glucose is rapidly broken down by glycolysis). See previous text for an explanation of random and fasting blood samples.

Note: The collection of blood for glucose tolerance tests is described at the end of this subunit.

Measuring c.s.f. glucose: The glucose oxidase method described in this subunit can also be used for measuring glucose in cerebrospinal fluid (see step 3).

Method

1 Take four or more tubes (depending on the number of tests) and label as follows:
    B   – Reagent bank
    S   – Standard, 10.0 mmol/l
    C   – Control serum (see 6.2)
    1, 2, etc   – Patients' tests

2 Pipette 1.5 ml of protein precipitant reagent into each tube.

3 Add to each tube as follows:
    Tube
    B .... 50 μl (0.05 ml) distilled water
    S .... 50 μl standard, 10 mmol/l
    C .... 50 μl control serum
    1, 2, etc .... 50 μl patient's plasma
    Mix well.

    Important: If a glucose request is urgent because a patient is thought to be in a hypoglycaemic (low glucose) coma, to avoid any possible delay set up an additional tube containing 100μl of plasma (divide the result by two).

    Measurement of glucose in cerebrospinal fluid (c.s.f.):

    Use 0.2 ml (200 μl) of c.s.f. and divide the result by four (a fasting lumbar c.s.f. glucose is normally 40–80% of the blood glucose). The glucose concentration will be lower when the c.s.f. contains bacteria and cells.

4 Centrifuge the control and patients' samples (tubes C, 1, 2, etc) for 3–5 minutes at medium to high speed to obtain clear supernatant fluids.

5 Transfer 0.5 ml from the blank, standard, control, and patients' samples to a second set of tubes (labelled as in step 1).

6 Add 1.5 ml of colour reagent to each tube and *mix well.*

    Incubate at 37 °C in a heat-block or water bath for 10 minutes. Shake occasionally to ensure adequate aeration of the samples.

7 Read the absorbances of the solutions in a col-orimeter using a green filter 520 nm (e.g. Ilford No. 604) or in a spectrophotometer set at wavelength 515 nm. Zero the instrument with the blank solution in tube B.

Note: For some colorimeters it may be necessary to use a modified cuvette holder to measure small volumes. No modification is required if using the Biochrom CO 7000 Colorimeter (see subunit 4.10).

8 Calculate the concentration of glucose in the control and patients' samples by:

    – Reading the values from the calibration graph providing the result of the 10 mmol/l standard agrees with the calibration or if not by

    – Using the following formula:

    $$\text{Glucose mmol/l} = \frac{AT}{AS} \times 10.0$$

    where: AT = Absorbance of test(s) or control
                AS = Absorbance of 10 mmol/l standard

Glucose results below 2.2 mmol/l
Repeat the assay using 0.1 ml (100 μl) of patient's plasma. Multiply the result by two.

Glucose results over 25.0 mmol/l
Repeat the assay after diluting the plasma 1 in 2, i.e. mix 50 μl plasma with 50 μl distilled water and use 50 μl of this diluted sample in the test.

9 Report the patients' results if the value of the control serum is acceptable.

Quality control

The principles of quality control in clinical chemistry are described in subunit 6.2.

TEST RESULTS
Approximate glucose reference (normal) range
Adults
– Fasting (plasma) 3.6–6.4 mmol/l (see *Note*)
– Random (plasma) 3.3–7.4 mmol/l (see *Note*)
Children
– Fasting (plasma) 2.4–5.3 mmol/l (see *Note*)
    Newborn values are slightly lower, i.e. 1.1–4.4 mmol/l

To convert from mmol/l to mg%, multiply by 18.

To convert from mg% to mmol/l, divide by 18.

Note: In current practice, reference ranges have little real use. Plasma glucose results are now compared to definitive numerical criteria as detailed below (see *Interpretation of results*).

Venous plasma values are about 15% higher than whole blood values (except in anaemia).

There is little difference between values obtained from venous plasma and capillary plasma when the glucose concentration is normal. When the glucose is raised however, the value obtained from capillary plasma will be slightly higher than that from venous plasma.

Interpretation of blood glucose results

Increases

A raised blood glucose level is called hyperglycaemia. When definite it is diagnostic of diabetes mellitus (see previous text). In an adult with symptoms of diabetes mellitus, a random venous plasma glucose of 11.1 mmol/l or more on two occasions or a fasting value of 7.0 mmol/l or more on two occasions is diagnostic.

VALUES DIAGNOSTIC OF DIABETES MELLITUS

	Fasting	Random
Plasma	mmol/l	mmol/l
Venous:	≥7.0 (126 mg%)	≥11.1 (200 mg%)
Capillary:	≥7.0 (126 mg%)	≥12.2 (220 mg%)
Whole blood		
Venous:	≥6.1 (110 mg%)	≥10.0 (180 mg%)
Capillary:	≥6.1 (110 mg%)	≥11.1 (200 mg%)

Note: The above are adult values obtained on two separate occasions.

Other causes of raised glucose levels:

Hyperglycaemia may accompany pancreatic disease and some endocrine disorders such as thyrotoxicosis and Cushings syndrome. Steroid therapy may also cause hyperglycaemia. Transient hyperglycaemia often occurs following severe stress, e.g. after surgery, injury, shock, infections, or severe burns.

These are essentially forms of transient diabetes (e.g. "stress diabetes", "steroid diabetes"). However, it is now recognized that a number of these patients may have pre-existing type 2 diabetes, therefore it is important to check that hyperglycaemia does resolve when the intercurrent illness resolves or steroid treatment is withdrawn.

Decreases

A low blood glucose level is called hypoglycaemia. Persistent occurrences of hypoglycaemia with glucose levels less than 2.2 mmol/l accompanied by symptoms such as fainting, fits, sweating, hunger, pallor, confusion, or violence, should be investigated.

Causes of hypoglycaemia include severe malnutrition, kwashiorkor, severe liver disease, alcoholic excess, insulin secreting tumours, Addison's disease, and certain drugs. Commonly, however, markedly reduced blood glucose levels occur following the overtreatment of diabetes.

Neonatal hypoglycaemia: Newborn infants may suffer hypoglycaemia when blood glucose levels fall below 1.1 mmol/l. Infants particularly at risk are underweight poorly nourished babies, twins, premature infants, and babies born of diabetic mothers. It is important to detect hypoglycaemia of the newborn because without treatment brain damage may occur.

Malaria associated hypoglycaemia: In severe malaria, hypoglycaemia is a common finding and can increase mortality particularly in young children. Hypoglycaemia can also occur in those being treated with quinine and quinidine.

False glucose values

A falsely high glucose level will result if a blood sample is collected from an arm receiving a glucose (dextrose) intravenous (i.v.) infusion. A falsely low value may be obtained if the plasma is markedly icteric.

GLUCOSE TOLERANCE TEST (GTT)

Glucose tolerance: A GTT measures the ability of the body to tolerate, or cope with, a standard dose of glucose. The degree of tolerance to the glucose, as shown by a change in the blood level, is mainly dependent on the rate of glucose absorption and on the insulin response. As the glucose is absorbed, the level of glucose in the blood rises and the normal response is for insulin to be released from the pancreas to lower the glucose level. Tolerance is reduced when insulin is insufficient or absent.

A glucose tolerance test (GTT) is usually requested to investigate glycosuria or when a random or fasting blood glucose is suggestive but not diagnostic of diabetes. It happens only rarely however that the result of a fasting or random blood glucose is difficult to interpret and a GTT is necessary. If glycosuria is found, measurement of fasting glucose should be performed before the patient is subjected to a GTT. A GTT should not be necessary in children.

Preparation of the patient
– Before the test the patient should be on a diet containing not less than 150 g of carbohydrate per day for at least 3 days. If the GTT is performed following starvation or a diet low in carbohydrate, glucose tolerance will be reduced which will make the results of the test difficult to interpret.
– Ideally the test should be performed in the morning. The patient should be instructed not to

Summary of Glucose Method

For detailed instructions, see text

• Pipette into tubes as follows:	BLANK B	STANDARD S	CONTROL C	TEST 1, 2, etc
Protein precipitant reagent	1.5 ml	1.5 ml	1.5 ml	1.5 ml
Distilled water	50 μl	–	–	–
Standard, 10.0 mmol/l	–	50 μl	–	–
Control serum	–	–	50 μl	–
Patient's plasma	–	–	–	50 μl

- Mix well.

- Centrifuge tubes C, and tests 1, 2, etc to obtain clear supernatant fluids.

- Take a second set of tubes and label B, S, C, 1, 2, etc.

• Transfer from first to second set of tubes	0.5 ml	0.5 ml	0.5 ml	0.5 ml
• Add colour reagent to second set of tubes	1.5 ml	1.5 ml	1.5 ml	1.5 ml

- Mix well.

- Incubate at 37 °C for 10 minutes. Shake occasionally.

- READ ABSORBANCES

  Colorimeter: Green filter 520 nm, e.g. Ilford No. 604
  Spectrophotometer: 515 nm

- Zero instrument with blank solution in tube B.

- Obtain values from the calibration graph if the result of 10 mmol/l standard agrees with calibration. If not, calculate the results as follows:

$$\text{Glucose mmol/l} = \frac{\text{Absorbance of test or control}}{\text{Absorbance of 10.0 mmol/l standard}} \times 10$$

- Report patients' results if control value is acceptable.

50 μl = 0.05 ml

eat, drink (except plain water), or smoke for 10–16 hours before the test.

- Patients should be reassured if anxious. Outpatients should be allowed to rest for about 20 minutes before starting the test especially if they have had to walk a considerable distance to reach the hospital. Excessive exercise, excitement, or fear may reduce glucose tolerance.

- During the test the patient should, if possible, be sitting up. If lying down the patient should be positioned on the right side to ensure rapid emptying of the stomach.

- Ideally the patient should have no other disease at the time a glucose test is performed. A note should be made of any drug treatments.

Method of performing a glucose tolerance test

1 Prepare a GTT chart for the patient on which to record collection times and test results.

2 Collect a fasting venous blood sample into a bottle or tube containing fluoride-oxalate. Label the container 'fasting blood'.

3 Give the patient 75 g of glucose (D-glucose monohydrate) in 250–300 ml water, to be drunk in 5 to 15 minutes. To reduce nausea a few drops of lemon juice may be added to the water.

4 Make a note of the time and enter on the GTT chart the time at which the next blood sample is to be collected, i.e. 2 hours after the glucose water has been drunk.

Collection times

Formerly blood samples were collected at 30 minute intervals but studies have shown that it is the fasting and 2 hour post glucose samples that are of major diagnostic value.

5 Instruct the patient to rest quietly and not to eat, drink, exercise, smoke, or leave the hospital during the test. Inform the patient when the test will be completed.

Important: If the patient should feel faint, very nauseated or begin to perspire excessively, call a medical officer.

6 Collect the second blood sample at the correct time, labelling the container with the collection time.

7 Measure the glucose concentration in each of the blood specimens.

8 Enter the patient's results on the GTT chart if the value of the control serum is acceptable.

Collection times	Plasma glucose results
Fasting	.... mmol/l
2 hours*	.... mmol/l

*After drinking the glucose water

Interpretation of GTT

The following diagnostic criteria (WHO) are for venous plasma glucose results:

Diabetic	Fasting	≥7.0 mmol/l
	2 hour specimen	≥11.1 mmol/l
Impaired glucose tolerance	Fasting	<7.0 mmol/l
	2 hour specimen	7.8–11.1 mmol/l

Note: For asymptomatic patients, two abnormal values (either fasting plasma glucose >7.0 mmol/l, or random plasma glucose >11.1mmol/l) are needed to establish a diagnosis of diabetes mellitus.

Glycated haemoglobin in monitoring blood glucose control in diabetes

Red cells normally contain some haemoglobin A in glycated form, i.e. attached to a glucose residue. Glycated (glycosylated) haemoglobin A is referred to as HbA_1. The main glycated fraction is HbA_{1c} (forms about 5% of circulating Hb). HbA_{1c} is specifically glycated by glucose. The glucose remains complexed to the haemoglobin molecule for the lifetime of the red cell and therefore the concentration of glycated haemoglobin circulating in red cells is a guide to the average blood glucose level over a period of the previous 8–12 weeks (lifespan of red cells).

Measurement of the glycated haemoglobin can help in assessing the control of diabetic patients, particularly patients with type 2 diabetes whose blood glucose levels do not change markedly. The test does not detect swings from high to low blood glucose levels, as it reflects an average of preceding glycaemia. Nevertheless, HbA_{1c} levels are closely related to the risk of complication development in diabetes. Levels of 7.0% or below are ideal, though these are often hard to achieve.

Microchromatographic and ion-exchange resin colorimetric methods for measuring glycated haemoglobin are available but expensive. HbA_{1c} results are expressed as a percentage of total Hb. In poorly controlled diabetes the level of HbA_{1c} may be greatly increased. Reference ranges are assay specific and to some extent are not relevant to the clinical situation, as "target levels" (based on previous clinical research) are of more use. With some assays, the presence of abnormal haemoglobins such as Hb S, C, D and increased levels of HbF can affect test results.

Glycosal Hb_{1c} *meter*

Glycosal is a compact portable meter that uses boronate affinity chromatography to measure Hb_{1c}. The test takes about 5 minutes to perform. It is unaffected by the presence of haemoglobin variants.

All the reagents needed to perform the test are contained in a circular disposable cartridge which fits in the meter. The test is easy to perform with the meter display indicating when to rotate the cartridge, add the 10µl capillary blood sample, and react it with the reagents in the central reaction well of the cartridge. HbA_{1c} is displayed as a percentage. The measuring range of the meter is 3–18% Hb_{1c}.

In a field study in northern Ethiopia, the *Glycosal* meter performed well and retained accuracy at high ambient temperature.[9] Although costly, the test offers the possibility of improved glycaemic control which is likely to reduce the costs involved in treating diabetic complications.[9] The *Glycosal* meter measures 200×110 mm and is available from Provalis Diagnostics (see Appendix 11).

Further reading: *Africa Health* special feature on care and management of diabetes in Africa, March, 2004, pp 9–16. Also, WHO booklet, *Laboratory diagnosis and monitoring of diabetes mellitus*, 2002, pages 27. This is a free of charge booklet, Order No 18503736. Can also be downloaded from WHO website www.who.int as a pdf file.

6.6 Measurement of serum or plasma bilirubin

Analyte: Bilirubin is formed from the breakdown of erythrocytes and other haem-containing proteins such as myoglobin and cytochromes. The haem (iron porphyrin) of the haemoglobin molecule is separated from the globin and the haem is converted mainly in the spleen to biliverdin which is reduced to bilirubin. This bilirubin is referred to as *unconjugated (indirect) bilirubin*. It is not soluble in water and cannot be excreted in the urine. It is bound to albumin and transported in the blood to the liver. In the liver cells, the enzyme glucuronosyltransferase joins (conjugates) glucuronic acid to bilirubin forming bilirubin glucuronides (mainly diglucuronides). This bilirubin is referred to as *conjugated (direct) bilirubin*. It is water-soluble.

Conjugated bilirubin passes into the bile canaliculi, through the bile duct and into the intestine. In the terminal ileum and colon, the bilirubin is deconjugated and reduced by bacteria to various pigments and colourless chromogens (urobilinogen) most of which are excreted in the faeces as stercobilinogen. Some of the bilirubin and urobilinogen from the intestine is reabsorbed into the portal circulation and reaches the liver where it re-enters the intestine in the bile and is excreted in the faeces.

A small amount of reabsorbed urobilinogen is carried in the blood through the liver and transported to the kidneys where it is excreted in the urine. When exposed to air urobilinogen is rapidly oxidized to the brown coloured pigment urobilin (and stercobilinogen to stercobilin).

Note: In a healthy individual about 5% of the total plasma bilirubin is conjugated and 95% or more, unconjugated. Urine contains a trace of urobilinogen and no bilirubin.

Value of test

The measurement of serum or plasma bilirubin is usually performed to investigate the causes of liver disease and jaundice, and to monitor a patient's progress, e.g. an infant with serious neonatal jaundice (high levels of unconjugated bilirubin).

Common causes of liver disease in tropical countries

- Hepatitis due to hepatitis viruses and less frequently to other viruses (e.g. yellow fever virus, Marburg and Ebola viruses, Epstein-Barr virus, cytomegalovirus), bacteria such as *Leptospira interrogans*, parasites including *Toxoplasma gondii*, and certain drugs and toxins.

- Cirrhosis caused by alcohol and dietary toxins. The ingestion of alkaloid toxins in 'bush teas' is a cause of veno-occlusive disease (narrowing of central and sublobular hepatic veins) in the West Indies, parts of Africa and the Middle East. An excess of hepatic copper is linked to infantile cirrhosis in India.

- Hepatoma, especially in areas where there is a high incidence of viral hepatitis.

- Parasitic diseases, especially visceral leishmaniasis, hepatic amoebiasis, hepatosplenic schistosomiasis, hepatic hydatid disease, repeated infection with malaria parasites, and severe infections with *Opisthorchis* and *Fasciola* species.

Liver disorders are often associated with jaundice (icterus). Visible jaundice occurs when the concentration of bilirubin in the plasma rises to more than twice its normal limit, i.e. about 34 μmol/l (2 mg%). The whites of the eyes appear yellow and the skin and body fluids also become pigmented.

Types of jaundice

Haemolytic jaundice
In haemolytic (prehepatic) jaundice, more bilirubin is produced than the liver can metabolize, e.g. in severe haemolysis (breakdown of red cells). The excess bilirubin which builds up in the plasma is mostly of the unconjugated type and is therefore not found in the urine.

Hepatocellular jaundice
In hepatocellular (hepatic) jaundice, there is a build up of bilirubin in the plasma because it is not transported, conjugated, or excreted by the liver cells because they are damaged, e.g. in viral hepatitis. The excess bilirubin is usually of both the unconjugated and conjugated types with bilirubin being found in the urine.

Obstructive jaundice
In obstructive (posthepatic) jaundice, bilirubin builds up in the plasma because its flow is obstructed in the small bile channels or in the main bile duct. This can be caused by gall stones or a tumour obstructing or closing the biliary tract. The excess bilirubin is mostly of the conjugated type and is therefore found in the urine. The term cholestasis is used to describe a failure of bile flow.

Note: Jaundiced patients often have both hepatocellular and obstructive features. It is usual to find some obstruction when there is damage to liver cells and following obstruction there is usually some liver cell damage.

TEST SELECTION AND CALIBRATION

A method based on that developed by Jendrassik and Grof is recommended as a manual colorimetric method for measuring serum or plasma bilirubin.[10] Compared with methods such as Malloy and Evelyn, Lathe and Ruthven, Watson and Powell, the Jendrassik and Grof method can be performed with greater precision and is more rapid, sensitive and specific. Methods that use methanol are not recommended.[11]

Methods for measuring both total and conjugated bilirubin are described but for most purposes the measurement of total bilirubin is sufficient, particularly when results are interpreted with clinical findings and the results of urine bilirubin and urobilinogen tests (see chart 6.3 at the end of this subunit).

Bilirubin meters
Bilirubin photometric analyzers are available for the rapid, direct measurement of total bilirubin in neonates, but most are very expensive. The absorbance of undiluted plasma is measured at two wavelengths i.e. 454 nm which is the absorbance of bilirubin and haemoglobin, and 540 nm which is the absorbance of haemoglobin alone. The instrument subtracts the 540 nm reading from the 454 nm reading and compares the difference with that from a standard. The bilirubin value is digitally displayed.

Principle of the Jendrassik and Grof bilirubin method
Sulphanilic acid is diazotized by the nitrous acid produced from the reaction between sodium nitrite and hydrochloric acid.

Bilirubin reacts with the diazotized sulphanilic acid (diazo reagent) to form azobilirubin. Caffeine is an accelerator and gives a rapid and complete conversion to azobilirubin. The pink acid azobilirubin is converted to blue azobilirubin by an alkaline tartrate reagent and the absorbance of the blue-green solution is read in a colorimeter using an orange filter 590 nm (Ilford No. 607) or in a spectrophotometer at wavelength 600 nm. Measurement of the azobilirubin in an alkaline medium removes turbidity and increases specificity. There is very little interference by other pigments at 600 nm wavelength.

Conjugated (direct) bilirubin: This is measured in the absence of the caffeine-benzoate catalyst and at an acid pH. Under these conditions only the conjugated bilirubin will react. The reaction is terminated by ascorbic acid and alkaline tartrate is added. The

concentration of unconjugated bilirubin can be calculated by subtracting the conjugated bilirubin value from the total bilirubin value.

Calibration
The bilirubin assay is most easily calibrated from a control serum of high bilirubin concentration, e.g. *Seronorm Bilirubin Paediatric* lyophilized control serum (value around 340 μmol/l, manufactured by Sero AS (see Appendix 11). It is supplied lyophilized in a 6 × 3 ml pack. In lyophilized form, *Seronorm Bilirubin Paediatric* has a shelf-life of at least 3 years when stored in the dark at 2–8 °C. After reconstitution (with distilled water) it is stable for 4 days in the dark at 2–8 °C. However, when stored frozen (in amounts ready for use) at −20 °C or below, the serum can be kept for several weeks. There is a 3% decrease in value per week at −20 °C.

Bilirubin standards
1 Reconstitute the Seronorm Bilirubin Paediatric serum (or other control serum) exactly as instructed by the manufacturer.
   Important: Bilirubin is unstable. It is rapidly destroyed by ultraviolet light, therefore protect the serum from daylight and fluorescent light.
2 Prepare five standards by taking five small containers and numbering them 1 to 5. Pipette accurately into each as follows:

Container	Control serum	Physiological saline
1	0.1 ml	0.9 ml
2	0.2 ml	0.8 ml
3	0.5 ml	0.5 ml
4	0.8 ml	0.2 ml
5	Neat serum	–

Mix well the contents in each container.
Important: Protect the bilirubin from direct light by wrapping black paper or aluminium foil around each container.
3 Calculate the concentration of bilirubin in each standard by multiplying the concentration of bilirubin in the serum (as given by the manufacturer) by the following factors:
   Standard, 1: multiply by 0.1
   　　　　　　2:　　　„　　　0.2
   　　　　　　3:　　　„　　　0.5
   　　　　　　4:　　　„　　　0.8
   　　　　　　5:　　　„　　　1.0 (neat serum)

Example

If the control serum contains 340 μmol/l bilirubin, the concentration in each of the standards would be 34 μmol/l, 68 μmol/l, 170 μmol/l, 272 μmol/l, and 340 μmol/l.

Note: The manufacturer's calibration instructions which accompany the serum can also be followed but these usually recommend the use of four instead of five standards.

Preparation of bilirubin calibration graph

1 Take ten tubes and label them 1 to 5 and B1 to B5 (each standard requires its own blank (B) solution as in the test method).

2 Pipette 1 ml of caffeine-benzoate reagent (see *Reagents*) into each tube.

   Caution: Caffeine is a harmful chemical, therefore handle with care and *do not* mouth-pipette.

3 Add to each tube as follows:

   Tube
   1 and 1B .... 0.1 ml (100 μl) standard No. 1
   2 and 2B .... 0.1 ml standard No. 2
   3 and 3B .... 0.1 ml standard No. 3
   4 and 4B .... 0.1 ml standard No. 4
   5 and 5B .... 0.1 ml standard No. 5

4 Add 0.5 ml of diazo reagent (see *Reagents*) to tubes 1, 2, 3, 4, 5 and mix well.

5 Add 0.5 ml of sulphanilic acid, 5 g/l reagent (see *Reagents*) to tubes 1B, 2B, 3B, 4B, 5B and mix well.

6 Leave for 5 minutes at room temperature (20–28 °C).

   Note: A variety of waiting times are recommended for the Jendrassik and Grof method. Using caffeine-benzoate, 99.5% of the colour is developed within 30 seconds.

7 Continue as described in steps 7 to 8 of the total bilirubin method.

8 Take a sheet of graph paper and plot the absorbance of each standard (vertical axis) against its concentration in μmol/l (horizontal axis) as described in subunit 4.10.

   The useful working limit (linearity) of the Jendrassik and Grof method is about 350 μmol/l.

Important: Check the calibration graph by measuring a control serum as described in the total bilirubin method. A new calibration graph should be prepared and checked against controls whenever stock reagents are renewed.

TEST METHOD

Reagents

– Sulphanilic acid, 5 g/l	Reagent No. 65
– Sodium nitrite, 5 g/l	Reagent No. 61
– Caffeine-benzoate reagent	Reagent No. 16
– Alkaline tartrate reagent	Reagent No. 7

All the reagents except the sodium nitrite reagent are stable at room temperature (20–28 °C) for about 6 months. The sodium nitrite reagent must be stored at 2–8 °C. It is stable for at least 1 month when kept tightly stoppered.

Diazo reagent

Mix: 20.0 ml suphanilic acid reagent
      0.5 ml sodium nitrite reagent

When kept tightly stoppered at 2–8 °C, the diazo reagent is stable for about 5 hours.

Total bilirubin
Specimen

The method requires 0.2 ml (200 μl) of patient's serum or plasma from EDTA or heparin anticoagulated blood. The specimen should be as fresh as possible (not more than 24 hours hold).

Samples from infants: Icteric plasma from infants can be diluted 1 in 2 (0.1 ml plasma and 0.1 ml physiological saline) or if highly icteric 1 in 4 (50 μl plasma and 0.15 ml physiological saline). Multiply the result by two or by four according to which dilution is used.

Important: Protect the specimen from daylight and fluorescent light because bilirubin is *rapidly* destroyed by ultraviolet light.

Method

1 Take six or more tubes (depending on the number of tests) and label as follows:
   S .... Standard
   SB .... Standard blank
   C .... Control serum (see 6.2)
   CB .... Control blank
   1, 2, etc .... Patients' tests
   1B, 2B, etc .... Patients' blanks

2   Pipette 1 ml of caffeine-benzoate reagent into each tube.

3   Add to each tube as follows:

Tube

S, SB .... 0.1 ml standard serum (170–340 μmol/l)

C, CB .... 0.1 ml control serum

1, 1B, 2, 2B, etc.............. 0.1 ml patient's serum
.... or plasma

Mix well.

4   Add 0.5 ml of diazo reagent to tubes S, C, 1, 2, etc, and mix well.

5   Add 0.5 ml of sulphanilic acid, reagent to tubes SB, CB, 1B, 2B, etc and mix well.

6   Leave at room temperature (20–28 °C) for 5 minutes.

7   Add 1 ml of alkaline tartrate reagent to each tube and mix well.

Note: With the addition of this reagent any turbidity in the solutions will clear.

8   Read immediately the absorbances of the solutions (blanks first) in a colorimeter using an orange filter 590 nm (e.g. Ilford No. 607) or in a spectrophotometer set at wavelength 600 nm. Zero the instrument with distilled water.

Subtract the blank readings from the standard, control and patients' samples, i.e. subtract reading SB from S, CB from reading C, B1 from 1, etc.

Note: For some colorimeters it may be necessary to use a modified cuvette holder to read the small volumes. No modification is required if using the Biochrom CO 7000 Colorimeter (see subunit 4.10).

9   Calculate the concentration of total bilirubin in the control and patients' samples by:

–   Reading the values from the calibration graph providing the reading of the standard agrees with the calibration, or if not by:

–   Using the following formula:

Concentration of total bilirubin in μmol/l =

$$\frac{AT}{AS} \times \text{concentration of standard}$$

where: AT = Absorbance of test(s) or control
       AS = Absorbance of standard

Bilirubin values greater than 350 μmol/l (20 mg%)
Repeat the assay after diluting the serum or plasma 1 in 4 in physiological saline. Multiply the result by four.

10 Report the patients' results if the value of the control serum is acceptable.

Conjugated (direct) bilirubin
In addition to the measurement of total bilirubin, the measurement of conjugated (direct) bilirubin may occasionally be required. From these two values, the concentration of unconjugated (indirect) bilirubin can be calculated.

Reagents
–   Hydrochloric acid, 50 mmol/l. Reagent No. 35.
–   Sulphanilic acid, as for total bilirubin.
–   Alkaline tartrate reagent, as for total bilirubin.
–   Ascorbic acid, 40 g/l.
    Prepare daily by dissolving 0.2 g ascorbic acid in 5 ml of distilled or deionized water.
–   Diazo reagent. Prepare daily as described for total bilirubin method.

Method
1   Take two tubes and label one 'Test' and the other 'TB' (test blank). Pipette into each as follows:

	Test	TB
Hydrochloric acid, 50 mmol/l	1.0 ml	1.0 ml
*Patient's serum or plasma	0.1 ml	0.1 ml
Diazo reagent	0.5 ml	–
Sulphanilic acid, 5 g/l	–	0.5 ml

* *Icteric samples from infants:* Dilute as described for total bilirubin method.

2   Mix well and leave at room temperature for 5 minutes.
3   To each tube add:
    –   0.05 ml (50 μl) ascorbic acid reagent and mix.
    –   1.0 ml alkaline tartrate reagent and mix.
4   Read absorbances immediately using the same filter and wavelength as for total bilirubin. Zero the instrument with distilled water.
    Subtract the test blank (TB) reading from the test reading.
5   Calculate the concentration of conjugated bilirubin in μmol/l using the calibration graph or calculate the value from the formula:
    $$\frac{AT}{AS} \times \text{concentration of standard}$$

Note: Use the absorbance reading of the standard and standard concentration as used in the calculation for total bilirubin.

Summary of Total Bilirubin Method

For detailed instructions, see text

Pipette into tubes as follows:	STANDARD S	STANDARD BLANK SB	CONTROL C	CONTROL BLANK CB	TESTS 1, 2, etc	TEST BLANKS 1B, 2B, etc
Caffeine-benzoate reagent	1 ml	1 ml	1 ml	1 ml	1 ml	1 ml
Standard serum	0.1 ml	0.1 ml	–	–	–	–
Control serum	–	–	0.1 ml	0.1 ml	–	–
Patient's serum or plasma	–	–	–	–	0.1 ml	0.1 ml
Diazo reagent (fresh)	0.5 ml	–	0.5 ml	–	0.5 ml	–
Sulphanilic acid, 5 g/l	–	0.5 ml	–	0.5 ml	–	0.5 ml

- Mix well.

- Leave at room temperature for 5 minutes.

Pipette into tubes Alkaline tartrate reagent	1 ml	1 ml	1 ml	1 ml	1 ml	1 ml

- Mix well.

- READ ABSORBANCES (Blanks first):

  Colorimeter: Orange filter 590 nm, e.g. Ilford No. 607
  Spectrophotometer: 600 nm

- Zero the instrument with distilled water.

- Subtract blank readings.

- Obtain values from the calibration graph if the result of the standard agrees with the calibration. If not, calculate the result as follows:

$$\text{Total bilirubin } \mu\text{mol/l} = \frac{\text{Absorbance of test or control}}{\text{Absorbance of standard}} \times \text{Concentration of standard}$$

- Report patients' results if control value is acceptable.

Note: See text for conjugated bilirubin method.

0.1 ml = 100 μl
0.5 ml = 500 μl

Unconjugated (indirect) bilirubin

Subtract the conjugated value from the total bilirubin value.

Quality control

The principles of quality control in clinical chemistry are described in subunit 6.2.

TEST RESULTS

Approximate total bilirubin reference (normal) range

Adults: 3–21 μmol/l (0.2–1.3 mg%)
Newborns: 8–67 μmol/l (0.5–4.0 mg%)*

*Highest values in the first 3–5 days of life.

To convert μmol/l to mg%, multiply by 0.06.
To convert mg% to μmol/l, multiply by 17 or divide by 0.06.

Interpretation of serum or plasma bilirubin results

A rise in the level of bilirubin in the blood is called hyperbilirubinaemia. The main causes are as follows:

● Overproduction of bilirubin caused by an excessive breakdown of red cells (haemolytic jaundice). The bilirubin is of the unconjugated type. In tropical countries haemolysis is due mainly to:
  – Severe falciparum malaria.
  – Sickle cell disease haemolytic crisis.
  – Haemolysis associated with glucose-6-phosphate dehydrogenase deficiency and hereditary spherocytosis.
  – Antigen antibody reactions as in haemolytic disease of the newborn, autoimmune haemolytic anaemias, or following an incompatible blood transfusion.
  – Toxins from bacteria, snake venoms, drugs, or herbs.

● Liver cell damage in which there is usually an increase in both conjugated and unconjugated bilirubin (hepatocellular jaundice). The commonest causes are:
  – Hepatitis caused by hepatitis viruses and other viruses
  – Leptospirosis
  – Relapsing fever
  – Brucellosis
  – Typhoid
  – Chemicals, plant toxins and drugs

● Metabolic disturbances in the liver involving defective conjugation, transport and, or, excretion of bilirubin. Examples include:
  – type of neonatal jaundice, often referred to as 'physiological jaundice' (see following text)

  – rare inherited disorders of conjugation such as Gilbert's and Crigler-Najjar syndromes.

● Partial or complete stopping of the flow of bile through bile channels with a build up of conjugated bilirubin in the blood (obstructive jaundice). Cholestasis can be due to:
  – Obstruction of the extra-hepatic biliary ducts by gallstones, tumours (especially hepatomas and carcinoma of the pancreas), cholangitis (inflammation of the biliary ducts), or by helminths such as *Opisthorchis* and *Fasciola* species. Occasionally heavy *Ascaris* infections, especially in children, may result in blockage of the common bile duct.
  – Pressure on the small bile ducts as may occur in hepatitis or as a side effect of drugs.

Note: Mild to moderate hyperbilirubinaemia may also be found in association with any serious condition such as a terminal illness, or following major trauma, surgery, or blood transfusion.

Neonatal jaundice

As previously described, a type of neonatal jaundice known as 'physiological' jaundice may develop in a newborn baby if the conjugation mechanism of the infant is not fully developed. The jaundice begins to appear on the second day after birth and is of longer duration in premature infants.

Other common causes of neonatal jaundice in tropical countries are as follows:

  – Glucose-6-phosphate dehydrogenase deficiency, especially in Papua New Guinea, Malaysia, Singapore and other parts of South-East Asia. The jaundice develops soon after birth.

  – Infections, particularly septicaemia, congenital syphilis, toxoplasmosis, and viral infections. The jaundice usually develops 3–4 days after birth.

  – ABO haemolytic disease of the newborn in which jaundice occurs usually within 24 hours of birth.

In neonatal jaundice the level of unconjugated bilirubin is important. Levels in excess of 340 μmol/l (20 mg%) in the normal child may result in the unconjugated bilirubin being deposited in the basal ganglion of the brain, a condition known as kernicterus. This may cause permanent damage to the brain cells of the infant. It is therefore important to measure the serum or plasma bilirubin at regular intervals.

Even at bilirubin levels much lower than 340 μmol/l the premature child is especially at risk as is the child with acidosis or low serum or plasma albumin levels because the levels of 'free' bilirubin not bound to albumin are much higher and it is this type of bilirubin that causes kernicterus.

Note: In differentiating hepatocellular disease from obstructive jaundice, serum or plasma alkaline phosphatase and aspartate aminotransferase (AST) tests are of particular value. Alkaline phosphatase levels are lower and AST levels are usually much higher in hepatocellular disease than in obstructive jaundice. In viral hepatitis, AST levels are markedly raised.

Chart 6.3 Test results in haemolytic diseases, hepatitis, and biliary obstruction*

	URINE TESTS		PLASMA BILIRUBIN, μmol/l	
	Bilirubin	*Urobilinogen*	*Total*	*Conjugated*
Normal adult	–	Trace	3–21	About 5%
Haemolytic diseases	–	+	<60	Below 5%
Hepatitis:				
Onset	Trace	+	<35	Raised
Jaundice	+	–	<250	High
Recovery	Falling	Trace/+	Falling	Falling
Biliary obstruction	+	–	<400	High

* Information for the above chart has been taken from *Lecture Notes on Clinical Biochemistry*, Blackwell Scientific.

6.7 Measurement of serum albumin

Analyte: Albumin is produced entirely in the liver and constitutes about 60% of total serum protein. It is important in regulating the flow of water between the plasma and tissue fluid by its effect on plasma colloid osmotic pressure (oncotic pressure). When the concentration of albumin is significantly reduced, the plasma osmotic pressure is insufficient to draw water from the tissue spaces back into the plasma. This leads to a build-up of fluid in the tissues, referred to as oedema.

Albumin also has important binding and transport functions. It binds and inactivates substances including calcium, bilirubin, fatty acids, urate, hormones, and magnesium, and also drugs such as penicillin, salicylates, sulphonamides, and barbiturates. When albumin levels are reduced, toxic effects can develop from an increase in unbound substances.

Albumin diffuses easily through damaged membranes and is more readily filtered out by the kidneys than most globulins because its molecules are smaller.

Value of test

Serum albumin is mainly measured to investigate liver diseases, protein energy malnutrition, disorders of water balance, nephrotic syndrome, and protein-losing gastrointestinal diseases.

TEST SELECTION AND CALIBRATION

The bromocresol green (BCG) binding method is recommended as a manual colorimetric technique for measuring serum albumin.[12] The BCG reagent is best purchased ready-made (see later text).

Principle of the BCG albumin method

Bromocresol green is an indicator which is yellow between pH 3.5–4.2. When it binds to albumin the colour of the indicator changes from yellow to blue-green. The absorbance of the colour produced is measured in a colorimeter using an orange filter 590 nm (Ilford No. 607) or in a spectrophotometer at 632 nm wavelength.

Calibration

The bromocresol green method for albumin can be calibrated from a 50 g/l solution of albumin, e.g. Sigma 50 g/l albumin solution, code A4628 or purchased within an albumin BCG test kit, e.g. from Plasmatec (see later text).

Albumin standards 10, 20, 30, 40, 50 g/l

1 Take five small containers and number them 1 to 5. Pipette accurately into each as follows:

Container	Albumin 50 g/l	Protein Diluent Reagent No. 52
1	0.2	0.8
2	0.4	0.6
3	0.6	0.4
4	0.8	0.2
5	1.0	–

Note: To prevent the stock bottle of albumin becoming contaminated, use a sterile needle and syringe to remove the amount of albumin required, i.e. just over 3 ml.

2 Mix well the contents of each container. The concentration of albumin in each of the standards is as follows:

Container 1 = 10 g/l
2 = 20 g/l
3 = 30 g/l
4 = 40 g/l
5 = 50 g/l

3 Label and store at 2–8 °C. The standard solutions are stable for several months.

Preparation of the albumin calibration graph

1   Take six tubes and label them 'B' (reagent blank) and 1 to 5.

2   Pipette 4 ml of BCG reagent (see *Reagents*) into each tube.

Note: Allow the BCG reagent to come to room temperature before use.

3   Add to each tube as follows:

Tube
B .... 20 μl (0.02 ml) distilled water
1 .... 20 μl standard, 10 g/l
2 .... 20 μl standard, 20 g/l
3 .... 20 μl standard, 30 g/l
4 .... 20 μl standard, 40 g/l
5 .... 20 μl standard, 50 g/l

4   Mix well but avoid frothing of the reagent. If air bubbles are present the absorbance readings will be incorrect.

5   Continue as described in steps 5 and 6 of the test method.

6   Take a sheet of graph paper and plot the absorbance of each standard solution (vertical axis) against its concentration in g/l (horizontal axis), as described in subunit 4.10.

The useful working limit (linearity) of the bromocresol green method for albumin is about 50 g/l (5 g%).

Important: Check the calibration graph by measuring a control serum as described in the albumin method. A new calibration graph should be prepared and checked against controls whenever stock reagents are renewed.

TEST METHOD

Reagent

−   Bromocresol green (BCG) working reagent,

pH 4.2 (succinate buffered)

Purchase ready-made reagent*

* Ready-made BCG products
A suitable BCG working reagent is contained in the *Albumin BCG* test kit available from Plasmatec (see Appendix 11), catalogue No ALB0120. The test kit contains BCG reagent 2 × 125 and also 5ml of 5g/100ml albumin solution.

BCG working reagent (shelf-life 18 months) is also available from Span Diagnostics, code BO311 (see Appendix 11).

Note: Take precautions to prevent contamination of the BCG reagent. If it becomes cloudy it must not be used.

Specimen

The method requires 20 μl (0.02 ml) of non-lipaemic, non-icteric patient's serum. The blood must be collected with the *minimum of venous stasis and haemolysis should be avoided*. Bilirubin, haemoglobin, lipids and salicylates can interfere in the test. For the stability of albumin in serum refer to Chart 6.1 in subunit 6.2.

Method

1   Take four or more tubes (depending on the number of tests) and label as follows:
B   −   Reagent blank
S   −   Standard, 30 g/l (see *Calibration*)
C   −   Control serum (see subunit 6.2)
1, 2, etc   −   Patients' tests

2   Pipette 4 ml of BCG reagent into each tube.

3   Add to each tube as follows:

Tube
B.............................. 20 μl (0.02 ml) distilled water
S.............................. 20 μl standard, 30 g/l
C.............................. 20 μl control serum
1, 2, etc.................. 20 μl patient's serum

Note: If a patient's sample appears turbid, prepare a serum blank by mixing 20 μl of patient's serum in 4 ml of succinate buffer (Reagent No. 63).

4   Mix *well* but avoid frothing of the solutions. If air bubbles are present the absorbance readings will be incorrect.

5   Within 5 minutes read the absorbances of the solutions in a colorimeter using an orange filter 590 nm (e.g. Ilford No. 607) or in a spectrophotometer set at 632 nm. Zero the instrument with the reagent blank solution in tube B.

Note: If using a serum blank, read its absorbance after zeroing the instrument with distilled water. Subtract this reading from the reading of the patient's BCG sample (read against the reagent blank solution).

6   Calculate the concentration of albumin in the control and patients' samples by:

−   Reading the values from the calibration graph providing the reading of the 30 g/l standard agrees with the calibration, or if not by

−   Using the following formula:

$$\text{Albumin g/l} = \frac{AT}{AS} \times 30$$

where: AT = Absorbance of test(s) or control
AS = Absorbance of 30 g/l standard

7 Report the patients' results if the value of the control serum is acceptable.

Quality control
The principles of quality control in clinical chemistry are described in subunit 6.2.

TEST RESULTS

Approximate albumin reference (normal) range 30–45 g/l

To convert from g/l to g%, divide by 10.
To convert from g% to g/l, multiply by 10.

Note: Albumin levels are lower in infants and when individuals are lying down (by 10%).

Interpretation of serum albumin results

Increases
Serum albumin levels are rarely raised except in diarrhoea or prolonged vomiting and artefactually by prolonged venous stasis.

Decreases
Hypoalbuminaemia occurs whenever there is increased plasma volume (e.g. in pregnancy). Pathological causes include:
– Low protein intake as in protein energy malnutrition.
– Malabsorption as in chronic pancreatitis, coeliac disease, and sprue.

Summary of Albumin Method				
	BLANK B	STANDARD S	CONTROL C	TEST 1, 2, etc
● Pipette into tubes as follows:				
Bromocresol green (BCG) reagent	4 ml	4 ml	4 ml	4 ml
Distilled water	20 µl	–	–	–
Standard, 30 g/l	–	20 µl	–	–
Control serum	–	–	20 µl	–
Patient's serum	–	–	–	20 µl

● Mix *well* but avoid frothing.

● READ ABSORBANCES within 5 minutes.

   Colorimeter: Orange filter 590 nm, e.g. Ilford No. 607
   Spectrophotometer: 632 nm

● Zero instrument with blank solution in tube B.

● Obtain values from the calibration graph if the result of the 30 g/l standard agrees with the calibration. If not, calculate the results as follows:

   $$\text{Albumin g/l} = \frac{\text{Absorbance of test or control}}{\text{Absorbance of 30 g/l standard}} \times 30$$

● Report patients' results if control value is acceptable.   20 µl = 0.02 ml

- Loss of albumin from the body in urine as in the nephrotic syndrome. Albumin can also be lost from the skin following severe burns or from the bowel as in ulcerative colitis and other forms of protein-losing gastroenteropathy.
- Liver disease associated with a reduction in the production of albumin (total protein levels may be within the reference range because the albumin levels fall and the globulin levels rise at the same time). Several parasitic infections can also cause a reduction in albumin production.
- An increase in the body's need for protein, e.g. as a result of infection, malignant disease or following surgery or serious tissue damage when protein is required for energy and repair.
- In AIDS, hypoalbuminaemia is common and may be due to several of the above causes, e.g. malnutrition, malabsorption, high protein demands.

Note: The BCG method is not very accurate at low levels of serum albumin, giving results with positive bias when the albumin is less than 20 g/l. This is probably unimportant in clinical practice.

Measurement of total protein
The measurement of total plasma proteins (albumin, globulins, fibrinogen) or total serum protein (albumin and globulins) has only limited clinical value and is therefore not described. A fall in albumin concentration may be balanced by a rise in immunoglobulin concentration, e.g. in liver disease.

Most of the causes of low total protein levels (below 60 g/l) are due to reduced albumin concentrations or more rarely to severe immunoglobulin deficiency.

An increase in total protein concentration can occur (greater than 80 g/l) when there is prolonged venous stasis during venepuncture, or when a person is dehydrated.

Pathological causes are rare and usually associated with:

– increased globulin production as in chronic infections such as tuberculosis, kala-azar, and tropical splenomegaly.

– presence of abnormal globulins as in multiple myeloma, lymphoma, or macroglobulinaemia.

If required the measurement of total protein is best made using a refractometer similar to that used to measure urine specific gravity (see end of subunit 6.11).

Note: The investigation of disorders of immunoglobulin synthesis, myeloma and other malignant paraproteinaemias requires the facilities of a specialist laboratory able to perform urine and protein electrophoresis, immunological assays, bone marrow examinations, and other tests to diagnose and monitor patients with these conditions.

6.8 Measurement of serum or plasma alanine aminotransferase (ALT) activity

Analyte: The enzymes, aspartate aminotransferase (AST), previously known as glutamate oxaloacetate transaminase (GOT), and alanine aminotransferase (ALT), formerly known as glutamate pyruvate transaminase (GPT), are concerned with amino acid metabolism.

Large amounts of AST are present in the liver, kidneys, cardiac muscle, and skeletal muscle. Small amounts of the enzyme are present in the brain, pancreas, and lungs. ALT is found principally in the liver with only small amounts being present in other organs. When there is liver cell damage the serum or plasma levels of both enzymes are raised.

Value of test

Measurement of ALT activity is mainly performed to investigate liver disease. Increasingly ALT is being measured to monitor patients receiving anti-retroviral drugs associated with hepatotoxicity such as nevirapine (NVP) and stavudine (d47). While both ALT and AST are raised with hepatocellular injury, ALT is more specific for detecting liver cell damage.

TEST SELECTION AND CALIBRATION

Whenever possible, enzymatic continuous monitoring techniques should be used for measuring ALT (and AST). In district laboratories however, the equipment, reagents, and trained staff required to perform these techniques are often unavailable, necessitating the use of a colorimetric end-point technique such as the Reitman-Frankel method.[13] The use of a test kit is recommended. The reagents have good stability.

Reitman-Frankel ALT kit
A recommended kit is that manufactured by Span Diagnostics (see Appendix 11), Code No 25912. It contains all the reagents required, including the working pyruvate standard used to calibrate the assay. The Span Diagnostics ALT test method is described in this subunit. An AST test kit is also available from Span Diagnostics, code 25913.

Principle of Reitman-Frankel ALT method
ALT is incubated at 37 °C for exactly 30 minutes in a pH 7.4 buffered substrate containing alanine and α-ketoglutarate. ALT catalyzes the transfer of the amino group from alanine to ketoglutarate, forming pyruvate and glutamate.

The pyruvate reacts with 2,4-dinitrophenylhydrazine (DNPH) to form 2,4-dinitrophenylhydrazone which in an alkaline medium gives a red-brown colour. The absorbance of the colour produced is measured in a colorimeter using a green filter 520 nm (Ilford No. 604) or in a spectrophotometer at 505 nm wavelength.

Calibration
Span Diagnostics ALT Kit 25912
The ALT kit method is calibrated from a ready-made pyruvate calibration standard (Reagent 4).

The method of calibration is as follows:

1 Take 5 tubes and label them 1 to 5. Pipette accurately into each as follows:

Tube	Reagent 1	Reagent 4
1	0.5 ml	–
2	0.45 ml	0.05 ml
3	0.4 ml	0.1 ml
4	0.35 ml	0.15 ml
5	0.3 ml	0.2 ml

2 Add 0.1 ml (100 μl) of distilled water to each tube and mix well.
3 Add 0.5 ml Reagent 2 to each tube and mix well.
4 Leave for 20 minutes at room temperature (20–28 °C).
5 Add 5 ml Solution 1 to each tube and mix well.
6 Leave for 10 minutes at room temperature.
7 Read the absorbances of the pyruvate calibration standards in a colorimeter using a green filter 520 nm (e.g. Ilford No. 604) or in a spectrophotometer set at wavelength 505 nm. Zero the instrument with distilled or deionized water.
8 Take a sheet of graph paper and plot the absorbance of each standard (vertical axis) against its equivalent ALT activity in IU/l (horizontal axis). A non-linear (curved line) graph will be obtained, see subunit 4.10. This means that test results will need to be read from the graph.
The ALT activity in each standard is as follows:

Tube	IU/l
1	0
2	28
3	57
4	97
5	150

Important: A new calibration graph requires preparation whenever new reagents are used. Use a control serum to check the calibration graph.

TEST METHOD
Span Diagnostics ALT Kit 25912

Reagents
– Substrate reagent, pH 7.4. . . . . .Reagent 1
   Store at 2–8 °C
– Colour reagent (DNPH) . . . . .Reagent 2
   Protect from light. Discard if not clear and light yellow. Store at 2–8 °C.
– Sodium hydroxide, 4 mol/l (4N) . . . .Reagent 3
   Store at room temperature (20–28 °C).
– Working pyruvate standard. . . . . .Reagent 4
   Store at 2–8 °C.
– Solution 1 (0.4 mol/l sodium hydroxide). Dilute 1 ml Reagent 3 to 10 ml with distilled or deionised water.

Specimen
The method requires 0.05 ml (50 μl) of patient's *fresh* serum or plasma which must be free from haemolysis. For details of blood collection and the stability of ALT activity in serum and plasma, see Chart 6.1 in subunit 6.2. If the serum or plasma is lipaemic this should be reported.

Method
1 Take three or more tubes (depending on the number of tests) and label as follows:
   B   – Reagent blank
   S   – Standard (pyruvate 57 ALT IU/l)
   1, 2, etc – Patients' tests
2 Pipette 0.25 ml of Reagent 1 into patients' tubes (1, 2, etc). Transfer these tubes to a heat-block or water bath set at 37 °C.

   After 5 minutes add 0.05 ml (50 μl) of patient's serum. Mix and incubate at 37 °C for *exactly* 30 minutes. Start timing after adding serum to the first tube.
3 Just before 30 minutes is due, pipette into the blank and standard tubes as follows:
   B . . . . 0.1 ml distilled water
                             0.5 ml Reagent 1
   S . . . . 0.1 ml distilled water
                             0.4 ml Reagent 1
                             0.1 ml Reagent 4

4 At *exactly* 30 minutes, remove tubes 1, 2, etc from the heat-block or water bath and place them in the rack with tubes B and S.

5 Add *immediately* 0.25 ml Reagent 2 to each tube and mix well. Leave at room temperature (20–28 °C) for 20 minutes.

6 Add 2.5 ml Solution 1 to each tube and mix well. Leave at room temperature for 10 minutes.

7 Read the absorbances of the standard, and patients' samples in a colorimeter using a green filter 520 nm (e.g. Ilford No. 604) or in a spectrophotometer set at wavelength 505 nm. Zero the instrument with the reagent blank solution in tube B.

The colours of the solutions are stable for up to 1 hour.

8 Read off the ALT activity in IU/l in the patients' sample from the calibration graph, making sure that the reading of the standard which corresponds to ALT 57 IU/l agrees with the calibration curve.

ALT results over 150 IU/l:

Repeat the assay using a 1 in 5 physiological saline dilution of the patient's serum. Multiply the result by 5.

Quality control
The principles of quality control in clinical chemistry are described in subunit 6.2.

TEST RESULTS

Approximate ALT reference (normal) range

5–35 IU/l (Reitman Frankel method)

Note: Other ALT methods give much lower reference values, particularly UV methods in which incubation is carried out at 25 °C.

Interpretation of serum or plasma ALT results

Liver disease

The most important cause of raised ALT activity is hepatocelluar injuy. With acute hepatocellular injury, AST levels are usually higher than ALT levels. As damage continues, ALT activity becomes higher. In viral hepatitis, both enzymes are usually raised before the patient becomes jaundiced. In cirrhosis, ALT levels fall below AST levels. Both ALT and AST are raised in hepatitis caused by hepatotoxic antiretroviral drugs.

Obstructive liver disease is usually accompanied by only small or moderate ALT and AST rises especially in the early stages. With complete obstruction, enzyme levels fall.

Myocardial infarction

An important cause of elevated AST activity is myocardial infarction, i.e. destruction of an area of heart muscle because its blood supply has been cut off due to a blood clot in a coronary artery. The enzyme level rises soon after the coronary vessel becomes blocked, reaches its highest value 24–48 hours after the infarct and returns to normal usually within 3–5 days. In general, the more extensive the infarct, the higher the AST peak level.

Other causes of raised AST levels

Because AST is widely distributed in body tissues many other diseases involving cellular injury may be accompanied by increases in AST levels, e.g. severe bacterial infections, malaria, pneumonia, infectious mononucleosis, pulmonary infarcts, and tumours. AST activity is also increased in some muscle disorders and following surgery, injury, or blood transfusion.

Note: ALT and AST enzymes are artefactually increased when haemolysis is present or if the blood has been stored without separation of the serum or plasma.

6.9 Measurement of serum or plasma *alpha*-amylase activity

Analyte: The enzyme *alpha*-amylase is present in large amounts in pancreatic juice and saliva. Pancreatic amylase hydrolyzes starches not split by salivary amylase. Some of the pancreatic amylase is absorbed into the blood and is excreted in the urine. Acute inflammation of the pancreas (pancreatitis) causes the release of large amounts of amylase into the circulation.

Value of test

Measurement of serum or plasma amylase activity is usually requested to assist in the differentiation of acute pancreatitis from other acute abdominal disorders. It is an early indicator of acute pancreatitis.

TEST SELECTION

The Caraway Somogyi starch-iodine amylase method[14] is a simple inexpensive technique that can be performed in district laboratories providing a good quality starch is available to make the substrate reagent.

Summary of ALT Method

	BLANK B	STANDARD S	TEST 1, 2, etc
• Pipette into tubes as follows:			
Reagent 1 (substrate)...	–	–	0.25 ml

• Warm the substrate in tubes 1, 2, etc at 37°C for 5 minutes.

• Pipette as follows: Patient's serum...	–	–	0.05 ml

• Incubate tubes 1, 2, etc at 37°C for *exactly* 30 minutes.

• Just before 30 minutes is due, pipette:			
Distilled water...	0.1 ml	0.1 ml	–
Reagent 1 (substrate)...	0.5 ml	0.4 ml	–
Reagent 4 (pyruvate standard)	–	0.1 ml	–

• At *exactly* 30 minutes, pipette as follows: Reagent 2 (Colour reagent)	0.25 ml	0.25 ml	0.25 ml

• Mix well and leave at room temperature for 20 minutes.

• Pipette as follows: Solution 1 (0.4mol/NaOH)	2.5 ml	2.5 ml	2.5 ml

• Mix well and leave at room temperature for 10 minutes.

• READ ABSORBANCES
Colorimeter: Green filter 520 nm, e.g. Ilford No. 604
Spectrophotometer: 505 nm
• Zero instrument with blank solution in tube B.

• Obtain values in IU/l from the calibration graph.

• Standard (S) should read 57 ALT IU/l.

0.25 ml	= 250 µl
0.05 ml	= 50 µl
0.4 ml	= 400 µl
0.1 ml	= 100 µl

Note: The *Phadebas* tablet test is no longer manufactured. Test kits that measure amylase using the substrate *p*-nitrophenyl-maltoheptaside are available but very expensive and the technique is not appropriate for district laboratories.

Principle of the Caraway Somogyi amylase method

The test is based on the hydrolysis of starch by amylase and the blue-black complex that forms when iodine reacts with starch. Amylase is incubated at 37 °C for exactly $7\frac{1}{2}$ minutes in a pH 7.0 phosphate buffered starch substrate. The enzyme hydrolyzes the starch to maltose and other fragments. The amount of starch which remains at the end of the incubation period is shown by the addition of an iodine solution, which produces a blue-black colour.

A reagent blank is used which contains starch and iodine but no serum. The absorbances of the test and blank solutions are read in a colorimeter using a red filter 680 nm (Ilford No. 608) or in a spectrophotometer set at 660 nm.

The amylase activity is measured by the difference in absorbance of the starch-iodine complex of the test against that of the reagent blank in which there is no hydrolysis. The result is expressed in international units per litre (U/l).

Somogyi amylase units

A Somogyi unit of amylase is defined as the amount of amylase per 100 ml of serum or plasma that hydrolyzes 5 mg of starch in 15 minutes at 37 °C to the point at which it no longer gives a blue colour with iodine.

The factor of 1480 which is used to calculate amylase activity in U/l is derived from:

$$\frac{100}{0.02} \times \frac{0.4}{5} \times \frac{15}{7.5} \times 1.85$$

where:

Amount of serum or plasma used in the test is 0.02 ml.
Amount of starch used = 0.4 mg.
Incubation time = 7.5 minutes.

The figure 1.85 is the factor used to convert Caraway Somogyi units/100 ml to U/l, based on the formation of 0.185 μmol reducing group per minute so that 1 Somogyi unit/100 ml equals 1.85 U/l under these conditions.

TEST METHOD

Reagents

- Starch substrate, pH 7.0   Reagent No. 62
- Stock iodine solution   Reagent No. 39

Store the buffered starch substrate at 2–8 °C. Renew monthly. The stock iodine reagent when stored at 2–8 °C in a brown bottle is stable for about 2 months.

Working iodine reagent

Prepare by mixing 1 ml of stock iodine solution with 9 ml of distilled water.

Specimen

The method requires 20 μl (0.02 ml) of patient's *fresh* unhaemolyzed serum or heparinized plasma.

Note: Plasma from oxalated, EDTA, or citrated anticoagulated blood must *not* be used.

Method

1 Take two tubes and label as follows:

   T – Patient's test
   B – Reagent blank

2 Pipette 1 ml of *well-mixed* starch substrate into each tube.

3 Place tube T in a heat block or water bath at 37 °C for 3 minutes to warm the substrate.

4 Without removing the tube from the heat block or water bath, add 20 μl (0.02 ml) of patient's serum or plasma.

   Mix and incubate at 37 °C for *exactly* $7\frac{1}{2}$ minutes.

   Important: Avoid contaminating the samples with saliva from the mouth (*do not mouth-pipette*) or perspiration from the thumb or fingers. Both saliva and perspiration contain amylase.

5 After exactly $7\frac{1}{2}$ minutes, remove tube T from the water bath. *Immediately* add 1 ml of working iodine reagent.

   Note: If the substrate is colourless after adding the working iodine reagent to the patient's test sample this means that the amylase level is very high. Dilute the serum or plasma 1 in 6 with physiological saline (i.e. 20 μl patient's sample mixed with 0.1 ml saline) and repeat the test using 20 μl of the diluted sample. Multiply the result by 6.

6 Pipette 1 ml of working iodine reagent into tube B and mix.

7 Add 8 ml of distilled water to each tube and mix well.

8 Read *immediately* the absorbances of the test and reagent blank in a colorimeter using a red filter 680 nm (e.g. Ilford No. 608) or in a spectrophotometer set at 660 nm. Zero the instrument with distilled water.

9 Calculate the amylase activity in U/l in the patient's sample from the following formula:

$$\text{Amylase U/l} = \frac{AB - AT}{AB} \times 1480^*$$

where:
AB = Absorbance of reagent blank
AT = Absorbance of test

* For an explanation of this factor, see *Principle of test.*

Results over 735 U/l

Dilute the patient's serum or plasma 1 in 6 with physiological saline (20 µl and 0.1 ml saline) and repeat the assay using 20 µl of the diluted sample. Multiply the result by six.

Quality control

No commercially produced control serum is available for controlling the measurement of amylase activity by the Caraway Somogyi method. In the absence of a QC control, the reagents used in the test *must* be carefully prepared and monitored (starch used must be chemical grade soluble starch) and the test performed exactly as specified, e.g. the temperature of the water bath must be 37°C and the incubation time measured accurately.

TEST RESULTS

Approximate amylase reference (normal) range
70–340 U/l

Summary of Amylase Method

	TEST T	BLANK B
• Pipette into tubes as follows:		
Starch, substrate, *well-mixed*	1 ml	1 ml
• Warm tube T at 37°C for 3 minutes.		
• Add patient's serum or plasma	20 µl	–
• Mix well and incubate tube T at 37°C for *exactly* $7\frac{1}{2}$ mins.		
• Remove tube T from waterbath or heat block. • Immediately add working iodine reagent	1 ml	1 ml
• Mix well.		
• Add distilled water...	8 ml	8 ml
• READ ABSORBANCES *Colorimeter:* Red filter 680 nm, e.g. Ilford No. 608 *Spectrophotometer:* 660 nm • Zero instrument with distilled water.		

• Calculate as follows:

$$\text{Amylase U/l} = \frac{\text{Absorbance of blank} - \text{Absorbance of test}}{\text{Absorbance of blank}} \times 1480$$

20 µl = 0.02 ml
100 µl = 0.1 ml

To convert Caraway Somogyi units/100 ml to international units/litre (U/l), see previous text.

Interpretation of amylase results

Acute pancreatitis

Very high concentrations of serum or plasma amylase (over 1850 U/l) are virtually diagnostic of acute pancreatitis or acute episodes of chronic relapsing pancreatitis. When chronic pancreatitis has reached the stage of scarring and calcification, the serum amylase level is usually normal.

With acute pancreatitis, the rise in serum or plasma amylase is often very brief with the enzyme reaching its highest level within 12–24 hours and returning to normal within 3–5 days.

Slight to moderate increases of serum amylase must be interpreted carefully. They are not diagnostic of acute pancreatitis unless the blood has been collected too late to catch the peak level.

Note: It is useful to measure amylase both in serum and in urine. Amylase is quickly filtered into the urine, therefore a person suffering from acute pancreatitis may have normal serum amylase levels but high enzyme activity in the urine.

Other laboratory findings in pancreatitis

In acute pancreatitis the white cell count is raised. A serious condition is indicated if the serum or plasma albumin and calcium and blood haematocrit levels fall and the serum or plasma bilirubin and urea levels rise.

Other conditions giving raised amylase values

Serum or plasma amylase levels of approximately 740–1500 U/l may be due to:

- Renal failure
- Salivary gland obstruction or inflammation as with mumps
- Diabetic ketoacidosis
- Opiate drugs and some antiretroviral drugs
- Alcoholism
- Hypothermia
- Ectopic pregnancy
- Almost any acute abdominal emergency, and also cholecystitis, perforated peptic ulcer, or peritonitis.

Falsely raised amylase level

Falsely elevated amylase levels may result if the serum is markedly turbid or the sample has been contaminated with amylase during analysis (see previous text).

6.10 Measurement of sodium and potassium in serum or plasma

Analytes: The role of electrolytes is extensive, particularly that of the cations (positively charged ions) sodium and potassium which exist in the body fluids largely as free ions. As well as maintaining cellular tonicity and fluid balance between the various cellular components, they are involved in most metabolic processes, maintenance of pH, and regulation of neural and muscular function. Abnormal levels can be either the cause or result of a wide range of disorders.

Sodium is the main extracellular cation. The plasma sodium level is a major factor in the control of water homeostasis and extracellular fluid volume. An increase in plasma sodium normally results in three compensatory mechanisms coming into play:

- thirst prompts oral fluid intake,
- anti-diuretic hormone (ADH) secretion from the pituitary is increased, leading to renal water retention,
- there is a shift of water from intracellular to extracellular.

As the total intake of sodium chloride is almost completely absorbed from the gastrointestinal tract with no active control, regulation of the retained body sodium is maintained by the kidneys, with the excess excreted in the urine and fine control carried out by tubular reabsorption.

After initial glomerular filtration (see also the beginning of subunit 6.10):

- some 60% of the filtered sodium is recovered in the proximal tubules together with bicarbonate.
- 25% is reabsorbed in the Loop of Henle of the renal tubule with chloride.
- the remainder is reabsorbed in the distal tubules where, with aldosterone governing its reabsorption, it competes with potassium and hydrogen ions.

Potassium is the principal intracellular cation, 98% of which is maintained within the cells by the ATP dependent mechanism known as the sodium pump. Here, any sodium which diffuses into cells is actively excreted in exchange for potassium. Insulin also accelerates the cellular uptake of potassium and elevated levels of plasma potassium encourage secretion of insulin.

In addition to its role in intracellular osmolality, potassium is essential for many enzymatic reactions, the regulation of muscles (in particular heart muscle), and for the transmission of nerve impulses.

An important factor in the control of potassium cellular transport is the acid/base status. In acidosis the flow of hydrogen ions into cells causes the outflow of an equivalent number of potassium ions.

Dietary potassium intake is normally in excess of requirement and the surplus is excreted via the kidneys. Following potassium ingestion, aldosterone secretion is increased to enhance renal clearance and insulin levels rise to increase cellular absorption.

Value of tests

The measurement of sodium, potassium, or both electrolytes is usually requested in the assessment of renal function, to assist in the management of a patient that is unconscious or confused or a diabetic patient with ketoacidosis, to assess and monitor states of dehydration (particularly an infant losing fluid), to monitor diuretic therapy and to assist in fluid replacement therapy.[15]

Note: In the management of acid-base disorders, the measurement by blood gas analyzer of blood pH, carbon dioxide as PCO_2 and bicarbonate are required. These tests cannot be performed in district laboratories.

SELECTION OF TEST METHOD

The following techniques are available for measuring sodium and potassium in serum or plasma:

- Flame emission spectrometry using a flame photometer (more correctly termed flame emission spectrometer) which measures the concentration of sodium and potassium in mmol/l.

- Ion selective electrode (ISE) technology using an ISE analyzer which measures (senses) the activity of sodium and potassium ions and converts the activity measurements to mmol/l.

Choice of technique

Flame emission spectrometry using a flame photometer is widely used in clinical chemistry laboratories where the number of sodium and potassium tests performed justifies the cost of purchasing and running a flame photometer (see later text).

The measurement of sodium and potassium using an ISE analyzer is replacing the use of flame photometry in many laboratories because the technique is simpler and more rapid, whole blood can be used as well as serum or plasma and no gas supply is needed. Most ISE analyzers cost however, more than a basic flame photometer. ISE running costs can be high if only a few tests are performed. The electrodes require replacement every 4–12 months depending on the system.

To summarize: The ability of district laboratories to measure sodium and potassium and the method selected will depend on the number of test requests, whether the cost of purchasing, using, controlling and maintaining the electrolyte system can be afforded, and whether a local distributor is available for the purchase of essential consummables.

Flame photometry measurement of sodium and potassium

Principle of flame photometry: Using compressed air, diluted serum or plasma is sprayed as a fine mist of droplets (nebulized) into a non-luminous gas flame which becomes coloured by the characteristic emission of the sodium or potassium metallic ions in the sample. Light of a wavelength corresponding to

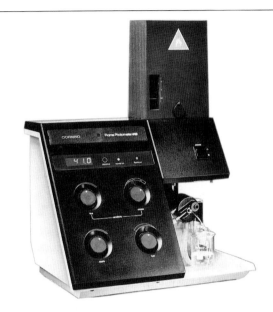

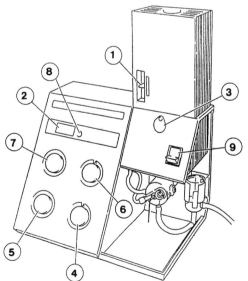

Plate 6.3 *410 Clinical Flame Photometer* for measuring sodium and potassium electrolytes.
Components shown in lower figure: 1 Filter selector, 2 Digital display, 3 Inspection flap, 4 Fuel adjustment control, 5 Blank control, 6 Coarse sensitivity control, 7 Fine sensitivity control, 8 Decimal push button, 9 Power switch.

the metal being measured is selected by a light filter or prism system and allowed to fall on a photosensitive detector system. The amount of light emitted depends on the concentration of metallic ions present. By comparing the amount of light emitted from the sample with that from a standard solution the amount of electrolyte in the sample can be measured.

Model 410 Clinical Flame Photometer

A basic flame photometer such as the *410 Clinical Flame Photometer* manufactured by Sherwood Scientific is suitable for use in district clinical chemistry laboratories. Sodium and potassium results are displayed in mmol/l.

The 410 photometer can be operated from butane, propane or Natural gas. It is supplied with filters, standard solutions and instruction manual. An air compressor and fuel regulator are essential to operate the flame photometer. A source of clean, dry, pulse-free compressed air at a pressure of 12–15 psi is required. To achieve this, the air compressor model 851 is recommended as this incorporates a moisture trap (needed in tropical climates).

With the *410 Clinical Flame Photometer*, measurements can be semi-automated by using model *805 Clinical Dilutor* which dilutes the samples 1 in 200 for the measurement of sodium and potassium. Further details of the *410 Clinical Flame Photometer*, price and local availability can be obtained from Sherwood Scientific (see Appendix 11). The manufacturer's instructions must be followed exactly regarding the use, cleaning and maintenance of the flame photometer.

Quality control when using a flame photometer

The following are important when measuring sodium and potassium using a flame photometer:

- Collect the specimen correctly. The blood must not be collected from an arm receiving an electrolyte or dextrose intravenous infusion. Haemolysis of the specimen must be avoided and the plasma or serum must be separated from the cells within $2\frac{1}{2}$ hours. A suitable anticoagulant is lithium heparin. An anticoagulant which contains sodium or potassium must not be used. If preferred, *fresh* serum can be used.
- Dilute the serum or plasma accurately preferably using model *805 Clinical Dilutor* when using the *410 Flame Photometer* A diluent recommended by the manufacturer of the instrument should be used. This must be free from bacteria and moulds. A suitable preservative to prevent the

growth of moulds is formalin (1–2 drops per litre of diluent). Commercially prepared diluents contain preservatives.

Note: Small strands of fibrin, bacteria, or moulds can cause inaccuracies by interrupting or blocking the flow of sample through the nebulizer.

- Prepare standards accurately or preferably use those supplied by the manufacturer. The standards should be stored in plastic (polypropylene) containers to prevent sodium contamination which can occur if glass bottles are used.
- Use chemically clean containers to prevent contamination of samples. Do not use the thumb to cover containers during mixing because perspiration from the thumb contains a high concentration of electrolytes.
- Clean the components of the flame photometer regularly and maintain it as instructed by the manufacturer. The nebulizer needs to be well rinsed after use.
- Make sure that the gas supply is of the correct pressure and of the type recommended for use with the flame photometer.
- Use an air supply that is clean, free from water, and at the correct pressure. If condensation in the air supply tubing (due to conditions of high temperature and humidity) is a problem, an air compressor with a water separator should be used such as that available for use with the *410 Clinical Flame Photometer*.
- Include control samples with each batch of tests.

ISE measurement of sodium and potassium

Principle of ISE analysis: Structurally an ISE analyzer is based on an electrochemical cell. ISE analyzers measure (sense) the electrochemical *activity* of ions whereas flame photometers measure the *concentration* of ions. Activity values are lower than concentration values, e.g. at a sodium concentration of 140 mmol/l in normal plasma the measured sodium activity would be about 105. To avoid confusion, most ISE analyzer manufacturers adjust the activity measurements of their instruments to give readings that are compatible with the concentration results given by flame photometers. The necessary adjustment is made by using specially formulated calibration solutions (produced by the manufacturers) and therefore these solutions *cannot* be interchanged between instruments.

Sodium ISE: This is made of special glass which is selective for sodium, i.e. only sodium ions are free to move to any extent.

Potassium ISE: This is usually constructed from polyvinyl chloride (PVC) in which the antibiotic valinomycin is immobilized. The valinomycin selectively transports potassium ions across the membrane.

Reference electrode: This is usually a calomel (Hg/Hg_2Cl_2) or silver chloride (Ag/AgCl) electrode. The electrical potential of the reference electrode must remain constant for long periods.

Note: The purchase price of an ISE analyzer and particularly its running costs can be very high.

Quality control when using an ISE analyzer

Regular maintenance of an ISE analyzer on a daily basis is *essential* to ensure its reliable performance. This includes cleaning the fluid transport system and other components, maintaining the electrodes, performing the required calibrations, and using controls as instructed by the manufacturer.

Interpretation of sodium and potassium test results

Approximate reference (normal) ranges

Sodium:
134–146 mmol/l (134–146 mEq/l)

Potassium:
Adults: 3.6–5.0 mmol/l (3.6–5.0 mEq/l)
Newborns: 4.0–5.9 mmol/l (4.0–5.9 mEq/l)
Values are highest immediately after birth.

Sodium
Increases
An elevated sodium level is known as hypernatraemia. It is nearly always due to dehydration with the rise in sodium (also chloride and urea) being due to a concentrating effect. It is usually brought about by a reduction of body water content by fluid loss without a compensatory reduction in sodium content, rather than a dietary overload, although excessive IV saline is a potential factor.

Typical causes of hypernatraemia are:
– Severe vomiting
– Prolonged diarrhoea
– Profuse sweating, fever
– Polyuria, as in diabetes
– Hyperaldosteroidism
– Cushing's syndrome
– Inadequate water intake
– Accidental ingestion of sea water.

Note: A high sodium level must be reported as soon as possible. Severe hypernatraemia (sodium level that has reached 155 mmol/l) is a serious finding which requires immediate correction to prevent coma and death.

Decreases
A low sodium level is known as hyponatraemia. It is a commoner finding than hypernatraemia. A greatly reduced level (as low as 125 mmol/l) indicates a dangerous condition and must be reported as soon as possible.

A low sodium level may accompany any severe illness including viral and bacterial infections, malaria, heart attacks, heart failure, strokes, and tumours of the brain and lung. Other causes of hyponatraemia include:
– Surgery or severe accident.
– Treatment with diuretics.
– Side effect of some drugs.
– When loss of salt and water (e.g. by vomiting, diarrhoea or excessive sweating) is replaced by water only.
– Loss of sodium in the urine as in severe renal impairment and salt-losing nephritis.
– Hypoadrenalism (Addison's disease). In tropical countries hypoadrenalism can be caused by tuberculosis of the adrenal glands.

Potassium
Increases
A raised potassium level is known as hyperkalaemia. Levels above 6.5 mmol/l are particularly dangerous and must be reported *immediately* because fatal disorders of heart rhythm can occur suddenly.

Typical causes of hyperkalaemia are:
– Excessive IV infusion, or increased ingestion of potassium.
– Reduced renal excretion, renal failure with oliguria, anuria, acidosis.
– Addison's disease.
– Hypoaldosteronaemia.
– Leakage of cellular potassium following: acute starvation, gross haemolysis, diabetic ketoacidosis, dehydration, severe tissue injury.

Falsely high potassium result: This can occur if a blood sample is haemolyzed due to poor venepuncture technique, a sample is left for a long time (e.g. overnight) without the plasma or serum being removed or if whole blood is refrigerated before it is centrifuged. Red cells contain a high concentration of potassium.

Decreases
A low potassium level is called hypokalaemia. The depletion of potassium can be masked by the

topping up of the plasma levels from intracellular sources and clinical symptoms may present in the face of apparently normal values. These include weakness, tetany, polyuria and ECG changes.

Causes of hypokalaemia include:
- Inadequate intake of potassium in the diet and long term starvation.
- Increased loss of potassium due to prolonged vomiting or diarrhoea, renal tubular failure, diuretics, hyperaldosteroidism.
- Redistribution from plasma into cells; insulin therapy, metabolic or respiratory alkalosis.

Note: In the management of patients with salt and water depletion a simple test for urine chloride may be of value when facilities are not available for measuring serum or plasma electrolytes (see following text).

Table 6.4 Laboratory test results in losses of body fluid

LOSS OF WATER ALONE*
* Literally dehydration caused by water deprivation, e.g. in the very young or unconscious person, or during drought.
Laboratory findings after about 36–48 h without water (12–24 h in infants) include:

Blood tests
- Increased sodium and chloride
- Increased total protein
- Increased urea
- Raised packed cell volume (haematocrit)
- Increased haemoglobin

Urine tests
- Raised specific gravity
- Increased sodium and chloride
- Ketones detected (late stages)
- Protein detected (late stages)
- Red cells and casts may be found (late stages)

LOSS OF WATER WITH ELECTROLYTES*
* Commonly caused by diarrhoea, vomiting, excessive sweating, or burns.
Laboratory findings in moderate to severe water and salt depletion include:

Blood tests
- Normal or reduced sodium and chloride
- Increased urea (late stages)
- Raised packed cell volume
- Increased haemoglobin

Urine tests
- Reduced specific gravity
- Absent or reduced sodium and chloride

SEMIQUANTITATIVE ESTIMATION OF CHLORIDE IN URINE

When unable to measure plasma electrolytes, a simple test to estimate chloride in urine may be of

value in the management of patients with salt and water depletion. Loss of water together with dissolved salts results in the conservation of sodium and chloride by the kidneys and therefore a lower concentration of sodium chloride in the urine.

Depending on the amount of sodium chloride excreted in the urine a patient can be classified as having mild, moderate, or severe salt and water depletion.

Principle of test

When acidified silver nitrate is added to urine, silver chloride is the only salt which is precipitated. The degree of precipitation (cloudiness) is therefore a measure of the chloride concentration in the urine.

Reagents
- Acidified silver nitrate   Reagent No. 5
- Standard solutions containing 150, 75, 50, 30, 7.5, 3.0 mmol/l sodium chloride

Preparation of sodium chloride standards 150, 75, 50, 30, 7.5, 3.0 mmol/l

1 Take six large tubes and label them 150, 75, 50, 30, 7.5, and 3.0.

2 Pipette into each tube as follows:

Tube	Distilled water	Physiological saline
150	–	10.0 ml
75	5.0 ml	5.0 ml
50	6.7 ml	3.3 ml
30	8.0 ml	2.0 ml
7.5	6.5 ml	0.5 ml
3.0	9.8 ml	0.2 ml

3 Stopper each tube and mix well.

4 Take six small tubes (2 to 5 ml capacity) and label them 150, 75, 50, 30, 7.5, and 3.0 mmol/l.

Transfer 1 ml from each of the larger tubes to the set of small tubes.

5 Add 1 ml of acidified silver nitrate reagent to each of the small tubes, stopper and mix.

Caution: Do not mouth-pipette the reagent because it is corrosive. Handle it with care because although colourless it will stain skin, clothes, bench surfaces, etc, and the brown colour is difficult to remove.

Note: The small standard tubes can be kept for 3 or 4 days providing they are kept tightly stoppered and in a cool place.

Method of estimating urinary chloride

1 Pipette 1 ml of clear urine into a test tube of the same size as the small standard tubes.

   If the urine is cloudy, filter or centrifuge it to obtain a clear sample for testing.

2 Add 1 ml of acidified silver nitrate reagent to the urine and mix.

   Caution: The reagent is corrosive. Also handle it with care because although colourless it will stain skin, clothes, bench surfaces, etc, and the brown colour is difficult to remove.

3 Examine the urine for a cloudiness. Estimate the approximate concentration of chloride in the urine by matching the cloudiness with the standards. Matching is best carried out against a dark background.

4 Report the approximate chloride concentration in the urine in mmol/l.

Note: If the urine remains clear after adding the reagent report the test as 'no chloride detected'. Use a 'normal' urine as a positive control.

Interpretation of results
The sodium chloride content in urine from a patient with moderate to severe salt and water depletion will be less than 10 mmol/l (or less than 20 mmol/l per 24 h). The salt deficiency will not be corrected until the amount of sodium chloride being excreted reaches 65 mmol/l or more.

6.11 Urine clinical chemistry tests

Urine production: Urine is produced and excreted by the kidneys. Each kidney contains over 1 million functional units called nephrons. The filtration part of each nephron consists of a cup-shaped structure called the Bowman's capsule which surrounds a mass of blood capillaries called the glomerulus. Each Bowman's capsule leads into a complex nephron tubule (renal tubule).

The pressure in the glomerulus is higher than that in the capsule and this results in water, glucose, electrolytes, amino acids and the waste products of metabolism (urea, creatinine, uric acid) passing from the blood into the capsule. The water and substances filtered from the blood as it passes through the kidneys is known as the glomerular filtrate. It passes from the Bowman's capsule into the renal tubule. About 2 ml of glomerular filtrate is normally produced per second. This is known as the glomular filtration rate (GFR).

As the filtrate passes through the tubule, the proximal tubular cells reabsorb most of the water and those substances which the body requires, e.g. glucose, amino acids, and electrolytes. These pass into the blood in the capillary network which surrounds the renal tubule and eventually re-enter the circulation. Further water is reabsorbed depending on the body's needs. If the plasma is concentrated the level of antidiuretic hormone (ADH) is increased which allows more water to pass through the wall of the tubule and into the circulation. When the body needs to excrete more water, ADH falls which results in more water being excreted in the urine.

In the proximal (beginning) tubules most of the sodium (Na^+) is reabsorbed. Reabsorption of the remainder of the sodium in the distal (furthest) convoluted tubules and collecting ducts depends mainly on the hormone aldosterone. When plasma volume is reduced, e.g. in dehydration, aldosterone secretion is increased which causes the distal tubules to reabsorb most or all of the sodium and return it to the extravascular fluid (plasma and fluid surrounding the tissues). Sodium is the most important osmotically active ion in the body's fluids. When plasma sodium increases, the extracellular fluid becomes hypertonic, causing water to pass (by osmosis) from the intracellular fluid to the stronger extracellular fluid until the osmotic pressure balance between the two fluids is restored.

Because the electrical charge of the ions retained and excreted must be kept balanced in the body, sodium reabsorption is associated with hydrogen (H^+) or potassium (K^+) excretion and the reabsorption of chloride (Cl^-) and bicarbonate (HCO_3^-).

Certain substances, e.g. drugs such as penicillin are not filtered from the blood as it passes through the glomerulus but are cleared from the blood by being secreted into the renal tubule. Hydrogen ions and ammonia are also secreted into the filtrate to maintain the correct acid-base balance in the body.

Urine changes in disease
As explained in the previous text, the production and composition of urine depend on glomerular filtration, tubular reabsorption and tubular secretion. Changes that can occur in the volume, appearance, constituents, and mass density (specific gravity) of urine in disease are as follows:

Volume

The volume of urine excreted daily depends on fluid intake, diet, climate, and other physiological factors. It is usually between 1–2 litres per 24 hours.

An increase in the volume of urine is called polyuria. It occurs in diabetes mellitus due to an increase in the osmolality of the filtrate preventing the normal reabsorption of water (osmotic diuresis). Polyuria also occurs when the secretion of the antidiuretic hormone is reduced, e.g. in diabetes insipidus.

A decrease in the volume of urine excreted is called oliguria. It occurs when the renal blood flow and, or, glomerular filtration rate are reduced. One of the causes of a reduced renal blood flow is low blood pressure (hypotension) caused for example by severe dehydration or cardiac failure. A fall in glomerular filtration rate occurs in acute glomerulonephritis (inflammation of the kidney glomeruli) and also in the early stages of acute tubular necrosis.

If severe oliguria progresses to a complete cessation of urine flow, this is called anuria and is usually due to severe damage to the renal tubules (acute tubular necrosis). Acute tubular necrosis may follow any of the conditions which cause severe hypotension or may be due to a direct toxic effect on the tubules by drugs or following an incompatible blood transfusion.

Appearance

Normal freshly passed urine is clear and pale to dark yellow in colour. A dilute urine appears pale in colour and a concentrated one has a dark yellow appearance. The yellow colour is due to the pigments urochrome, urobilin, and porphyrins.

When normal urine has been allowed to stand for some time, a white phosphate deposit may form if the urine is alkaline (dissolved by adding a drop of acetic acid) or a pink uric acid deposit may form if the urine is highly acidic or concentrated (disappears on warming). A 'mucus' cloud may also form if normal urine is left to stand.

The appearance of urine may be altered in many conditions including:

- Urinary tract infections in which the urine appears cloudy because it contains pus cells and bacteria.

- Urinary schistosomiasis in which the urine often appears red and cloudy because it contains blood (haematuria).

- Malaria haemoglobinuria (blackwater fever) and other conditions causing intravascular haemolysis in which the urine appears brown and cloudy because it contains free haemoglobin (haemoglobinuria).

- Jaundice in which the urine may appear yellow-brown or green-brown because it contains bile pigments or increased amounts of urobilin (oxidized urobilinogen).

- Bancroftian filariasis in which the urine may appear milky-white because it contains chyle.

Composition and pH

The composition of urine is greatly dependent on diet and the metabolic activities of the body's cells. In health, urine contains water which makes up about 95% of the urine, electrolytes including sodium, potassium, magnesium, chloride, and bicarbonate, and the waste products of metabolism including urea, uric acid, and creatinine. Urine also contains surplus acids and alkalis (in buffered form) to maintain the acid-base balance in the body.

The normal reaction of freshly passed urine is slightly acid, around pH 6.0.

Abnormal *chemical* constituents in urine include:

- Protein which can be found in the urine of persons with urinary schistosomiasis, urinary tract infections, nephrotic syndrome, renal diseases such as pyelonephritis and glomerulonephritis, and renal tuberculosis. It may also be found in urine from pregnant women and sometimes from healthy young individuals.

- Glucose which may be found in the urine of diabetic patients and occasionally in some healthy individuals.

- Ketones which can be found in the urine of untreated diabetic patients or persons suffering from starvation.

- Bilirubin which can be found in the urine of persons with hepatocellular jaundice or cholestatic (obstructive) jaundice.

- Urobilinogen (in increased amounts), which can be found in the urine of those with conditions causing abnormal haemolysis.

- Nitrite which can be found in the urine of patients with urinary tract infection caused by nitrate-reducing bacteria.

- Blood which can be found in the urine in urinary schistosomiasis, bacterial infections, acute glomerulonephritis (inflammation of the glomeruli of the kidneys), sickle cell disease, leptospirosis, infective endocarditis, calculi (stones) in the urinary tract, malignancy of the urinary tract, and haemorrhagic conditions.

  Free haemoglobin in urine can be found in malaria haemoglobinuria and other conditions that cause intravascular haemolysis.

Relative mass density (specific gravity)

The normal mass density (specific gravity) of urine varies from 1.002–1.025 depending on the state of hydration of the person and the time of day. It is highest at the beginning of the day. Normal mass density is mainly proportional to the urea and sodium concentrations in the urine.

In renal failure, the ability of the kidneys to concentrate and dilute urine is reduced. Normal concentrating power can be assumed if the mass density of a urine sample is 1.018 or over.

Unusually high mass density measurements may be found when the urine contains glucose, protein, or other heavy particles.

Urine clinical chemistry tests

This subunit describes the testing of urine for:

1 Protein
2 Glucose
3 Ketones
4 Bilirubin
5 Urobilinogen
6 Haemoglobin and whole blood
7 Nitrite and leukocyte esterase
8 Mass density (specific gravity)

---

1   TESTING URINE FOR PROTEIN

Proteinuria: Most plasma proteins are too large to pass through the glomeruli of the kidney. The small amount of protein which does filter through is normally reabsorbed back into the blood by the kidney tubules. Only trace amounts of protein (less than 50 mg per 24 h) can therefore be found in normal urine. These amounts are insufficient for detection by routine laboratory tests.

When more than trace amounts of protein are found in urine this is termed proteinuria. The condition is often referred to as albuminuria because when there is glomerular damage most of the protein which passes through the glomerular filter is albumin because this protein molecule is smaller than most of the globulins.

The following methods are used to test for proteinuria:

■ Protein reagent strip tests
■ Sulphosalicylic acid test

Note: The heat coagulation test (boiling test) is not recommended because it involves boiling urine specimens which can be dangerous.

Protein reagent strip tests

Urine protein strip tests detect mainly albumin. The test area is impregnated with the indicator tetrabromophenol blue (Bayer) or a tetrabromophenol-phthalein ethyl ester (Roche) and buffered to an acid pH. In the presence of protein there is a change in the colour of the indicator from light yellow to green-blue depending on the amount of protein

present. The urine specimen must be fresh.

The strips are very sensitive, detecting as little as 0.1 g/l (10 mg%) of albumin. The reaction is unaffected by turbidity in the urine. Proteins such as globulin, mucoprotein, haemoglobin, and Bence Jones protein give only weak reactions.

Commercially available protein test strips include:

● *Albustix* (Bayer) which measures albumin semi-quantitatively:
   Scale: Negative, trace, + 0.3 g/l, ++ 1 g/l, +++ 3 g/l, ++++ 20 g/l or more
● *Uristix* (Bayer) which measures protein semi-quantitatively and also detects glucose. *Combur 3 Test E* (Roche) measures protein semi-quantitatively and also detects glucose and blood. Other strips with protein testing areas can be found in Chart 6.3 at the end of this subunit.

False strip test reactions

False positive results may be obtained when the urine is contaminated with disinfectants which contain quaternary ammonium compounds or chlorhexidine. Strongly alkaline urine may also give false positives and overstated results, and also if the urine is contaminated with vaginal or urethral secretions.

Roche literature also mentions that false positive results may be obtained during or after an infusion with the plasma expander polyvinylpyrrolidone.

Note: The control of urine reagent strips is described at the end of this subunit.

Sulphosalicylic acid test

This test is based on the precipitation of protein, particularly albumin, by sulphosalicylic acid.

Reagent

– Sulphosalicylic acid, 200 g/l   Reagent No. 66 (20% w/v)

Method

1 Take two tubes and label one 'C' for comparison and the other 'T' for test.
2 Pour about 2 ml of clear urine into each tube.
   Note: If the urine is cloudy, filter or centrifuge it to obtain a clear sample.
3 Using pH papers or neutral litmus paper, test the reaction of the urine. If neutral or alkaline, add a drop of glacial acetic acid to each tube and mix.
   Caution: Glacial acetic acid is a corrosive and flammable chemical, therefore handle with care away from an open flame.

4   Add 2–3 drops of the sulphosalicylic acid reagent to tube 'T'.

5   Holding both tubes against a dark background, examine for any cloudiness in tube 'T' compared with tube 'C'. Report the appearance in tube 'T' as follows:

No cloudiness	Negative
Slight cloudiness	Protein +
Moderate cloudiness	Protein + +
Marked cloudiness	Protein + + +
Cloudiness with precipitate	Protein + + + +

False sulphosalicylic acid test reactions

False positive reactions may occur if the urine is tested while the patient is receiving tolbutamide (a hypoglycaemic drug), or intensive therapy with penicillin, *para*-aminosalicylic acid, or sulphonamides. False positive reactions may also occur if the specimen is collected following an intravenous pyelogram (IVP) or an intravenous infusion of the plasma expander polyvinylpyrrolidone.

A high concentration of urates in the urine may cause a false positive result due to precipitation of urate in an acidic urine.

Causes of proteinuria

– Glomerular or tubular urinary disease.
  Proteinuria accompanies acute glomerulonephritis and is due to increased permeability of the glomerular basement membrane. The degree of proteinuria reflects the severity of the condition and helps in assessing prognosis and response to treatment.

– HIV associated renal disease and treatment with nephrotoxic antiretroviral drugs.

– Pyogenic or tuberculous pyelonephritis.

– Severe lower urinary tract infection.

– Nephrotic syndrome which is a condition characterized by heavy proteinuria and oedema. The oedema is caused by a reduction in the colloid osmotic pressure due to a fall in the level of plasma albumin brought about when proteinuria rises to 5 or 10 g/l per day.

– Eclampsia when there is moderate to marked proteinuria.

– Urinary schistosomiasis which is usually accompanied by both proteinuria and haematuria.

– Severe febrile illnesses including malaria.

– Occasionally in diabetes (see also following text (*Microalbuminuria*). Diabetic nephropathy sometimes causes a nephrotic syndrome.

– Hypertension.

– Accompanying haematuria.

Note: Proteinuria should always be considered to indicate underlying disease until proved otherwise.

Important: Whenever proteinuria is found, the urine should be examined for bacteria, pus cells, red cells, and casts.

Microalbuminuria
In poorly controlled diabetic patients the finding of albumin in the urine often indicates the development of renal disease (diabetic nephropathy). Only a very small amount of albumin is excreted usually below that which can be detected by the routine protein reagent strip tests or chemical tests. An immunological test strip, to detect microalbuminuria called *Micral-Test* is available from Roche Diagnostics but the strip is very expensive. An alternative technique is to use the semi-quantitative nigrosin assay developed by Kutter *et al* which has a cut-off point of 50 mg/l of albumin.[16]

Bence Jones protein in urine

Bence Jones protein is an abnormal low molecular weight globulin consisting of monoclonal free light chains of immunoglobulins. It may be found in the urine of patients with multiple myeloma which is a malignant disease of the plasma cells, mainly affecting bone.

If myeloma is suspected, urine protein electrophoresis is required to demonstrate Bence Jones protein, and serum electrophoresis to detect the paraprotein 'M' (monoclonal immunoglobulin). Haematological investigations are also required, including a bone marrow examination.

Heat-precipitation test: This test is based on demonstrating a protein in urine which precipitates at 40–60 °C and redissolves upon cooling. The test lacks sensitivity and specificity and should not be used as a screening test for myeloma.

---

2   **Testing urine for glucose**

Glycosuria: Almost all the glucose which passes from the blood into the glomerular filtrate is normally reabsorbed back into the circulation by the kidney tubules. Usually less than 0.8 mmol/l (15 mg%) is excreted in the urine. The term glycosuria (or more correctly glucosuria) refers to the presence of more than the usual amount of glucose in the urine.

Renal threshold for glucose
The highest level that the blood glucose reaches before glycosuria occurs is referred to as the renal threshold for glucose. In health it is about 9–10 mmol/l (160–180 mg%) which represents the normal maximum reabsorptive capacity of the kidney tubules. The threshold is lower in persons suffering from renal insufficiency

Requests for tests to detect glycosuria are usually made to screen for diabetes mellitus. The semiquantitative estimation of glucose in a series of urine specimens from a known diabetic patient can provide information on the degree of blood glucose control.

The following methods are used to test for glycosuria:

- Glucose reagent strip tests
- Benedict's test

Glucose reagent strip tests

A reagent strip test is recommended in preference to Benedict's test for detecting glycosuria because it is specific and more sensitive for glucose.

Several urine glucose strip tests are commercially available. They are based on a glucose oxidase reaction. Glucose is oxidized to gluconolactone by the enzyme glucose oxidase (specific for glucose) with the release of hydrogen peroxide. A chromogen is then oxidized by the hydrogen peroxide and a peroxidase enzyme is used to convert the chromogen from a reduced colourless state to a coloured oxidized state.

The various glucose reagent strips differ from one another chemically as regards the type of chromogen and buffer system used. There are also differences in the stability and sensitivity of the different strips and the degree of interference from substances other than glucose which may be present in the urine. The manufacturers' literature must therefore be read carefully.

Strips that measure glucose semiquantitatively in urine are recommended. These include:

- *Diastix* (Bayer) which detects 5.5 mmol/l of glucose and measures it semiquantitatively up to 111 mmol/l (2%).

  Scale: Negative, 5.5, 14, 28, 55, 111 mmol/l or more.

- *Diabur-Test 5000* (Roche) which detects 5.5 mmol/l of glucose and measures it semiquantitatively up to 280 mmol/l (5%).

  Scale: Negative, 5.5, 14, 28, 56, 111, 167, 280 mmol/l.

Note: The Bayer strip test *Clinistix* only detects glucose (qualitative test), it does not measure it semiquantitatively like *Diastix* and *Diabur-Test 5000*.

Note: Glucose test areas can also be found with ketones on the test strips *Keto-Diastix* (Bayer) and *Keto-Diabur-Test* (Roche) and also on several other test strips as listed in Chart 6.3 at the end of this subunit.

False strip test reactions

A number of urinary or contaminating substances may give false negative or false positive glucose strip test results. The most commonly occurring of these interfering substances are as follows:

- Oxygen receptors in the urine, i.e. substances which (when present in moderate to large amounts) can be oxidized by the hydrogen peroxide in preference to the chromogen. This can lead to a loss in sensitivity of the strip. Such substances include ascorbic acid* and certain drug metabolites.

  * The effect of ascorbic acid on Roche manufactured strips has been largely eliminated so that at glucose concentrations of 5.5 mmol/l (100 mg/dl) and above, even high ascorbic acid concentrations are not likely to give false negative test results.

- Moderate to large amounts of acetoacetate in urine as can be found in specimens from out-of-control diabetic patients, may interfere and give misleading results with some strips (read the manufacturer's literature).

- Catalase, when present in high concentration in the urine (as in severe *E. coli* infections) can destroy hydrogen peroxide and so cause a false negative result.

- Disinfectants such as bleach which oxidize the chromogen directly and therefore cause a false positive reaction.

Note: The control of urine reagent strips is described at the end of this subunit.

Benedict's test

When boiled in alkaline copper sulphate, glucose and other sugars, reduce cupric (copper II) ions to red-brown cuprous (copper I) oxide, the degree of reduction corresponding to the concentration of reducing substance present.

Benedict's test can be performed using:

- a solution reagent
- dry reagents

The dry reagent method uses chemicals to generate the heat necessary for boiling the mixture whereas in the solution reagent method heat is applied to boil the mixture.

Note: Whenever possible the Benedict's test should be replaced by a glucose-specific strip test. Benedict's test is described for those laboratories unable to obtain urine strip tests.

SOLUTION REAGENT METHOD

The following reagents are required:

- Benedict's reagent   Reagent No. 11
- Glucose control solution, equivalent to 1.0% of reducing substance.*

*Prepare by dissolving 1 gram of glucose in 100 ml of 1 g/l benzoic acid (see Reagent No. 12). The solution is stable for several months at room temperature (20–28 °C).

Method

1 Take three or more (depending on the number of tests) heat-resistant glass tubes and label as follows:

POS   – Positive control
NEG   – Negative control
1, 2, etc – Patients' tests

2 Dispense 2.5 ml of Benedict's reagent into each tube.

A plastic 2.5 ml syringe or graduated plastic bulb pipette can be used to dispense the reagent. It is not necessary to use a calibrated pipette.

3 Add to each tube as follows:

Tube
POS .... 0.2 ml glucose control solution
NEG .... 0.2 ml of distilled or boiled filtered water
1, 2, etc ..... 0.2 ml of fresh patient's urine
Mix the contents of each tube.

4 Place the tubes in a heat-block set at 100 °C or in a container of boiling water for *exactly* 5 minutes.

5 Remove the tubes and examine the solution in each tube for precipitate and change of colour. Report the sugar concentration as follows:

Appearance of solution	Sugar concentration
Blue, clear or cloudy	Nil
Green, no precipitate	Trace
Green, with precipitate	About 0.5 g%
Brown and cloudy	About 1.0 g%
Orange and cloudy	About 1.5 g%
Red and cloudy	2.0 g% or more

Controls: The negative control (tube NEG) should show the *Nil* reaction. The positive control (tube POS) should show the reaction equivalent to 1.0% of reducing substance.

Note: For the causes of glycosuria, see later text.

Substances which may also reduce Benedict's reagent

These include other sugars which may occasionally be present in urine such as galactose, lactose, fructose, and pentose. Lactose may be present during late pregnancy or lactation.

False positive reactions may also be obtained if certain drugs are present, e.g. salicylates, penicillin, streptomycin, isoniazid, and *p*-aminosalicyclic acid.

Chemicals present in a concentrated urine which may reduce Benedict's reagent include creatinine, urate, and ascorbic acid (reduction is slight).

DRY REAGENT METHOD

Then following reagents are needed:

– Benedict's dry reagent, prepared by grinding and mixing together:

Copper 11 sulphate, 5-hydrate .... 10 g
($CuSO_4.5H_2O$), analytical grade
Citric acid .... 150 g

Store the reagent in a screw-cap container. It is stable indefinitely. It is not hygroscopic.

– Sodium hydroxide or potassium hydroxide pellets

In between use make sure the container cap is completely closed because the chemical is deliquescent.

– Glucose control solution. Prepare as previously described for the solution reagent method.

Method

1 Take three or more (depending on the number of tests) heat-resistant glass tubes, measuring about 12 mm in diameter, and label as follows:

POS   – Positive control
NEG   – Negative control
1, 2, etc – Patients' tests

2 Add a pea-size amount of *well-mixed* dry Benedict's reagent to each tube, i.e. to a depth of about 10 mm in each tube.

3 Using a plastic bulb pipette or glass dropper, add to each tube as follows:

POS .... 3 drops glucose control solution
NEG .... 3 drops of distilled or boiled filtered water
1, 2, etc .... 3 drops of fresh patient's urine
Note: 3 drops should measure about 0.2 ml

4 To each tube in turn, add 1 pellet of sodium hydroxide and shake the tube gently. The mixture will begin to boil. Continue shaking until the boiling stops, observing for any the change of colour or precipitate.

Report the sugar concentration as follows:

Appearance	Sugar concentration
Blue clear or cloudy	Nil or less than 0.2 g%
Slight orange precipitate with blue supernatant	About 0.2 g%
Persistent orange precipitate	About 0.5 g%
Orange precipitate turning brown during boiling	About 1.0 g%
Green-brown precipitate, rapidly turning dark brown	2.0 g% or more

Controls: The negative control (tube NEG) should show the *Nil* reaction. The positive control (tube POS) should show the reaction equivalent to 1.0 g% reducing substance.

Note: See previous text for substances other than glucose that can reduce Benedict's reagent.

Clinitest

Clinitest (Bayer) is a modification of the Benedict's dry reagent test method in tablet form. Each tablet contains copper sulphate, sodium carbonate, sodium hydroxide, and citric acid. As the diluted urine acts upon the tablet, the citric acid is neutralized by the sodium carbonate and sodium hydroxide with the production of intense heat and the release of carbon dioxide. The heat produced brings the mixture to the boil and the copper ions are reduced by the glucose, the degree of reduction corresponding to the concentration of reducing substance present.

In humid tropical climates, *Clinitest* tablets are not stable. They become rapidly unfit for use.

Interpretation of results: Follow the manufacturer's instructions for reporting the test. The reaction is not specific for glucose. Substances which reduce copper ions in the *Clinitest* are similar to those listed for Benedict's test (see previous text). Because the reaction is not specific for glucose, it is possible for a urine to give a positive *Clinitest* but a negative reagent strip test (glucose-specific).

It is also possible to obtain a positive strip test and a negative *Clinitest*. This is because *Clinitest* is unable to detect less than 13.8 mmol/l (250 mg%) of glucose in the urine whereas the strip tests are more sensitive, detecting as little as 5.5 mmol/l (100 mg%) or less of glucose.

Causes of glycosuria

– A rise in the concentration of blood glucose with the kidney tubules being unable to reabsorb the increased amount of glucose in the glomerular filtrate, e.g. in untreated diabetes mellitus.

Raised renal threshold for glucose

If the blood glucose level is high but the filtration rate is slow or the flow of blood to the kidneys is reduced as in heart failure, sodium depletion, or shock, there will be a rise in the renal threshold for glucose. Glucose will not appear in the urine until the blood glucose is well over 10 mmol/l (180 mg%). With diabetes mellitus the renal threshold for glucose is often raised, especially in elderly diabetic patients, those with cardiac failure, or those in diabetic coma with shock.

– A reduced rate of reabsorption of glucose by the kidney tubules as occurs in serious tubular damage or an inherited defect of tubular absorption causing a lowering of the glucose renal threshold. Glucose appears in the urine when the blood glucose level is well below 10 mmol/l (180 mg%). This is often referred to as renal glycosuria.

Fanconi syndrome

When glucose, amino acids, phosphate, and other substances are excreted due to impaired reabsorption this is termed the Fanconi syndrome.

– An increase in the rate of glomerular filtration as may sometimes occur during pregnancy.

Important: The blood glucose level should be measured whenever glucose is found in urine and the patient is not a known diabetic receiving glucose intravenously.

---

3   TESTING URINE FOR KETONES

Ketonuria: Acetoacetate, *beta*-hydroxybutyrate and acetone are collectively referred to as ketone bodies or simply ketones. The excretion of more than a trace of these substances in the urine is called ketonuria.

Formation of ketones: The metabolism of glucose normally provides the body with its energy requirements. If, however, the intake of glucose is insufficient as in starvation, or glucose metabolism is defective due to a lack of insulin as occurs in untreated or uncontrolled diabetes, the body obtains its energy by breaking down fats. It is this increase in fat metabolism which leads to a build up of ketones in the body. An accumulation of ketones in the body is called ketosis.

Ketones are toxic to the brain and if present in sufficiently high concentration in the blood they can contribute to the coma found in diabetic ketoacidosis. Metabolic acidosis is caused by a variety of non-volatile acids accumulating in the plasma of patients with diabetic coma. With coma due to ketoacidosis, ketonuria is always present.

Urine ketone tests detect acetoacetate and acetone. *Beta*-hydroxybutyrate is not detected.

The following methods are used to test for ketonuria:

■ Ketone reagent strip tests
■ Nitroprusside tube or tile test

The reactions of these tests are similar. Acetoacetate and acetone react with sodium nitroprusside* in an alkaline medium to give a violet dye complex. The strips are more sensitive to acetoacetate than acetone.

* The accepted international name for sodium nitroprusside is sodium pentacyanonitrosylferrate.

Important: The urine must be tested soon after it is passed before the acetoacetate is carboxylated to acetone.

Ketone reagent strip tests

Several ketone strip tests are available commercially. They include:

● *Ketostix* (Bayer) which will detect 0.5–1.0 mmol/l of acetoacetate. It is less sensitive to acetone.

    Scale: Negative, + (small), ++ (moderate), +++ (large)

● Similar ketone test areas can also be found with glucose on *Keto-Diastix* (Bayer), and

Keto-Diabur-Test (Roche). The latter strip is particularly useful because it measures urine glucose from 5.5 mmol/l to 280 mmol/l (i.e. up to 5%). Ketone test areas are also included on most of the multiple strip tests (see Chart 6.3 at the end of this subunit).

False reactions

Bayer literature mentions that some high specific gravity/low pH urine samples may give trace positive reactions. False positive reactions (trace) may also occur with highly pigmented urine especially specimens that contain large amounts of L-dopa metabolites.

Roche literature advises that phenylketones and phthanlein compounds give an orange-red colour reaction which is easy to distinguish from the mauve-purple reaction due to ketones. Substances containing sulfhydryl groups may produce false positive results.

Nitroprusside tube or tile test

The nitroprusside tube or tile test is a sensitive technique for detecting ketones in urine. Fresh urine is reacted with a dry reagent containing sodium nitroprusside, ammonium sulphate and sodium carbonate. In an alkaline medium, sodium nitroprusside reacts with acetoacetate and acetone to give a mauve-purple colour.

Reagent

– Nitroprusside dry reagent   Reagent No. 44
The reagent is stable for several months when it is stored in a tightly capped container.

Method

1 Transfer about 0.5–1.0 g (pea-size) of well-mixed nitroprusside reagent to the bottom of a small test tube or to the well of a white porcelain tile.
2 Add 1 drop of fresh urine, sufficient to moisten the reagent.
3 For 1 minute observe the moistened reagent for the development of a mauve-purple colour.
Note: If using a tube, any change in colour can be seen more easily if the tube is held against a white piece of paper.
4 Report the test as follows:

No colour change	Ketones not detected
Slight purple colour	Ketones +
Moderate purple	Ketones + +
Dark purple	Ketones + + +

False reactions

Weak false positive reactions may occur if the urine contains L-dopa or large amounts of phenyl-pyruvic acid (found in the rare disorder phenyl-ketonuria).

Causes of ketonuria

– Untreated diabetes. The finding of ketonuria in a diabetic patient being treated usually indicates an out-of-control state.
– Conditions of starvation when fat metabolism is increased.
– Eating a diet that is very low in carbohydrates.
– Severe dehydration following prolonged vomiting or diarrhoea.
– Glycogen storage disease.

Testing of serum or plasma for ketones

The testing of serum or plasma for ketones can assist in the investigation of hyperglycaemic patients. The same tests that are used to detect ketones in urine can be used to test for ketones in serum or plasma. Results can be interpreted as follows:

● *Negative or weakly positive serum/plasma ketones in hyperglycaemic patient:* This indicates hyperglycaemia with no ketoacidosis (hyperosmolar non-ketotic coma).

● *Strongly positive serum/plasma ketones (ketonuria also present) in hyperglycaemic patient:* This indicates hyperglycaemia with ketoacidosis.

4   TESTING URINE FOR BILIRUBIN

Bilirubinuria: Bilirubin is not normally detected in the urine. When it is found, the condition is referred to as bilirubinuria. Urine containing 8.4 μmol/l (0.5 mg%) or more of bilirubin has a characteristic yellow-brown colour (hepatocellular jaundice) or a yellow-green appearance (obstructive jaundice).

Note: The formation of bilirubin is described in subunit 6.6.

The following methods are used to test for bilirubin in urine:

■ Fouchet's test
■ Bilirubin strip tests

Specimen:

Freshly passed urine is required. It should be protected from daylight and fluorescent light because bilirubin is rapidly oxidized by ultraviolet light to biliverdin which is not detected by the reagents used in the tube or strip tests.

Fouchet's test

This test is recommended for detecting bilirubin in urine because it is sensitive, easy to perform, inexpensive and stable when compared with the strip tests.

Barium chloride is used to precipitate the sulphates in the urine. Any bilirubin present becomes attached to the precipitated barium sulphate. When Fouchet's reagent is added to the precipitate, the iron III (ferric) chloride oxidizes the bilirubin to green-blue biliverdin.

Reagents

– Barium chloride, 0.48 mol/l   Reagent No. 9
  (10% w/v)
– Fouchet's reagent   Reagent No. 30

Method

1 Dispense about 5 ml of *fresh* urine into a tube or small bottle.

    A 5 ml (5 cc) syringe can be used to dispense the specimen. It is not necessary to use a calibrated pipette.

    Note: If the urine is alkaline, acidify it by adding one or two drops of glacial (concentrated) acetic acid.

2 Add 2.5 ml of barium chloride reagent and mix well. The sample will become cloudy.

    A syringe or graduated 3 ml plastic bulb pipette can be used to add the reagent.

3 Filter or centrifuge to obtain a precipitate which will contain any bilirubin that is present. Unfold the filter paper and place it, precipitate upwards, on a piece of absorbent paper.

4 Add 1 drop of Fouchet's reagent to the precipitate on the filter paper or to the sediment in the tube (after discarding the supernatant urine).

5 Report as follows:

Immediate blue-green colour around the drop	Bilirubin positive
No blue-green colour	Bilirubin negative

Note: Any pink-mauve colour which develops is due to salicylates in the urine.

Bilirubin strip tests

Commercially produced strip tests to detect bilirubinuria are expensive and mostly available as multiple test strips (see Chart 6.3 at the end of this subunit). The bilirubin reaction is based on the coupling of bilirubin with 2,6-dichlorobenzenediazonium fluoroborate in an acid medium to give a reddish-violet azo dye. Strip tests have a sensitivity of 7–14μmol/l bilirubin.

False reactions

Sensitivity of urine bilirubin strip tests is reduced by nitrite which may be present with some bacterial urinary infections. Rifampicin and phenazopyridine may mask a small reaction.

False positive reactions may be produced by drugs that colour the urine red or turn red in an acid environment, e.g. phenazopyridine and chlorpromazine metabolites.

Causes of bilirubinuria

Bilirubin can be found in the urine whenever there is an increase of conjugated bilirubin in the blood (see also subunit 6.6). Bilirubinuria occurs therefore in obstructive jaundice and also in hepatocellular jaundice when the blood usually contains both conjugated and unconjugated bilirubin.

Bilirubin is not found in the urine in haemolytic jaundice or in other conditions in which the excess bilirubin in the blood is of the unconjugated type.

In the early stages of viral hepatitis, bilirubinuria together with raised aminotransferase levels can be found before a patient becomes clinically jaundiced.

Note: A chart summarizing the serum and urine findings in the different forms of jaundice can be found in subunit 6.6.

---

5   TESTING URINE FOR UROBILINOGEN

Urobilinogen in urine: As explained in subunit 6.6 it is normal to find small amounts of urobilinogen in the urine derived from that which is reabsorbed from the intestine. The concentration of urobilinogen in the urine is therefore dependent on the amount of bilirubin being produced and entering the intestine and on the ability of the liver to excrete the urobilinogen coming to it from the intestine.

Urine is often tested for increases in urobilinogen when investigating haemolysis or liver disorders in which liver function is impaired.

The following methods are used to test for increased urobilinogen in urine:

■ Ehrlich's test
■ Urobilinogen strip tests

Specimen: Freshly passed urine is required because urobilinogen which is colourless is rapidly oxidized to the orange pigment urobilin which is not detected by Ehrlich's test or by urobilinogen strip tests.

Note: If a delay in testing urine is unavoidable a technique must be used which detects urobilin in urine such as the

Schlesinger test. Details of this test can be found in textbooks of clinical biochemistry.

Ehrlich's test (Watson's modification)

Urobilinogen reacts with *p*-dimethylaminobenzaldehyde to form a red condensation product. The intensity of colour produced corresponds to the concentration of urobilinogen present. Bilirubin interferes with the reaction and therefore if present it must first be removed by reacting the urine with barium chloride.

Reagents

- Hydrochloric acid, 50% v/v   Reagent No. 36
- Ehrlich's reagent   Reagent No. 24
- Chloroform or amyl alcohol

Method

1 Take two small tubes and label one 'T' (test) and the other 'C' (comparison).

2 Dispense 5 ml of *fresh* urine into each tube.

     A 5 ml (5 cc) syringe can be used to dispense the specimen. It is not necessary to use a calibrated pipette.

     Note: If the urine contains bilirubin, mix equal volumes of the specimen with 0.48 mol/l barium chloride (Reagent No. 9). Centrifuge or filter to obtain a clear supernatant or filtrate to test for urobilinogen.

3 Add 0.5 ml of Ehrlich's reagent to tube 'T' and mix.

     Add 0.5 ml of 50% v/v hydrochloric acid to tube 'C' and mix.

4 Leave both tubes at room temperature (20–28 °C) for 5 minutes.

5 *Looking down through the tubes,* examine for a definite red colour in tube 'T' as compared with tube 'C'.

Results

Red colour in tube 'T'	Increased urobilinogen
Pink colour in tube 'T'	Normal urobilinogen
'T' and 'C' appear similar	No urobilinogen

How to check that the red colour is due to urobilinogen and not to porphobilinogen*:

- Add 1–2 ml of chloroform or amyl alcohol. Mix well and allow to settle.

- Look for a red colour in the chloroform or amyl alcohol layer, indicating the presence of urobilinogen. If the red colour is not in this layer it is due to porphobilinogen.*

* Porphobilinogen is excreted in the urine of patients with acute idiopathic porphyria, a rare inherited disease that affects nerves and muscles.

False reactions

A false negative reaction may occur if the urine contains nitrite as in some bacterial urinary infections. The nitrite will oxidize the urobilinogen to urobilin which is not detected by Ehrlich's reagent. A negative reaction may also occur if a patient is receiving intensive antimicrobial therapy. The antimicrobials will reduce the number of bacteria in the intestine and so prevent urobilinogen being formed.

     Besides porphobilinogen, other substances which react with Ehrlich's reagent include the metabolite indican and drugs such as *p*-aminosalicylic acid and sulphonamides.

Note: Heating the test solution, as is sometimes recommended, does not intensify the reaction. The increase in colour produced by heat is due to the presence of indole derivatives.

Urobilinogen strip tests

Commercially produced strip tests to detect and measure urobilinogen in urine are expensive and mostly available as multiple test strips (see Chart 6.3 at the end of this subunit). For strips manufactured by Bayer, the urobilinogen reaction is based on the Ehrlich reaction (as used in the chemical test). For Roche strips, a pink-red azo dye is formed by 4-methoxybenzene-diazonium fluoroborate when it combines with urobilinogen. The strips cannot be used to demonstrate the absence of urine urobilinogen.

False reactions

The strips manufactured by both Roche and Bayer do not react with porphobilinogen within the time specified for the urobilinogen reaction. With phenzaopyridine (found in some disinfectants), a rapid red colour is formed due to the acidity of the buffers impregnating both strips.

     A momentary yellow coloration of the test area is indicative of large amounts of bilirubin but this does not affect the test reading. PAS metabolites may give atypical colours.

Note: The control of reagent strip tests is described at the end of this subunit.

Interpretation of urine urobilinogen results

Increases

- Haemolytic disease when the amount of bilirubin being produced is increased leading to greater amounts of urobilinogen being formed.
- Paralytic ileus or enterocolitis when there is an increase in the production of urobilinogen in the intestine.

– Hepatocellular damage or hepatic congestion, resulting in less of the absorbed urobilinogen being excreted by the liver. The urobilinogen then passes into the general circulation leading to more being excreted by the kidneys.

– Cirrhosis of the liver.

Note: A chart summarizing the serum and urine findings in the different forms of jaundice can be found in subunit 6.6.

Decrease or absence of urine urobilinogen

– Obstruction of bile ducts preventing the flow of bilirubin to the intestine for conversion to urobilinogen.

– Hepatocellular damage preventing the conjugation and excretion of bilirubin for conversion to urobilinogen.

– Absence or reduction of the normal intestinal bacterial flora (necessary to convert conjugated bilirubin to urobilinogen), leading to little or no urobilinogen being produced. This may occur in neonates or following intensive antimicrobial therapy.

Note: In viral hepatitis, urine urobilinogen is at first increased but as liver cell damage increases the small biliary ducts become obstructed leading to a reduction or even an absence of urobilinogen in the urine.

In the recovery stages, urine urobilinogen again increases due to the bilirubin, now in excess, being able to pass through the biliary ducts into the intestine.

---

6   TESTING URINE FOR HAEMOGLOBIN

Haemoglobinuria: The presence of free haemoglobin in urine is called haemoglobinuria. It occurs with severe intravascular haemolysis when the amount of haemoglobin being released into the plasma is more than can be taken up by haptoglobin (the plasma protein that binds free haemoglobin to prevent it being lost from the body). The renal threshold for free haemoglobin is 1.0–1.4 g/l.

The following methods can be used to test for haemoglobinuria:

■ Reagent strip tests
■ Guaiac test

Specimen:
Urine containing haemoglobin appears brown or brown-grey in colour and is usually cloudy. It should be tested as soon as possible after it has been passed.

Urine haemoglobin strip tests

A strip test is a sensitive and simple method of testing for free haemoglobin in urine. The strip tests are based on the ability of haemoglobin and myoglobin (rare) to catalyze the oxidation of a colour indicator by an organic peroxide to give a blue-green complex. A uniform green colouring of the test area indicates the presence of free haemoglobin, or haemolyzed erythrocytes or myoglobin in the urine. A green spotting of the yellow test area indicates the presence of intact red cells in the urine. Differentiation between haemoglobinuria and haematuria is not possible when the urine contains visible amounts of blood. The strips are more sensitive to free haemoglobin than intact red cells.

Commercially produced strip tests that detect haemoglobin in urine include:

● *Hemastix* which is capable of detecting 150–620 µg/l free haemoglobin or up to 5–20 intact red blood cells per microlitre in urines with a relative mass density of 1.005. The test is less sensitive to urine with a high relative mass density.

● Several multiple strip tests also contain areas for detecting free haemoglobin and intact red cells as listed in Chart 6.3 at the end of this subunit. Roche strips have separate colour scales for intact red cells and haemoglobin.

False reactions

False positive reactions can result from the presence of contaminating oxidizing detergents in the urine such as bleach. Heavy proteinuria (i.e. over 5 g/l protein) may reduce the colour reaction. High concentrations of ascorbic acid reduce sensitivity. Captopril may cause decreased reactivity.

Note: The control of reagent strips is described at the end of this subunit.

Guaiac test

This test is described for those laboratories unable to use a reagent strip test. The guaiac test is based on the pseudo-peroxidase property of haemoglobin. Unlike those tests that use carcinogenic benzidine or a o-toluidine chemicals, the reagents used in the guaiac test are not carcinogenic.

Reagents

– Gum guaiac reagent   Reagent No. 33
– Hydrogen peroxide, 30%   Reagent No. 37

Both the above reagents must be freshly prepared.

Method

1 Dispense 5 ml of fresh urine into a heat-resistant glass tube.
2 Add freshly made gum guaiac reagent until a turbidity forms.
3 Add about 10 drops of freshly prepared hydrogen peroxide.
4 Look for a blue colour. If a blue colour develops, boil the urine in a container of boiling water for 15–20 seconds.

Results

Blue colour remains after boiling	Positive test for haemoglobin
Blue colour disappears after boiling	Negative test

Causes of haemoglobinuria

Haemoglobinuria occurs with severe intravascular haemolysis. It is associated with:

– Severe falciparum malaria.
– Typhoid fever.
– Glucose-6-phosphate dehydrogenase (G6PD) deficiency following the ingestion of certain drugs.
– *Escherichia coli* septicaemia.
– Incompatible blood transfusion.
– Snake bites that cause acute haemolysis.
– Sickle cell disease crisis with severe haemolysis.
– Thalassaemia
– Severe viral haemorrhagic fever accompanied by intravascular haemolysis.

Myoglobinuria: This can be found in severe muscle crush injuries.

Note: The microscopical examination of urine for red cells is described in subunit 7.12 in Part 2 of *District laboratory practice in tropical countries.*

7 TESTING URINE FOR NITRITE AND LEUKOCYTES

Nitrite and leukocytes in urine: Urine from a healthy person does not contain nitrite. The detection of nitrite in urine is a useful test in the investigation of urinary tract infections caused by nitrate-reducing bacteria, particularly when cultural facilities are not available. Most pathogenic bacteria reduce the nitrate normally found in urine to nitrite (see later text). The presence of leukocytes in urine indicates inflammation of the urinary tract, the commonest cause of which is a urinary tract infection (see subunit 7.12 in Part 2).

Specimen:
The most suitable specimen for testing is urine that has remained in the bladder for 4–8 hours such as the first passed urine of the morning.

Nitrite and leukocyte strip tests

A nitrite reagent strip which also detects leucocyte esterases is the *Combur 2 Test LN*, manufactured by Roche.

● *Combur 2 Test LN (leukocytes and nitrite)*
The nitrite reaction uses the same principle as the Griess test reaction in which sulphanilamide reacts with nitrite in an acid buffer medium to form a diazonium compound. Together with a coupling component, the diazonium produces a red azo dye, changing the colour of the test area from white to pink. The test detects nitrite in a concentration as low as 11 μmol/l. When first morning urine is tested, the nitrite reaction is positive in about 90% of all urinary tract infections. When testing urine collected at other times, up to 70% of infections will be detected where there is significant bacteriuria.

The leukocyte reaction detects the presence of esterases that occur in granulocytic leukocytes. Esterase enzymes cleave an indoxyl ester. The indoxyl reacts with a diazonium salt to produce a violet colour. Both intact and lyzed leukocytes are detected. The reaction is not affected by bacteria or red cells in the urine. The detection limit is 10–25 leukocytes/μl.

● Nitrite and leukocyte testing areas can also be found on several of the multiple strip tests as listed in Chart 6.3 at the end of this subunit.

False nitrite reactions

A negative reaction will be obtained if an infection is caused by bacteria that do not reduce nitrite. False negatives can occur if the urine has been in the bladder too short a time or the urine is not fresh and the nitrite has decomposed. A false negative reaction may also occur if the urine contains insufficient nitrate. High concentrations of ascorbic acid in the urine can also cause a false negative result with some nitrite strips (check the manufacturer's literature). Sensitivity is reduced when the urine has a high mass density (specific gravity).

False positive results are rare. Drugs containing phenazopyridine can colour the test area pink-red.

Note: Nitrite reagent strip tests deteriorate rapidly in humid conditions. The strips *must* be kept dry.

False leukocyte reactions
Medication with antibiotics containing imipenem, meropenem or clavulanic acid may cause false positive reactions. If the urine is strongly coloured, the colour reaction may be masked. Urinary protein in excess of 500 mg/dl and glucose in excess of 2g/dl may reduce the intensity of the reaction colour as also high daily doses of cephalexin or gentamicin.

Modified Griess tests to detect nitrite in urine
The test is specific for nitrite. The reaction is similar to that described for nitrite reagent strip tests. The method described uses a dry reagent.

Reagent
The Griess test dry reagent is made by grinding and mixing together:

alpha-Naphthylamine .... 6.2 g
Sulphanilic acid .... 1.0 g
Citric acid .... 25.0 g

Caution: Sulphanilic acid is a harmful chemical, therefore handle with care.

Store the reagent in a screw cap container in a cool place. Renew every 3 months.

Method
1 Transfer 0.5–1.0 g (pea-size) of *well mixed* Griess dry reagent to the well of a white porcelain tile or to a small test tube.
2 Moisten the reagent with a fresh sample of urine, preferably the first passed urine of the morning.
3 Look for the immediate development of a red colour and report as follows:

Red colour	Nitrite positive
No red colour	Nitrite negative

Note: The modified Griess test is positive in over 80% of urinary tract infections caused by nitrite forming bacteria.

False reactions with Griess test
These are the same as those described for nitrite strip tests.

Causes of nitrite and leukocytes in urine
Bacteria that produce the enzyme nitrate reductase are able to reduce nitrate in urine to nitrite.

Nitrate-reducing bacteria include:

Escherichia coli	*Aerobacter* species
Proteus species	*Citrobacter* species
Klebsiella species	*Salmonella* species

A negative test cannot rule out a urinary tract infection because the causative organism may be one that does not reduce nitrate to nitrite, e.g. *Enterococcus faecalis*, *Staphylococcus albus*, *Staphylococcus saprophyticus*, *Pseudomonas* species, or *Candida* species. A negative reaction will occur if the nitrate-reducing bacteria are too few in the urine or if the intake of nitrate is insufficient, e.g. a diet lacking in vegetables.

A positive leukocyte esterase reaction indicates inflammation of the urinary tract. The commonest cause is urinary tract infection (see subunit 7.12 in Part 2).

Note: In most cases the leukocyte esterase reaction will still be positive in the urine of a patient suffering from infection of nitrate non-reducing bacteria.

8 MEASURING URINE DENSITY (SPECIFIC GRAVITY)

Mass density of urine: The relative mass density (d), formerly known as specific gravity (SG), of any liquid is its density compared with distilled water which has a density of 1.000. By measuring the mass density of urine, information can be obtained regarding the concentrating and diluting ability of the kidneys.

The following methods are commonly used to test the mass density of urine:
- Urinometer
- Refractometer
- Reagent strip tests

Specimen: This should be the first urine passed at the beginning of the day with the patient having taken no fluid for 10 hours. The testing of random urine specimens has little clinical value.

Urinometer method
This technique uses a specially calibrated hydrometer. The lower the concentration of solutes the further the urinometer will sink in the urine.

A new urinometer must be checked for accuracy by being floated in distilled water. The reading should be 1.000 at the temperature specified on the urinometer. If the reading is not 1.000, subtract the difference in value from each urine reading. For example, if the density of the distilled water is 1.002, subtract 0.002 from each urine reading.

Method
1 Obtain at least 50 ml of urine. Transfer the urine to a cylinder.

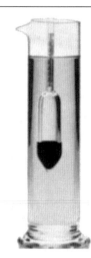

Plate 6.5 Urinometer for measuring urine mass density (specific gravity).

Note: The cylinder and urine must be detergent-free because even a trace of detergent will lower the surface tension of the urine and give an incorrect reading.

2 Immerse the urinometer in the urine and make sure that it floats centrally and does not touch the bottom or sides of the cylinder (see Plate 6.5).

3 Take the reading at the lowest point of the meniscus. This must be done at eye level.
The scale of the urinometer is calibrated from 1.000–1.060 with each division being equal to 0.001.

Adjustment for temperature

Most urinometers are calibrated for use at 15 °C or 20 °C. For each 3 °C difference, 0.001 must be added if above or subtracted if below the calibration temperature.

Example: If the mass density reading of the urine is 1.022 at 23 °C, and the urinometer has been calibrated at 20 °C, the corrected reading is 1.022 + 0.001 = 1.023.

Adjustment for protein

Subtract 0.001 from the mass density reading for every 4 g protein per litre (0.4 g %) of urine.

Adjustment for glucose

Subtract 0.001 from the mass density reading for every 15 mmol/l glucose per litre of urine.

Refractometer method

A refractometer measures refractive index. The measurement is based on the number of dissolved particles in the urine. The higher the concentration of particles, the greater the increase in refractive index (refraction). From refractive index measurements a scale of relative mass density (specific gravity) values can be prepared.

Several models of clinical refractometer for measuring urine relative density (specific gravity) are available, including digital readout models. The most useful, however, are those instruments that also measure serum total proteins such as the bench model Atago T2-NE clinical refractometer shown in Plate 6.6. Urine specific gravity and serum or plasma protein scales of a clinical refractometer are shown in Plate 6.7. The serum protein scale reads 0.0 to 12.0g/100ml and the urine mass density (specific gravity) scale reads 1.000 to 1.050. The T2-NE refractometer measures 150 × 100 × 210 mm and weighs 840g.

Availability: The Atago T2-NE clinical refractometer is available from Atago USA Inc. (see Appendix II).

Method (based on Atago refractometer T2-NE)

1 Check that the instrument scale is correctly adjusted by placing a few drops of distilled water on the face of the prism. Gently close the cover plate. With the refractometer facing the light, bring the scale into focus by turning the eyepiece.

If the boundary line does not coincide with the Wt (water) line, make the necessary adjustment by rotating the scale adjustment knob.

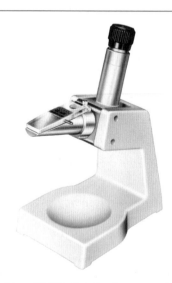

Plate 6.6 Atago T2-NE clinical refractometer for measuring urine specific gravity. Can also be used for measuring serum total proteins.

2 To measure urine specific gravity, place one or two drops of urine on the prism surface as shown in Plate 6.7, and gently close the cover plate.

3 Rotate the eyepiece until the scale becomes clearly visible.

Observe the point on the urine specific gravity scale where the dark part of the field meets the light area (see Plate 6.7). Read off the urine specific gravity value.

Urine specific gravity strip tests

The specific gravity reagent test area responds to the concentration of ions in the urine. It contains certain pretreated polyelectrolytes, the pKa of which changes depending on the ionic concentration of the urine. The indicator bromothymol blue is used to detect the change. Colours range from deep blue-green when the urine is of low ionic concentration, through green to yellow-green when the specimen is of high ionic concentration.

The strip specific gravity test does not indicate the amount of non-ionic urinary constituents present such as urea, creatinine, or glucose.

Specific gravity test areas are found mostly on multiple test strips as shown in Chart 6.3 at the end of this subunit. They are therefore expensive.

The specific gravity (SG) scale covers the range 1.000 to 1.030 in steps of 0.005. Increased accuracy can be obtained by adding 0.005 to the reading if the pH of the urine is pH 7.0 or more.

False reactions

In general the accuracy of reagent strip tests in measuring urine specific gravity is poor compared with urinometer and refractometer methods. Falsely high readings may be obtained if more than 0.1 g/l of protein is present. Highly buffered alkaline urines may cause low readings. Large quantities of divalent cations such as Ca^{2+} produce raised readings.

Note: The control of reagent strips is described at the end of this subunit.

Interpretation of urine relative mass density results

The reference (normal) range for urine relative mass density is 1.010–1.030.

Low values

A consistently low urine mass density usually indicates poor tubular reabsorption.

Excessive fluid intake, however, will also result in a low mass density. In general, the greater the volume of urine excreted the lower is its density and the lighter its colour.

High values

A high urine mass density may be the result of heavy perspiration, dehydration, or to the presence of substances not normally found in urine such as glucose or protein (if not corrected for in the test method).

Concentration of urine expressed as osmolality/kg

This is the best way of expressing the concentration of urine because it depends on the number of osmotically active solute particles per unit of solvent whereas mass density depends on the type as well as the number of solute particles. It is however, much simpler to measure the mass density of urine rather than its osmolality. A mass density of 1.002 is equivalent approximately to an osmolality of 100

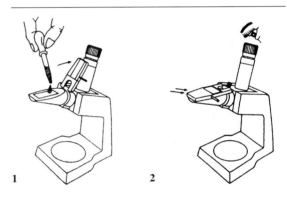

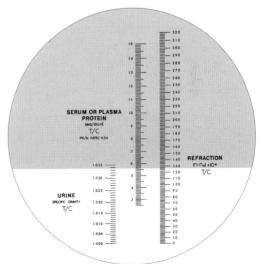

Plate 6.7 *Upper:* How to use the Atago T2-NE clinical refractometer. *Lower:* Left hand lower scale used to measure urine specific gravity. Central scale used to measure serum or plasma total protein in g/100ml (cannot be used for measuring urine total protein).

mosmol/kg and a mass density of 1.025 to about 1000 mosmol/kg.

CONTROL AND SELECTION OF URINE REAGENT STRIP TESTS

A wide range of urine reagent strip tests is available. The strips provide rapid test results and the simpler stable strips are often less expensive than performing chemical tests. The reliability of reagent strip test results depends on the correct urine sample being used, the correct storage, use, and control of the strips, and a knowledge of the causes of false reactions. It is therefore essential to read carefully the literature supplied by the manufacturer which will be found in each strip container.

Correct storage of reagent strips

Read carefully the expiry date and the storage instructions supplied with the strips. To prevent the deterioration of reagent strips the following are important precautions:

- Protect the strips from moisture and excessive heat and light, but do not refrigerate.

  A desiccant (drying agent) is supplied either in the lid of the container (Roche strips) or as a sachet in the container (Bayer strips).

- Remove strips only as required. After removing a strip, replace the container top immediately and tightly to prevent moisture from the air entering. This is particularly important in humid climates. The reagents impregnating the test areas deteriorate rapidly if they become damp. This can happen after only a few minutes of exposure in humid conditions.

Correct use and quality control of reagent strips

The instructions supplied must be followed exactly as regards the urine specimen, use of individual strips, timing of reactions, and reading of test results.

The following general guidelines apply:

- Collect urine samples in clean, dry, detergent-free containers. The urine should be as fresh as possible and well mixed. First-voided morning urine is best (most concentrated). Do not add any preservative/stabilizer.

- Before removing a strip, read how to test the urine. Become familiar with the test areas and possible reactions.

- Do not use strips that show any discoloration of the test areas.

- Do not contaminate a strip by touching the test areas with the fingers or by laying it down on the bench. Avoid using the strips in the presence of chemical fumes.

- Dip the strip *briefly* in the urine making sure that the test areas are fully immersed. Avoid prolonged contact with the urine because this may result in a dissolving out of the reagents from the test areas.

- Remove excess urine from the strip by running the edge of the strip along the rim of the urine container.

- Read carefully the reactions in a good light at exactly the times stated by the manufacturer, particularly when using multiple test strips. Compare the reactions by holding the strip close to the colour chart on the container label, but avoid contaminating the container with urine.

- Be aware of any substances or conditions which can cause a false reaction as described in the manufacturer's literature.

- Do not use strips beyond their expiry date.

Control reference solutions are available from manufacturers for multiple strip tests. The performance of strip tests can also be controlled by checking regularly the strip reactions against those obtained by standard chemical tests. Control urines of known negative and positive reactions should also be prepared and tested with patients' specimens.

Up-to-date manufacturers' literature must always be consulted regarding the quality control of different strips and the substances which may interfere with the various reactions.

Note: A list of the urine strip tests available from Roche and Bayer can be found in the following Chart 6.3. With the exception of *Combur 7 Test, Combur 9 Test* and *Combur 10 Test*, Roche strip tests are available 50 strips per vial. The other three are packaged 100 strips per vial. Bayer multiple (*Multistix*) strips are packaged 100 strips per container. Other strips are available 50 strips per container.

Further information: Up-to-date information about the chemical reactions, use and control of commercially available urine strip tests can be obtained upon request from Bayer Diagnostics and Roche Diagnostics (see Appendix II)

Chart 6.3   **Roche and Bayer reagent strip tests for urine testing**

Reagent strips	Com-pany	Nitrite	pH	Protein	Glu-cose	Ket-ones	Urobil-inogen	Bili-rubin	Blood	Leuko-cytes	SG
Albustix	B			§ Qn							
Clinistix	B				§						
Diabur-Test 5000	R				§ Qn						
Diastix	B				§ Qn						
Ketur-Test	R					§					
Ketostix	B					§					
Combur 2 Test LN	R	§								§ Qn	
Hemastix	B								§		
Uristix	B			§ Qn	§						
Keto-Diabur-Test	R				§ Qn	§					
Combur 3 Test E	R			§ Qn	§				§		
Keto-Diastix	B				§ Qn	§					
Combur 3 Test	R		§ Qn	§ Qn	§						
Hema-Combistix	B		§ Qn	§ Qn	§				§		
Combur 4 Test	R			§ Qn	§ Qn				§	§ Qn	
Combur 4 Test N	R	§	§ Qn	§ Qn	§						
Combur 5 Test	R	§		§ Qn	§ Qn				§	§ Qn	
Combur 5 Test D	R		§ Qn	§ Qn	§	§			§		
Labstix	B		§ Qn	§ Qn	§	§			§		
N Labstix	B	§	§ Qn	§ Qn	§	§			§		
Combur 6 Test	R	§		§ Qn	§		§ Qn		§	§	
Labstix SG	B		§ Qn	§ Qn	§	§			§		§
Combur 7 Test	R	§	§ Qn	§ Qn	§	§			§	§	
Multistix SG	B		§ Qn	§ Qn	§	§	§ Qn	§	§		§
Combur 9 Test	R	§	§ Qn	§ Qn	§	§	§ Qn	§	§	§	
N-Multistix SG	B	§	§ Qn	§ Qn	§	§	§ Qn	§	§		§
Combur 10 Test	R	§	§ Qn	§ Qn	§	§	§ Qn	§	§	§	§
Multistix 8 SG*	B	§	§ Qn	§ Qn	§	§			§	§	§
Multistix 10 SG	B	§	§ Qn	§ Qn	§	§	§ Qn	§	§	§	§

* Also available in 25 pack size, called *Multistix GP*.

Key: B = Bayer Diagnostics (see Appendix II)
R = Roche Diagnostics (see Appendix II)

§ = Substance or reaction tested
Qn = Semi-quantitative result
SG = Specific gravity (relative mass density)

BAYER URINE TABLET TESTS

Name	Substance tested
Clinitest	Glucose and other sugars

Note: Ictotest and *Acetest* are no longer produced.

Note: Strips which contain more than a few test areas are considerably more expensive than the simpler strips and require more skill to read correctly.

6.12 Cerebrospinal fluid chemical tests

The biochemical testing of cerebrospinal fluid (c.s.f.) is performed to assist in the diagnosis of meningitis and other disorders of the central nervous system. It usually includes:

- Measurement of total protein
- Occasionally, measurement of glucose

Other c.s.f. investigations
The testing of c.s.f. for pathogens and cells is included in subunit 7.13 in the microbiology chapter of Part 2 *District laboratory practice in tropical countries*.

Specimen

It is usual to collect two samples of c.s.f. in sterile containers. Sample No. 1 (about 1 ml) is used for culture and sample No. 2 (2–3 ml) is used for microscopy, cell count, and chemical testing.

Sample No. 2 is used for the measurement of glucose and protein because there is less chance of it containing blood if the lumbar puncture is traumatic. If blood is present in the c.s.f. it is unsuitable for cell counting and the measurement of glucose and protein.

---

1   MEASUREMENT OF C.S.F. PROTEIN

Total protein in c.s.f. can be measured by the following methods:

- Colorimetrically using a trichloroacetic acid method.
- Visual comparative semiquantitative method when a colorimeter is not available.

Pandy's test
This is a simple technique that is sometimes used to screen for increases in c.s.f. globulin when it is not possible to measure c.s.f. total protein.

Colorimetric trichloroacetic acid c.s.f. total protein method
Required
- Trichloroacetic acid, 50 g/l   Reagent No. 67

   (5% w/v)

– Protein standards prepared from a protein solution or serum of known protein concentration.

Preparation of protein standards using a serum of known protein concentration

1   Dilute the serum 1 in 10 by mixing 1 ml of serum with 9 ml of physiological saline. Calculate the protein value of the diluted serum by dividing its original value by 10.

   Example: If the protein value of the serum is 78 g/l (7.8 g%), the protein value after dilution will be 7.8 g/l (780 mg%).

2   Take five tubes and number them 1 to 5. Pipette into each tube as follows:

Tube No.:	1	2	3	4	5
ml of saline:	1.9	1.8	1.7	1.6	1.5
ml of diluted serum:	0.1	0.2	0.3	0.4	0.5

Mix well the contents of each tube.

3   Calculate the concentration of protein in each of the five standards as follows:

   No. 1:   Divide value of *diluted* serum   by 20
   2:                                  by 10
   3:                                  by 6.6
   4:                                  by 5.0
   5:                                  by 4.0

Preparation of a calibration graph

1   Take five tubes and label them 1 to 5.

2   Pipette 2.4 ml of the trichloroacetic acid reagent into each tube.

   Caution: The trichloroacetic acid solution is corrosive and has an irritating vapour, *do not* mouth-pipette.

3   Add 0.8 ml of standard solution to each tube (standard No. 1 to tube No. 1, etc). Mix the contents of each tube and leave for 5 minutes.

4   Remix each standard solution taking care not to introduce air bubbles. Read the absorbance of each in a colorimeter using a blue filter (e.g. Ilford No. 602) or in a spectrophotometer at wavelength 450 nm. Zero the instrument with distilled water.

5   Take a sheet of graph paper and plot the absorbance of each standard (vertical axis) against its concentration in g/l (horizontal axis). Draw a straight line passing through zero and the points plotted (see subunit 4.10).

Specimen

The method requires 0.8 ml of c.s.f. (usually the supernatant fluid from No. 2 sample). Fluoride-oxalate c.s.f. can also be used.

Method

1   Pipette 2.4 ml of the trichloroacetic acid solution into a tube.

2   Add 0.8 ml of c.s.f. Mix and leave for 5 minutes.

Note: If after adding the c.s.f. a heavy precipitate forms, set up the test again using a 1 in 5 dilution of the c.s.f. (0.2 ml c.s.f. mixed with 0.8 ml of physiological saline gives a 1 in 5 dilution; use 0.8 ml of the diluted fluid). Multiply the result by 5.

Blank solution: If the c.s.f. is coloured yellow or red, prepare a blank solution by adding 0.8 ml of c.s.f. to 2.4 ml of physiological saline.

3   Remix the contents of the tube, taking care not to introduce air bubbles. Read the absorbance of the precipitated protein in a colorimeter using a blue filter (e.g. Ilford No. 602) or in a spectrophotometer set at wavelength 450 nm. Zero the instrument with distilled water or with a blank solution.

4   Read off the concentration of c.s.f. protein in grams per litre (g/l) from the previously prepared calibration graph.

    Note: If the concentration is over 1.5 g/l (150 mg%), repeat the test using a 1 in 5 dilution of the c.s.f. (see previous text). The calibration graph should be linear for values up to 1.5 g/l.

Visual comparative method for measuring c.s.f. total protein

Required

–   Trichloroacetic acid, 50 g/l   Reagent No. 67
    (5% w/v)

–   Protein standards containing 0.44 g/l (44 mg%), 0.88 g/l (88 mg%), and 1.10 g/l (110 mg%) protein

Preparation of protein standard solutions
The standards may be easily prepared from a 22% albumin solution (as used in blood transfusion work), as follows:

1   Take three screw-cap bottles of 50 ml capacity and label them 0.44 g/l, 0.88 g/l, and 1.10 g/l.

    Pipette into each bottle as follows:

Bottle	22% albumin solution*
0.44 g/l (44 mg%)	0.1 ml
0.88 g/l (88 mg%)	0.2 ml
1.10 g/l (110 mg%)	0.25 ml

*If only a 30% albumin solution is available, obtain a 22% solution by mixing 1.6 ml of distilled water with 4.4 ml of the 30% solution.

2   Add 50 ml of distilled water (sterile if possible) to each bottle, stopper, and mix well.

    Store the solutions at 2–8 °C. Renew every month or before they become contaminated.

Method

The method requires 0.5 ml of c.s.f. (usually the supernatant fluid from No. 2 sample).

1   Take four tubes and label them 1, 2, 3, and P (Patient).

2   Pipette into each tube as follows:

Tube:	1	2	3	P
ml of trichloroacetic acid, 50 g/l	1.5	1.5	1.5	1.5
ml of 0.44 g/l standard:	0.5	–	–	–
ml of 0.88 g/l standard:	–	0.5	–	–
ml of 1.10 g/l standard:	–	–	0.5	–
ml of c.s.f.:	–	–	–	0.5

Caution: *Do not* mouth-pipette the trichloroacetic acid or c.s.f. Use a pipette with pipette-filler, a plastic bulb pipette, or a dispenser.

3   Mix the contents of each tube, and leave for 5 minutes.

4   Remix the solutions in each tube, and make an estimate of the approximate amount of protein in the c.s.f. by comparing the cloudiness in the patient's tube (P) with that in each of the three standard tubes.

    Report the approximate protein concentration in grams per litre (g/l).

    Note: It is easier to match the turbidity in the patient's tube with that in the standard tubes if a printed card is held behind the tubes.

Values greater than 1.10 g/l (110 mg%)

If the turbidity in the patient's tube is greater than 1.10 g/l, repeat the test after diluting the c.s.f. 1 in 5 in physiological saline (0.1 ml of c.s.f. added to 0.4 ml of saline will give a 1 in 5 dilution). Multiply the result by 5.

Pandy's globulin test
This screening test detects rises in c.s.f. globulin. It is only of value when it is not possible to perform a total protein estimation.

Required
–   Phenol, saturated solution   Reagent No. 45

Method
Specimen: The test requires one drop of c.s.f. or supernatant c.s.f. sample.

1   Pipette about 1 ml of saturated phenol solution into a small tube.

    Caution: Phenol is a highly corrosive and harmful chemical, therefore *do not* mouth-pipette. Use a graduated plastic bulb pipette or a pipette with pipette-filler.

2 Use a glass dropper or a plastic bulb pipette and holding the tube at eye level against a dark background, add 1 large drop of c.s.f. (supernatant fluid from centrifuged No. 2 sample). Do *not* mix.

3 Look for an immediate cloudiness around the drop of c.s.f., indicating the presence of excess globulin.

Report the test as:

Immediate cloudiness	Pandy's test positive
No cloudiness	Pandy's test negative

Note: After a few minutes the cloudiness may disappear.

Interpretation of c.s.f. protein results
The c.s.f. total protein is normally 0.15–0.40 g/l (15–40 mg%). The range for ventricular fluid is slightly lower. Values up to 1.0 g/l (100 mg%) are normal for newborn infants. Only traces of globulin are found in normal c.s.f. (insufficient to give a positive Pandy's test).

An increase in total protein and a positive Pandy's test occurs in all forms of meningitis, in amoebic and trypanosomiasis meningoencephalitis, cerebral malaria, brain tumours, cerebral injury, spinal cord compression, poliomyelitis, the Guillain-Barré syndrome (often the only abnormality), and polyneuritis. Increases in c.s.f. protein also occur in diseases which cause changes in plasma proteins such as multiple myeloma.

When the total protein exceeds 2.0 g/l (200 mg%), the fibrinogen level is usually increased sufficiently to cause the c.s.f. to clot. This may occur in severe pyogenic meningitis, spinal block, or following haemorrhage.

2 MEASUREMENT OF C.S.F. GLUCOSE

The measurement of c.s.f. glucose may be required to give supportive evidence of meningitis. To help interpret c.s.f. glucose results a serum or plasma glucose test should ideally also be performed. The concentration of glucose in c.s.f. is a half to two thirds of that found in serum or plasma.

Glucose in c.s.f. can be measured as follows:

■ Colorimetrically using a glucose oxidase method.
■ Semiquantitatively using Benedict's reagent if a colorimeter is not available.

Important: c.s.f. glucose must be measured as soon as possible (within 20 minutes) after it has been withdrawn otherwise a false low result will be obtained due to glycolysis. If a delay is unavoidable, sample No. 2 must be collected into fluoride-oxalate

preservative (Reagent No. 27). This will prevent glycolysis. The fluoride-oxalate will not interfere with the measurement of protein.

Note: A reagent strip test that measures blood glucose should not be used for measuring c.s.f. glucose. The blood glucose strips are not calibrated for c.s.f. glucose levels.

Glucose oxidase method for measuring c.s.f. glucose
This is the same method as described for measuring serum or plasma glucose in subunit 6.5 except four times the amount of c.s.f. (fresh or fluoride-oxalate c.s.f. is used (i.e. 0.2 ml) and the result is divided by four. More c.s.f. is used because the concentration of glucose in c.s.f. is much less than that found in serum or plasma and markedly reduced levels occur in meningitis.

Benedict's semiquantitative c.s.f. glucose method
Benedict's method for measuring c.s.f. glucose requires 1 ml of *fresh* or fluoride-oxalated c.s.f. (usually the supernatant fluid from centrifuged No. 2 sample).

Reagent
– Benedict's reagent*　　　Reagent No. 11

　*This is the same reagent solution as used for urine testing.

Method
1 Take five tubes and label them 1, 2, 3, 4, and C (Control). Pipette into each tube as follows:

Tube	1	2	3	4	C
ml of Benedict's reagent:	2.0	2.0	2.0	2.0	2.0
ml of c.s.f.	0.1	0.2	0.3	0.4	–

Caution: Do not mouth-pipette the reagent or c.s.f. A 2 ml syringe or graduated plastic bulb pipette can be used to dispense the reagent, and a pipette with pipette-filler can be used to dispense the c.s.f.

2 Mix the contents of each tube and place all five tubes in a container of *boiling* water for 5 minutes.

3 Remove the tubes and compare the colour of the solutions in tubes 1 to 4 with that in the control tube. Make a note of the tubes in which reduction (R) has occurred. Reduction of the reagent is indicated by a change in colour from blue (as seen in the control tube) to blue-brown.

4 Interpret and report the results as follows:

Reactions					c.s.f. Glucose	
Tube	1	2	3	4	mmol/l	mg%
	–	–	–	–	0–1.1	0–20
	–	–	–	R	1.2–1.7	21–30
	–	–	R	R	1.8–2.2	31–40
	–	R	R	R	2.3–2.8	41–50
	R	R	R	R	>2.8	>50

Key
R = Reduction reaction (blue-brown solution)
– = No reduction (blue solution, like control)
> = Greater than

Interpretation of c.s.f. glucose results
Decreases
Low c.s.f. glucose levels are found in most forms of meningitis, particularly pyogenic meningitis when glucose may even be absent. In viral meningitis however, the c.s.f. glucose is often normal.

Increases
A raised c.s.f. glucose is found when there is a raised blood glucose and sometimes with encephalitis or following damage to cerebral capillaries.

Note: c.s.f. chemical and microbiological findings in meningitis and other diseases of the central nervous system are summarized in subunit 7.13 in the microbiology Chapter of Part 2 of *District laboratory practice in tropical countries*.

6.13 Faecal clinical chemistry tests

Clinical chemistry faecal tests that may be requested in district laboratories include:

■ Testing faeces for occult blood
■ Testing faeces for lactase deficiency
■ Examining faeces for excess fat

---

1 TESTING FAECES FOR OCCULT BLOOD

Bleeding into the gastrointestinal tract may be rapid with the vomiting of blood (haematemesis) or the passage of blood through the rectum (melaena).

When the bleeding is chronic with only small amounts of blood being passed in the faeces, the blood (or its breakdown products) is not recognized in the faeces and is referred to as occult (hidden) blood.

Requests for occult blood testing are usually made to investigate the cause of iron deficiency anaemia or to assist in the diagnosis of bleeding lesions of the gastrointestinal tract, e.g. peptic ulcer, carcinoma, or diverticulosis.

Occult blood can be detected in faeces:

■ Chemically using guaiac based reagents prepared in the laboratory, e.g. aminophenazone test, or ready-made reagent in kit tests, e.g. *Hema-Screen*.

■ Immunologically using a haemoglobin specific cassette or strip test such as the *Instant-View Faecal Occult Blood* test manufactured by Alfa Scientific Designs Inc. (see Appendix 11). Immunological tests are more expensive than chemical tests.

Specificity of occult blood tests: Chemical tests are not specific for haemoglobin. They are based on the principle that haemoglobin and its derivatives react in a similar way to peroxidase enzymes, i.e. they catalyze the transfer of an oxygen atom from a peroxide such as hydrogen peroxide to a chromogen such as guaiacum, 2,6-dichlorophenolindophenol or aminophenazone. Oxidation of the chromogen is shown by the production of a blue, blue-green, or pink colour.

In chemical tests, non-haemoglobin substances with peroxidase activity can therefore cause false positive reactions. Other substances can interfere with peroxidase activity resulting in false negative results. The specificity of chemical tests can be improved by dietary restrictions (see later text).

Immunological occult blood tests are specific for the detection of human haemoglobin in faeces. A monoclonal antibody directed against human haemoglobin is used. This selectively binds to human haemoglobin present in the faeces.

Sensitivity of occult blood tests: Considerable variation of sensitivity is shown by both chemical and immunological occult blood tests. Highly sensitive tests can be misleading because they detect trace amounts of blood which can be found in normal faeces. Highly sensitive chemical tests can give false positive reactions when faeces contain dietary substances which have peroxidase-like activity. Tests of low sensitivity can also be misleading because they may fail to detect small amounts of blood which are pathological.

Choice of occult blood test

In district laboratories the use of an adequately sensitive chemical occult blood test (with dietary restrictions two days before the collection of faeces) is suitable. The aminophenazone chemical test which uses reagents that can be prepared in the laboratory is described.

Alternatively, a kit test which uses guaiac impregnated paper slides, such as the *Hema-Screen* manufactured by Immunostics Inc (see Appendix II) is recommended. *Hema-Screen* is packaged as single tests and the results are easy to interpret with a positive control being incorporated adjacent to the test area.

Benzidine and o-tolidine chemical tests
Tests which use benzidine or *o*-tolidine are not recommended because both these chemicals are known to have carcinogenic properties.

Aminophenazone test

Haemoglobin and its derivatives catalyze the transfer of oxygen from hydrogen peroxide to aminophenazone. Oxidation of the amino-phenazone produces a purple red colour.*

Reagents

– Acetic acid, 10% v/v	Reagent No. 1
– Alcohol, 95% v/v	Reagent No. 6
– Hydrogen peroxide (H_2O_2) 10 vols solution*	Reagent No. 37

* A 10 vols (volume) hydrogen peroxide solution means that 1 volume will give 10 volumes of oxygen at NTP on complete degradation. If the solution available is 100 vols, dilute 1 in 10 with distilled water to obtain a 10 vols solution. Store in a tightly stoppered dark bottle away from light and heat.

Working aminophenazone reagent

The amounts given are sufficient for 1 test with positive and negative controls. Prepare fresh as follows:

Alcohol, 95% v/v .... 15 ml
Acetic acid, 10% v/v .... 1 ml
4-Aminophenazone* (4-aminoantipyrine) ...... 0.4 g

* Accurate weighing is not necessary. For easy preparation, mark a small tube to hold 0.4 g of the chemical. Between use keep the marked tube attached to the bottle of chemical with an elastic band.

Dissolve the aminophenazone in the alcohol solution and *immediately before use* add the acetic acid. Mix well.

Specimen
Two days before collecting the faeces, instruct the patient not to ingest red meat, fish, turnips, spinach, horseradish. Also withdraw drugs, vitamins, and fruit juices that contain ascorbic acid, iron, barium sulphate, cimetidine, and also cough medicine. The patient should eat plenty of vegetables, corn, and non-citrus fruit.

Method

1 Dispense about 7 ml of distilled water into a wide bore test tube.

   A 10 ml syringe may be used to dispense the water.

2 Add a sample of faeces about 10–15 mm in diameter (taken from various parts of the specimen). Using a glass or plastic rod, emulsify the faeces in the water.

3 Allow the faecal particles to settle or centrifuge the emulsified specimen.

4 Take three *completely clean* tubes and label them:

   T   – Patient's test
   Neg – Negative control
   Pos – Positive control

5 Add to each tube as follows:

   T .... 5 ml supernatant fluid from emulsified faeces
   Neg .. 5 ml distilled water
   Pos .... 5 ml distilled water in which about 50 μl of whole blood has been mixed

   A 5 ml syringe may be used to dispense the faecal super-natant fluid and distilled water. It is not necessary to use a calibrated pipette.

6 Layer 5 ml of working aminophenazone reagent on top of the fluid in each tube (i.e. pipette down the side of each tube). Do *not* mix.

7 Add 10 drops of the 10 vols hydrogen peroxide solution. Do *not* mix. Allow to stand for 1 minute.

8 Look for the appearance of a blue colour where the aminophenazone reagent meets the sample or control solutions.

   Report the results as follows:

No colour change	Negative test
Pale red	Positive +
Dark red	Positive + +
Dark red purple	Positive + + +

Negative control: This should show no colour change.

Positive control: This should show a positive reaction.

False reactions
A false positive reaction may occur if the faeces contains peroxidase-like substances. Such reactions may be avoided by dietary restrictions (see *Specimen*).

A false negative reaction may be obtained if the faeces contains a high concentration of ascorbic acid.

Note: If the test is negative but there is high clinical suspicion, two further specimens should be tested to detect bleeding which may be intermittent.

Interpretation of results

The commonest causes of positive occult blood tests in tropical and other developing countries are hookworm infection, peptic ulcer, colitis and bleeding from oesophageal varices due to cirrhosis of the liver.

Other causes include carcinoma in the gastrointestinal tract, erosive gastritis due to alcohol or drugs, or swallowed blood from recurrent nosebleeds.

2   TESTING FAECES FOR LACTASE DEFICIENCY

Lactase is an enzyme which converts lactose to glucose and galactose. If lactase is deficient, lactose is not digested or absorbed but ferments to lactic acid with the production of gas. This causes abdominal pain and diarrhoea which may be persistent and severe especially in young children.

When there is lactase deficiency faecal specimens usually contain lactose and have low pH due to the presence of lactic acid.

Testing lactose in faeces

The simplest method of detecting lactose in a fluid faecal specimen is to use Benedict's reagent or *Clinitest*.

If using Benedict's reagent, the specimen is tested in the same way as described for urine in subunit 6.11 except that 8 drops of freshly passed fluid faecal specimen are used instead of urine.

If using *Clinitest*, add 5 drops of freshly passed fluid specimen to 10 drops of clean water. After boiling has stopped mix the contents of the tube and note the colour of the fluid. A yellow-brown colour indicates the presence of $++$ sugar (lactose).

Testing pH of faeces

The pH of a faecal fluid specimen can be tested using a pH meter or narrow range pH papers.

Interpretation of results

Lactase deficiency is indicated if a faecal specimen:

−   Contains $++$ or more of sugar (lactose).
−   Has a pH of 6.0 or below.

3   EXAMINATION OF FAECES FOR EXCESS FAT

Most dietary fat is absorbed in the small intestine with very little being excreted in the faeces. Normal fat absorption requires the presence of bile salts, pancreatic and intestinal lipase, and a normal intestinal mucosa.

Steatorrhoea

Disorders of fat absorption cause excessive amounts of fat to be excreted in the faeces. The condition is referred to as steatorrhoea.

In tropical countries, steatorrhoea can occur with post-infective tropical malabsorption (tropical sprue), giardiasis, strongyloidiasis, chronic pancreatitis, and less commonly pancreatic or biliary obstruction.

Microscopical examination of faeces for fat

Fatty stools are pale in colour, bulky, float on water, and are often frothy with an offensive odour.

Excess fat in faeces may occur as:

■   Neutral fat globules
■   Fatty acid crystals
■   Soapy flakes

Method

1   Make a thin preparation of the faeces in physiological saline on a slide. Cover with a cover glass (avoid trapping air bubbles).

2   Examine the preparation for excess neutral fat globules, fatty acid crystals, and soapy fats using the 10× and 40× objectives with the condenser iris closed sufficiently to give good contrast.

Note: Constant focusing is necessary because fat does not sediment but tends to float in the preparation.

Neutral fat globules

These are easily recognized because they are highly refractile, colourless, and variable in size and shape with an oily look (see Fig. 6.6). They can be stained orange-red with a concentrated alcoholic solution of Sudan III or a saturated solution of oil red 0 in isopropanol (the stain can be run under one end of the cover glass).

If a drop of ethanol or diethyl ether is added, the fat globules will dissolve. Patients taking liquid paraffin excrete droplets of oil which are identical in appearance to the fat globules present in steatorrhoea.

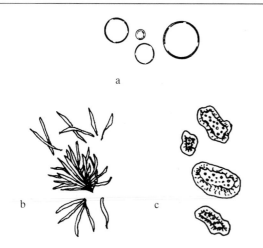

Fig. 6.6 *a* Neutral fat globules. *b* Fatty acids. *c* Soapy plaques.

Fatty acids

Fatty acids usually appear as groups of needle-like colourless crystals (see Fig. 6.6). They do not stain with Sudan III or oil red 0, but melt easily if *gentle* heat is applied to the preparation. Fatty acid crystals dissolve in ethanol and diethyl ether.

Soapy fats

Soaps also form masses of needle-like colourless crystals. They can be distinguished from fatty acid crystals because they do not melt with heat and they do not dissolve in ethanol or diethyl ether unless first treated with acetic acid. Soapy fats occur as flakes (soapy plaques) as shown in Fig. 6.6.

Interpretation of microscopical findings
- The presence of excess neutral fat globules in the faeces of a person taking a normal diet suggests lipase deficiency due to pancreatic disease. Neutral fat is the unsplit form of fat which is found in food before it is digested.

- The presence of excess fatty acids and soapy fats (split fats that have not been absorbed) in faeces suggests malabsorption.

REFERENCES
1 *Production of basic diagnostic laboratory reagents.* World Health Organization, Alexandria, 1995 (WHO Regional Publication, Eastern Mediterranean Series No. 11). Obtainable from WHO Regional Office, PO Box 7608, Nasr City, Cairo 11371, Egypt. Email: emro@who.sci.eg, Website: emro.who.int
2 *Use of anticoagulants in diagnostic laboratory investigations, and stability of blood, plasma and serum samples.* World Health Organization, WHO/(DIL/LAB/99.1. Revised 2004.
3 *Methods recommended for essential clinical chemical and haematological tests for intermediate hospital laboratories.* World Health Organization, WHO LAB/86.3, 1986.
4 **Browning DM, et al.** *Preparation of stabilized liquid quality control serum to be used in clinical chemistry.* World Health Organization, 1983. Document LAB/86.4.
5 **Slot C.** *Scandinavian Journal of Clinical Laboratory Investigation,* 1965, 17, pp. 381–387.
6 **Wybenga D, et al.** *Clinical Chemistry,* 1971, 17, pp. 891–895.
7 *Definition, diagnosis and classification of diabetes mellitus and its complications. Part 1 Diagnosis and classification of diabetes mellitus.* Report of a World Health Organization Consultation, Geneva, 1999.
8 **Trinder P.** *Annals of Clinical Biochemistry,* 1969, 6, pp. 24–27.
9 **Gebrekidan A et al.** An accurate and portable system for glycated haemoglobin measurement in the tropics. *Tropical Doctor,* 2004, 34, pp 94–95.
10 *Selected Methods for the Small Clinical Chemistry Laboratory.* American Association for Clinical Chemistry Inc, 1982.
11 **Doumas BT, et al.** Standardization in bilirubin assays: Evaluation of selected methods and stability of bilirubin solutions. *Clinical Chemistry,* 1973, 19, 9, pp. 984–993.
12 **Spencer K and Price CP.** *Annals of Clinical Biochemistry,* 1977, 14, pp. 105–115.
13 **Reitman S and Frankel S.** *American Journal of Clinical Pathology,* 1957, 28, pp. 56–63.
14 **Caraway WT.** *American Journal of Clinical Pathology,* 1959, 32, pp. 97–99.
15 **Healy T.** Electrolytes: their role and management. *Africa Health,* 1995, January, pp. ix-xi.
16 **Kutter D et al.** A simple and inexpensive screening test for low protein levels in urine. *Clin. Chim. Acta,* 1997, 258, pp 231–239.

RECOMMENDED READING
Basics of quality assurance for intermediate and peripheral laboratories. World Health Organization, Alexandria, 2nd edition 2002 (WHO Regional Publication, Eastern Mediterranean Series No. 2). Obtainable from WHO Regional Office, PO Box 7608, Nasr City, Cairo 11371, Egypt.

Production of basic diagnostic laboratory reagents. World Health Organization, Alexandria, 1995 (WHO Regional Publication, Eastern Mediterranean Series No. 11). Obtainable from WHO Regional Office, PO Box 7608, Nasr City, Cairo 11371, Egypt.

Whitby LG, et al. *Lecture notes on clinical biochemistry,* 6th edition, Blackwell Scientific, 1998.

Reinauer H et al. *Laboratory diagnosis and monitoring of diabetes mellitus,* 2002. World Health Organization. Free of charge booklet. Order from Dept Blood and Safety and Clinical Technology, WHO, 1211 Geneva, 27 Switzerland, Order No 18503736.

Gaw A et al. Clinical Biochemistry – An Illustrated Colour Text, 3rd edition. Churchill Livingstone (Esevier Science), 2004.

Gaskin G. Signs and symptoms of renal disease. *Africa Health*, Jan 2005, pp 9–12.

Neill G H. Urinary tract infection. *Africa Health*, Jan 2005, pp 13–18.

Africa Health special feature on care and management of diabetes in Africa. Africa Health, March 2004, pp 9–16. Available from FSG Communications, Vine House, Fair Green, Reach, Cambridge, CB5 0JD, UK. Website www.fsg.co.uk

Appendix I

Preparation of Reagents

PREPARING REAGENTS

Guidelines on the preparation of stains and reagents can be found in subunit 2.6. The safe handling of chemicals and the use of hazard symbols are described in subunit 3.5.

Note: Deionized water can be used instead of distilled water. The term 'room temperature' as used in this Appendix refers to 20–28 °C.

Acetic acid, 10% v/v   No. 1
To make 100 ml:

Acetic acid, glacial .... 10 ml
Distilled water .... 90 ml

1   Fill a 100 ml cylinder to the 90 ml mark with water.

2   Add 10 ml of glacial acetic acid, i.e. to the 100 ml mark.

     Caution: Glacial acetic acid is a corrosive chemical with an irritating vapour, therefore use in a well ventilated room. *Do not* mouth-pipette.

3   Transfer to a leak-proof bottle, and mix well.

4   Label the bottle and store at room temperature. The reagent is stable indefinitely.

Acetic acid, 60% v/v   No. 2
To make 100 ml:

Acetic acid, glacial .... 60 ml
Distilled water .... 40 ml

1   Fill a 100 ml cylinder to 40 ml mark with water.

2   Add 60 ml of glacial acetic acid, i.e. to the 100 ml mark.

     Caution: See text under Reagent No. 1

3   Transfer to a leak-proof bottle, and mix well.

4   Label the bottle, and mark it *Corrosive* and *Harmful*. Store the reagent at room temperature in a safe place. It is stable indefinitely.

Acid alcohol, 3% v/v   No. 3
This is a 3% v/v hydrochloric acid solution in 70% v/v alcohol.

To make 1 litre:

Ethanol or methanol, absolute* .... 680 ml
Distilled water .... 290 ml
Hydrochloric acid, concentrated .... 30 ml
* Technical grade is suitable.

1   Measure the ethanol or methanol and transfer to a 1 litre capacity leak-proof container.

     Caution: Ethanol and methanol are highly flammable, therefore use well away from an open flame.

2   Measure the water, add to the alcohol, and mix.

3   Measure 30 ml of concentrated hydrochloric acid, add to the solution, and mix well.

     Caution: Concentrated hydrochloric acid is a corrosive chemical with an injurious vapour, therefore handle with great care in a well ventilated room.

4   Label the bottle, and mark it *Flammable*. Store at room temperature in a safe place. The reagent is stable indefinitely.

     For use: Transfer a small amount of the reagent to a dispensing container that can be closed when not in use.

Acid pepsin solution   No. 4
To make about 100 ml:

Pepsin .... 0.5 g
Hydrochloric acid, concentrated .... 0.7 ml
Distilled water .... 100 ml

1   Weigh the pepsin and transfer it to a leak-proof bottle of 100 ml capacity.

2   Measure 100 ml of water and add about half of it to the bottle. Dissolve the pepsin in the water. Add the remainder of the water.

3   Add 0.7 ml of concentrated hydrochloric acid and mix well.

     Caution: Concentrated hydrochloric acid is a corrosive chemical with an injurious vapour, therefore handle it with great care in a well ventilated room. Do *not* mouth-pipette.

4   Label the bottle and store at 2–8 °C. The reagent is stable for several months.

Acidified silver nitrate   No. 5
To make 500 ml:

Silver nitrate .... 14.5 g
Nitric acid, 7.7 mol/1 (50% v/v)* .... to 500 ml
* Prepare by mixing 250 ml of concentrated nitric acid with 250 ml of distilled water. Add the acid to the water.

Caution: Concentrated nitric acid is a highly corrosive chemical, therefore handle it with care.

1   Weigh the silver nitrate and transfer it to a 500 ml volumetric flask.

     Caution: Silver nitrate is an oxidizing and corrosive chemical, therefore handle it with care.

2   Half fill the flask with the nitric acid solution

(7.7 mol/l), and mix until the silver nitrate is completely dissolved.

3 Make up to the 500 ml mark with the nitric acid solution (7.7 mol/l), and mix well.

Caution: Make sure the flask is tightly stoppered. Although the solution appears colourless, silver nitrate will stain skin, clothing, the laboratory bench, etc. The brown stain is very difficult to remove.

4 Transfer to a dark glass bottle.

5 Label the bottle and mark it *Corrosive*.

6 Store at room temperature out of direct sunlight. The reagent is stable for several months.

Alcohol (Ethanol), 95% v/v   No. 6
To make 100 ml:

Ethanol, absolute .... 95 ml
Distilled water .... 5 ml

1 Using a 100 ml cylinder, measure 95 ml of absolute ethanol.

Caution: Absolute ethanol is highly flammable, therefore use it well away from an open flame.

2 Add 5 ml of water, i.e. to the 100 ml mark.

3 Transfer to a leak-proof bottle and mix well.

4 Label the bottle and mark it *Flammable*. Store at room temperature in a safe place. The reagent is stable indefinitely.

Alkaline tartrate reagent   No. 7
To make 100 ml:

Potassium sodium tartrate .... 35.0 g
Sodium hydroxide .... 7.5 g
Distilled water .... to 100 ml

1 Weigh the potassium sodium tartrate and sodium hydroxide and transfer to a 100 ml volumetric flask.

Caution: Sodium hydroxide is a corrosive deliquescent chemical, therefore handle it with care and make sure the stock bottle of chemical is tightly stoppered after use.

2 About half fill the flask with water and mix until the chemicals are fully dissolved.

3 Make up to the 100 ml mark with water and mix well.

4 Transfer to a leak-proof bottle. Label the bottle and mark it *Corrosive*. Store at room temperature. The reagent is stable for at least 6 months.

Ammonium chloride, 0.87% w/v   No. 8
To make 1 litre:

Ammonium chloride .... 8.7 g
Distilled water .... to 1 litre

1 Weigh the chemical and transfer it to a 1 litre capacity container, previously marked to hold 1 litre.

Caution: Ammonium chloride is a harmful chemical. Do not ingest or inhale the chemical. Wear eye protection.

2 Add about half the volume of water and mix to dissolve the chemical. Make up to the 1 litre mark and mix.

3 Label the bottle and store at room temperature. Renew if the reagent becomes cloudy.

Barium chloride, 0.48 mol/l (10% w/v)   No. 9
To make 500 ml:

Barium chloride .... 50 g
Distilled water .... to 500 ml

1 Weigh the barium chloride and transfer it to a 500 ml volumetric flask.

Caution: Barium chloride is a poisonous chemical which is injurious to health when inhaled or swallowed.

2 Half fill the flask with water and mix to dissolve the chemical.

3 Make up to the 500 ml mark with water and mix well.

4 Transfer to a leak-proof bottle. Label the bottle and mark it *Toxic*. Store at room temperature. The reagent is stable for several months.

Bayer's stock solution   No. 10
To make about 107 ml:

Copper II chloride dihydrate .... 0.7 g
($CuCl_2.2H_2O$)
Acetic acid, glacial .... 7 ml
Formalin solution, 20% v/v* .... 100 ml

* Prepare by mixing 20 ml of concentrated formaldehyde solution (37–40% v/v) with 80 ml of distilled or filtered water.

Caution: Formaldehyde solution is a toxic chemical with an irritating and harmful vapour, therefore handle it with care in a well ventilated room.

1 Weigh the copper II chloride and transfer it to a leak-proof bottle.

2 Measure the formalin solution and acetic acid, and add to the bottle. Mix until the copper II chloride is completely dissolved.

Caution: Glacial acetic acid is corrosive and flammable. It is also irritating to the eyes, therefore handle it with care away from any open flame and in a well ventilated room. Do *not* mouth-pipette.

3 Label the bottle and mark it *Corrosive* and *Toxic*. Store at room temperature in a safe place. The reagent is stable indefinitely.

Working Bayer's solution
Dilute the stock solution 1 in 10 in distilled water, e.g. mix 2 ml of stock solution with 18 ml of water.

Benedict's reagent (qualitative)   No. 11
Purchase ready-made, or prepare as follows:
To make 500 ml:

Copper II sulphate, 5-hydrate* .... 8.6 g
* Use analytical grade
Sodium carbonate, anhydrous .... 50.0 g
tri-Sodium citrate .... 86.4 g
Distilled water .... to 500 ml

1 Weigh the copper sulphate, and transfer it to a clean beaker. Measure about 75 ml of water, add to the beaker, and stir to dissolve the chemical.

2 Weigh the sodium carbonate and sodium citrate. Transfer these to a 500 ml volumetric flask.

3 Half fill the flask with water and mix to dissolve the chemicals (placing the flask in a container of hot water for a few minutes will help to dissolve the chemicals. Allow to cool).

4 Add the copper sulphate solution to the volumetric flask, a little at a time, mixing after each addition. Rinse out the beaker with distilled water to make sure all the copper sulphate is transferred to the flask.

5 Make up to the 500 ml mark with water, and mix well.

6 Transfer to a leak-proof plastic bottle. Label the bottle. Store at room temperature. When kept tightly stoppered the reagent is stable indefinitely.

Benzoic acid, 1 g/l (0.1% w/v)   No. 12
To make 1 litre:
Benzoic acid .... 1 g
Distilled water .... to 1 litre

1 Heat about 500 ml of distilled water to 50–70 °C.

2 Weigh the benzoic acid, and transfer it to a

1 litre volumetric flask.

3 Half fill the flask with the hot water, and mix to dissolve the chemical. Allow to cool.

4 When cool, make up to the 1 litre mark with water and mix well.

5 Transfer to a leak-proof bottle. Label the bottle. Store at room temperature. The solution is stable indefinitely.

Buffered saline, pH 7.0–7.1   No. 13
This can be prepared by adding 0.4–0.7 ml of 10 g/l *di*-sodium hydrogen phosphate* to every 500 ml of physiological saline (Reagent No. 50). Check the pH using narrow range pH papers or a pH meter.
* Prepare by dissolving 1 g *di*-sodium hydrogen phosphate in 100 ml distilled water.

Buffered water, pH 7.1–7.2   No. 14
This is best prepared from stock phosphate buffer solutions A and B as follows:

Stock phosphate solution A
Sodium dihydrogen phosphate, ... 27.6 g
1-hydrate ($NaH_2PO_4.H_2O$)
Distilled water .... to 1 litre

1 Accurately weigh the chemical and transfer it to a 1 litre volumetric flask.

2 Half fill the flask with water, and mix to dissolve the chemical. Make up to the 1 litre mark with distilled water, and mix well. Transfer to a leak-proof bottle.

3 Label the bottle 'Stock phosphate solution A'. Store in a cool place or preferably at 2–8 °C. The solution is stable for several months.

Stock phosphate solution B
di-Sodium hydrogen phosphate, ... 28.39 g
anhydrous (Na_2HPO_4)
Distilled water .... to 1 litre

Prepare as described above for solution A. Label the bottle 'Stock phosphate solution B'. Store in a cool place or preferably at 2–8 °C. The solution is stable for several months.

To make 1 litre buffered water, pH 7.2:
Stock phosphate solution A .... 140 ml
Stock phosphate solution B .... 360 ml
Distilled water .... 500 ml

1 Accurately measure the stock phosphate solutions and water, transfer to a clean leak-proof bottle, and mix well. Check the pH using narrow range pH papers or a pH meter.

Alternatively, measure the stock phosphate

solutions, transfer to a litre volumetric flask, and make up to the mark with water. Transfer to a leak-proof bottle, and mix well. Check the pH using narrow range pH papers or a pH meter.

2 Label the bottle and store it at room temperature. The buffer is stable for several months.

Burrow's stain   No. 15
To make 100 ml:

Thionin .... 0.02 g
Ethanol, absolute (absolute alcohol) .... 3 ml
Acetic acid, glacial .... 3 ml
Distilled water .... 94 ml

1 Weigh the thionin* and transfer it to a leak-proof bottle of 100 ml capacity.

   * If an accurate balance is not available to weigh the 0.02 g (20 mg) of thionin, transfer a small amount of the powdered stain to a small tube and dip the end of a wet swab stick (or unburnt end of a match stick) in the powder. This will give approximately 20 mg.

2 Measure the ethanol and acetic acid and add these to the bottle. Mix until the thionin is completely dissolved.

   Caution: Ethanol is highly flammable and glacial acetic acid is corrosive, flammable, and has an irritating vapour, therefore handle these chemicals with care, well away from any open flame, in a well ventilated room. Do *not* mouth-pipette.

3 Add the water and mix well.

4 Label the bottle and store preferably at 2–8 °C. Renew every 3 months.

Caffeine-benzoate reagent   No. 16
To make 500 ml:

Sodium acetate, trihydrate .... 46.5 g
Sodium benzoate .... 28.0 g
di-Sodium EDTA* .... 0.5 g
(* ethylenediamine tetra-acetic acid, *di*sodium salt)
Caffeine .... 19.0 g
Distilled water .... to 500 ml

1 Weigh the sodium acetate, sodium benzoate, and *di*-sodium EDTA, and transfer these to a 500 ml volumetric flask.

2 About half fill the flask with water and mix to dissolve completely the chemicals.

3 Add the caffeine and mix to dissolve.

4 Make up to the 500 ml mark with water and mix well.

5 Filter the reagent into a leak-proof bottle. Label the bottle and store it at room temperature. The reagent is stable for at least 6 months.

Carbol fuchsin   No. 17
This is the same as the carbon fuchsin stain used in the Ziehl-Neelsen technique to detect AFB in sputum smears.

To make about 1115 ml:

Basic fuchsin .... 10 g
Ethanol or methanol, absolute* .... 100 ml
Phenol .... 50 g
Distilled water .... 1 litre
* Technical grade is adequate.

1 Weigh the basic fuchsin on a piece of clean paper (preweighed), and transfer the powder to a bottle of at least 1.5 litre capacity.

2 Measure the ethanol (ethyl alcohol) or methanol (methyl alcohol), and add to the bottle. Mix at intervals until the basic fuchsin is fully dissolved.

   Caution: Methanol and ethanol are highly flammable, therefore use well away from an open flame.

3 With great care, weigh the phenol in a beaker. Measure the water, and add some of it to the beaker to dissolve the phenol. Transfer to the bottle of stain, and mix well.

   Caution: Phenol is a highly corrosive, toxic, and hygroscopic chemical, therefore handle it with *great care*. To avoid spilling phenol on the balance pan, remove the beaker when adding or subtracting the chemical.

4 Add the remainder of the water, and mix well.

5 Label, and store at room temperature. The stain is stable indefinitely.

For use: Filter a small amount of the stain into a dropper bottle or other suitable stain dispensing container.

Citric acid-Tween solution   No. 18
To make 1 litre:

Citric acid .... 12.91 g
di-Sodium hydrogen phosphate, ... 27.61 g
hydrated ($Na_2HPO_4.12H_2O$)
Tween 80 .... 50 ml
Merthiolate .... 0.1 g
Distilled water .... to 1 litre

1 Weigh the citric acid and *di*-sodium hydrogen phosphate and transfer these to a 1 litre volumetric flask.

2 Half fill the flask with warm water and mix

until the chemicals are completely dissolved.

3 Add 50 ml of Tween 80 and make up to the 1 litre mark with water.

4 Transfer to a leak-proof bottle. Add 0.1 g merthiolate (preservative) and mix gently but well.

5 Label the bottle and store at room temperature. The solution is stable for several months.

Colour reagent for glucose assay   No. 19
To make 230 ml:

4-Aminophenazone, 5 g/l† .... 16 ml
Fermcozyme 952 DM‡ .... 4 ml
Phosphate buffer (Reagent No. 47) .... 60 ml
Distilled water .... 150 ml

† Prepare by dissolving 0.5 g of 4-aminophenazone* (4-aminoantipyrine) in 100 ml of distilled water.

* Obtainable from Merck Chemicals or other chemical manufacturer.

‡ Obtainable from Hughes and Hughes or other agent. For the addresses of these companies, see Appendix II.

Fermocozyme 952 DM contains 1250 U/ml of glucose oxidase and 1 mg/ml of peroxidase. It is available in 50 ml bottles. It is a stable product with a shelf-life from manufacture in excess of 2 years. It requires storage at 2–8 °C.

1 Measure the aminophenazone, *Fermcozyme*, phosphate buffer, and water, and transfer these to a dark coloured leak-proof bottle. Mix well.

2 Label the bottle and store at 2–8 °C. When refrigerated the colour reagent is stable for about 3 months.

Delafield haematoxylin   No. 20
It is recommended that this stain be bought ready-made. For those laboratories wishing to make their own stain the following formula can be used:

Haematoxylin .... 4.0 g
Ammonium alum .... 8.0 g
Potassium permanganate .... 0.2 g
Ethanol, absolute .... 125 ml
Distilled water .... 400 ml

1 Weigh the haematoxylin and transfer it to a bottle or flask.

2 Measure the absolute ethanol and add it to the haematoxylin. Stopper the flask or bottle and stand it in a container of hot water to help the haematoxylin to dissolve. Do not heat

over an open flame (ethanol is highly flammable). Mix well and when cool, filter.

3 Weigh the ammonium alum and transfer to a bottle or flask. Add 400 ml of hot water (40–50 °C) to help the ammonium alum to dissolve. When dissolved, add the solution to the filtered haematoxylin solution and mix well.

4 Dissolve the potassium permanganate in about 10 ml of distilled water and add this to the stain (this will 'ripen' the stain, i.e. enable it to be used immediately). Mix well.

5 Label the bottle and store it at room temperature. The stain is stable for several months.

Diacetyl monoxime, 4 g/l   No. 21
To make 500 ml:

Diacetyl monoxime .... 2 g
Distilled water .... to 500 ml

1 Weigh the diacetyl monoxime and transfer it to a 500 ml volumetric flask.

2 Half fill the flask with water and mix until the chemical is completely dissolved.

3 Make up to the 500 ml mark with water and mix well.

4 Transfer to a leak-proof bottle and label. Store preferably at 2–8 °C. The reagent is stable for at least 6 months.

Dobell's iodine
See Reagent No. 38

EDTA (seqestrene) anticoagulant   No. 22
Obtain ready-prepared anticoagulated bottles, or prepare as follows:

Di-potassium ethylene- .... 2.5 g
diamine-tetra-acetic acid
Distilled water .... 25 ml

1 Weigh the chemical, and transfer it to a small glass bottle.

2 Measure 25 ml of water, add to the chemical, and mix to dissolve. Label the bottle.

3 For use, pipette 0.04 ml of the reagent into small bottles marked to hold 2.5 ml of blood.

4 Place the small bottles without tops, on a warm bench for the anticoagulant to dry. Protect from dust and flies.

5 When dry, replace the bottle tops, and store ready for use.

Eosin stain, 5 g/l (0.5% w/v)   No. 23
To make about 100 ml:

Eosin powder .... 0.5 g
Distilled water .... 100 ml

1 Weigh the eosin on a clean piece of paper (pre-weighed), and transfer the powder to a leak-proof, brown bottle of 100 ml capacity.

2 Add 100 ml of water, and mix to dissolve the stain.

3 Label the bottle, and store it at room temperature. The stain is stable indefinitely.

For use: Transfer a small amount of the stain to a bottle with a cap into which a dropper can be inserted.

Erhlich's reagent   No. 24
To make about 200 ml:

4-Dimethylaminobenzaldehyde .... 4 g
Hydrochloric acid, concentrated .... 40 ml
Distilled water .... 160 ml

1 Weigh the 4-dimethylaminobenzaldehyde, and transfer it to a leak-proof brown bottle.

2 Measure the water and add to the chemical. Mix to dissolve.

3 Add the concentrated hydrochloric acid, and mix well.

   Caution: Concentrated hydrochloric acid is a corrosive chemical with an injurious vapour, therefore handle it with great care in a well ventilated room.

4 Label the bottle and mark it *Corrosive*. Store at room temperature. The reagent is stable for several weeks if protected from daylight.

Field's stain A   No. 25
To make 500 ml:

Field's stain A powder* .... 10 g
Distilled water (hot) .... 500 ml

* Obtain from HD Supplies, Merck/BDH Chemicals, or other reliable supplier.

1 Weigh the powder on a piece of clean paper (pre-weighed), and transfer it to a large Pyrex beaker or high density polyethylene reagent bottle.

2 Measure the water and heat to boiling.

3 Add the hot water to the stain and mix to dissolve the powder.

4 When cool, filter the stain into a storage bottle.

5 Label the bottle and store it at room temperature. The stain is stable indefinitely.

Field's stain B   No. 26
To make 500 ml:

Field's stain powder B* .... 10 g
Distilled water (hot) .... 500 ml

* Obtain from HD Supplies, Merck/BDH Chemicals, or other reliable supplier.

Prepare as described for Field's stain A (Reagent No. 25). Label the bottle and store at room temperature. The stain is stable indefinitely.

Fluoride-oxalate reagent   No. 27
To make 100 ml:

Sodium fluoride .... 1 g
Potassium oxalate .... 3 g
Distilled water .... to 100 ml

1 Weigh the sodium fluoride and potassium oxalate and transfer these to a 100 ml volumetric flask.

2 Half fill the flask with water and mix until the chemicals are completely dissolved. Make up to the 100 ml mark with water and mix well.

3 Transfer to a leak-proof bottle, and label. Store at room temperature. The reagent is stable for several months.

Preparation of containers
Dispense 0.1 ml of reagent into small containers and allow the water content to evaporate (cover the containers with a thin cloth). When dry, stopper the containers.

For use: The amount of fluoride-oxalate in each tube is sufficient to preserve 1 ml of blood. After adding the blood, mix gently. The fluoride prevents glycolysis and the oxalate prevents clotting of the blood. Fluoride-oxalated blood or c.s.f. can also be used in protein and urea tests.

Formol detergent solution   No. 28
To make 500 ml:

Formaldehyde, concentrated solution .... 10 ml
Detergent solution* .... 10 ml
Clean water .... 480 ml

* This can be *Lipsol, Fairy Liquid, Decon, Teepol*, or other washing-up detergent.

1 Measure the water and transfer to a storage bottle.

2 Measure the detergent solution and add to the water.

3 Measure the formaldehyde solution and add to the bottle. Mix well.

Caution: Concentrated formaldehyde solution is a toxic chemical with a vapour that is irritating to the eyes and mucous membranes, therefore handle it with great care in a well ventilated room.

4 Label the bottle and store at room temperature. The solution is stable indefinitely.

Formol saline, 10% v/v   No. 29
To make 500 ml:

Physiological saline .... 450 ml
(Reagent No. 50)
Formaldehyde solution, concentrated .... 50 ml

1 Measure the physiological saline and transfer it to a leak-proof bottle.

2 Measure the formaldehyde solution and add to the saline. Mix well.

Caution: Concentrated formaldehyde solution is a toxic chemical with a vapour that is irritating to the eyes and mucous membranes, therefore handle it with great care in a well ventilated room.

3 Label the bottle and store at room temperature in a safe place. The reagent is stable indefinitely.

Fouchet's reagent   No. 30
To make 100 ml:

Trichloroacetic acid (TCA) .... 25 g
Iron III chloride (ferric chloride), ... 10 ml
100 g/l (10% w/v)*
Distilled water .... to 100 ml
* Prepare by dissolving 10 g of the chemical in 100 ml of distilled water.

1 Rapidly weigh the TCA in a beaker. Add 30–40 ml of distilled water, and stir to dissolve the chemical.

Caution: TCA is a strongly corrosive and deliquescent chemical, therefore avoid contact with the eyes and skin and make sure the stock bottle of chemical is tightly stoppered after use.

2 Using a funnel, transfer the dissolved acid to a 100 ml volumetric flask or if unavailable, a measuring cylinder.

3 Add the iron III chloride solution, and mix. Make up to the 100 ml mark with distilled water, and mix well.

4 Transfer the reagent to a small brown bottle (one in which a dropper can be inserted).

5 Label the bottle, and mark it *Corrosive*. Store at room temperature. The reagent is stable for several months.

Giemsa stain   No. 31
Purchase ready-made or prepare using the following formula.

To make about 500 ml:

Giemsa powder .... 3.8 g
Glycerol (glycerine) .... 250 ml
Methanol (methyl alcohol) .... 250 ml

1 Weigh the Giemsa on a piece of clean paper (preweighed), and transfer to a *dry* brown bottle of 500 ml capacity which contains a few glass beads.

Note: Giemsa stain will be spoilt if water enters the stock solution during its preparation or storage.

2 Using a *dry* cylinder, measure the methanol, and add to the stain. Mix well.

Caution: Methanol is toxic and highly flammable, therefore handle it with care and use well away from an open flame.

3 Using the same cylinder, measure the glycerol, and add to the stain. Mix well.

4 Place the bottle of stain in a water bath at 50–60 °C, or if not available at 37 °C, for up to 2 hours to help the stain to dissolve. Mix well at intervals.

5 Label the bottle, and mark it *Flammable and Toxic*. Store at room temperature in the dark. If kept well-stoppered, the stain is stable for several months.

For use: Filter a small amount of the stain into a *dry* stain dispensing container.

Glycerol jelly   No. 32
To make about 310 ml:

Gelatin .... 15 g
Glycerol (glycerine) .... 50 ml
Distilled water .... 250 ml

1 Measure the water and heat to boiling.

2 Weigh the gelatin and add to the hot water. Stir until the gelatin is completely dissolved.

3 Measure the glycerol and mix with the gelatin water.

4 Dispense in 10–20 ml amounts in screw-cap bottles, and allow to gel. Label each bottle and store at 2–8 °C.

For use: Liquefy a container of glycerol jelly by placing it in hot water (about 50 °C).

Gum guaiac   No. 33
Prepare fresh before use:

Gum guaiac .... 0.1 g
Ethanol, 95% v/v* .... 6.0 ml

* See Reagent No. 6.

1 Weigh the chemical and transfer it to a bottle of 10 ml capacity (alternatively, measure the chemical in a narrow tube pre-marked to hold 0.1 g).

2 Add the ethanol, stopper the bottle and mix until the chemical is fully dissolved.

   Caution: The ethanol (alcohol) reagent is flammable, therefore handle it well away from any open flame.

Note: Use the reagent on the same day it is prepared.

Hydrochloric acid, 100 mmol/l   No. 34
(0.1 mol/l)
To make 500 ml:

Hydrochloric acid, concentrated .... 4.5 ml
Distilled water .... to 500 ml

1 Half fill a 500 ml volumetric flask with water.

2 Measure 4.5 ml of concentrated hydrochloric acid and add this to the water.

   Caution: Concentrated hydrochloric acid is a corrosive chemical with an injurious vapour, therefore handle it with great care in a well ventilated room. Do *not* mouth-pipette.

3 Make up to the 500 ml mark with water and mix well.

4 Transfer to a leak-proof bottle and label. Store at room temperature. The reagent is stable indefinitely.

Hydrochloric acid, 50 mmol/l   No. 35
To make 100 ml:

Hydrochloric acid, concentrated .... 4.2 ml
Distilled water .... to 100 ml

Prepare as described in Reagent No. 34.

Hydrochloric acid, 50% v/v   No. 36
To make 100 ml:

Hydrochloric acid, concentrated .... 50 ml
Distilled water .... 50 ml

1 Using a cylinder, measure 50 ml of water and transfer to a leak-proof screw cap bottle.

2 Measure 50 ml of concentrated hydrochloric acid and add to the water. Cap the bottle and mix well.

   Caution: See Reagent No. 34.

3 Label the bottle and mark it *Corrosive*. Store at room temperature in a safe place. The reagent is stable indefinitely.

Hydrogen peroxide (3%) 10 vols solution No. 37
Prepare fresh before use. To make 10 ml:

Hydrogen peroxide, 30% v/v* .... 1 ml
Distilled water .... 9 ml

* A 30% hydrogen peroxide solution is available from Merck/BDH and other suppliers of chemicals. It contains 100 volumes.

1 Measure the water and transfer it to a chemically clean bottle of 10–15 ml capacity.

2 Add 1 ml of 30% hydrogen peroxide solution. Cap the bottle and mix.

   Caution: Hydrogen peroxide is a corrosive and oxidizing chemical, therefore handle it with care. Always store it in a cool dark place, preferably at 2–8 °C because exposure to warmth and light causes oxygen to be evolved with a build up of pressure, which may lead to an explosion.

Note: Use the reagent on the same day it is prepared.

Iodine (Dobell's) for faecal preparations No. 38
To make about 100 ml:

Potassium iodide .... 4 g
Iodine .... 2 g
Distilled water .... 100 ml

1 Weigh the potassium iodide and dissolve *completely* in about 50 ml of the water.

2 Weigh the iodine and add to the potassium iodide solution. Mix well to dissolve.

   Caution: Iodine is injurious to health if inhaled or allowed to come in contact with the eyes, therefore handle with care in a well ventilated room.

3 Add the remainder of the water, and mix. Transfer to a brown bottle.

4 Label the bottle, and mark it *Harmful*. Store in the dark at room temperature. The reagent is stable for several months.

   For use: Transfer to a small brown bottle with a cap into which a dropper can be inserted.

Iodine, stock solution, 50 mmol/l   No. 39
To make 1 litre:

Potassium iodate .... 3.57 g
Potassium iodide .... 45.00 g
Hydrochloric acid, concentrated .... 9.0 ml
Distilled water .... to 1 litre

1 Weigh the potassium iodate and potassium iodide, and transfer these to a 1 litre volumetric flask.

2 Add about 800 ml of water and mix until the chemicals are completely dissolved.

3 Measure the concentrated hydrochloric acid and *slowly*, with mixing, add this to the flask.

   Caution: Concentrated hydrochloric acid is a corrosive chemical with an injurious vapour, therefore handle it with care and use in a well ventilated room. Do *not* mouth-pipette.

4 Make up to the 1 litre mark with water and mix.

5 Transfer to a leak-proof brown bottle and label. Store at room temperature away from sunlight. The reagent is stable for about 1 year.

Working iodine solution
Prepare as described in subunit 6.9.

Lactophenol solution   No. 40
To make about 110 ml:

Phenol .... 25 g
Lactic acid .... 25 ml
Glycerol .... 50 ml
Distilled water .... 25 ml

1 Rapidly weigh the phenol in a preweighed beaker.

2 Measure the water and add to the phenol. Mix to dissolve the phenol. Transfer to a leak-proof brown bottle.

   Caution: Phenol is a highly corrosive, toxic, and hygroscopic chemical, therefore handle it with great care. To avoid damaging the balance pan, remove the beaker when adding or subtracting the chemical. Make sure the stock bottle of phenol is tightly stoppered after use.

3 Measure the lactic acid and glycerol and add to the bottle. Cap the bottle and mix well.

4 Label the bottle and mark it *Toxic* and *Corrosive*. Store at room temperature in a safe place. The reagent is stable for many months.

Malachite green, 5 g/l (0.5% w/v)   No. 41
To make 1 litre:

Malachite green .... 5 g
Distilled water .... to 1 litre

1 Weigh the malachite green on a piece of clean paper (preweighed), and transfer to a bottle of 1 litre capacity.

2 Measure the water, and add about a quarter of it to the bottle. Mix until the dye is fully dissolved.

3 Add the remainder of the water, and mix well.

4 Label the bottle and store at room temperature. The stain is stable for several months.

   For use: Transfer a small amount of the stain to a dropper bottle or other stain dispensing container.

Methylene blue-saline, 1% w/v   No. 42
To make 100 ml:

Physiological saline (Reagent No. 50) ..... 100 ml
Methylene blue .... 1.0 g

1 Weigh the methylene blue and transfer it to a leak-proof bottle.

2 Measure the saline and add to the dye. Mix until the methylene blue is completely dissolved.

3 Label the bottle and store it at room temperature. Discard the stain if it becomes contaminated.

For use: Filter a small amount of the stain into a dropper bottle.

Nigrosin stain   No. 43
To make about 120 ml:

Acetic acid, glacial .... 10 ml
Methanol, absolute .... 50 ml
Nigrosin, saturated aqueous solution* ...... 10 ml
Distilled water .... 50 ml

* Prepare by dissolving sufficient *water-soluble* nigrosin in about 12 ml of warm distilled water until no more can be dissolved. Filter 10 ml.

1 Measure the water and transfer it to a leak-proof brown bottle.

2 Measure the acetic acid and methanol and add these to the water.

   Caution: Glacial acetic acid is a corrosive and flammable chemical with an irritating vapour and methanol is highly flammable. Handle, therefore, these chemicals with care, well away from any open flame and in a well ventilated room.

3 Add the nigrosin stain and mix well. Label the bottle and store it at room temperature. The reagent is stable for many months.

Nitroprusside dry reagent   No. 44
To make about 153 g:

Ammonium sulphate .... 100 g
Sodium carbonate, anhydrous .... 50 g
Sodium nitroprusside* .... 3 g

* The accepted international name for sodium nitroprusside is sodium nitrosopentacyanoferrate III.

1 Weigh the sodium nitroprusside, and transfer it to a wide-necked, plastic, screw-cap container.

   Caution: Sodium nitroprusside is a poisonous chemical, therefore handle it with care.

2 Using a pestle or the end of a clean test tube (made of thick glass), grind the crystals to a powder.

3 Weigh the sodium carbonate and ammonium sulphate, and transfer these to the container.

4 Cap the container and mix the powders by shaking.

5 Label the container and mark it *Toxic*. Store at room temperature. The reagent is stable for several months. Mix the reagent before use.

Phenol, saturated solution   No. 45
To make about 30 ml:

Phenol crystals .... 2 g
Distilled water .... 30 ml

1 Weigh the phenol in a beaker (preweighed). Add the water, and stir to dissolve the chemical. Transfer to a leak-proof bottle and mix well.

   Caution: Phenol is a highly corrosive, toxic, and hygroscopic chemical, therefore handle it with great care. To avoid damaging the balance pan, always remove the beaker when adding or subtracting the chemical. Make sure the stock bottle of phenol is tightly stoppered after use.

2 Label the bottle, and mark it *Corrosive*. Store at room temperature in a safe place. The reagent is stable indefinitely.

Phosphate borate buffer, pH 12.8   No. 46
To make 500 ml:

tri-Sodium orthophosphate .... 9.5 g
di-Sodium tetraborate .... 9.5 g
Distilled water .... to 500 ml

1 Accurately weigh the sodium orthophosphate and sodium tetraborate, and transfer these to a 500 ml volumetric flask.

2 Half fill the flask with water and mix to dissolve the chemicals.

3 Measure the pH and adjust to pH 12.8 by adding 1 mol/l sodium hydroxide (Reagent No. 60). About 110 ml will be required.

4 Make up to the 500 ml mark with water and mix well.

5 Transfer to a leak-proof bottle and label. Store at room temperature. The reagent is stable indefinitely.

Phosphate buffer for glucose colour reagent   No. 47
To make 500 ml:

di-Sodium hydrogen orthophosphate .... 10 g
anhydrous (Na_2HPO_4)
Potassium dihydrogen orthophosphate .... 10 g
(KH_2PO_4)
Sodium azide .... 2 g
Distilled water .... to 500 ml

1 Accurately weigh the chemicals and transfer these to a 500 ml volumetric flask.

2 Half fill the flask with water and mix to dissolve the chemicals. Make up to the 500 ml mark with water and mix well.

3 Transfer the reagent to a leak-proof bottle (preferably plastic), and label. Store at room temperature. The reagent is stable for several months.

Phosphate buffered saline, pH 7.0   No. 48
To make about 200 ml:

Stock phosphate solution A* .... 39 ml
Stock phosphate solution B* .... 61 ml
Distilled water .... 100 ml
Sodium chloride .... 1.7 g

* See Reagent No. 14.

1 Mix the phosphate solutions with the water. Add the sodium chloride and mix to dissolve.

2 Check the pH using narrow range pH papers or a pH meter. Store the reagent in a cool place or preferably at 2–8 °C. The reagent is stable for several weeks. Renew if it becomes contaminated (cloudy).

Phosphate buffered saline, pH 7.2   No. 49
To make about 200 ml:

Stock phosphate solution A* .... 28 ml
Stock phosphate solution B* .... 72 ml
Distilled water .... 100 ml
Sodium chloride .... 1.7 g
* See Reagent No. 14.

1   Mix the phosphate solutions with the water. Add the sodium chloride, and mix well to dissolve.

2   Check the pH using narrow range pH papers or a pH meter. Store the reagent in a cool place or preferably at 2–8 °C. The reagent is stable for several weeks. Renew if it becomes contaminated (cloudy).

Physiological saline, 8.5 g/l   No. 50
(0.85% w/v)
To make 1 litre:

Sodium chloride .... 8.5 g
Distilled water .... to 1 litre

1   Weigh the sodium chloride, and transfer it to a leak-proof bottle premarked to hold 1 litre.

2   Add distilled water to the 1 litre mark, and mix until the salt is fully dissolved.

3   Label the bottle, and store it at room temperature. The reagent is stable for several months. Discard if it becomes contaminated.

Picric acid reagent (13 g/l)   No. 51
This reagent is a saturated solution of picric acid, i.e. it contains 13 g of the chemical per litre. It is best purchased in this form (Merck/BDH, No. 22035) because picric acid is not available as a dry chemical for weighing like other chemicals. It is always supplied containing about 50% water (*dry* picric acid is explosive).

If saturated picric acid cannot be obtained, a saturated solution can be prepared from picric acid containing 50% water as follows:

1   Weigh about 11 g of the well mixed moist picric acid in a beaker.

2   Add the chemical to 500 ml of distilled water and mix at intervals for several hours to produce a saturated solution.

3   Transfer to a leak-proof brown bottle. Label the bottle and mark it *Harmful*. Store at room temperature. The reagent is stable indefinitely.

Protein diluent   No. 52
To make 1 litre:

Sodium chloride .... 9 g
Sodium azide .... 1 g
Distilled water .... to 1 litre

1   Weigh the sodium chloride and sodium azide, and transfer these to a 1 litre volumetric flask or leak-proof bottle pre-marked to hold 1 litre.

    Caution: Sodium azide is a toxic chemical. Do not inhale or ingest it. Wear eye protection.

2   Half fill the flask or bottle with water and mix until the chemicals are completely dissolved.

3   Make up to the 1 litre mark with water and mix well.

4   Label the bottle and store at room temperature. The reagent is stable indefinitely.

Protein precipitant reagent   No. 53
To make 500 ml:

Sodium tungstate, dihydrate .... 5 g
di-Sodium hydrogen phosphate, ... 5 g
anhydrous (Na_2HPO_4)
Sodium chloride .... 4.5 g
Phenol .... 0.5 g
Hydrochloric acid, 1 mol/1* .... 62 ml
Distilled water .... to 500 ml
* Prepare by diluting concentrated hydrochloric acid 1 in 10.

1   Weigh the sodium tungstate, di-sodium hydrogen phosphate, and sodium chloride. Transfer these to a 500 ml volumetric flask.

2   Half fill the flask with distilled water and mix until the chemicals are completely dissolved.

3   Add 62 ml of 1 mol/1 hydrochloric acid solution and mix.

4   Weigh the phenol and add to the flask. Mix to dissolve.

    Caution: Phenol is a highly corrosive and hygroscopic chemical, therefore take great care when weighing the chemical and transferring it to the flask. After use, make sure the stock bottle of phenol is tightly stoppered.

5   Make up to the 500 ml mark with distilled water and mix well.

6   Transfer the reagent to a leak-proof bottle and label. Store at room temperature. The reagent is stable indefinitely.

Saline
See Reagent No. 50.

Saponin solution
See Reagent No. 54.

Saponin-saline solution — No. 54
This is a 1% w/v solution of saponin in physiological saline.

To make about 500 ml:

Saponin (white, pure grade) .... 5 g
Physiological saline (Reagent No. 50) ..... 500 ml

1 Weigh the saponin and transfer this to a leak-proof bottle.

   Caution: Saponin powder is a harmful chemical, therefore handle it with great care. Do not inhale or ingest the powder.

2 Measure the saline and add about half of it to the bottle. Mix gently (by swirling) to dissolve the chemical (standing the bottle in hot water will help the saponin to dissolve).

3 Add the remainder of the saline and mix gently but well (avoid excess frothing).

4 Label the bottle and store it preferably at 2–8 °C. The reagent is stable for several months.

For use: Transfer a small amount to a dropper bottle.

Sargeaunt stain — No. 55
To make 100 ml:

Malachite green .... 0.2 g
Glacial acetic acid .... 3 ml
Ethanol, 95% v/v* .... 3 ml
*See Reagent No. 6
Distilled water .... 94 ml

1 Weigh the malachite green and transfer it to a container of 100 ml capacity.

2 Measure the ethanol and glacial acetic acid and add to the stain. Mix until the stain is fully dissolved.

   Caution: The ethanol reagent is flammable, therefore use well away from any open flame. Glacial acetic acid is a corrosive chemical with an irritating vapour, therefore use in a well ventilated area. Do *not* mouth-pipette.

3 Add the water and mix well. Label the bottle and store at room temperature. The stain is stable indefinitely.

Sodium citrate, 6% w/v — No. 56
To make about 100 ml:

tri-Sodium citrate .... 6.0 g
Distilled water .... 100 ml

Prepare as described for Reagent No. 57.

Sodium citrate anticoagulant — No. 57
To make about 100 ml:

tri-Sodium citrate .... 3.8 g
Distilled water .... 100 ml

1 Weigh the sodium citrate and transfer it to a leak-proof bottle.

2 Add 100 ml of water and mix to dissolve the chemical.

3 Label the bottle and store preferably at 2–8 °C. Renew every 6 weeks or sooner if it becomes contaminated (cloudy).

Sodium dodecyl sulphate, 40 g/l — No. 58
To make 500 ml:

Sodium dodecyl sulphate .... 20 g
Distilled water .... to 500 ml

1 Weigh the sodium dodecyl sulphate and transfer it to a 500 ml volumetric flask.

   Caution: Sodium dodecyl sulphate is a harmful chemical, therefore handle it with care.

2 Half fill the flask with water and mix until the chemical is completely dissolved.

3 Make up to the 500 ml mark with water and mix.

4 Transfer to a leak-proof bottle. Label and mark the bottle *Harmful*. Store at room temperature in a safe place. The reagent is stable indefinitely but should be discarded if it becomes turbid.

Sodium hydroxide, 0.4 mol/l (0.4N) — No. 59
To make 1 litre:

Sodium hydroxide .... 16 g
Distilled water .... to 1 litre

1 Weigh the sodium hydroxide and transfer it to a 1 litre volumetric flask.

   Caution: See Reagent No. 60.

2 Half fill the flask with distilled water and mix until the chemical is fully dissolved.

3 Make up to the 1 litre mark with distilled water and mix well.

4 Transfer to a leak-proof bottle (preferably plastic). Label the bottle and mark it *Corrosive*. Store at room temperature. The reagent is stable indefinitely.

Note: A 0.4 mol/l solution of sodium hydroxide can also be prepared from a 1 mol/l volumetric solution of sodium hydroxide (dilute 400 ml of

1 mol/l sodium hydroxide to 1 litre with distilled water).

Sodium hydroxide, 1 mol/l (4% w/v)　　No. 60

Purchase ready-made as a 1 mol/l volumetric solution or prepare as follows:

To make 1 litre:

Sodium hydroxide .... 40.01 g
Distilled water .... to 1 litre

1　Weigh the sodium hydroxide, and transfer it to a 1 litre volumetric flask.

　Caution: Sodium hydroxide is a corrosive deliquescent chemical, therefore handle it with care, and make sure the stock bottle of chemical is tightly stoppered after use.

2　Half fill the flask with water, and mix to dissolve the chemical. Make up to the 1 litre mark with water, and mix well.

3　Transfer to a leak-proof bottle (preferably plastic). Label the bottle, and mark it *Corrosive*. Store at room temperature. The reagent is stable indefinitely.

Sodium nitrite, 5 g/l (0.5% w/v)　　No. 61

To make 100 ml:

Sodium nitrite .... 0.5 g
Distilled water .... to 100 ml

1　Weigh the sodium nitrite, and transfer it to a 100 ml volumetric flask.

　Caution: Sodium nitrite is a toxic and oxidizing chemical, therefore handle it with care.

2　Half fill the flask with distilled water, and mix until the chemical is fully dissolved. Make up to the 100 ml mark, and mix well.

3　Transfer to a brown bottle. Label the bottle and mark it *Toxic*. Store at 2–8 °C, and renew every 2 weeks.

Starch substrate, pH 7.0　　No. 62

To make 500 ml:

di-Sodium hydrogen phosphate, ... 13.3 g
anhydrous (Na$_2$HPO$_4$)
Sodium chloride .... 0.9 g
Benzoic acid .... 4.3 g
Soluble starch* .... 0.2 g
Distilled water .... to 500 ml

* Use a *good quality* chemical grade starch such as Sigma Soluble starch (product S 9765, 100 g).

1　Weigh the *di*-sodium hydrogen phosphate, sodium chloride, and benzoic acid. Transfer these chemicals to a heat resistant beaker or flask.

2　Add about half the water and mix. Place the beaker or flask in a container of water and heat to boiling. Mix at intervals to dissolve the chemicals.

3　Accurately weigh the starch and dissolve it in about 10 ml of cold distilled water.

4　With *mixing*, stir in the starch suspension to the hot solution in the beaker. Continue mixing until the solution reaches 100 °C. Allow to boil for 1 minute.

5　Cool to room temperature. Transfer to a 500 ml volumetric flask and make up to the 500 ml mark with water. Mix well.

6　Transfer to a leak-proof bottle and label. Store at 2–8 °C. Renew monthly.

Important: Before use, mix the reagent *well*.

Succinate buffer, pH 4.2　　No. 63

To make 1 litre:

Succinic acid .... 5.6 g
Sodium hydroxide .... 1.0 g
Sodium azide .... 0.1 g
Distilled water .... to 1 litre

1　Weigh the chemicals and transfer them to a 1 litre volumetric flask.

2　Half fill the flask with distilled water and mix until the chemicals are completely dissolved.

3　Make up to the 1 litre mark with distilled water and mix well.

4　Check that the pH of the buffer is pH 4.2 ± 0.05 at room temperature. If the pH is not 4.2, adjust it using 10 g/l (1% w/v) sodium hydroxide or 50 g/l (5% w/v) succinic acid. Add drop by drop.

5　Transfer to a leak-proof bottle and label. Store at 2–8 °C. The buffer is stable for several months.

Sucrose solution　　No. 64

Sucrose .... 200 g
Phenol .... 2.6 g
Distilled water .... 128 ml

1　Weigh the sucrose and transfer it to a container of about 200 ml capacity.

2　Measure the water and add to the sucrose. Mix until the chemical is dissolved.

3　Weigh the phenol and add to the solution. Mix well.

　Caution: Phenol is a highly corrosive, toxic, and hygroscopic chemical, therefore handle it with great care. Weigh the chemical in a beaker and remove the beaker from the balance pan when adding or subtracting the chemical. Make sure the stock bottle of phenol is tightly stoppered after use.

4 Label the bottle and store at room temperature. The reagent is stable indefinitely.

Sulphanilic acid, 5 g/l   No. 65
To make 500 ml:

Sulphanilic acid .... 2.5 g
Hydrochloric acid, concentrated .... 7.5 ml
Distilled water .... to 500 ml

1 Weigh the sulphanilic acid and transfer to a 500 ml volumetric flask.

Caution: Sulphanilic acid is a harmful chemical, therefore handle it with care.

2 Half fill the flask with water.

3 Measure the hydrochloric acid and add to the flask.

Caution: Concentrated hydrochloric acid is a corrosive chemical with an injurious vapour, handle it with great care in a well ventilated area. Do *not* mouth-pipette.

4 Mix until the sulphanilic acid is completely dissolved. Make up to the 500 ml mark with water and mix well.

5 Transfer to a leak-proof bottle. Label the bottle and mark it *Harmful*. Store at room temperature. The reagent is stable for about 6 months.

Sulphosalicylic acid, 200 g/l (20% w/v)   No. 66
To make 250 ml:

Sulphosalicylic acid .... 50 g
Distilled water .... to 250 ml

1 Weigh the acid, and transfer to a 250 ml volumetric flask (or bottle premarked to hold 250 ml).

2 Half fill the flask with distilled water, and mix to dissolve the acid.

3 Make up to the 250 ml mark with distilled water, and mix well. Transfer to a storage bottle.

4 Label the bottle, and store at room temperature. The reagent is stable for several months.

Trichloroacetic acid, 50 g/l (5% w/v)   No. 67
To make 100 ml:

Trichloroacetic acid (TCA) .... 5 g
Distilled water .... to 100 ml

1 Weigh the TCA in a beaker (preweighed). Add about 30 ml of the water, and stir to dissolve the TCA.

Caution: TCA is a strongly corrosive and deliquescent chemical with an irritating vapour, therefore handle it with care in a well ventilated room. Make sure the stock bottle of chemical is tightly stoppered after use.

2 Transfer to a 100 ml volumetric flask. Make up to the mark with distilled water, and mix well.

3 Transfer to a leak-proof bottle. Label, and mark it *Corrosive*. Store at room temperature. The reagent is stable indefinitely.

Urea acid reagent   No. 68
To make 500 ml:

Thiosemicarbazide .... 0.05 g
Cadmium sulphate .... 1.60 g
Sulphuric acid, concentrated .... 44.0 ml
ortho-Phosphoric acid .... 66.0 ml
Urea working standard, 2.5 mmol.l* .... 1.5 ml
Distilled water .... to 500 ml

* See subunit 6.4.

1 About half fill a 500 ml volumetric flask with water.

2 Measure the sulphuric acid and *slowly*, with mixing, add it to the water. Considerable heat will be evolved.

Important: The acid *must* be added to the water. Concentrated sulphuric acid is a highly corrosive and deliquescent chemical, therefore handle it with *great care*.

3 Measure the phosphoric acid and slowly with mixing, add it to the flask.

Caution: Concentrated phosphoric acid is a *highly corrosive* acid, therefore handle it with great care.

4 Allow the solution to cool to room temperature.

5 Measure the thiosemicarbazide and cadmium sulphate and add these to the solution. Mix to dissolve (make sure the stopper of the flask is tight fitting).

6 Measure the urea standard solution, and add it to the flask.

7 Make up to 500 ml mark with water and mix.

8 With care, transfer the reagent to a dark, leak-proof bottle. Label, and mark the bottle *Corrosive* and *Toxic*. Store at room tempera-

ture. The reagent is stable for at least 6 months.

Zinc sulphate solution, 33% w/v   No. 69
To make approximately 500 ml:

Zinc sulphate .... 165 g
Distilled water .... 500 ml

1 Weigh the zinc sulphate and transfer it to a leak-proof bottle of about 1 litre capacity.

2 Measure the water and add it to the chemical.

3 Stopper the bottle, and mix well.

4 Stand the bottle in a container of hot water to dissolve the zinc sulphate. Mix until the chemical is completely dissolved.

5 Allow the solution to cool to room temperature.

6 Using a hydrometer, check the relative density of the solution. If the density is not within 1.180–1.200, add more chemical or water to bring the solution within the correct density range.

7 Label the bottle and store at room temperature. When stored with the bottle top tightly stoppered, the solution is stable for several weeks. The relative density should be checked periodically.

Appendix II

Useful Addresses

Adam Equipment Co Ltd (UK)
Bond Avenue
Milton Keynes
MK1 1SW, UK
Phone: +44 (0) 1908 274545
Fax: +44 (0) 1908 641339
E-mail: sales@adamequipment.co.uk
Website: www.adamequipment.co.uk

Adam Equipment, South Africa
7 Megawatt Road
Spartan EXT 22
Kempton Park
Johannesburg
SOUTH AFRICA
Phone: +27 (0) 11 9749745
Fax: +27 (0) 11 3922587
E-mail: sales@adamequipment.co.za
Website: www.adamsequipment.com

Alfa Scientific Designs Inc.
12330 Stowe Dr.
Poway
CA 92064
USA
Phone: +1 858 513 3888
Fax: +1 858 513 8388
Website: www.alfascientific.com

Almedica AG
Haupstrasse 76
3285 Galmiz
SWITZERLAND
Phone: +41 26 672 90 90
Fax: +41 26 672 90 99
E-mail: office@almedica.ch
Website: www.almedica.ch

Alpha Laboratories Ltd
40 Parham Drive
Eastleigh, Hampshire
SO50 4NU, UK
Phone: +44 (0) 238 048 3000
Fax: +44 (0) 238 064 3701

Antec International
Windham Road
Chilton Industrial Estate
Sudbury, Suffolk
CO10 2XD, UK
Phone: +44 (0) 1787 377305
Fax: +44 (0) 1787 375391
E-mail: humanhealth@antecint.com
Website: www.antechh.com

Atago USA Inc.
12011 Bel-Red Road
Suite 101 Bellevue
WA 98005
USA
Phone: +1 425 637 2107
Fax: +1 425 637 2110
E-mail: customerservice@atago-usa-com
Website: www.atago.net

Azlon Products, see **Bibby Sterilin**

Bayer Diagnostics UK
Bayer House, Strawberry Hill
Newbury
RG14 1JA, UK
Phone: +44 1635 563000
Fax: +44 1635 563393
Website: www.bayer.co.uk
or   www.bayer.poct.co.uk

Bayer HealthCare AG
51368 Leverkusen
GERMANY
Phone: +49 214 3010
Fax: +49 214 3066328
Website: www.bayer.ag.de

Becton Dickinson (BD Diagnostic Systems)
7 Loveton Circle
Sparks
MD 21152
USA
Phone: +1 410 771 0100
Fax: +1 201 847 6475
Website: www.bd.com

Bibby Sterilin Ltd
Beacon Road,
Stone, Staffordshire
ST15 OSA, UK
Phone: +44 (0) 1785 812 121
Fax: +44 (0) 1785 813 748
E-mail: sterilin@bibby-sterilin.com
Website: www.bibby-sterilin.com

Binax Inc.
217 Read Street
Portland, ME04103
USA   *continued above*

Phone   +1 207 772 3988
Fax: +1 207 761 2074
E-mail: Info@binax.com
Website: www.binax.com

Binder, see **WTB Binder Labortechnik**

Biochemical Systems International
Via G. Ferraris, 220
52100 Arezzo
ITALY
Phone: +39 0575 984164
Fax: +39 0575 984238
E-mail: biosys@biosys.it
Website: www.biosys.it

Biochrom Ltd
22 Cambridge Science Park
Cambridge
CB4 0FJ, UK
Phone: +44 (0) 1223 423723
Fax: +44 (0) 1223 420164
E-mail: enquiries@biochrom.co.uk
Website: www.biochrom.co.uk

Browne Group Ltd
Chancery House
190 Waterside Road
Hamilton Industrial Park
Leicester
LE5 1QZ, UK
Phone: +44 (0) 116 276 8636
Fax: +44 (0) 116 276 8639
Website: www.thebrownegroup.co.uk

Cole-Parmer
Unit 3
River Brent Business Park
Trumpers Way, Hanwell
London
W7 2QA, UK
Phone: +44 (0) 20 8574 7556
Fax: +44 (0) 20 8574 7543
E-mail: sales@coleparmer.co.uk
Website: www.coleparmer.co.uk

Cope A J & Sons
The Oval
Hackney Road
London
E2 9DU, UK
Phone: +44 (0) 20 7729 2405
Fax: +44 (0) 20 7729 2657

E-mail: nigelc@ajcope.co.uk
Website: www.thelabwarehouse.com

Coris BioConcept
Science Park Crealys-Cassiopée
Rue Phocas Lejeune
30 Bte 9-5032 Gembloux
BELGIUM
Phone: +32 8171 9917
Fax: +32 8171 9919
E-mail: info@corisbio.com
Website: www.corisbio.com

Cortex Diagnostics
23961 Craftsman Road
Suite E/F
Calabasas, CA 91302
USA
Phone: +1 818 591 3030
Fax: +1 818 591 8383
E-mail: onestep@rapidtest.com
Website: www.rapidtest.com

Developing Health Technology (DHT)
Gordon-Keeble GP Head Office
Bridge House
Worlington Road
Barton Mills, Suffolk
IP28 7DX, UK
Phone: +44 (0) 1638 510055
Fax: +44 (0) 1638 515599
E-mail: dht@gordon-keeble.co.uk
Website: www.gordon-keeble.co.uk

Diamedica Ltd
Grange Hill
Bratton Fleming
North Devon
EX31 4UH, UK
Phone   +44 (0) 1598 710 066
Fax   +44 (0) 1598 710 055
E-mail: info@Diamedica.co.uk
Website: www.Diamedica.co.uk

Dixons Surgical Instruments Ltd
1 Roman Court
Hurricane Way
Wickford Business Park
Wickford, Essex
SS11 8YB, UK
Phone: +44 (0) 1268 764 614
Fax: +44 (0) 1268 764 615
E-mail: info@dixons-uk.com
Website: www.dixons-uk.com

Durbin plc
Unit 5
Redlands Business Centre
Coulsdon, Surrey
CR5 2UN, UK
Phone: +44 (0) 208 6455851
Fax: +44 (0) 208 6680751
E-mail: cataloguesales@durbin.co.uk

Eiken Chemical Company
1–33–8 Hongo
Bunkyo-ku
Tokyo 113-8408
JAPAN
Phone: +81 3381 35401
Website: www.eiken.co.jp

Elcomatic/Gillett & Sibert
Kirktonfield Rd
Neilston, Glasgow
Scotland
G78 3PL UK
Phone: +44 (0) 141 881 5825
Fax: +44 (0) 141 881 5828
E-mail: user@elcomatic.co.uk
Website: www.elcomatic.co.uk

Fairey Industrial Ceramics Ltd
Lymedale Cross
Lower Milehouse Lane
Newcastle-Under-Lyme
Staffordshire
ST5 9BT, UK
Phone: +44 (0) 1782 664420
Fax: +44 (0) 1782 664490
E-mail: enquiries@faireyceramics.com
Website: www.faireyceramics.com

FAKT Consult for Training and Technologies
Gänsheidestrasse 43
D-70184 Stuttgart
GERMANY
Phone: +49 711 210 95 0
Fax: +49 711 210 95 55
E-mail: fakt@fakt-consult.de
Website: www.fakt-consult.de

Fumouze Diagnostics
110–114 rue Victor Hugo
B.P. 314
92303 Levallois Perret Cedex
FRANCE
Phone: +33 14968 4100
Fax: +33 14968 4142

Graticules Ltd, see **Pyser-SGI**

GTZ (German Agency for Technical Cooperation)
Post Box 5180
D-65726 Eschborn
GERMANY
Phone: +49 6196 790
Fax: +49 6196 7911 15
Website: www.gtz.de

Guest Medical Trading Limited
Enterprise Way
Edenbridge, Kent
TN8 6EW, UK
Phone: +44 (0) 1732 867 466
Fax: +44 (0) 1732 867 476
E-mail: enquiries@guest-medical.co.uk
Website: www.guest-medical.co.uk

Hanna Instruments Ltd
Eden Way
Pages Industrial Park
Leighton Buzzard
Bedfordshire
LU7 4AD, UK
Phone: +44 (0) 1525 850 855
Fax: +44 (0) 1525 853 668
E-mail: sales@hannainst.co.uk
Website: www.hannainst.co.uk

HD Supplies
44 Rabans Close
Rabans Lane Ind Estate
Aylesbury, Bucks
HP19 3RS, UK
Phone: +44 (0) 1296 431920
Fax: +44 (0) 1296 392121
E-mail: hdsupplies@tiscali.co.uk

Healthlink Worldwide
56–64 Leonard Street
London
EC2A 4JX, UK
Phone: +44 (0) 20 7549 0240
Fax: +44 (0) 20 7549 0241
E-mail: info@healthlink.org.uk
Website: www.healthlink.org.uk

Hermle Labortechnik GmbH
Gosheimer Strasse 56
D-78564 Wehingen
GERMANY
Phone: +49 7426 96220

Fax: +49 7426 962249
E-mail: hermle@hermle.biz
Website: www.hermle.biz

Hughes & Hughes Ltd
Unit 1F Lowmoor Industrial Estate
Tonedale
Wellington
Somerset
TA21 0AZ, UK
Phone: +44 (0) 1823 660 222
Fax: +44 (0) 1823 660 186
E-mail: sales@hughesandhughes.co.uk
Website: www.hughesandhughes.co.uk

Immunostics Inc
3505 Sunset Avenue
Ocean, New Jersey
07712, USA
Phone: +1 732 918 0770
Fax: +1 732 918 0618
E-mail: sales@immunostics.com
Website: www.immunostics.com

InBios International Inc.
562 First Avenue South
Suite 600
Seattle, WA 98104
USA
Phone: +1 206 344 5821
Fax: +1 206 344 5823
Website: www.inbios.com

Kalon Biological Ltd
8 Enterprise Estate
Station Road West
Ash Vale
Aldershot
GU12 5QJ, UK
Phone: +44 (0) 1252 522 635
Fax: +44 (0) 1252 523 851
E-mail: info@kalonbio.co.uk
Website: www.kalonbio.co.uk

KIT (Royal Tropical Institute) Biomedical Research
Parasitology
Meibergdreef 39
1105 AZ Amsterdam
The NETHERLANDS
Phone: +31 20 566 5441
Fax: +31 20 697 1841
E-mail: h.schallig@kit.nl

Lab-Plant Ltd
Cliffe End Firs
Longwood Road
Huddersfield, West Yorkshire
HD3 4EL, UK
Phone: +44 (0) 1484 657 736/650 111
Fax: +44 (0) 1484 460 048
E-mail: sales@labplant.com
Website: www.labplant.com

Labnet International Inc.
PO Box 841
Woodbridge
NJ, 07095
USA
Phone: +1 (732) 417 0700
Fax: +1 (732) 417 1750
E-mail: labnet@labnetlink.com
Website: www.labnetlink.com

Mast Diagnostics
Mast House, Derby Road
Bootle, Merseyside
L20 1EA, UK
Phone: +44 151 933 7277
Fax: +44 151 944 1332
E-mail: sales@mastgrp.com
Website: www.mastgrp.com

Millipore UK Ltd
Units 3 and 5, The Courtyards
Hatters Lane, Watford
WD18 8YH, UK
Phone: +44 (0) 870 900 4445
Fax: +44 (0) 870 900 4644
Website: www.millipore.com

National Diagnostic Products Pty Ltd
7–9 Merriwa Street, Sidney
Gordon NSW 2072
AUSTRALIA
Phone: +61 2 9418 1100
Fax: +61 2 9418 1181
E-mail: info@betachek.com
Website: www.ndp.com.au

Nickel-Electro Ltd
Oldmixon Crescent
Weston-super-Mare
North Somerset
BS24 9BL, UK
Phone: +44 (0) 1934 626 691
Fax: +4 (0) 1934 630 300
E-mail: clifton@nickel-electro.co.uk
Website: www.nickel-electro.co.uk

Ohaus Corporation
19A Chapin Road
PO Box 2033
Pine Brook, NY 07058
USA
Phone: +1 973 377 9000
Fax: +1 973 593 0359
Website: www.ohaus.com

Orchid Biomedical Systems
Plot Nos 88/89, Phase 11C
Verna Industrial Estate
Verna
Goa 403 722
INDIA
Phone: +91 832 2783140
Fax: +91 832 2783139
E-mail: orchid-goa@sancharnet.in
Website: www.tulipgroup.com

Pacific Paramedical Training Centre
PO Box 7013
Wellington
NEW ZEALAND
Phone: +64 4 389 6295
Fax: +64 4 389 6295

PATH (Program for Appropriate Technology in Health)
1455 NW Leary Way
Seattle
WA 98107
USA
Phone: +1 206 285 3500
Fax: +1 206 285 6619
E-mail: info@path.org
Website: www.path.org

Plasmatec Laboratory Products
Unit 29 Dreadnought Trading Estate
Bridport, Dorset
DT6 5BU, UK
Phone: +44 (0) 1308 421829
Fax: +44 (0) 1308 421846
E-mail: admin@plasmatec.demon.co.uk
Website: www.plasmatec.uk.com

Portable Medical Laboratories Inc
PO Box 667
Solana Beach
California 92075
USA
Phone: +1 (858) 755 7385
Fax: +1 (858) 259 6022
E-mail: wsanborn@portmedtech.com
Website: www.portable-medical-lab.com

Poulten and Graf
1 Alfreds Way
Barking, Essex
IG11 0AS, UK
Phone: +44 (0) 208 5944 256
Fax: +44 (0) 208 5948 419
E-mail: volacjpl@aol.com
Website: www.poulten-graf.com

Prestige Medical
PO Box 154
Clarendon Road
Blackburn, Lancashire
BB1 9UG, UK
Phone: +44 (0) 1254 682 622
Fax: +44 (0) 1254 682 606
E-mail: info@prestigemedical.co.uk
Website: www.prestigemedical.co.uk

Prince Leopold Institute of Tropical Medicine
Applied Technology and Production Unit
Nationalestraat 155
B–2000 Antwerpen
BELGIUM
Phone: +32 (0) 3247 6368
Fax: +32 (0) 3247 6373
E-mail: emagnus@itg.be

Provalis Diagnostics Ltd
Newtech Square, First Avenue
Deeside Industrial Park
Deeside
CH5 2NT, UK
Phone: +44 (0) 1244 288 888
Fax: +44 (0) 1244 280 320
E-mail: enquiries@provalis.plc.uk
Website: www.provalis.com

Purolite Company
Cowbridge Road
Pontyclun
CF12 8YL, UK
Phone: +44 (0) 1443 235411
Fax: +44 (0) 1443 231113
E-mail: sales@purolite.com
Website: www.purolite.com

Pyser-SGI Ltd
Fircroft Way
Edenbridge
TN8 6HA, UK
Phone: +44 (0) 1732 864111
Fax: +44 (0) 1732 865544
E-mail: sales@pyser-sgi.com
Website: www.pyser-sgi.com

Radleys
Shire Hill
Saffron Walden, Essex
CB11 3AZ, UK
Phone: +44 (0) 1799 513320
Fax: +44 (0) 1799 513283
E-mail: sales@radleys.co.uk
Website: www.radleys.co.uk

Randox Laboratories Ltd
55 Diamond Road
Crumlin, Co Antrim
BT29 4QY, UK
Phone: +44 (0) 2894 422413
Fax: +44 (0) 2894 452912
E-mail: marketing@randox.com
Website: www.randox.com

Roche Diagnostics GmbH
Sandhoferstrasse 116
68305 Mannheim
GERMANY
Phone: +49 621 759 0
Fax: +49 621 759 28 90
Website: www.roche.de/diagnostics

Sartorius AG
Weender Landstrasse 94–108
D-37075 Goettingen
GERMANY
Phone: +49 551 3080
Fax: +49 551 308 3289
Website: www.sartorius.com

Scientific Industries Inc.
70 Orville Drive
Bohemia
NY 11716
USA
Phone: +1 (631) 567 4700
Fax: +1 (631) 567 5896
E-mail: info@scientificindustries.com
Website: www.scientificindustries.com

Sero AS
PO Box 24
N-1375 Billingstad
NORWAY
Phone: +47 6685 8900
Fax: +47 6698 2201
E-mail: sales@sero.no
Website: www.sero.no

Sherwood Scientific Ltd
1 The Paddocks
Cherry Hinton Road
Cambridge
CB1 8DU, UK
Phone: +44 (0) 1223 243444
Fax: +44 (0) 1223 243300
E-mail: info@sherwood-scientific.com
Website: www.sherwood-scientific.com

SKAT
Vadianstrasse 42
CH 9000 St Gallen
SWITZERLAND
Phone: +41 71 228 5454
Fax: +41 71 228 5455
E-mail: info@skat.ch
Website: www.skat.ch

Span Diagnostics Ltd
173-B New Industrial Estate
Udhna, Surat – 394 210
INDIA
Phone: +91 261 227 7211
Fax: +91 261 227 9319
E-mail: span@spandiag.com
Website: www.span.co.in

Stuart Scientific Co Ltd, see **Bibby Sterlin**

TDR World Health Organization
1211 Geneva 27
SWITZERLAND
Phone: +41 22791 3725
Fax: +41 22791 4854
E-mail: tdr@who.int
Website: www.who.int/tdr

Techlab Inc
2001 Kraft Drive
Blacksburg, VA 24060–6358
USA
Phone: +1 (540) 953 1664
Fax: +1 (540) 953 1665
E-mail: techlab@techlab.com
Website: www.techlab.com

Trinity Biotech
IDA Business Park
Bray, Co Wicklow
IRELAND
Phone: +353 1 276 9800
Fax: +353 1 276 9881
E-mail: info@trinitybiotech.ie
Website: www.trinitybiotech.com

Tropical Health Technology (THT)
PO Box 50
Fakenham
NR21 8XB, UK
Phone: +44 (0) 1328 855805
Fax: +44 (0) 1328 853799
E-mail: thtbooks@tht.ndirect.co.uk
Website: www.thtbooks.ndirect.co.uk

UNICEF Supply Division
Unicef Plads, Freeport
DK-2100 Copenhagen OE
DENMARK
Phone: +45 3527 3800
Fax: +45 3527 3810
E-mail: unicefdk@unicef.dk
Website: www.unicef.org

World Health Organization (WHO)
1211 Geneva
27-SWITZERLAND
Phone: +41 22 791 21 11
Fax: +41 22 791 0746
Website: www.who.int

WPA, see **Biochrom Ltd**

WTB Binder Labortechnik GmbH
Postfach 102
D-78502
Tuttlingen
GERMANY
Phone: +49 7461 1792 0
Fax: +49 7461 1792 10
E-mail   info@binder-world.co
Website: www.binder-world.com

Appendix III

Useful Tables and Figures

SI Units

Prefix	Symbol	Function
femto	f	10^{-15}
pico	p	10^{-12}
nano	n	10^{-9}
micro	μ	10^{-6}
milli	m	10^{-3}
* ⎡ centi	c	10^{-2} ⎤
deci	d	10^{-1}
⎣ deca	da	10^{1} ⎦
hecto	h	10^{2}
kilo	k	10^{3}
mega	M	10^{6}
giga	G	10^{9}
tera	T	10^{12}

*Use not recommended

Mass

$$1 \text{ kg} = 10^{3} \text{ g (1000 g)}$$
$$1 \text{ mg} = 10^{-3} \text{ g (0.001 g)}$$
$$1 \text{ } \mu\text{g} = 10^{-6} \text{ g (0.000 001 g)}$$
$$1 \text{ ng} = 10^{-9} \text{ g (0.000 000 001 g)}$$
$$1 \text{ pg} = 10^{-12} \text{ g (0.000 000 000 001 g)}$$
$$1 \text{ kg} = 1000 \text{ g}$$
$$1 \text{ g} = 1000 \text{ mg}$$
$$1 \text{ g} = 1 \text{ 000 000 } \mu\text{g}$$
$$1 \text{ g} = 1 \text{ 000 000 000 ng}$$
$$1 \text{ g} = 1 \text{ 000 000 000 000 pg}$$
$$1 \text{ mg} = 0.001 \text{ g}$$
$$1 \text{ mg} = 1000 \text{ } \mu\text{g}$$
$$1 \text{ kg} = 2.205 \text{ lb}$$

Amount of substance

$$1 \text{ mmol} = 10^{-3} \text{ mol (0.001 mol)}$$
$$1 \text{ } \mu\text{mol} = 10^{-6} \text{ mol (0.000 001 mol)}$$
$$1 \text{ nmol} = 10^{-9} \text{ mol (0.000 000 001 mol)}$$
$$1 \text{ mol} = 1000 \text{ mmol}$$
$$1 \text{ mol} = 1 \text{ 000 000 } \mu\text{mol}$$
$$1 \text{ mol} = 1 \text{ 000 000 000 nmol}$$
$$1 \text{ mmol} = 1000 \text{ } \mu\text{mol}$$
$$1 \text{ mmol} = 1 \text{ 000 000 nmol}$$
$$1 \text{ } \mu\text{mol} = 1000 \text{ nmol}$$

Pressure

Approx. conversion: $\dfrac{\text{mm Hg} \times 2}{15} = \text{kPa}$

lb/sq inch x 6.895 = kPa

Length

$$1 \text{ dm} = 10^{-1} \text{ m (0.1 m)}$$
$$1 \text{ cm} = 10^{-2} \text{ m (0.01 m)}$$
$$1 \text{ mm} = 10^{-3} \text{ m (0.001 m)}$$
$$*1 \text{ } \mu\text{m} = 10^{-6} \text{ m (0.000 001 m)}$$
$$1 \text{ nm} = 10^{-9} \text{ m (0.000 000 001 m)}$$
$$1 \text{ km} = 1000 \text{ m (10}^{3} \text{ m)}$$
$$1 \text{ m} = 10 \text{ dm}$$
$$1 \text{ m} = 100 \text{ cm}$$
$$1 \text{ m} = 1000 \text{ mm}$$
$$1 \text{ m} = 1 \text{ 000 000 } \mu\text{m}$$
$$1 \text{ m} = 1 \text{ 000 000 000 nm}$$
$$1 \text{ cm} = 10 \text{ mm}$$
$$1 \text{ cm} = 10 \text{ 000 } \mu\text{m}$$
$$1 \text{ mm} = 1000 \text{ } \mu\text{m}$$
$$1 \text{ m} = 3.281 \text{ feet}$$
$$1 \text{ km} = 0.62137 \text{ mile}$$
$$1 \text{ inch} = 2.54 \text{ cm}$$

Volume

$$1 \text{ dl} = 10^{-1} \text{ l (0.1 l)}$$
$$1 \text{ cl} = 10^{-2} \text{ l (0.01 l)}$$
$$1 \text{ ml} = 10^{-3} \text{ l (0.001 l)}$$
$$1 \text{ } \mu\text{l} = 10^{-6} \text{ l (0.000 001 l or 1 mm}^{3}\text{)}$$
$$1 \text{ nl} = 10^{-9} \text{ l (0.000 000 001 l)}$$
$$1 \text{ pl} = 10^{-12} \text{ l (0.000 000 000 001 l)}$$
$$1 \text{ l} = 10 \text{ dl}$$
$$1 \text{ l} = 1000 \text{ ml}$$
$$1 \text{ l} = 1 \text{ 000 000 } \mu\text{l}$$
$$1 \text{ l} = 1 \text{ 000 000 000 nl}$$
$$1 \text{ dl} = 100 \text{ cm}^{3}\text{, formerly 100 ml}$$
$$1 \text{ ml} = 1000 \text{ } \mu\text{l}$$
$$1 \text{ pint} = 0.568 \text{ l}$$
$$1 \text{ l} = 1.760 \text{ pints}$$
$$1 \text{ l} = 0.22 \text{ gallons}$$

Temperature conversion

To convert °C to °F:
multiply by 9, divide by 5, and add 32.

To convert °F to °C:
subtract 32, multiply by 5, and divide by 9.

0 °C	= 32 °F
10 °C	= 52 °F
20 °C	= 68 °F
30 °C	= 86 °F
36.9 °C	= 98.4 °F
40 °C	= 104 °F
50 °C	= 122 °F
100 °C	= 212 °F

Element	Symbol	Relative Atomic Mass	Valence
Aluminium	Al	26.9815	3
Antimony	Sb	121.75	3, 5
Barium	Ba	137.34	2
Cadmium	Cd	112.40	2
Calcium	Ca	40.08	2
Carbon	C	12.011	2, 4
Chlorine	Cl	35.453	1, 3, 5, 7
Chromium	Cr	51.996	2, 3, 6
Cobalt	Co	58.9332	2, 3
Copper	Cu	63.546	1, 2
Fluorine	F	19.9984	1
Gold	Au	196.8665	1, 3
Hydrogen	H	1.0079	1
Iodine	I	126.9045	1, 3, 5, 7
Iron	Fe	55.847	2, 3, 6
Lead	Pb	207.2	2, 4
Lithium	Li	6.941	1
Magnesium	Mg	24.305	2
Manganese	Mn	54.9380	2, 3, 4, 6, 7
Mercury	Hg	200.59	1, 2
Molybdenum	Mo	95.94	2, 3, 4, 5, 6
Nickel	Ni	58.7	2, 3
Nitrogen	N	14.0067	3, 5
Oxygen	O	15.9994	2
Phosphorus	P	30.9738	3, 5
Platinum	Pt	195.09	2, 4
Potassium	K	39.098	1
Selenium	Se	78.96	2, 4, 6
Silicon	Si	28.086	4
Silver	Ag	107.868	1
Sodium	Na	22.9898	1
Sulphur	S	32.06	2, 4, 6
Tin	Sn	118.69	2, 4
Tungsten	W	183.85	2, 4, 5, 6
Zinc	Zn	65.38	2

Note: The atomic weights quoted are the 1973 values* based on carbon 12.
*IUPAC. *Atomic weights of the elements,* 1973.

MOLE PER LITRE SOLUTIONS OF SOME CONCENTRATED ACIDS

Acetic acid, glacial, 99.6% w/w:	Approx. 17.50 mol/l
Hydrochloric acid, 1.16, 32% w/w:	Approx. 10.20 mol/l
Hydrochloric acid, 1.18, 36% w/w:	Approx. 11.65 mol/l
Nitric acid, 1.42, 70% w/w:	Approx. 15.80 mol/l
Sulphuric acid, 1.84, 97% w/w:	Approx. 18.00 mol/l

To make approx. 1 mol/l solutions from concentrated acids

Concentrated acids	*ml diluted to 1 litre*
Acetic acid, (glacial), 99.6% w/w	57 ml
Hydrochloric acid, 32% w/w	98 ml
Hydrochloric acid, 36% w/w	86 ml
Nitric acid, 70%, w/w	63 ml
Sulphuric acid, 97% w/w	56 ml

RELATIVE MOLECULAR MASSES OF SOME SUBSTANCES

Substance	Symbol	Relative Molecular Mass (taken to two decimal places)
Acetic acid	CH_3COOH	60.08
Ammonium carbonate	$(NH_4)_2CO_3$	96.09
Ammonium chloride	NH_4Cl	53.50
Ammonium molybdate	$(NH_4)_2MoO_4$	196.03
Ammonium nitrate	NH_4NO_3	80.05
Ammonium oxalate	$(NH_4)_2C_2O_2 \cdot H_2O$	142.12
Barium chloride	$BaCl_2$	208.27
Barium hydroxide	$Ba(OH)_2 \cdot 8H_2O$	315.51
Boric acid (boracic acid)	H_3BO_3	61.84
Calcium chloride	$CaCl_2$	110.98
CopperII sulphate (cupric)	$CuSO_4$	159.61
	$CuSO_4 \cdot 5H_2O$	249.69
Hydrochloric acid	HCl	36.47
Iron III chloride	$FeCl_3$	162.22
(Ferric chloride)	$FeCl_3 \cdot 6H_2O$	270.32
Lead nitrate	$Pb(NO_3)_2$	331.23
Lithium carbonate	Li_2CO_3	73.89
Magnesium chloride	$MgCl_2 \cdot 6H_2O$	203.33
Mercury II chloride	$HgCl_2$	271.52
(Mercuric chloride)		
Molybdic acid	H_2MoO_4	161.97
	$H_2MoO_4 \cdot H_2O$	179.98
Nitric acid	HNO_3	63.02
Phosphoric acid	H_3PO_4	98.00
Potassium carbonate	K_2CO_3	138.20
	$K_2CO_3 \cdot 1\frac{1}{2}H_2O$	165.24
Potassium chloride	KCl	74.55
Potassium cyanide	KCN	65.11
Potassium dichromate	$K_2Cr_2O_7$	294.21
Potassium ferricyanide	$K_3Fe(CN)_6$	329.25
Potassium ferrocyanide	$K_4Fe(CN)_6 \cdot 3H_2O$	422.39
Potassium hydrogen phosphate	K_2HPO_4	174.18
Potassium dihydrogen phosphate	KH_2PO_4	136.09
Potassium hydroxide	KOH	56.10
Potassium hypochlorite	$KClO$	90.55
Potassium iodate	KIO_3	214.02
Potassium iodide	KI	166.02
Potassium nitrate	KNO_3	101.10
Potassium nitrite	KNO_2	85.10
Potassium oxalate	$K_2C_2O_4 \cdot H_2O$	184.23
Potassium permanganate	$KMnO_4$	158.03
Potassium phosphate	K_3PO_4	212.27
Potassium sulphate	K_2SO_4	174.26
Potassium tartrate	$K_2C_4H_4O_6 \cdot \frac{1}{2}H_2O$	235.27
Potassium thiocyanate	$KSCN$	97.18
Silver nitrate	$AgNO_3$	169.89
Sodium azide	NaN_3	65.02
Sodium barbital (Sodium diethyl barbiturate)	$NaC_8H_{11}N_2O_3$	206.18
Sodium benzoate	$NaC_7H_5O_2$	144.11
Sodium carbonate	Na_2CO_3	106.00
	$Na_2CO_3 \cdot H_2O$	124.02
Sodium chlorate	$NaClO_4$	106.45
Sodium chloride	$NaCl$	58.45

Substance	Symbol	Relative Molecular Mass (taken to two decimal places)
Sodium chromate	Na_2CrO_4	162.00
Sodium citrate	$Na_3C_6H_5O_7 \cdot 2H_2O$	294.12
Sodium cyanide	$NaCN$	49.02
Sodium dithionite	$Na_2S_2O_4 \cdot 2H_2O$	210.16
Sodium ferricyanide	$Na_3Fe(CN)_6 \cdot H_2O$	298.97
Sodium ferrocyanide	$Na_4Fe(CN)_6 \cdot 10H_2O$	484.11
Sodium fluoride	NaF	42.00
Sodium bicarbonate	$NaHCO_3$	84.02
Sodium hydroxide	$NaOH$	40.01
Sodium metabisulphite	$Na_2S_2O_5$	190.13
Sodium molybdate	$Na_2MoO_4 \cdot 2H_2O$	241.98
Sodium nitrate	$NaNO_3$	85.01
Sodium nitrite	$NaNO_2$	69.01
Sodium nitroprusside	$Na_2(NO)Fe(CN)_5 \cdot 2H_2O$	297.97
Sodium oxalate	$Na_2C_2O_4$	134.01
Sodium perchlorate	$NaClO_4 \cdot H_2O$	140.47
Sodium phosphate	$Na_3PO_4 \cdot 12H_2O$	380.16
Sodium sulphate	Na_2SO_4	142.06
Glauber's salt	$Na_2SO_4 \cdot 10H_2O$	322.22
Sodium sulphite	Na_2SO_3	126.06
Sodium thiosulphate	$Na_2S_2O_3 \cdot 5H_2O$	248.21
Sodium tungstate	$Na_2WO_4 \cdot 2H_2O$	329.95
Sulphuric acid	H_2SO_4	98.08
Zinc acetate	$Zn(C_2H_3O_2)_2 \cdot 2H_2O$	219.50
Zinc chloride	$ZnCl_2$	136.29

SQUARE ROOTS OF 0.1 TO 4.00

	0.00	0.01	0.02	0.03	0.04	0.05	0.06	0.07	0.08	0.09
0.1	0.32	0.33	0.35	0.36	0.37	0.39	0.40	0.41	0.42	0.44
0.2	0.45	0.46	0.47	0.48	0.49	0.50	0.51	0.52	0.53	0.54
0.3	0.55	0.56	0.57	0.57	0.58	0.59	0.60	0.61	0.62	0.62
0.4	0.63	0.64	0.65	0.66	0.66	0.67	0.68	0.69	0.69	0.70
0.5	0.71	0.71	0.72	0.73	0.73	0.74	0.75	0.76	0.76	0.77
0.6	0.77	0.78	0.79	0.79	0.80	0.81	0.81	0.82	0.82	0.83
0.7	0.84	0.84	0.85	0.85	0.86	0.87	0.87	0.88	0.88	0.89
0.8	0.89	0.90	0.91	0.91	0.92	0.92	0.93	0.93	0.94	0.94
0.9	0.95	0.95	0.96	0.96	0.97	0.97	0.98	0.98	0.99	0.995

	0.00	0.01	0.02	0.03	0.04	0.05	0.06	0.07	0.08	0.09
1.0	1.00	1.01	1.01	1.02	1.02	1.03	1.03	1.03	1.04	1.04
1.1	1.05	1.05	1.06	1.06	1.07	1.07	1.08	1.08	1.09	1.09
1.2	1.10	1.10	1.11	1.11	1.11	1.12	1.12	1.13	1.13	1.14
1.3	1.14	1.15	1.15	1.15	1.16	1.16	1.17	1.17	1.18	1.18
1.4	1.18	1.19	1.19	1.20	1.20	1.20	1.21	1.21	1.22	1.22
1.5	1.23	1.23	1.23	1.24	1.24	1.25	1.25	1.25	1.26	1.26
1.6	1.27	1.27	1.27	1.28	1.28	1.29	1.29	1.29	1.30	1.30
1.7	1.30	1.31	1.31	1.32	1.32	1.32	1.33	1.33	1.33	1.34
1.8	1.34	1.35	1.35	1.35	1.36	1.36	1.36	1.37	1.37	1.38
1.9	1.38	1.38	1.39	1.39	1.39	1.40	1.40	1.40	1.41	1.41
2.0	1.41	1.42	1.42	1.43	1.43	1.43	1.44	1.44	1.44	1.45
2.1	1.45	1.45	1.46	1.46	1.46	1.47	1.47	1.47	1.48	1.48
2.2	1.48	1.49	1.49	1.49	1.50	1.50	1.50	1.51	1.51	1.51
2.3	1.52	1.52	1.52	1.53	1.53	1.53	1.54	1.54	1.54	1.55
2.4	1.55	1.55	1.56	1.56	1.56	1.57	1.57	1.57	1.58	1.58
2.5	1.58	1.58	1.59	1.59	1.59	1.60	1.60	1.60	1.61	1.61
2.6	1.61	1.62	1.62	1.62	1.63	1.63	1.63	1.63	1.64	1.64
2.7	1.64	1.65	1.65	1.65	1.66	1.66	1.66	1.67	1.67	1.67
2.8	1.67	1.68	1.68	1.68	1.69	1.69	1.69	1.69	1.70	1.70
2.9	1.70	1.71	1.71	1.71	1.72	1.72	1.72	1.72	1.73	1.73
3.0	1.73	1.74	1.74	1.74	1.75	1.75	1.75	1.75	1.76	1.76
3.1	1.76	1.76	1.77	1.77	1.77	1.78	1.78	1.78	1.78	1.79
3.2	1.79	1.79	1.79	1.80	1.80	1.80	1.81	1.81	1.81	1.81
3.3	1.82	1.82	1.82	1.83	1.83	1.83	1.83	1.84	1.84	1.84
3.4	1.84	1.85	1.85	1.85	1.86	1.86	1.86	1.86	1.87	1.87
3.5	1.87	1.88	1.88	1.88	1.88	1.88	1.89	1.89	1.89	1.90
3.6	1.90	1.90	1.90	1.91	1.91	1.91	1.91	1.92	1.92	1.92
3.7	1.92	1.93	1.93	1.93	1.93	1.94	1.94	1.94	1.94	1.95
3.8	1.95	1.95	1.95	1.96	1.96	1.96	1.97	1.97	1.97	1.97
3.9	1.98	1.98	1.98	1.98	1.99	1.99	1.99	1.99	2.00	2.00
4.0	2.00	2.00	2.01	2.01	2.01	2.01	2.02	2.02	2.02	2.02

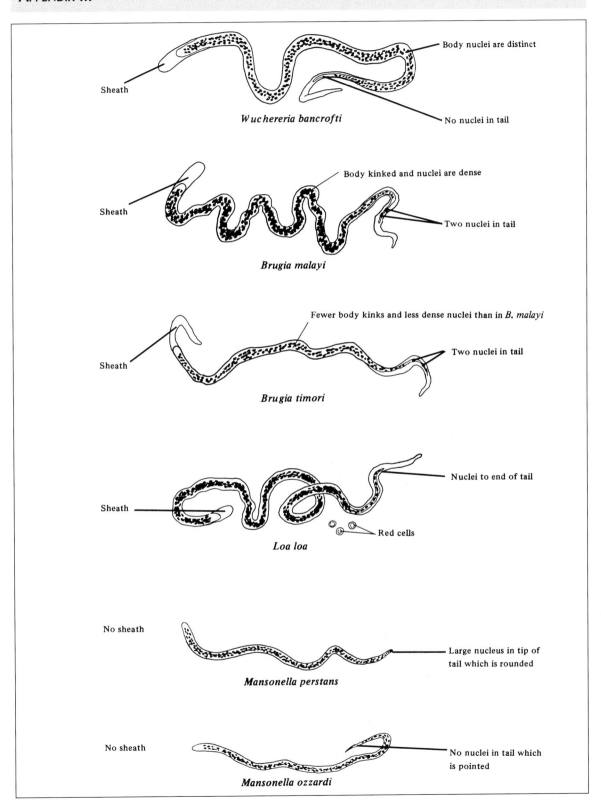

Microfilariae which can be found in blood.

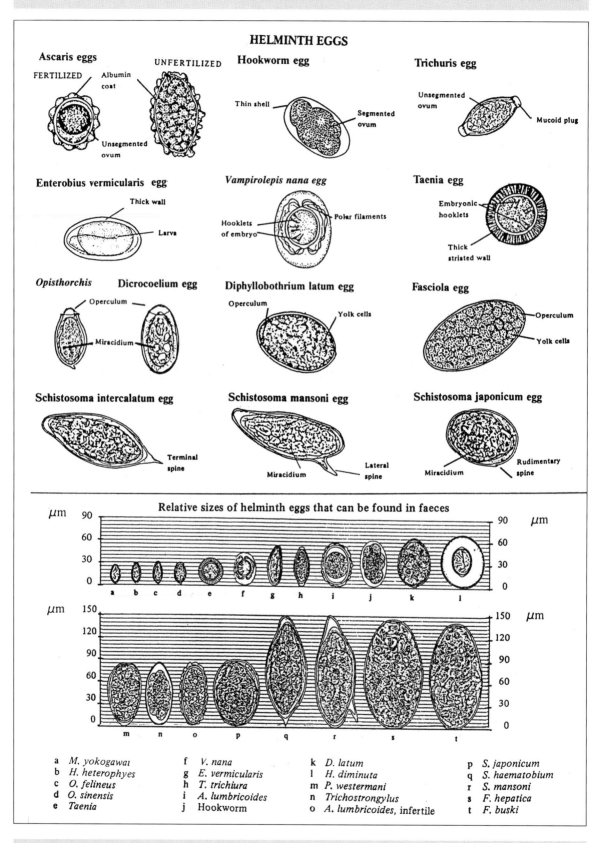

HELMINTH EGGS

Ascaris eggs
FERTILIZED — Albumin coat
UNFERTILIZED
Unsegmented ovum

Hookworm egg
Thin shell
Segmented ovum

Trichuris egg
Unsegmented ovum
Mucoid plug

Enterobius vermicularis egg
Thick wall
Larva

Vampirolepis nana egg
Hooklets of embryo
Polar filaments

Taenia egg
Embryonic hooklets
Thick striated wall

Opisthorchis   Dicrocoelium egg
Operculum
Miracidium

Diphyllobothrium latum egg
Operculum
Yolk cells

Fasciola egg
Operculum
Yolk cells

Schistosoma intercalatum egg
Terminal spine

Schistosoma mansoni egg
Miracidium
Lateral spine

Schistosoma japonicum egg
Miracidium
Rudimentary spine

Relative sizes of helminth eggs that can be found in faeces

a	*M. yokogawai*	f	*V. nana*	k	*D. latum*	p	*S. japonicum*
b	*H. heterophyes*	g	*E. vermicularis*	l	*H. diminuta*	q	*S. haematobium*
c	*O. felineus*	h	*T. trichiura*	m	*P. westermani*	r	*S. mansoni*
d	*O. sinensis*	i	*A. lumbricoides*	n	*Trichostrongylus*	s	*F. hepatica*
e	*Taenia*	j	Hookworm	o	*A. lumbricoides*, infertile	t	*F. buski*

Supplement

Training curriculum for district laboratory personnel

TRAINING CURRICULUM FOR DISTRICT LABORATORY PERSONNEL

Developing a training curriculum involves more than making a list of the topics to be taught and learned. This is what is meant by a syllabus. A curriculum is needed because it details:

- The learning objectives of a course, i.e. the tasks the student must learn.
- Facts, skills, and attitudes laboratory officers need to learn to do their tasks competently and provide a quality service.
- Methods used to help students learn.
- Time and place where the students will learn, i.e. timetable.
- The resources available for training, e.g. teachers, workrooms, laboratories, equipment, learning materials, books.
- Methods used to assess students.

Designing the curriculum

Designing a competency-based training curriculum for district laboratory personnel involves:

1 Performing a situation analysis, i.e. studying the work and working environment of district laboratory staff and making a list of the technical and management tasks that make up the job.

2 Performing a task analysis to identify those facts, skill, and attitudes that are *essential* to perform each task.

3 Deciding what training is required after considering the educational background and qualifications of students.

4 Writing the learning (educational) objectives.

5 Selecting the most appropriate ways to help students learn.

6 Organizing the learning.

7 Assessing whether students can perform their tasks competently, i.e. whether the learning objectives have been achieved.

8 Evaluating and modifying the course as required.

Note: Each of these stages requires careful planning.

---

1 Situation analysis

The first and most important requirement in designing a competency-based curriculum for district laboratory personnel is for those in charge of training, and the district laboratory coordinator, to visit as many as possible of the laboratories in which trainees will work after qualifying:

- getting to know the working situation in district laboratories and understanding the problems laboratory staff experience.
- identifying accurately the technical and management tasks needed.
- discussing with laboratory staff and laboratory users, which tests are required, what type of service is needed, and what resources are available.
- assessing how long the training programme should be.

Consultations will also need to be held with the district health management team. The information obtained will determine what district laboratory students should learn.

Working situation in district laboratories

- District laboratory officers work closely with the community and need to have a clear understanding of the clinical and public health functions of district laboratories, i.e. an awareness of individual and community health needs.
- Many test requests will be from outpatients with results needed as soon as possible, i.e. during the patient's visit.
- District laboratories may not have a regular water supply or stable mains electricity and laboratory equipment service engineers are rarely available.
- Community-based laboratories need to be as self-reliant as possible.
- District laboratory officers are responsible for health and safety in their place of work, the efficient management of resources, and the quality of laboratory service provided.

Only by getting to know the job, working environment, and responsibilities of district laboratory staff, can the learning objectives of a training programme be identified. The list of technical and management tasks produced at the end of the situation analysis is the list of learning objectives for the course.

2 Task analysis

This is best carried out by observing and noting in detail how a competent district laboratory officer performs the tasks identified in the situation analysis. For each task tutors will need to decide the facts, skills, and attitudes that are essential for the task to be performed competently, intelligently, and safely.

What facts are essential?

A particular fact should be considered essential information if it is needed by the student:

– to understand why a test is required, e.g. clinical and public health indications for a test request.
– to perform and control a test in a certain way, i.e. follow a standard operating procedure (SOP).
– to perform a task safely.
– to perform a task efficiently without waste.
– to calculate, report, and record a test result correctly.
– to understand the meaning of a test result.

When knowing a fact does not influence the way a task is performed, it usually means such information is not essential. The teaching of irrelevant information should be avoided, particularly if it reduces the time a student may have for performing skills. Useful and interesting to learn facts can be added at a later stage, if time permits, and when *basic competency has been achieved*.

The teaching of non-essential facts by tutors to fill time or impress students indicates poor planning of a training programme and a misunderstanding by tutors of competency-based learning objectives. Any unplanned spare time that arises in a training session, e.g. due to a power failure, is better spent in using realistic problem-solving exercises to assess whether trainees can apply what they have learned (district laboratory practice is not short of problems that trainees will need to know how to address).

What skills are essential?

Identifying accurately which skills are necessary to perform different tasks is of utmost importance in designing a job related curriculum. Many tasks will involve similar skills, others will require specific skills as follows:

- Basic skills such as:
  - use and care of a microscope and other equipment.
  - accurate and precise pipetting, dispensing, and measuring fluids.
  - weighing and handling chemicals.
  - preparing and staining slide preparations.
  - safety skills and personal hygiene.

- Specific technical skills which require a longer period to learn and more personal tuition such as:
  - reporting microscopical examinations.
  - reporting cultures.
  - interpreting water-testing results.

- Numerical and accountancy skills such as:
  - use of SI units in laboratory work.
  - calculating test results from formulae.
  - working out dilutions and percentages.
  - using quality control charts.
  - calculating volumes and preparing calibrants and reagents.
  - estimating laboratory operating costs.
  - keeping basic accounts and preparing a budget.

- Management, problem-solving, and decision-making skills, such as:
  - organizing and coordinating work activities and staff duties.
  - monitoring standard operating procedures.
  - requisitioning supplies and keeping an inventory.
  - monitoring health and safety regulations.
  - helping to formulate laboratory policies.
  - organizing quality assurance of test procedures.
  - monitoring decontamination and cleaning procedures.
  - maintaining patient confidentiality and the security of patient information and reports.
  - arranging equipment maintenance.
  - organizing mobile laboratory work and assisting in epidemiological surveys.
  - managing problems such as work overload, incorrect requesting of laboratory tests, too many urgent test requests, delayed test reports, laboratory errors, staff disagreements, problems due to equipment failure, shortage of reagents, constant interruptions, deteriorating working conditions, and managing laboratory accidents.

■ Communication skills such as:
- communicating appropriately with patients, patient's relatives, professional colleagues, blood donors, and others.
- using the telephone and other channels of communication.
- writing work reports, collating laboratory data, and using tables and charts.
- presenting information at meetings and participating in discussions.
- using the laboratory in health education.
- reporting problems affecting work performance and staff welfare.

Important: Skills need to be learned in the context of both routine and emergency working conditions.

What attitudes are essential?

Attitudes and personal qualities influence the way an individual thinks, behaves, and works. They can also affect the performance of others. Having the correct attitudes and qualities for the job are important if district laboratory practice is to be accepted and respected by the community.

The following are among the attitudes and qualities most frequently identified in laboratory task analyses:

■ Responsibility, reliability, and a professional approach.
■ Thoroughness with attention to detail.
■ Alertness.
■ Coordinated approach to the work with correct attitudes to accuracy and precision.
■ Honesty and integrity with an ability to act appropriately when errors are made.
■ Correct attitudes towards patients, relatives of patients, fellow workers and those requesting laboratory tests. These include respect, thoughtfulness, patience, kindness, approachability, and helpfulness.
■ Correct attitudes to health, safety, and security.
■ Neatness of work and appearance.

Important: Students need to learn the correct approach to different working conditions, e.g. ability to perform reliably and consistently when working alone or the need to work quickly, competently, and calmly under emergency conditions, heavy workload, or when unforeseen situations develop such as a power failure or equipment breakdown.

3 Deciding what training is required

Deciding what needs to be taught will depend on what the students enrolling for the course know and can do. Most laboratory training programmes accept as students those with a proven knowledge of basic mathematics, science and biology, and ability to understand, communicate, and write in the language of the course.

Depending therefore on the educational background and experiences of the students, tutors may be able to reduce the time spent learning some of the basic facts and skills. It must be remembered, however, that passing school examinations does not guarantee that students will possess the adequate skills or be able to apply their knowledge and experience in medical laboratory work.

4 Writing the learning objectives

Well written learning objectives are dependent on performing an accurate situation analysis and a careful task analysis to identify the tasks that are needed and the facts, skills, and attitudes a student needs to learn. Learning objectives state what a course is trying to achieve and the standard of work required. Some teachers prefer the term learning goals.

The learning objectives are important because they determine:

- what is taught.
- how the teaching is done.
- how the students are tested.

Learning objectives must be achievable, observable, and above all relevant to the job that students are being trained to do.

5 Selecting appropriate ways to help students learn their objectives

When helping students to learn, tutors need to remember that students learn best by *doing.* 'What I hear I forget, what I see I remember, WHAT I DO, I KNOW. Tutors should teach theory, practice, and attitudes together because this reflects the working situation.

Active learning

This helps to prevent theory overload and students

simply listening to lectures and learning very little. Active learning is always more interesting and helps students to remember better and more quickly achieve competence in performing their tasks. Active learning teaching methods include:

- Practising skills following demonstrations.
- Problem-solving and decision-making exercises which will help students to apply what they have learned and cope with difficulties in their job.
- Question and answer sessions and discussions.
- Role play exercises which are particularly helpful when teaching attitudes and skills.
- Project work to encourage students to learn by their own efforts.
- Active use of effective visual aids.

Dividing a class into groups and involving each group in a different learning method, not only gives students the opportunity to learn a task more comprehensively but also helps to ensure all students receive 'hands on' experience when equipment is in short supply, e.g. microscopes.

It is particularly important to give laboratory students exercises that will help them to work economically and efficiently with good coordination, accuracy, and precision. Students must be taught how to work systematically with attention to detail so that they can follow standard operating procedures.

Other ways to help students learn

Besides making learning active, other ways in which tutors can help students learn include:

- providing feedback to students by frequent testing.
- teaching clearly by making sure students can hear what is said and see what is written and demonstrated.
- using simple language, incorporating easy to understand examples, and using good visual aids.
- checking that *all* students can perform the necessary tasks.
- reviewing whether students have remembered what they have been taught.
- allowing enough free time for individual study and project work.
- using a variety of teaching methods.
- tutors showing that they care whether their students learn.

Note: Teaching methods are well described in the WHO book *Teaching for better learning* (see end of *Supplement* for details).

6 Organizing the learning

This stage involves:
- Identifying appropriate locations for the teaching and learning. Lecturing in a classroom about laboratory techniques will not help students to learn or become competent in their tasks. 70–80% of the teaching for district laboratory students should be practical active learning.
- Deciding on how long teaching sessions and study periods should be and the time of day when learning should take place (particularly important in tropical countries).
- Deciding the sequence of learning, taking note of what has been learned previously upon which the learning of a new knowledge or skill can be based. When initial tuition is carried out in a training centre with practical work performed in the working laboratory, it is particularly important for tutors to teach a technique before students are expected to perform it in the laboratory.
- Identifying appropriate resources and facilities to use during teaching sessions and study periods to motivate students to learn.

Note: Whenever possible teaching aids should be prepared nationally. Manuals, charts, posters, bench aids, slide sets, tapes or videos that are produced outside the country should be evaluated carefully by laboratory tutors for their appropriateness and effectiveness. Consideration will need to be given to the educational background of trainees and resources available.

Importance of work experience during training

During their training, students must spend sufficient time in a district laboratory as similar as possible to the one in which they will work after qualifying, e.g. health centre laboratory or district hospital laboratory. Only in the working situation can students:

- appreciate the importance of laboratory practice in district health care.
- practice their *Code of Professional Conduct.*
- gain work experience under supervision.
- learn to work in a coordinated way, meeting target turnround times for test results.
- experience working under pressure and how to manage difficult situations.

- learn what action to take if a mistake is made.
- learn to respond appropriately when tests are requested urgently.
- develop communication skills and the correct approach to patients, patient's relatives, fellow workers, medical officers, and other health staff.

Note: Adequate work experience during training is also necessary so that tutors, supervizors, and the district laboratory coordinator can assess the suitability of students for district medical laboratory work. On-site job experience is usually best carried out towards the end of training when students can benefit most from their experience and still have the opportunity to return to their training centre for further tuition if required. Tutors *must* ensure that the time a student spends in the working laboratory is adequately supervized and assessed.

7 Assessing students

Testing students is required for the following reasons:

- To assess whether students have learned what is needed and can perform their tasks to the standard required for qualification and registration.
- To help students learn.
- To assess whether the learning objectives of the course have been achieved and what changes to the curriculum are indicated.
- To provide tutors with feedback to help them improve their teaching methods.
- To provide employing health authorities with the assurance that a student who has been assessed as competent and holds a *Certificate of Qualification* is fit to work in a district laboratory.

To meet these requirements the method(s) selected for assessing students must be:

- effective and appropriate to the task and standard of performance being assessed, e.g. practical skills require testing in a practical way.
- workable, affordable, and achievable for tutors and students.
- sufficiently informative, precise and objective to be of help to students and tutors and avoid significant differences in marking between tutors.
- acceptable to the health authority and those in charge of the training and registration of laboratory personnel.

Assessment methods for laboratory students

The traditional methods of assessing laboratory students by using written, practical, and oral examinations at the end of the training course have been largely replaced by methods which test learning objectives more appropriately and are less stressful to students.

Poor assessment of laboratory students by written, practical, and oral examinations

From surveys reported by McMinn,[6] it was estimated that:

- 80% of all written questions tested only recall of information. Very few questions tested the ability of the student to use the information to solve problems.
- 67% of question papers sampled less than 20% of the syllabus.
- 90% of practical examinations tested only 15% of the practical skills expected of trained technical officers.
- 37% of the questions on written examinations asked students to describe how to perform specific practical skills.

Oral examinations were equally poor at assessing the performance of students with 78% of questions simply testing recall information.

Effective methods of assessing the performance of laboratory students include:

- continuous, or frequent, testing.
- the use of logbooks.

Continuous assessment: This involves testing the facts, skills, and attitudes of students throughout their training. When qualification is dependent on the results of these tests, continuous assessment makes students work harder. Guidance is provided both to students and tutors. Students are shown throughout the course what standard is expected.

Use of logbooks: This helps to personalize the learning for students and makes sure students are able to carry out *all* the required tasks competently. Each student is given a logbook which lists all the technical *and* management tasks which require assessment. When the student is ready, the tutor or head of the department in which the training is taking place, records in the logbook when a student is able to perform a particular task.

Assessment of tests should include how well a method is performed, the correctness of the result, how results are presented and interpreted, and the attitudes of the student to the patient and their work. Assessment of many of the management tasks can take the form of a problem-solving exercise. If the student fails the assessment, he or she is able to try again at a later stage after discussion with the tutor.

The logbook system helps to identify at an early stage any learning difficulties or inadequate teaching. The tasks in the assessment logbook should form the basis of a Certificate of Qualification.

Certificate of Qualification for district laboratory personnel

The *Certificate of Qualification* awarded to successful trainees at the end of their basic training must state *exactly what the person is qualified to do.* It should list the tests, test methods, and the management tasks the person is qualified to perform. This type of certificate is of far greater value to the student and employers than one which simply states that a person is qualified as a district laboratory officer with a certain grade.

The Certificate should show the name and address of the Training School (qualifying centre), duration of training, and date of qualification. It must be signed by the person in charge of training.

Important: Newly qualified staff require supervision and support in the workplace if they are successfully to put into practice what they have learned and remain motivated.

8 Evaluating and modifying the course

A training programme will develop as experience is gained in using it. With experience the good points and less good features of the course will become apparent. Almost always the teaching methods and the ways students learn can be improved and often also the learning locations, sequence of learning, resources used, and assessment methods.

Evaluating the quality of a training programme involves reviewing the learning patterns and performances of students, the teaching effectiveness of tutors, and how well the curriculum is achieving its learning objectives.

Encouragement to tutors to change to job related training

Changing to job related competency-based training is a challenge for any tutor. No one should expect the new training to be perfect to begin with. What matters is that a commitment to job-related training is made and a curriculum is developed which is as relevant as possible to the work and as practically orientated as possible. Do not make it too complex in the beginning.

Try to avoid introducing too much theory, particularly in a non-integrated way. This will only lead to students 'not seeing the wood for the trees'. Spend more time making sure students can do the tests correctly and will be able to run their laboratories efficiently and safely. This is what will benefit patients and the health service and lead to job satisfaction, staff motivation, and better resourcing of district laboratories.

Index